Textbook of PAIN

Dr. PRAMOD KUMAR
M.D., D.A.
Sr. Professor & Head,
Dept. of Anaesthesiology,
M.P. Shah Medical College,
Jamnagar, Gujarat (India)

CBS

CBS PUBLISHERS & DISTRIBUTORS
NEW DELHI • BANGALORE (INDIA)

ISBN : 978-81-239-1567-8

First Edition : 2005
Reprint : 2008

Publishing Director : Vinod K. Jain

Published by :
Satish Kumar Jain for CBS Publishers & Distributors,
4596/1-A, 11 Darya Ganj, New Delhi - 110 002 (India)
E-mail: cbspubs@vsnl.com • Website: www.cbspd.com

Branch Office :
2975, 17th Cross, K.R. Road, Bansankari 2nd Stage, Bangalore-70
Fax : 080-26771680 • E-mail : cbsbng@vsnl.net

Printed at: Asia Printograph, Delhi

DEDICATED

TO

MY PARENTS

PREFACE

I have the honour of presenting my book "A Textbook of Pain" for students and Pain clinicians. I hope this book will go a long way in increasing the knowledge and treatment of pain, which is incidentally the most common complaint of any living being. The pain as a subject has been included in the Medical Council of India curriculum for medical undergraduates and specially the postgraduate curriculum of anaesthesiology. This book will be useful for anaesthesiologists, who are managing pain during and after operations and treating acute and postoperative pain in the Pain Clinic, and for physicians, rheumatologists, psychiatrists, surgeons *e.g.*, general, ENT, cancer, radiotherapists, gynaecologists. The basic scientists (*e.g.*, Physiologists, anatomists, pharmacologists, biochemists) will also be benefited by this book. It is appropriate to say that all doctors in teaching or in the practice of medical science are beneficiaries of this book.

There is presently no textbook on the subject of Pain in India. The author has already started an effort by publishing "Handbook of Management of Cancer Pain and Related Symptoms" and "An Atlas on Peripheral Nerve Blocks" earlier, with a tremendous response from postgraduates of Anaesthesiology and pain clinicians of various specialities.

There is a definite scope for this book in the medical sciences in India as the textbooks available are from the West and are very costly and written according to their context. This book relevantly point out to the Indian scenario, so is more useful and also easily affordable. The language and contents of the book are kept simple so that the postgraduates can understand the basics of the pain mechanisms easily. The treatment part is well supported by figures specially in case of peripheral nerve blocks. This helps in understanding the procedure of nerve blocks, direction of the needle, the structures penetrated.

The reader can thus understand the subject of pain and is involved in the specialty of pain as a whole. The basic idea of writing this book is to make more and more physicians and postgraduates interested in pain. Once involved, they can be stimulated to practice pain relief in their patients.

The present day status of pain relief services can be summarised as under.

- To wait for the magic pill which will solve the problem of pain at one go.
- To forget about the pain of the patient altogether.
- To organise pain relief services with proper understanding and definite protocols.

This book believes in the last option and gives a clarion call to all physicians to arise, awake and act.

—Dr. Pramod Kumar

ACKNOWLEDGEMENTS

I acknowledges the moral support of Mrs. Aparna Kumar, Neha P. Kumar and Dr. Prasanna Vadhnan; and Dr. Sidharth Goswami and Dr. Harsha for their help in preparing the manuscript.

I thank **Mr. M.L. Pandey, (Executive Vice-President),** Modern Publishers for cheerfully meeting all my demands to present this book.

I will be failing in my duty if I don't thank **Mr. Brijesh Singh (Editor),** Modern Publishers for sparing his valuable time in helping me out with the correction of the mistakes and making the volume perfect as far as possible. It is a matter of pride that the publisher of this book ***(MBD Group of Publishers)*** is an ISO 9001–2000 certified.

No book is the result of one person's effort and therefore my sincere thanks are due to all those members of the staff of Modern Publishers whom I have not mentioned by names but who are involved in the production of this book. I thank all those persons who have been so courteous, tolerant and helpful throughout.

—Dr. Pramod Kumar

CONTENTS

SECTION–I

History

HISTORY OF PAIN RELIEF

1

Pain is as old as the mankind or even animals also have knowledge of plants *e.g.*, grass used by dogs to produce vomiting. Although some of the enthusiasts claim that first operation and anaesthesia was performed by God who breathed onto the Adam's mouth and putting him to sleep and then took out his left rib that was made into Eve (Oldtestament). However, in the history of modern medicine operation like trephining of skull in the Stone Age is well documented in California, Arizona, Peru, Africa, India, Arab and Mexico natives 7000 years ago.[1] In South Pacific tribes the operations are performed by an Abicidian glass and a herbal ointment application is still a common practice. Peru natives 2000 years ago, were using coca leaves which were chewed by the patient before trephining procedures. Egyptians were using opium for pain relief in trephining as per Eber's Papyrus 7,000 years ago.[1] Even in Stone Age there has been knowledge of various herbal medicines apart from taboo.[2] South African Stone Age excavations revealed 137 herbal medicines in 1888, while Bantu tribes catche was found to include 164 plants with 42 having medicinal value. In this collection Opium, Coca, Cinchona, Ephedrine, Hashish, Hemp, Eucalyptus, Tobacco types of pain reducing herbs were found. These herbs were used as ointments, fumes or enema by Stone Age man. Apart from herbs, splints were used to prevent bone pain apart from massage and hot water fomentations. There had been existence of pain in the life of Stone Age man, who was looking for pain relief methods and using them with success, partially or completely.[2]

In the later ages as the social structure was well defined. The old "medicine man" was replaced by a physician or 'Vaidya'. The era before Christ leads to a successful Greek, Indian and Chinese medicines which was led by Hippocrates, Charak and Sushruta. The disease process was well documented; treatises written and basic cause of disease was explained to imbalance of Air, Phlegm and Bile. Probably there was a good exchange of medical knowledge between these systems. The knowledge of pulse leading to diagnosis of the disease may have travelled from one continent to the other.

GREEK MEDICINE

Homer's Iliad during Hellenic periods records the physicians applying ointments and herbal preparations used for wounds and pain caused during war. A physician was essential part of an army. The Hippocrates, the father of medicine, used mandragora. Later Greek physicians wrote treatises on medicine.

INDIAN MEDICINE

In India the treatises by Charak and Shushruta were written describing various diseases, their diagnosis and treatment. Even Atharva Veda has clearly documented various diseases clearly. Shushruta, who was a disciple of king of Kashi Dhanvantri (not the originator of Ayurveda) was doing surgery using herbal fumes to reduce pain during operation and various herbs were well documented in Shushruta and Charak Samhitas for pain relief. There might be a controversy about the times of Sushruta and Charak, who seem to be almost contemporaries 2500 years ago. Physicians had a rightful place in the social structure who were training their pupils in the art of treatment; pain naturally was most common complaint of all diseases, as always. In fact in India the knowledge of herbal medicine reached its zenith in this period. There is a story how Jivaka a pupil of Charak was asked to locate a plant without any medicinal value within a sphere of 3–5 km. He came back empty handed showing the depth and extent of the knowledge of herbs. There is another story when the king under whom Jivaka was serving had severe pain in the forehead, Jivaka diagnosed it to be due to a worm in the nasal bone and gave him the medicine. The effect of medicine was to start after a while and the process of removal of worm was excruciatingly painful. Meanwhile Jivaka, wise as he was, anticipated the king's reaction during removal of worm and went away. The king when in pain ordered death sentence for Jivaka and sent his commander to carry out the death sentence. The commander found that Jivaka was eating an apple on the wayside. Jivaka offered him his apple which was impregnated with a drug which caused temporary paresis of the commander's body. Since Jivaka knew that after the worm is out, the king's pain will be relieved and then he will repent his order of death sentence. Hence he bought time by using medicated apple to his commander. The story ends happily as the king revoked his death sentence and Jivaka was reinstated. Jivaka was serving Emperor Bimbsar as a state physician. There were great universities like Nalanda in east and Taxila in west India (present day Islamabad in Pakistan), where knowledge was disseminated to the scholars from India, China, Arab and Europe. This knowledge must have travelled to Europe through Arabia.

CHINESE MEDICINE

From China in east, the knowledge travelled through scholars like Huen-T sang and Fie-Han. Various herbal medicines, ointments, potions and even surgical methods were used for relief of various diseases and the pain related to them. Emperor Shen Nung (2300 BC) was an authority on herbs. Huang Ta (2600 BC) originated Nei Ching, which described acupuncture with the concept that when spirit is bad, pain ensues and when body, is the hurt swellings occur. Virtually every disease was treated by acupuncture which tried to rectify imbalance of Yang and Yin by introducing needles into any of the 355 points along the 12 meridians traversing the body. In the second century Huo T'O used wine with an anaesthetic powder for surgical pain.

The Arab world acted as a torch bearer to the Greek medicine and kept the flame active till medieval period. Before this time the whole Europe especially Great Britain was inhabited by forest tribes without any significant contribution to medical sciences as a whole. Roman Galen's influence was observed, who used upto 100 ingredients to treat a disease.

HISTORY OF MODERN MEDICINE[2] (B.C. TO C. 1500)

A locally applied technique may have been used for circumcision, certainly freezing with ice was used during the medieval period. Oral and rectal preparations including cannabis, opium and mandragora were applied from the first century and throughout the medieval period.

Renaissance Period (C 1500 to C 1750)

Surgeons were wary of using understandardized herbal preparations because of the possibility of fatal accidents and association with the capital crime of witchcraft. Pare (France), used nerve compressions during amputations, condemning the use of potions to control pain.

The Age of Enlightment

Priestley in UK discovered oxygen and analgesic uses of nitrous oxide gas. Beddoes attempted to treat disease by inhalation of gases and vapours. His assistant Humphrey Davy demonstrated the inebriating and analgesic properties of nitrous oxide.

C 1800 to 1842

Many techniques to control surgical pain *e.g.*, nerve compression, asphyxiation, hypnosis and local refrigeration has been documented.

MODERN ANAESTHESIA[2]

Ether was independently given by William Clarke and Crawford Long without publishing their result. After failure of Horace Wells with nitrous oxide for surgical pain, WTG Morton, a Boston dentist, successfully used ether in the first public demonstration on 16th October 1846, bringing about a revolution in surgical pain relief. Mandragora and opium have been used since long for pain relief since medieval times. Wine and Hemlock extract was combined with these drugs.

Witchcraft and Mandrake

The roots of mandrake plant resembled a human form and plant was supposed to scream when uprooted and for a human, it was fatal to hear the screams, so the leaves were tied to a dog or horse's tail and herbalist keeping out of the hearing, leading to the death of the animal. However, in later thirteenth century use of mandrake was a capital crime. Further discovery and isolation of active agents, morphia and hyoscine by syringe in nineteenth century completely obviated the use of mandragora[2].

Mysterious Somnifera Spongia

Less used between 9–16th centuries. The soporific sponge was soaked in extracts of opium, mandragora and other herbs. The sponge was held close to patient's nose and inhaled. The fluid from sponge was absorbed through nasal mucosa and even ingested. In spite of above techniques used, the surgery was conducted under great agony. The surgeons were tying the patients with stakes under the sun, in open space, since there were no operational theatres or electricity. The patient was given a heavy draught of alcohol or opium and made drunk[1]. The concept of antisepsis was simply not there, surgeons using variety of instruments in the various pockets of their clothes and even over the ears and between teeth. The operations like amputations, caesarian sections were performed with a fast speed. In the later part of the operation the poor patient was already unconscious due to pain following surgery, making surgeons to satisfactorily complete the closure of the wound. The poor patients could not even run as he was tied well and held by 3–4 muscular men. If there was a heavy rain during operation, the abdomen was receiving plentiful of rainfall.

Hypnosis

Was used to relieve pain of surgery during early part of nineteenth century. Later this technique was popularized by Mesmer (1734–1815) in the mid nineteenth century. However, Mesmer himself had a cautious note about the therapeutic use of hypnosis because of the mystery surrounding it and was forced to resign his appointment at North London Hospital[2].

The advent of ether inhalation for surgical pain was a revolution in the field of pain relief. Since steam engine was installed within that week, the news spread to Europe within a fortnight, the fast speed at which a steam boat crossed the Atlantic Ocean. This idea was fast taken up by the physicians of the continent and ether anaesthesia was well established. In India, the news reached within a fortnight and ether was used successfully in surgical pain at Secunderabad. John Snow's Chloroform anaesthesia on a handkerchief to Queen Victoria during the birth of prince Leopold, lead to its official recognition throughout the world.

NUMBING EFFECTS OF COCAINE

Coca leaves were used by aborigines, American Indians to relieve stress and it was in 1860; the extract of Coca leaves was purified by Albert Nieman. In 1844, Carl Koller an intern, first published the numbing effect of cocaine on mucus membrane on the suggestion of his friend Sigmund Freud, who at the time was away on his honeymoon. This anaesthetic property of cocaine was recognized worldwide leading to local anaesthetic use in eye surgery[3]. The advent of anaesthesia marked a triumph of mankind over pain. However, the pain mechanism and anatomy was not much known. The cartesian concept of pain pathway was prevelant in seventeenth century (Fig. 1.1). The contribution of Professor Bonica, P.D Wall and Tony Yaksha greatly influenced the treatment of pain with their basic and clinical research. Their findings and wisdom guided the medical fraternity, anaesthesiologists in particular. Dr. Rowenstein, till his death in 1960, was famous for his research on his special course in anatomy, physiology and therapy of pain. Cancer pain remains a global problem. WHO estimated 3.5 million people suffering from pain (95% in terminal stage) without adequate pain relief. The reasons for inadequate treatment cited were over regulation of opioids and their under use in treating cancer pain.

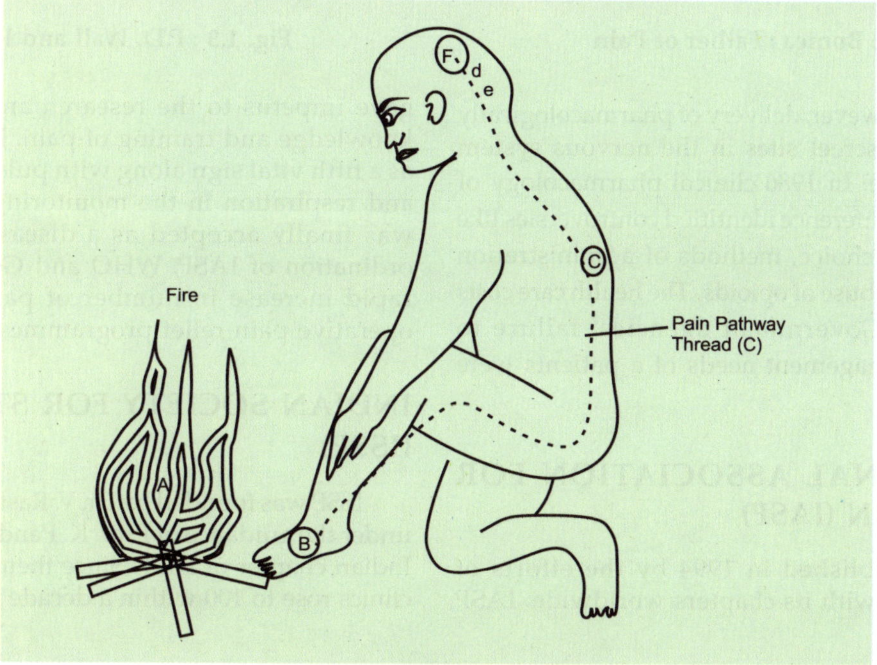

Fig. 1.1 : Descartes' (1664)

Concept of the pain pathway (When fire (A) comes near foot (B) the minute particles of the fire have the power to set in motion the spot of the skin of foot where it touched. This pulls a delicate thread (C) which is connected from (B) to end at (*d,e*). This pulling of C with a rapid force strikes a bell (F) which hangs at the other end.

RESEARCH

With the discovery of opiate receptors and endogenous opiates, the knowledge of pain was enhanced. The Gate control theory of pain proposed by Melzack and Wall was a landmark in the advancement

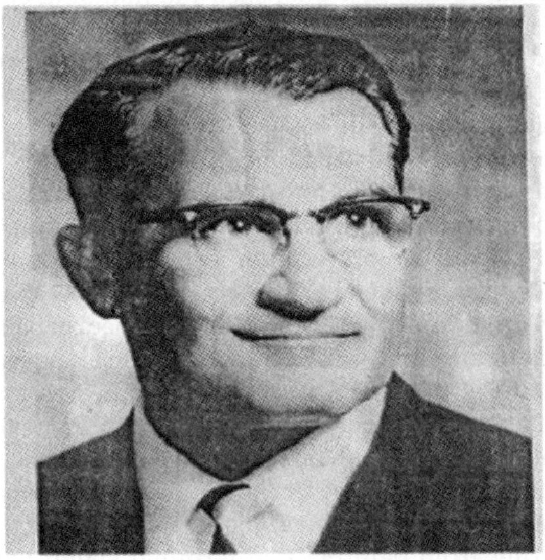

Fig. 1.2 : Bonica : Father of Pain

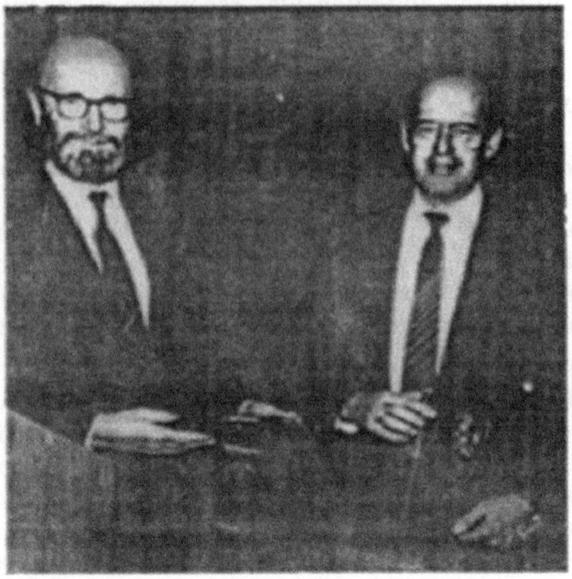

Fig. 1.3 : P.D. Wall and R. Melzack

of pain research. However, delivery of pharmacologically active agents to discreet sites in the nervous system remains a challenge. In 1986 clinical pharmacology of opioid analgesics conference identified controversies like controlled studies, choice, methods of administration tolerance and drug abuse of opioids. The health care costs and private and Government agencies' failure to recognize pain management needs of a patients were realized.

INTERNATIONAL ASSOCIATION FOR STUDY OF PAIN (IASP)

IASP was established in 1994 by the efforts of Dr. Bonica in USA with its chapters worldwide. IASP gave impetus to the research and dissemination of knowledge and training of pain. Pain was advocated as a fifth vital sign along with pulse, B.P., temperature and respiration in the monitoring. The chronic pain was finally accepted as a disease in itself. The co-ordination of IASP, WHO and Governments lead to rapid increase in number of pain clinics and post operative pain relief programmes.

INDIAN SOCIETY FOR STUDY OF PAIN (ISSP)

ISSP was founded by Dr. V. Rastogi and Dr. P. Kumar under the guidance of Prof. K. Pandey in 1984 and made Indian chapter of IASP. Since then the number of pain clinics rose to 100 within a decade in India.

REFERENCES

1. Mehta BS. History of Medicine. 1st edition, New Delhi. Parimal publications. 1999;1–48.
2. Boueton TB, Wilkinson DJ. The origins of Modern Anaesthesia. In Healy TEJ, Cohen RJ (Eds). A practice of Anaesthesia. 6th Edn, London, Arnold Edward, 1995;3–55.
3. Morris LE. Pain and analgesia for operative interventions (1847 to 1997). In History of Anaesthesia. Proceedings of Fourth International Symposium on History of Anaesthesia. Schulte AM, Goerig M (Eds). Luebeck dragger, 1998;57–72.

•••

SECTION–II

Basic Mechanism

PAIN–BASIC MECHANISM

2

Pain is a complex perception that has profound affective and cognitive features. Pain is not a stimulus. There are no pain fibres and no pain pathways within brain. Whether or not a particular stimulus will be perceived as painful depends on the nature of the stimulus, the situation in which it is experienced, memories, emotions etc. Pain serves an essential function to guarantee immediate awareness about actual or threatening injury warning the individual to adapt a protective behaviour. The experience of pain is subjective and involves sensory, cognitive and motivational components. The variability of human pain suggests that there are neural mechanisms that modulate transmission in pain pathways and modify individual's reaction to pain.

Descartes in 17th century described the pain pathway, whereby he proposed, the body works like a machine and that it can be studied by using experimental methods of physics. According to this theory injury activates pain fibres which in turn project pain impulses through a spinal pain pathway to a pain centre in the brain. Since then the emphasis has shifted from the central role of dorsal horn in spinal cord, then on to the role of brain as modulator, inhibitor and exciter of pain pathways as suggested by the concept of neuromatrix.

TWO TYPES OF PERSISTENT PAIN

Nociceptive / Inflammatory Pain[1]

The most peripheral apparatus for pain pathway is nociceptors which are present all over the body. On application of natural stimuli of adequate intensity to the skin, two sequential pain sensations are elicited. They are related to the activation of myelinated A-delta fibres (>2 m/sec) and unmyelinated C fibres (<2 m/sec). Most studies used heat and mechanical stimuli to study nociception and, therefore, nomenclature of CMH and AMH is used to refer to C fibre mechano-heat sensitive receptors and A fibre mechano-heat sensitive receptors respectively. Activity in nociceptor induces an increase in sympathetic discharge but the converse is not true under usual circumstances. Sympathetic nervous system pain dependent activity is referred to as sympathetically maintained pain (SMP), which is seen in acute herpes zoster, soft tissue trauma. Tissue damage results in a cascade of events leading to enhanced pain to natural stimulus.

Neuropathic Pain

Examples include post-herpetic neuralgia, complex regional pain syndrome (CRPS) and Phantom limb pain. This type of pain arises from injury to the peripheral / central nervous system. It is burning in quality. It is less responsive to opioids, but responds to local anaesthetics, anticonvulsants and tricyclic antidepressants[2].

Mechanism of Sensitization at Primary Afferent Nociceptors

Although there are no pain fibres in peripheral or central nervous system, there are anatomically and physiological specialized peripheral afferent fibres that responds to noxious stimuli. These thinly myelinated A-delta and unmyelinated C-afferents terminate as free unencapsulated peripheral nerve endings.

Physiological specificity of primary afferent is indicated from the following :

1. Nerve compression first blocks large fibres and nonpainful mechanical sensation, then the sensation mediated by small fibres and later the perception of noxious stimuli.
2. Local anaesthetics block small diameter fibres first and abolish pain.
3. Electrical stimulation of single primary afferents in the conscious human subject evokes pain only when thresholds for A-delta and C-fibres are reached. The former do not respond to painful stimuli but are necessary for normal quality of pain perception. In the absence of these large fibres all sensations are perceived as burning, indicating the breakdown of specificity when large fibres are

blocked. Convergence of large and small diameter afferents at the level of the dorsal horn underlies this phenomenon.

Allodynia

The stimuli that normally are not painful *e.g.*, movement and light touch become painful. The pain produced by touching sun burnt skin or movement of an arthritic joint[3].

Hyperalgesia

Hyperalgesia is an exacerbated pain produced by a noxious stimulus *e.g.*, slapping, sun burnt skin or reaction to noxious stimuli in a subject, whose large fibres in the arm are blocked by compression.

NSAIDs are effective through cyclooxygenase inhibition. COX-2 enzyme inhibitors, Celecoxib and Rofecoxib have a better utility without GIT side effects of Aspirin and NSAIDs.

Substance-P

An 11 amino acid peptide neurotransmitter synthesized by primary afferent nociceptors, substance-P is released in the dorsal horn and activates second order "pain" transmission neuron in the dorsal horn. It is released from the peripheral terminals of C-fibres and contributes to local, neurogenic inflammatory mechanisms, including vasodilatation, warmth, redness and swelling.

Capsaicin, an irritant is the pungent ingredient in the hot pepper. It stimulates C-fibres, because they express

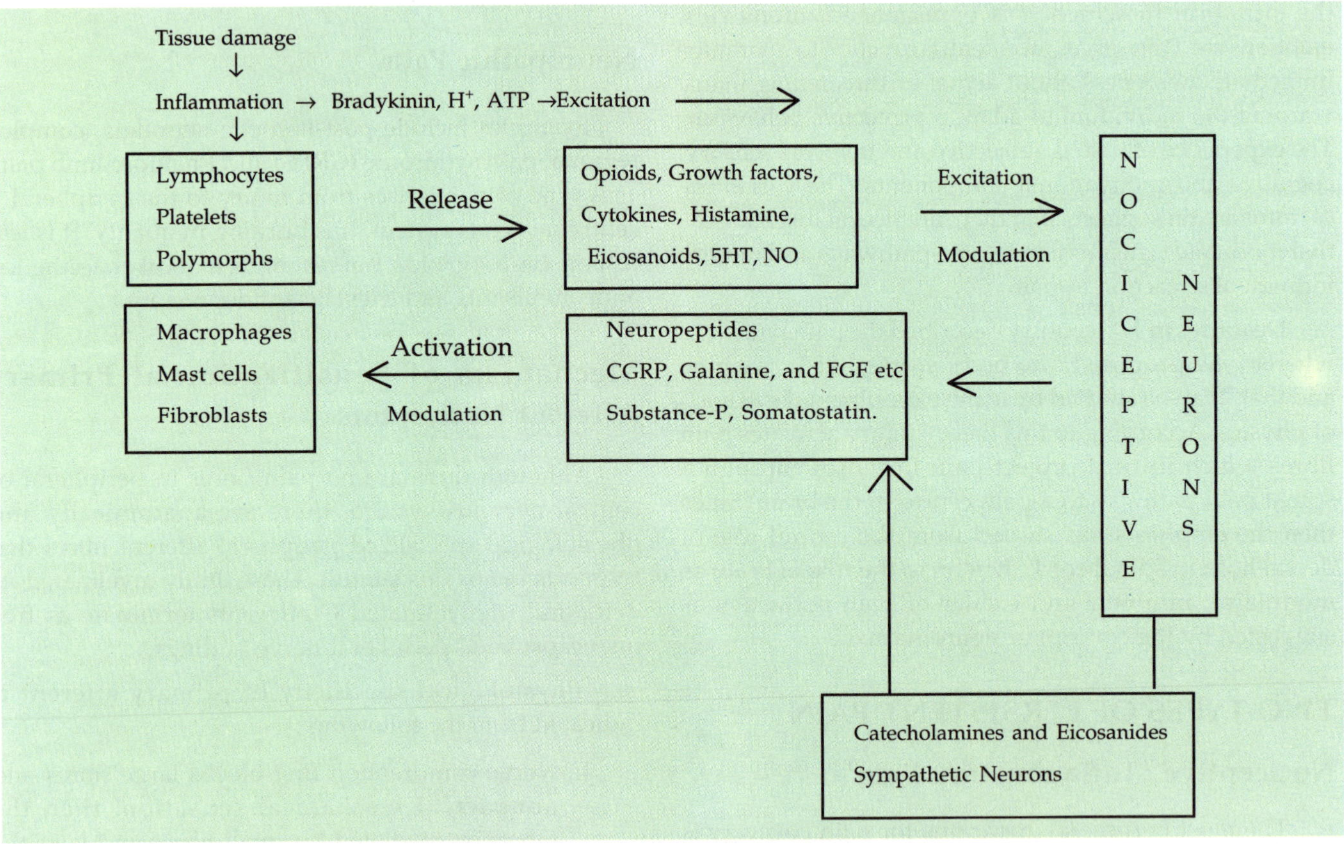

Fig. 2.1 : Mediators produced by injury, inflammation at the terminal neurons

Primary Sensitization Mechanism

After a tissue injury, the threshold for firing of A-delta and C-nociceptive afferent are lowered to a non-noxious range. Mechanism involves synthesis of arachidonic acid from membrane lipids via steroid sensitive phospholipase A2 enzyme. Arachidonic acid is acted upon by cyclooxygenase enzyme to produce prostaglandins which act directly on the peripheral terminals of A-delta and C-fibers, while their electrical activity remains unchanged. Light touch can now activate a C-fibre and produce pain. Aspirin and the venilloid (VR1) / capsaicin receptor. VR1 receptor also responds to noxious heat and is gated by pH. The acidity of injured tissue may enhance pain via VR1. Topical Capsaicin creams have been introduced to control a variety of pains. Their efficacy remains to be established.

Onward Transmission of Pain Impulse[4]

When the depolarization at the junction of the receptor and the axon to which it is attached reaches threshold level, an impulse is propagated along the surface of the axon. The nociceptive information is relayed by A-delta and C-fibres through posterior roots into the spinal cord. The grey matter in the spinal cord is divided into 10 layers (Laminae). The skin afferents terminate in Laminae-I, II, and V of the dorsal horn, while those from viscera, muscles and the other deep tissues terminate in Laminae-I, V and X. The neurons in the spinal cord are classified as those specific to nociceptive specific neurons and nonspecific or wide dynamic range. These axons pass from dorsal horn to the contra lateral side of the spinal cord. They further travel up with anterolateral region of the cord to form synapse with neurons in Thalamus, Mesencephalon or Reticular formation. N-methyl-D-aspartate receptor is activated in response to tissue damage along with other neuro–peptides *e.g.*, substance-P. Dorsal horn is the seat of control, excitatory and inhibitory influences (Fig. 3). These alterations in the functional performance of the cord will alter sensory processing and are likely to account both for failure to react to tissue damage on some occasions and the generation of pain in reaction to low intensity stimuli in others. Understanding the factors controlling or determining in which mode the

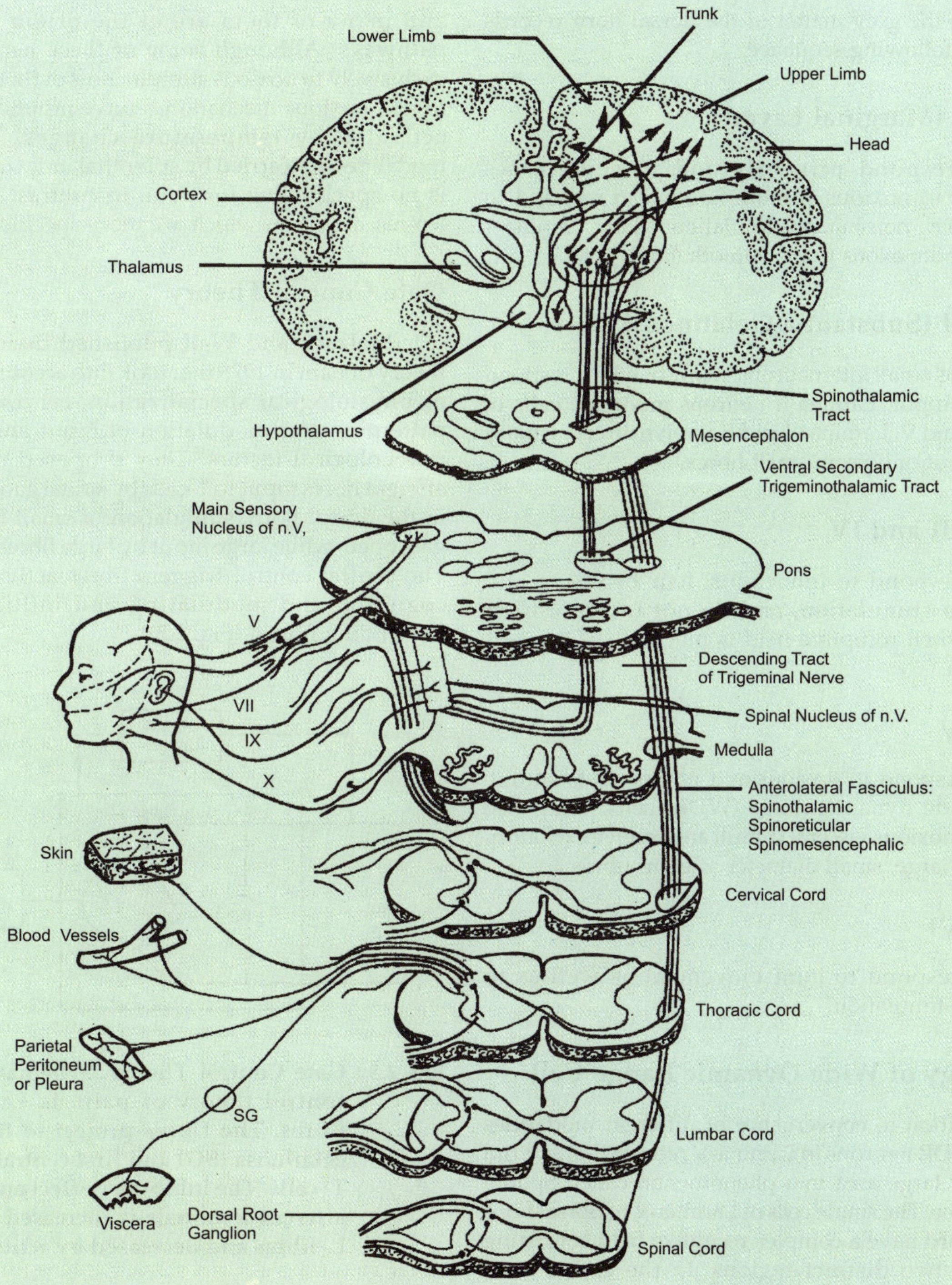

Fig. 2.2 : Scheme of nociceptive receptors from various part of the body to the brain

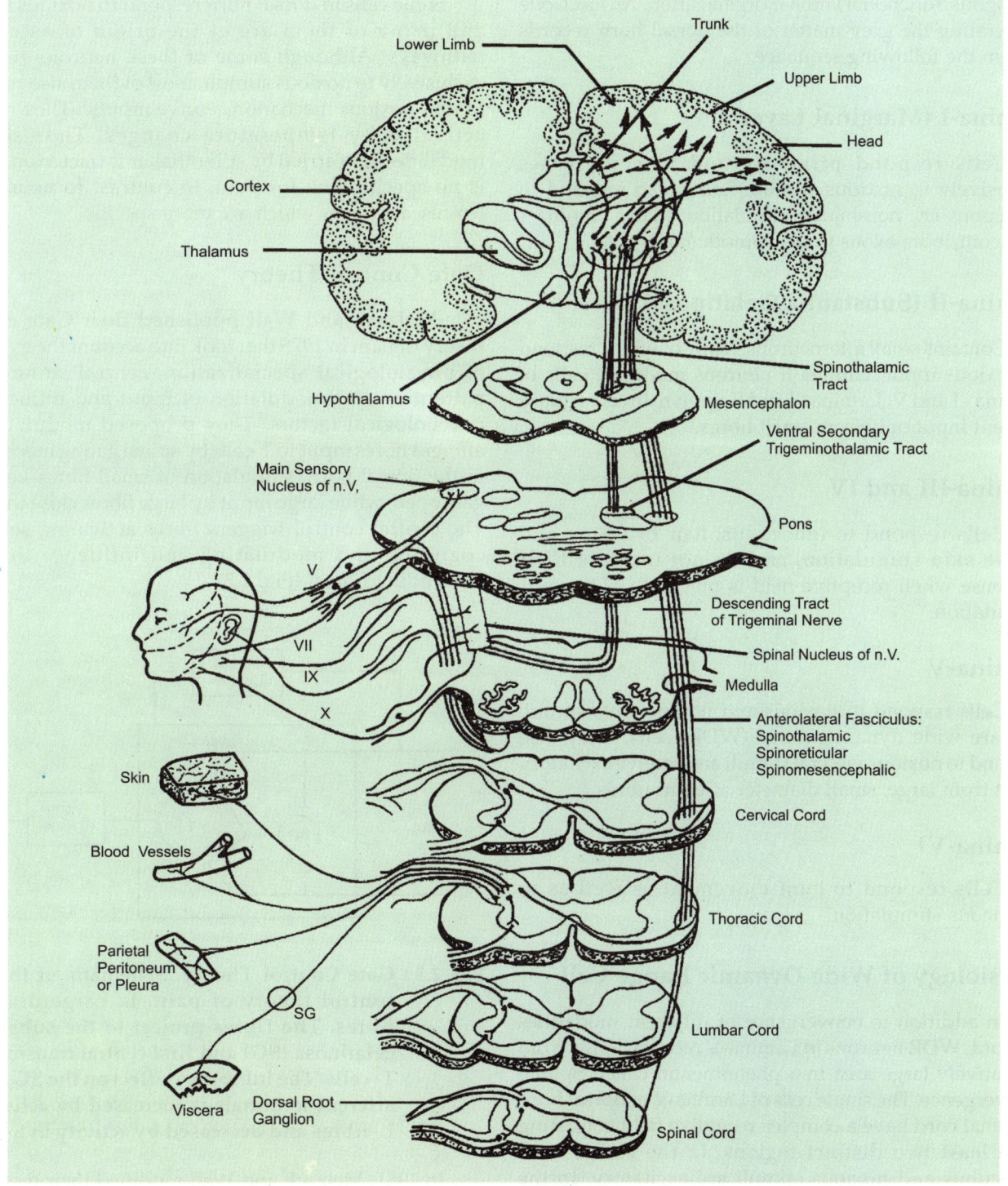

spinal cord is essential in order to understand the pathogenesis of pain. A damage to peripheral or CNS may alter or result in irreversible changes in sensory processing and disorders.

Spinal Cord Laminar Organization[1]

In 1954 Rexed demonstrated that the grey matter of the spinal cord could be divided into distinct laminae or layers. Physiological studies too have demonstrated an analogous, functional laminar organization. An electrode penetrating the grey matter of the dorsal horn records cells in the following sequence.

Lamina-I (Marginal Layer)

Cells respond primarily and in some cases exclusively to noxious stimuli. Some also respond to innocuous *i.e.,* non-injury stimulation. Many Lamina-1 cells contribute axons to the spinothalamic tract.

Lamina-II (Substantia Gelatinosa)

Contains small interneurons, many of which respond to noxious input. Lamina-II neurons modulate cells of Lamina - I and V. Lamina - I and II receive direct primary afferent input only from small fibres.

Lamina-III and IV

Cells respond to innocuous, hair brushing and tactile skin stimulation, and do not increase their response when receptive field is pinched *i.e.,* noxious stimulation.

Lamina-V

Cells respond to noxious and non-noxious stimuli and are wide dynamic range (WDR) cells. They also respond to noxious visceral stimuli and receive excitatory input from large, small diameter afferent fibres.

Lamina-VI

Cells respond to joint movement as well as to cutaneous stimulation.

Physiology of Wide Dynamic Range Cell

In addition to convergence of different modalities of input, WDR neurons in Lamina-V receive inputs from a relatively large area in a phenomenon called Spatial Convergence. The single cells of Lamina-V of dorsal horn of spinal cord have a complex receptive field consisting of at least two distinct regions. In the centre both innocuous and noxious stimuli are excitatory. In the surrounding regions, non-noxious stimuli (carried by large fibres) are inhibitory. This factor accounts for pain relieving effects of TENS. On the other hand, removal of the inhibitory components of the receptive field as in nerve injury might increase the response of a WDR cell to a noxious stimulus. The lesion causing selective damage to sources of inhibitory inputs to WDR neurons can produce pain.

Spinal Cord Neurons do not Transmit Pain

Some cells in dorsal horn respond to noxious stimuli and many of them are at the origin of ascending pathways. Although some of these neurons respond exclusively to noxious stimuli, most of them also respond to non-noxious mechanoreceptive inputs. They may be activated by temperature changes. Thus several modalities are carried by spinothalamic tract axon. There is no specific line for pain, in contrast to neurons in lemniscal system which are more specific.

Gate Control Theory

Melzack and Wall published their Gate control theory of pain in 1975 that took into account the evidence of physiological specialization, central summation, patterning and modulation of input and influence of psychological factors. They proposed modulation of afferent fibres input to T-cells by spinal gating mechanism in the dorsal horn, stimulation of small fibres keep the gate open, while large input by large fibres close the gate. The central control triggers fibres activating selective cognition and modulating and influence through descending fibres[5] (Fig. 2.3).

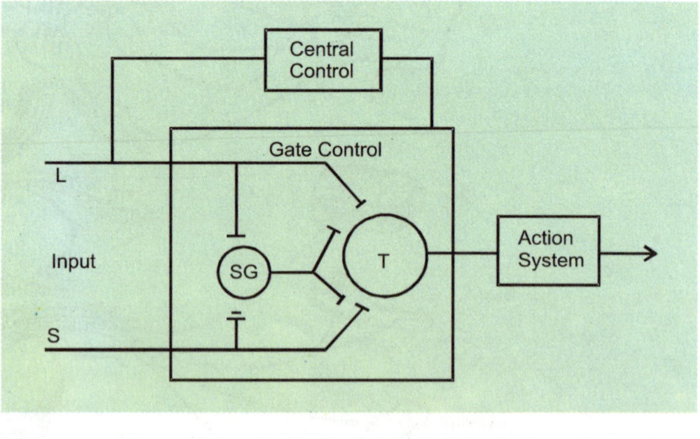

Fig. 2.3 : Gate Control Theory. Schematic of the gate control theory of pain. L. Large diameter fibres. The fibres project to the substancia gelatinosa (SG) and first central transmission T- cells. The inhibitory effect on the SG on the afferent terminals is increased by activity in L -fibres and decreased by activity in S-fibres

In 1981, Melzack and Wall modified their theory by taking into account the information acquired in the

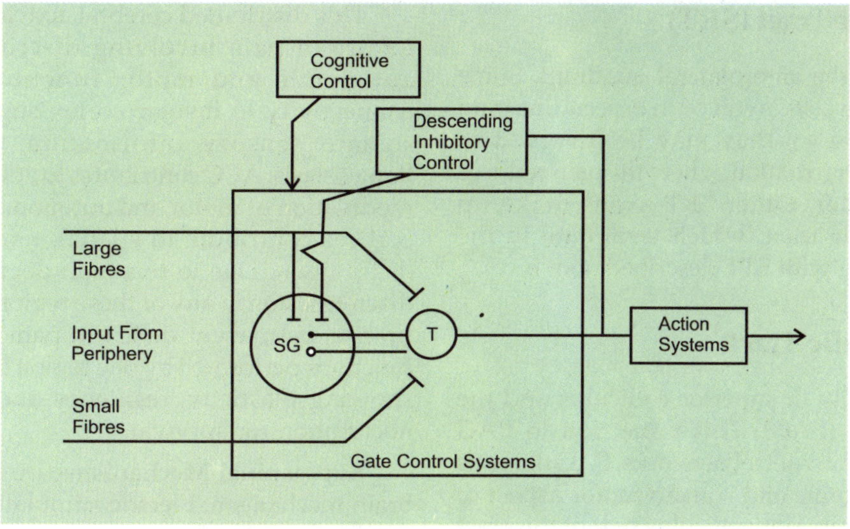

Fig. 2.4 : Modified Gate Control Theory

original proposal. Their model includes excitatory and inhibitory links from substantia gelatinosa to the transmission cells as well as the descending inhibitors of control from brain stem. These theories have provoked the development of new approaches to pain therapy[6].

Secondary Hyperalgesia (Central Sensitization)

Acute pain is brief, while post operative pain may be considered as extended acute pain. Unfortunately noxious stimuli may sometimes evoke long-term, persistent changes in the excitability of dorsal horn neurons leading to a greater response to subsequent impulse. This phenomenon is called secondary hyperalgesia in contrast to primary sensitization described earlier. Glutamate acting via N-methyl-D-aspartate (NMDA) receptor has a role in this condition. The secondary hyperalgesia can be prevented by pre-emptive analgesia using local anaesthetic blockade of afferents from a surgical site, in order to prevent the spinal cord from experiencing the noxious stimulus associated with surgery. Under general anaesthesia, patient is unaware of the stimulus, but the spinal cord and the memory of injury can still be established.

Referred Pain

The WDR cells that receive input from somatic nociceptive primary afferents in the skin and deep tissue also receive input from nociceptors in the viscera. This phenomenon presumably underlies the referral of visceral pain to somatic structures. For example, inflammation of the peritoneal surface of the diaphragm may cause referred pain of right shoulder. The afferents that innervates diaphragm arise from C3–C5 segments and run with phrenic nerve.

Ascending Pathways

Since surgical section of anterolateral spinothalamic tract relieves pain in the contralateral side, it has been thought earlier that spinothalamic tract is pain tract. But cutting the anterolateral quadrant does not selectively cut spinothalamic tract. Recently many ascending pathways have been found to transmit nociceptive messages to brain.

Spinothalamic Tract (STT)

Cells of origin are located in Rexed's Laminae I and V, majority of these axons cross locally in anterior commissure and ascend in the contralateral anterolateral column, terminating in ventro posterior thalamic nucleus. From there the axons go to somato sensory cortex in post central gyrus. Some of the spinothalamic tract axons terminate within medial thalamus in the intralaminar nuclei, having large receptive fields with little topographic organization. Firing of neurons in medial thalamus is influenced by behavioural state as reduced pain in humans who are destructed.

The inputs from medial thalamus are projected to many cortical, subcortical sites including limbic and motor regions. The diversity of these projections may reflect the variety of emotional and motor responses which pain evokes. The posterior nucleus of thalamus where majority of spinothalamic axons terminate, recently has been identified to receive specific information about noxious and temperature stimuli from Lamina-I of dorsal horn. This region of thalamus sends projection to the insular cortex.

The Spinoreticular Tract (SRT)

SRT is located in the anterolateral quadrant. Some SRT axons terminate on cells involved in descending pain modulation pathways so, they may be involved in phenomenon of counter irritation, where the pain reduces the severity of another. Other SRT axons make up spinoreticulo-thalamic tract, which terminate in the medial thalamus along with STT described above.

Spinomesencephalic Tract

Terminate primarily in superior colliculus and the peri aqueductal grey (PAG). This projection to PAG activates descending pain control networks. PAG neurons are involved in autonomic and somato motor aspect of defense reaction. The superior colliculus part of this tract is involved in multi sensory integration, behavioural reactions and orientation.

Postsynaptic Dorsal Horn Column Pathways

Mostly axon collaterals of large diameter, primary afferents and some of the Lamina-V axons project axons in this column, terminating in Cuneate and Gracile Nuclei. These may be responsible for transmission of the visceral pain.

Spino-ponto-amygdala System

Originates in Laminae-I and V of the dorsal horn, ascending in the dorso lateral funiculus. It projects to the para brachial area of the pons and from there to amygdala. This system may be involved in fear and memory of pain, as well as behavioural and autonomic reactions to noxious events *e.g.*, vocalization, flight, pupil dilatation and cardio respiratory responses.

Cortical Processing of Pain

Early observations by Kead and Holmes (1911) in soldiers who had extensive injuries of cerebral cortex continued to perceive pain. Penfield and Boldrey (1937) reached a similar conclusion, when patients rarely reported pain sensation after electrical stimulation of their cerebral cortex during surgery for removal of epileptic foci. They concluded that cerebral cortex played only a minimal role in pain perception despite nociceptive information reaching a number of cortical areas.[4]

Recently, Positron Emission Tomography (PET) to measure regional cerebral blood flow and use of Functional Magnetic Resonance Imaging (fMRI) to show changes in blood oxygenation, showed that several cortical regions are activated during pain. The heat, touch, capsaicin stimulus activated primary and secondary somatosensory cortices (S1, S2), anterior cingulate cortex (ACC) and Insular Cortex (IC).

This distributed cerebral activation reflects complex nature of pain involving discrimination, affective, autonomic and motor function. The anatomical connectivity to insular cortex suggests integration of somato sensory information with memory and homeostasis. ACC contributes to affective component and modulation of motor and autonomic reactions. S_1 and S_2 cortices contribute to spatial, temporal and intensity distribution. Due to this high degree of connectivity, a discrete lesion in any of these regions does not produce a precise, permanent deficit in pain perception. It shows functions performed by one region taken over by another, showing plasticity, resiliency and essential nature of nociception for survival.

Supraspinal Mechanisms are inhibitory part of the brain mechanism. Electric stimulation of midbrain PAG produces analgesia in humans along with inhibition of firing of dorsal horn neurons that respond to pain. The descending control is mediated via an excitatory connection from the PAG to Serotonin (5-HT) containing neurons of the nucleus Raphe Magnus of Medulla. The 5-HT axons from there inhibit the firing of neurons in Laminae-I and V. There also exist parallel descending noradrenergic inhibitory controls acted upon by Tricyclic antidepressant. The circuit from PAG to spinal cord constitutes brain's end organ pain control system.

Descending Inhibitory Pathways (DIP)

Begins in cerebral cortex and descends to thalamus and Peri Aqueductal Grey (PAG) of midbrain which is rich in opiate receptors, responsible for secreting enkephalin and endorphins. Fibres from PAG descend to Nucleus Raphe Magnus (NRM) in brainstem, responsible for secretion of 5-HT alleviating pain threshold and contributing depression. Then fibres descend to spinal cord, exciting other inhibitory neurons to secrete transmitter gamma-aminobutyric acid (GABA). These lower fibres of DIP synapse with interneurons, communicating pain signals entering spinal cord via A-delta and C-fibres as well as second order neurons in lateral spinothalamic tract. Thus DIP acts at all levels where pain signals first enter the CNS. In addition to pain and depression, neurotransmitters also enhance tissue healing, increasing quality of sleep time and in general increasing the quality of life.

Neuromatrix Theory

Proposed by Melzack where brain processes a neural network and it integrates multiple inputs to produce output pattern which produces pain. The synaptic architecture is determined by genetic and sensory influences. The inputs acting on neuromatrix or sensory, cognition and emotional inputs, intrinsic inhibitory and body stress regulation activity *e.g.*, cytokines, autonomic, immune and opioid system. Glial activation and its associated proinflammatory cytokine release are being implicated in exaggerated pain states, thus linked to acute peripheral inflammation, chronic nerve trauma and infection.[1]

Opiates, Opioids and Endorphins

PAG and dorsal horn have high opiate receptor concentration which bind morphine and naloxone and intrinsic endorphin peptides. The latter has been cloned providing future development of newer analgesics. The placebo activates the endorphins and reversed by naloxone. TENS, acupuncture also does the same. Hypnosis does not involve endorphin release. The morphine injection inhibits Laminae-I, V and blocks release of neurotransmitters *e.g.*, substance-P from small fibres.

Mechanism Underlying Progression of Acute to Chronic Pain State

Acute and chronic pain states have been identified as two markedly different entities from all aspects of their pathophysiology to manifestations, diagnosis and management. While acute pain serves a definitive protective and reparative function, easy to identify and treat chronic pain has been recognized as a disease state which persists beyond the usual course of an acute disease or healing process or recurs for months or years. An understanding of mechanisms underlying the development of chronic pain is important for its management and prevention of progression of acute to chronic pain.

Elegant neurophysiological experiments on inflammatory and arthritic pain models have supported clinical studies reporting peripheral as well as central sensitization following persistent stimulation of primary nociceptors.[7] Liberation of allogenic substance (serotonin, histamine, bradykinin, prostaglandins) alter the micro environment around the nociceptors causing their further stimulation and increased capillary permeability adding more mediators and increased sensitivity of nociceptors, development of oedema, allodynia and hyperalgesia. Peripheral sensitization is followed by spinal sensitization. Studies have revealed increased excitability of dorsal horn neurons and their receptive field, elevated levels of Glutamate, PGE_2, NO along with Neuropeptides (substance-P, calcitonin gene related peptide), upgrading of receptors followed by expression of genes coding neurotransmitters, if stimulation continues. The increased excitability spreads to lateral and ventral horn neurons activating sympathetic nervous activity and skeletal muscle spasm. This in turn creates a vicious cycle maintaining abnormal spinal neuron activity which may spread to suprasegmental and higher brain regions evoking neuroendocrinal responses.[6]

Pain resulting from nerve injuries, phantom limb and post herpetic neuralgia has been explained through hypothesis proposed by Wall and colleagues[4], which essentially suggests loss or imbalance of sensory input into the somatosensory system leading to inhibition of inhibitory mechanisms within neuraxis.

Role of sympathetic nervous system in several pain states is well documented. However, the studies revealed a significant hyperalgesia with cholinergic blockers and the effect was seen even in the spinal animals. An inhibitory role of acetylcholine on nociceptors and a link between cholinergic discharge noradrenergic receptors on peripheral nociceptors is suggested.[8]

Studies conducted on acute and chronic pain patients to evaluate acupuncture analgesia revealed varying degrees of pain relief and also basal autonomic status of these patients. Do the autonomic changes contribute to pain states or are just accompanying responses is not clear. It, however, seems that evaluation of autonomic status of pain patients may help identifying acute pain, patients likely to progress to chronic pain state.[4] Chronic pain affects 10% of the pain patients for more than 100 days. Examples are cancer pain, low back ache, arthritis, migraine with a history of multiple episodes.

REFERENCES

1. Basbaum A, Bushnell C. Pain, basic mechanism. In an updated review, refresher course syllabus, Giamberardino MA(Ed), Seattle, IASP Press, 2002;3–7.
2. Basbaum AJ, Jessel T. The perception of pain. In Kendel ER, Schwatz J, Jessel T (Ed). Principles of Neuro science, New York, Appleton and Lange, 2000;472–491.
3. Koltzernburg M. Neural mechanisms of cutaneous nociceptive pain. Clin. J. Pain, 2000;16:131–138.
4. Wall PD and Melzack R. Textbook of Pain, 3ed chapter-3, Edinburgh, Churchill Livingstone, 1996;57–78.
5. Renfield W, Boldrey E. Somatic motor and sensory representation in the cerebral cortex of man as studied by electrical stimulation, Brain;1937,60:389–443.
6. Melzack R, Wall PD. Pain mechanism a new theory. Science 1965;150:971–979. Head H, Holms G. Sensory disturbances from cerebral lesions. Brain, 1911:84:102–254.
7. Woolf CJ, Wall PD. The relative effectiveness of C-primary afferents on facilitation of flexor reflexes in rats. J. Neuro; Sci. 1986.1433–7.
8. Iggo A, Guilband G, Tegner R. Sensory mechanism in arthritic rat's joints. In: Kruger L, Libo-kins JC, (Ed). Advances in pain research and therapy.Volum 6, New York, Raven press, 1984;83–93.

•••

DEVELOPMENT OF FOETAL AND NEONATAL PAIN BEHAVIOUR

3

Few things stimulate a caregiver's helping instinct more than the pain cry of a child. Organized pain relief for children, however, historically has been hampered by societal and medical misinformation and by the slow and deliberate nature of good basic research. The fields of developmental biology, pain assessment, and treatment have seen tremendous gains. Progress is reflected in the fact that treatment for the pain of infants and children in both acute and chronic settings has become safe and effective. Assessment and measurement of pain in infants and preverbal children continue to be difficult. On the other hand, cognitive-behavioural treatments can be used quite effectively for children undergoing medical procedures as well as in the treatment of a range of acute and chronic pain problems. For many children, fear and anxiety dominate their thought processes during medical encounters.

Developmental Neurobiology of Pain

The study of pain in infancy and of the longer-term implications of noxious stimuli has intensified over the past 20 years. Pain plays an important role in learning and neurologic development. Thus, it would be expected that the afferent pathways for pain sensation and perception would develop early in life.[1]

At the time of birth, the nociceptive pathways and connections are well established. In fact, thalamo-cortical projections begin synapse formation with cortical neurons by 20 to 24 weeks' gestational age, and myelination of afferent pathways to the thalamus is generally complete by 30 weeks. Myelination of thalamocortical fibres is complete by roughly 37 weeks' gestational age. Although afferent nociceptive paths appear well developed by birth, descending control of pain is slower to develop.

Primary afferent nerve fibres project to peripheral targets midway through foetal life in rats and in humans. Infant rats show lower-impulse thresholds and more prolonged discharges in primary afferent C and A fibres when exposed to noxious stimuli than do adult rats. In addition, newborn rat pups respond to skin wound with extensive proliferation of A and C fibers in the region of the wound. Functionallly, the rat pups display hyperalgesia manifested by decreased flexion withdrawl thresholds. These behavioural and neuroanatomic responses appear to decrease in magnitude with advancing age.

The flexion withdrawl reflex is well developed in neonatal rats and human newborns. Interestingly, younger premature infants exhibit sensitization to repeated noxious stimuli. The closer the infants are to full-term gestational age, the more likely they are to habituate to the stimuli, a reponse characteristic of children and adults. Human newborns receiving repeated heel lancing for blood sampling develop secondary hyperalgesia, a manifestation of spinal plasticity.

In a number of studies, the protooncogene *C-fos* has been used as a marker of neuronal activity. In adult animals, noxious stimulation evokes *C-fos* expression in the superficial dorsal horn laminae. Fitzgerald showed that even nonnoxious stimulation evokes prominent *C-fos* expression in laminae 1 and 2 in neonatal rats. The neonatal rats have A-fibre light-touch afferent projections to synaptic targets on laminae 1 and 2 dorsal horn neurons. The light-touch A-fibre afferents of the adult rat normally synapse in deeper laminae of the dorsal horn, not in the superficial laminae that receive projections from C-and A-delta-fibre afferent fibres that are involved in nociception. In addition, dorsal horn neurons in neonatal animals often show quite prolonged firing after noxious stimulation.

It is unclear how to interpret what the experiments regarding flexion withdrawal reflexes, *C-fos* expression, and A-fibre projection to superficial laminae mean in terms of pain *experience* in the neonate. It would be an over interpretation to conclude that the neonate is inherently hyperalgesic.

Advances in the neurosciences have shown that infant nervous system is not simply an immature adult nervous system. Complex changes at the molecular, cellular and organizational levels result in a series of transient functional stages until the adult pattern is achieved.

During Prenatal Life

The reaction of foetal nervous system can be distinguished by different reflex responses, in place of pain perception "feeling", reflex response to somatic stimuli begins at 7.5 weeks in the human foetus[1]. The first area to become sensitive is perioral region which when touched results in contralateral bending of the head. The palms of hands, body and later hind limbs are sensitive. There are spontaneous reflex movements in the absence of any external stimuli *e.g.,* stretching hand to face contact, startle, sucking, continuing into the postnatal life[2]. The cortex is not functioning at this stage, so these movements are not conscious reaction to stimuli.

In Postnatal Life

The somatosensory reflexes in the foetal life are still present, but a prick on the hind foot brings about the whole body movement. With maturity this response is restricted to an isolated leg or foot movement, thus becoming more individualized due to an inhibitory process where total patterns tend to go into the background, lying dormant from where they may be aroused at any time later on by appropriate stimulation[3]. The cutaneous reflexes in newborn are exaggerated compared to adult, thresholds are lower and reflex muscle contractions are synchronized and long lasting. Repeated skin stimulation brings about hyper excitability and non-specific whole body movements upto 10 days and later flexor response in neonates. However, in adults this flexor response has a classic biphasic pattern, an early response followed by a reduced response (fade) and then reappearance of a longer lasting response that declines over the next hour[5].

Development of Peripheral and Central Nerves

In the postnatal phase and early neonatal period enormous changes take place in the nervous system of a newborn. The penetration of skin by nerve fibres and the maturation of C-fibre synaptic connections in the dorsal horn, intraneuronal development in the substantia gelatinosa and the functional development of descending inhibition from the brainstem, displaying late maturity which means a clear response to pain stimulus, but this response is not organized or predictable. The specific pain responses require convergent inputs building up over time to become apparent.

Development of Neurotransmitters

Many transmitters L-glutamate, substance-P, CGRP and somatostatin, thiamine and acid phosphates appear in the primary afferents in early development of nervous system. The other signaling molecules involved *e.g.,* opioid, peptides, monoamines (adrenaline), GABA are also present in early development stages, but adult levels are not reached for a considerable time. The receptors are frequently transiently over expressed or expressed in areas not seen in the adults. Low levels of neurotransmitters mean reduced functions, but wide spread and high density receptor distribution results in nonspecific or quite different function in the neonate as compared to the adult[7].

Gene Expression in Developing Pain Pathways

The *C-fos* gene, one of the immediate early genes is induced in P1 neonatal rat dorsal horn cells by subcutaneous capsaicin and formalin injections. This finding is consistent with *C-fos* induction by high threshold afferents in adults. The selective mutation of particular gene and studying changes of CNS development allows one to isolate the normal function of a gene. One such mutant lacking low affinity NGF receptor is viable and shows important changes in pain processing. The skin of this animal lacks SP and CGRP containing nerves and gradually become ulcerated with epidermal thinning. Another approach allows relevant gene construct along with a selective promoter to be induced into transgenic mice, allowing over expression of the gene in the resulting phenotype[8].

Mothers who treat their unborn children to classical music may be wasting their time. New research suggests that human babies and other animals are locked in a deep sleep until they are born—and gain little from such experiences.

The research flies in the face of the modern idea that foetuses become conscious while still in the womb. Such beliefs have doctors and vets to use relaxant drugs on foetuses when overseeing late-stage abortions or miscarriages.

Professor David Mellor, the physiologist who carried out the research, believes such concerns are unwarranted and that foetuses cannot feel anything before or during birth. Mellor suggest that in mammals the foetal brain is kept in a deep sleep throughout pregnancy by a combination of natural sedatives secreted by the brain and placenta. "Consciousness appears for the first time after birth. The foetus cannot suffer before or during birth. Suffering can only occur in the newborn when the onset of breathing oxygenates its tissues,"

The research on which Mellor—director of the Animal Welfare, Science and Bioethics Centre at Massey University in New Zealand —based his findings, was carried out on animals, mainly sheep, because it would have been too risky to test on humans. In the tests, pregnant animals were anaesthetised and operated on to expose their foetuses. Electrical leads that measure brain activity were attached to the foetuses' heads and they were replaced in the womb.

The researchers recorded brain activity for the rest of the pregnancy—with startling results. "The electrical activity of the brain was very low early on in pregnancy. Around halfway, occasional spikes suggested small bursts of activity. The electrical activity is never showing a conscious state. It is a sleep-like state."

"There was some thought that the foetus had an awake state but this is not so. There is a period of physical responsiveness in the last weeks when they move around but it is just a form of intermediate sleep."

Experts on human foetal development, however, are cautious about Mellor's findings. (The Sunday Times London).

REFERENCES

1. Bradley RM, Mistretta CM. Final sensory receptors, Physiological reviews, 1975;55:352–382.
2. DeVries JIP, Visser GHA, Precht HFR. The emergence of fetal behavior. Qualitative aspect. Early human development, 1982;12:302–322.
3. Angillo, Gonzalez AW. The prenatal development of behavior in the albino rat. Journal of Comparative Neurology, 1932;55:395–442.
4. Fitzgerald M. The development of activity evoked by fine diameter cutaneous fibres in the spinal cord of the newborn rat. Neuroscience. letters, 1988;86:161–166.
5. Dubuisson D, Dennis SG. The formalin test – a quantitative study of the analgesic effects of morphine, meperidine and brain stimulation in rats and cats. Pain, 1977;4:161–174.
6. Fitzgerald M, Gibson S. The physiological and neurochemical development of peripheral sensory C fibers. Neuroscience, 1984;13:933–944.
7. Fitzgerald M. Neurobiology of fetal and neonatal pain. In Textbook of PAIN, Wall PD and Melzack RM, Edinburgh, Churchill Livingstone, 1994;153–161.
8. Leek F, Lie A Huber L. Fetal, targeted mutation of gene encoding the low affinity NGF receptor, P75 leads to deficits in the peripheral sensory nervous system. Cell, 1992;69:737–749.

•••

4

CYTOKINES

Originating from a single fertilized egg cell, the mature human body contains some 85 trillion cells. This huge assembly of individual cells must act collectively and in harmony for the body to be in perfect health and this necessitates an efficient and reliable system for intercellular communication. The fundamental elements of this complex network are cytokines and their cellular receptors.

Cytokines are a diverse group of small secreted, protein mediators produced and released by activation of most or all of the cells of the immune system. Each cell produces its distinct set of cytokines. Secreted primarily from the leucocytes, cytokines stimulate the humoral and cellular immune responses, as well as activate the phagocytes. It is through the cytokines that the brain and the immune system communicate with each other, by sharing signal molecules and receptor mechanisms.

Originally called **lymphokines** and **monokines** to indicate their cellular sources, it became clear that cytokine is the best description, since all nucleated cells are capable of synthesizing these proteins and, in turn, responding to them. Many of the lymphokines are also known as **interleukines (ILs)**, since they are not only secreted by leucocytes but are also able to affect the cellular responses of leucocytes[1]. Cytokines have a role to play in essentially all the physiological processes in the human body. These biological activities have been identified in four different areas.

(A) Cellular immunology
(B) Virology
(C) Cell biology
(D) Haematology

Nomenclature

There is still no unifying system for the nomenclature of cytokines. For cytokine to be labelled as an IL, there are certain established criteria. The various names currently designated to the cytokines are given in Table. 4.1.

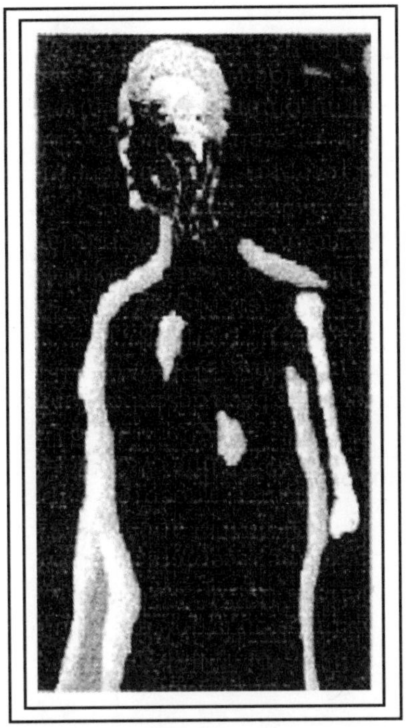

Fig. 4.1 : The organs of the immune system (thymus, spleen, and lymph nodes) and the organs of the neuro-immune system (adrenal gland, hypothalamus and the cortical and subcortical brain)

Table 4.1 : A functional grouping of the major cytokines.

Group	Cytokine (CK)	Abbreviation
Antiviral CK	Interferon-α (13 subtypes)	IFN-α
	Interferon-β	IFN-β
	Interferon-ω	IFN-ω
	Interferon-γ	IFN-γ
Pro-inflammatory CK	Interleukin-1α	IL-1α
	Interleukin-1β	IL-1β

	Interleukin-6	IL-6
	Tumour necrosis factor-α	TNF-α
Anti-inflammatory CK	Interleukin-I receptor antagonist	IL-Ira
	Interleukin-10	IL-10
	Transforming growth factors	TGF-β
	Interleukin-13	IL-13
Immunological CK	Interleukin-2	IL-2
	Interleukin-4	IL-4
	Interleukin-5	IL-5
	Interleukin-6	IL-6
	Interleukin-9	IL-9
	Interleukin-12	IL-12
	Interleukin-13	IL-13
	Interleukin-15	IL-15
	Interleukin-16	IL-16
	Interleukin-17	IL-17
	Interleukin-18	IL-18
	Interleukin-γ	IL-γ
Cytotoxic CK	Tumour necrosis factor-α	TNF-α
	Tumour necrosis factors-β	TNF-β
	Lymphotoxin-β	LT
	Fas ligand	Fas ligand
	CD40 ligand	CD40 ligand
	TNF-related apoptosis inducing ligand	TRAIL
Haematopoixic CK	Colony stimulating factor	CSF-I
	Granulocyte colony stimulating factor	G-CSF
	Granulocyte-monocyte stimulating factor	GM-CSF
	Stem cell factor	SF
	Erythropoietin	EPO
	Flt3 -ligand	Flt3-ligand
	Leukemia inhibitory factor	LIF
	Interleukin-1	IL-1
	Interleukin-3	IL-3
	Interleukin-6	IL-6
	Interleukin-7	IL-7
	Interleukin -11	IL-11
Growth factors	Epidermal growth factor	EGF
	Fibroblast growth factor (9 subtypes)	FGF-a, b, 3-9
	Transforming growth factors β (3)	TGF-β
	Bone morphogenetic proteins (9)	
	Insulin-like growth factor-I and II	IGF-I and II
	Nerve growth factor	NGF
	Oncostatin-M	osm
	Platelet-derived growth factor-A, B	PDGF-A,B
	Transforming growth factor-α	TGF-α
	Vascular-endothelial cell growth factor	VEGF
	Hepatocyte growth factor	HGF

Chemo-attractant CK GRO-α, β, γ	C-X-C chemokines (11) C-C chemokines (25) C chemokines (1) C-X,-C chemokines (1) Interleukin-16	*e.g.*, IL-8, NAP-2, *e.g.*, RANTES, cotaxin Lymphotactin Fractalkine IL-16 (1)
Functions not yet possible to assign	Interleukin-14 Interleukin-19 Interleukin-20	IL-14 IL-19 IL-20

Some cytokines (CK) are listed in more than one group because of their multiple activities.

Characteristic Features of Cytokines

The cytokines share a variety of features[3] :

- They are all simple proteins or glycoproteins with a molecular weight of less than 40 kDa.
- Most are not produced constitutively by cells, but are induced by a stimulus.
- Induction is at the level of transcription or translation.
- They are produced in very small quantities and have a short half-life.
- They bind to the specific receptors on the cell surface.
- Interaction of the cytokines (ligand) with its specific receptor leads to transduction of the signal to the nucleus and this induces an altered pattern of gene expression.
- Most cytokines tend to be paracrine or autocrine, rather than endocrine. Most cytokines are synthesized as they are needed and not stored. Alternatively, some cytokines (tumour necrosis factor, transforming growth factor, endothelial growth factor 4) are presynthesized and stored in cytoplasmic granules.

Action of Cytokines In Vivo

In vivo, a cell will rarely, if ever, encounter one cytokine in isolation at a time they may show the following features :

(A) Pleiotropy

(B) Ambiguity

(C) Redundancy

(D) Synergy

(E) Antagonism

(F) Transmodulation of Cytokine Receptors

Cytokine Receptors

Many cytokine receptors can be grouped into families with shared structural features. The largest group is—class I cytokine receptor family or haematoprotein family of receptors. Class II cytokine receptors are also known as the IFN family receptors. The other families are the TNF receptor family, IL-1 receptor family, TGF β receptors and chemokine receptors. The mechanism by which the cytokine signal is delivered from the receptor to the nucleus (signal transduction), is determined largely by the structural features of the cytokines receptors[4].

Cytokine Inhibitors

Inhibition of cytokines can be done in the following ways :

1. **Inhibitors of cytokines production :**
   - (*a*) Production of cytokines may be inhibited by cyclosporines and corticosteroids.
   - (*b*) Agents that increase cellular cAMP levels and PGE_2 production may lead to decrease in IL-1 and TNF-α synthesis and secretion through both transcriptional and post-transcriptional mechanisms.[5]
   - (*c*) Agents that inhibit IL-1β or TNF-α processing enzymes, comprise another potential mechanism of reducing the production of bioactive cytokines. The drugs pentoxifylline and thalidomide both inhibit TNF-α release and are being evaluated in clinical trials in a few human diseases. The antiosteoporotic effects of estrogen may be mediated, at least in part, by inhibition of IL-6 production.
   - (*d*) Lastly, some cytokines themselves block the production of other cytokines.
2. **Opposing effects of cytokines :** The stimulatory effects of a cytokine on a particular target cell may be specifically opposed by another cytokine. Knowledge about opposing effects of cytokines has been applied in the treatment of scleroderma, where IFN-γ is being evaluated as an agent to reduce collagen production by dermal fibroblasts.

3. **Antibodies to cytokines :** Antibodies to cytokines represent another mechanism to interfere potentially with the effects of specific cytokines.
4. **Protein binding of cytokines :** Both autoantibodies to cytokines and soluble receptors may comprise a large part of this binding activity. Uromodulin and α_2-macroglobulin, also may bind cytokines in vivo with mixed biologic consequences.
5. **Regulation of receptor expression :** Cell surface receptors for TNF-α are up-regulated by IL-1, IL-2, IL-4, IL-6, IFN-γ or TNF-α itself. In constrast, TNF-α receptor expression is down – regulated by bacterial liposaccharides (LPS).
6. **Soluble cytokine receptors :** This group has recently received a great deal of attention. The generation of soluble cytokines receptors appears to be a mechanism for regulating cytokines activities in vitro, since their levels are often raised in certain disease states. They have been described for most of the major cytokines including TNF-α, (sTNFR I and II), IL-1 (sIL-1R I and II), IL-2 (sIL-2R), IL-4 (sIL-4R), IL-6 (sIL-6R) and IFN-γ (sIFN-γR). The soluble cytokine receptors bind a cytokine in solution and prevent it from interacting with the cellular receptors and exerting its biological activities.
7. **Cytokine receptors antagonists :** Both TNF-α and IL-1 may be of central pathophysiologic importance in human autoimmune and chronic inflammatory diseases. The identification of a specific receptor antagonist for IL-1, termed IL-1ra, represents the first description of a naturally occurring receptor antagonist of any cytokine or hormone-like molecule. Clinical trials with IL-1ra have commenced in sepsis syndrome, rheumatoid arthritis, and other human chronic inflammatory diseases.

A Functional Grouping

Knowledge of the structure of the cytokines and their receptors has allowed the division of cytokines into families based on the homology of their pattern.

It is a description of the major cytokines with an emphasis on their biological activities. This knowledge is based on in vivo studies.

Antiviral Cytokines

The antiviral cytokines are the type I IFNs and include many subtypes of IFN-α, IFN-β and IFN-ω The type I IFNs are all derived from the same ancestral gene and have structural homology in between 165–172 amino acids. The type I IFNs can be produced by any cell type in the body. The induced IFNs stimulate the production of a range of proteins which produce many antiviral effects. This prevents the replication of majority of viruses in the target cell.

The other functions : Inhibition of replication of cells, modulation of expression of MHC class I molecules and upregulation of macrophage, cytotoxic T-cell and natural killer T-cell activity.

Pro-Inflammatory Cytokines[6]

Although the pleiotropic activities of pro-inflammatory cytokines may directly result in disease symptoms, such as elevated temperature, muscle loss and weight loss, all these activities are in fact important in the host defence against infection.

The pro-inflammatory cytokines, sometimes referred to as primary cytokines include two members of the interleukin family, (IL-1α and IL-Iβ), TNF-α and IL-6. These cytokines are multifunctional and have effects on numerous cell types. The most important source is the macrophage.

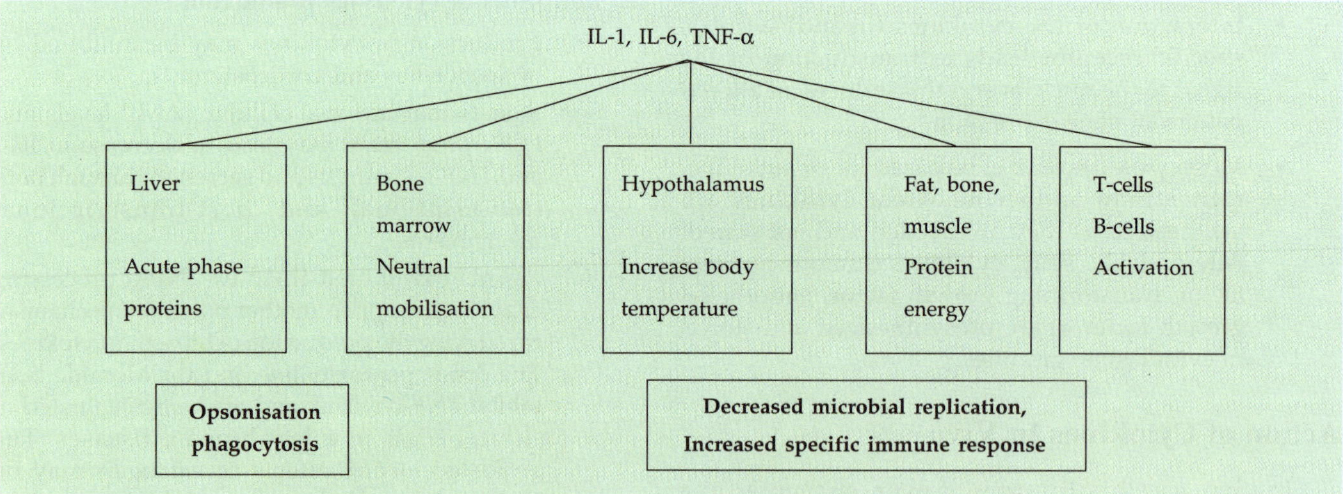

Fig. 4.2 : Pro-inflammatory cytokines in host defence

Essentially all the effects mediated by these cytokines have some antimicrobial activity. The metabolic activities of the cytokines provide fuel in the form of amino acids, fatty acids and glucose. This enables the specific immune system to mount an effective immune response against the stimulating microbe.

Interleukin-1

There are three members of the IL-1 family. The IL-1α and IL-β are the agonists and IL-1ra the antagonist.

Agents that stimulate the production of IL-1 in macrophages include most micro-organisms and their products; non-microbial substances can also induce synthesis of IL-1 proteins. Prostaglandin E_2 is a major inhibitor of IL-synthesis.

Interleukin-6

IL-6 is produced by cells of the immune system and cells of non-lymphoid origin. IL-6 has a role to play in the regulation of immune responses, haematopoiesis, and acute phase reactions. IL-6 is a glycoprotein of 21–28 kDa. The major cell types involved in IL-6 production are T-cells, macrophages and fibroblasts. The production of IL-6 is stimulated by lipopolysaccharides, numerous viruses and other cytokines such as IL-1, TNF-α IFN-β and PDGF. The IL-6 receptor consists of two molecules, an IL-6 binding protein and a signal transducing molecule gp 130 free IL-6. In inflammatory, infectious, or autoimmune disease, elevation of serum IL-6 is more consistent than elevation of TNF-alpha or IL-1 beta. There is evidence that serum IL-6 reflects the severity of injury and among all cytokines, IL-6 is considered to be the most reliable prognostic indication of outcome, particularly in sepsis.

Tumour Necrosis Factor-α[7]

TNF-α also known as cachectin, is a primary mediator of the inflammatory response and is also involved in the regulation of immunity. TNF-α can be synthesised by all types of white blood cells and a variety of mesenchymal and epithelial cells including fibroblasts, smooth muscles, cells, osteoblasts, neuronal cells and keratinocytes. Many tumour cells also synthesise TNF. TNF synthesis can be induced by a whole lot of stimuli like bacteria and their products, viruses, parasites and their products and chemical and physical stimuli. Cleavage of macrophage TNF receptors is stimulated by IL-1 and LPS.

ANTI-INFLAMMATORY CYTOKINES

The major anti-inflammatory cytokine is IL-1ra. The other anti-iflammatory cytokine is IL-10. IL-10 is produced by T-cells, B-cells, macrophages, epithelial cells and human placental cytotrophoblasts. Lymphocytes secrete IL-10 upon appropriate antigenic stimulation. IL-13 also has anti-inflammatory effects on macrophages, and inhibits IL-1 and TNF production by these cells, although the primary function of this cytokine is believed to be in regulation of IgE production by B-cells. Another cytokine with anti-inflammatory effects is TGF-β. TGF-β has completely opposite effect on the cells. It can decrease the expression of pro-inflammatory cytokines and enhance the expression of IL-1ra by macrophages.

CYTOTOXIC CYTOKINES

These include members of the TNF-α family. These cytokines are produced by the $CD4^+$ Th 1 cells or cytotoxic $CD8^+$ T-cells and interact with receptors on target cells that mediate death by apoptosis.

HAEMATOPOIETIC CYTOKINES

These are known as colony stimulating factors (CSF-1, GM-CSF, G-CSF) and these together with other haematopoietic factors are concerned with the growth and differentiation of cells in the bone marrow. Stem cell factor, is a growth factor for primitive lymphoid and myeloid haematopoietic stem cells and is produced by bone marrow stromal cells and fibroblasts. Erythropoietin is the erythroid growth factor concerned in the differentiation of erythroid precursor cells into mature red blood cells.

CHEMOATTRACTANT CYTOKINES

The chemokines constitute a super family of small cytokines that play a critical role in inflammatory and immune responses. There are more than 60 different human chemokines, the first one to be identified was IL-8. Most of the chemokines cause attraction of leucocytes, but these cytokines also affect angiogenesis, collagen production and the production and proliferation of haematopoietic precursors.

GROWTH FACTORS

The growth factors now encompass a large number of cytokines including families such as the TGF-beta family that has 30 members including the bone morphogenetic proteins. The primary action of these cytokines is to activate cellular proliferation and or differentiation.

CYTOKINE NETWORK CASCADE

Pro-inflammatory cytokines set the cascade into motion. Immunological cytokines regulate the specific response, ensuring (in most instances) that the appropriate response is mounted. Haematopoietic cytokines provide the leukocytes needed for defence against the exogenous agent. Chemokines attract the cells to the tissue site and, when the agent has been eliminated, growth factors stimulate tissue repair and regeneration.

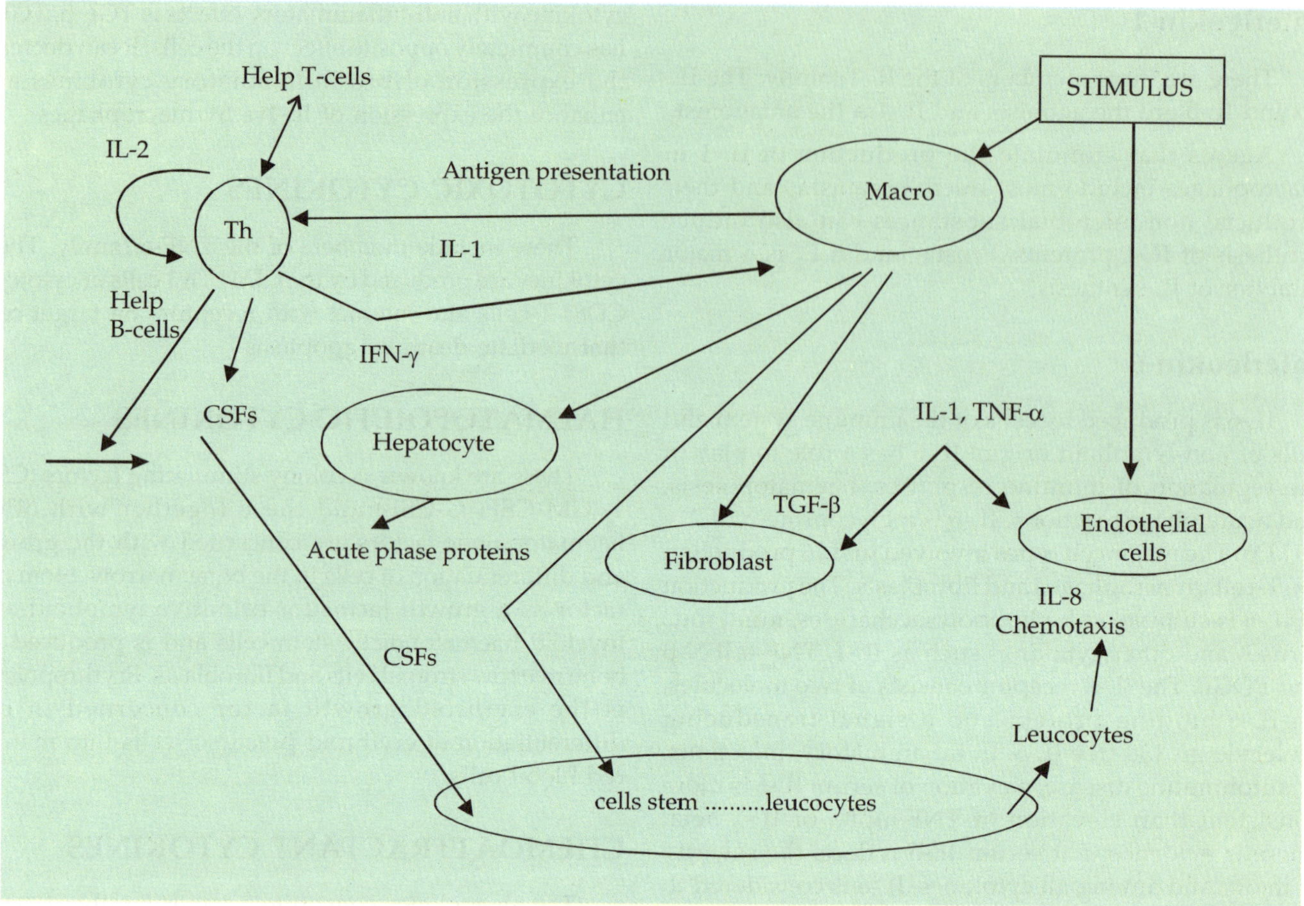

Fig. 4.3 : How the cytokine network operates in the immune defence of the body to an exogenous stimulus

Perhaps the most pertinent example of this is to consider how cytokines from all the functional groups may be involved in the host response to infection. The initial pro-inflammatory cytokine response activates the endothelial cells to allow recruitment of leukocytes to the tissue site. Their migration is guided by chemokines. Colony stimulating factors released by macrophages during the inflammatory response act to increase the production of leukocytes from the bone marrow. The pro-inflammatory cytokines prepare the blood stream for the invasion by the organism by providing acute phase reactants and a supply of amino acid building blocks and fatty acids and lipid stores to fuel the host response[8]. The elevated temperature is antimicrobial. The macrophages also form a link between the nonspecific and specific immune response. The appropriate Th-cell response is initiated and the immunological cytokines regulate the generation of appropriate type of response. The cytokines produced by Th-cells activate the appropriate cells and the organism is eliminated. Growth factors and chemokines produced by the macrophages regulate the wound healing response to restore homeostasis. Anti-inflammatory cytokines work to modulate the response to prevent excess immunopathology.

Although this is a gross over simplification, it serves to illustrate how the cytokine network may function in vivo. This example also demonstrates the potential pitfalls of attempting to understand cytokines in isolation.

CLINICAL APPLICATIONS

The discovery of new cytokines and the elucidation of their role in health and disease has become an area of extensive investigation in which remarkable advances have been made.

Role in Pain

Within the past few years, it has become recognized that the immune system communicates to the brain. "The central nervous system and the immune system are the two systems the body uses to 'sense' and respond to the environment," says Joyce, De- Leo neuropharmacologist from Dartmouth Medical School.[9] Substances released from activated immune cells (cytokines) stimulate peripheral nerves, thereby signalling the brain and spinal cord that infection/inflammation has occurred.[5] Immune cells contain opioid peptides that are released within inflamed tissue and act as opioid receptors on peripheral sensory nerve endings.[2] Additionally, peripheral infection/inflammation leads to de novo synthesis and release of cytokines within the brain and spinal cord. Thus, cytokines affect neural activation both peripherally and centrally. Through this communication pathway, cytokines such as interleukin-1, interleukin-6 and tumour necrosis factor markedly alter brain function, physiology and behaviour. One important but under recognized aspect of this communication is the dramatic impact that immune activation has on pain modulation. Current research is focussing on identifying the cells that produce various cytokines in the central nervous system such as microglia, the macrophages of the nervous system, astrocytes, the star-shaped cells long thought to function chiefly as structural support for nerve cells, and neurons. Astrocytes, which produce proteins that change the function of cells, appear to play a key role in the production and maintenance of pain.

There is ample evidence from experimental studies that pro-inflammatory cytokines induce or increase neuropathic pain as well as inflammatory pain.[6] Direct actions of cytokines on afferent nerve fibres have been shown as well as actions involving further mediators such as prostaglandins or nerve growth factor. Inhibition of pro-inflammatory cytokines, either by synthesis inhibitors, inhibitors of cleavage from the cell membrane, by direct antagonists, or by anti-inflammatory antibodies, reduce pain and hyperalgesia in most models studied. Preliminary data from human studies are encouraging in so far as in the future, cytokine inhibition may add to the panel of treatment modalities for neuropathic pain.

To date, the most thoroughly investigated pathway begins with NALC (nerve associated lymphoid cells), which release pro-inflammatory cytokines in response to infection, inflammation and/or tissue damage. These cytokines bind to and activate sensory cells in vagal paraganglia which, in turn, synapse with and activate sensory nerves of the vagus. Within the central nervous system, the vagal afferents activate the nucleus tractus solitarius – nucleus raphe magnus – spinal cord pathway.[9] At the level of the spinal cord, microglia and astrocytes are activated and this glial activation is key to the production of hyperalgesia. Spinal blockade by nitric oxide, excitatory amino acids, interleukin-1, substance-P, or nerve growth factor can each block the expression of sickness induced hyperalgesia. Recent studies, using the AIDS-related HIV-1 goat glycoprotein gp 120 strongly supports the role of spinal cord glia in mediating the exaggerated pain states. Intrathecal delivery of gp 120 both immunologically activates spinal cord glia, releases spinal cord interleukin-1, and produces hyperalgesia.

It is also apparent that different types of lymphocytes contain beta-endorphin, memory T-cells containing more β-endorphin than naive cells. These findings highlight an integral link between immune cell migration and inflammatory pain. Full-length mRNA transcripts for opioid precursor proteins are expressed in immune cells. Increased expression of pro-opiomelanocortin mRNA and β-endorphin has been demonstrated in stimulated lymphocytes and lymphocytes from animals with inflammation. Cytokines and corticotropin-releasing factor (CRF) release opioids from immune cells. Potent peripheral analgesia due to direct injection of CRF can be blocked by antagonists to CRF, antibodies to opioid peptides, antisense to CRF and opioid receptor specific antagonists. The release of opioid peptides from lymphocytes is calcium dependent and opioid receptor specific. Furthermore, endogenous sources of opioid peptides produce potent analgesia when implanted into the spinal cord. Activated immune cells migrate directly to inflammed tissue using cell adhesion molecules to adhere to the epithelial surface of the vasculature in inflamed tissue. Lymphocytes that have been activated can express opioid peptides. Memory type T-cells that contain opioid peptides are present within inflamed tissue; naive cells are not present in inflamed tissue and do not contain opioid peptides. Inhibiting the migration of memory type T-cells into inflamed tissue by blocking selectins results in reduced numbers of β-endorphin containing cells, a reduced quantity of β-endorphin in inflamed paws and reduced stress and CRF induced peripheral analgesia. Immunosuppression is associated with increased pain in patients. Immunosuppression results in decreased lymphocyte numbers as well as decreased analgesia in animals models.

As these neuroimmune mechanisms are further elucidated, new targets for drug delivery may be realized.

Burns and Sepsis

Cytokines may have a role in anticatabolic and anabolic strategies after burns and sepsis. Pro-inflammatory cytokines–TNF, IL-1, IL-6 have been shown to be associated with proteolytic activity. The production of these factors is markedly increased after burn injury. Since these factors appear to be involved with post-burn (trauma catabolism), blockade or attenuation would appear to be of benefit. Although promising, to date, this approach has not been shown to be effective in burn patients in decreasing catabolism. However, current available agents will be described since more research in this area may show some benefits.

Table 4.2 : Currently available pro-inflammatory cytokines

Interleukin-1 (IL-1) Antagonist
Blocks IL-1 receptors
Given parentally
Unable to reverse catabolism used alone
Very expensive, short half-life

Pentoxifylline A phosphodiesterase inhibitor, will inhibit TNF, IL-1 Given orally 400 mg /tid Decreases cytokines but has minimal effect on catabolism in studies to date
Thalidomide Anticytokine (TNF) activity Given 200 mg a day Appears to have modest anticatabolic and some anabolic activity Not been studied in burns and trauma

Rheumatoid disease and Psoriatic Arthritis

TNF is a major cytokine that is overproduced in rheumatoid joints and psoriatic arthritis. It is largely responsible for inflammation in rheumatoid arthritis patients. Etanercept blocks TNF activity by competitively inhibiting the binding of TNF to receptors of target cell surfaces.

Table 4.3 : Mechanism of action of ant. Rheumatoid drugs.

Drug	Mechanism
Etanercept	Binds to and inactivates TNF-alpha and TNF-beta
Infliximab	Neutralises soluble TNF-alpha and blocks membrane-bound cytokine
Thalidomide	Increases the degradation of mRNA for TNF-alpha

Inflammatory Bowel Disease with Colitis

IL-1 and other cytokines have been localized to the inflamed bowel in patients with colitis. Administration of IL-1ra reduced bowel oedema and suppresses the production of arachidonic acid metabolites in animal studies.

Reproductive System

(*a*) Normal Physiology : IL-1 may be an intermediary in the ovulatory process.

(*b*) Normal Pregnancy : High levels of IL-1ra are present in amniotic fluid throughout the duration of pregnancy, possibly preventing IL-1 induced premature labour.

Diabetes Mellitus

IL-1 has been implicated as an important effector molecule in the early stages of pancreatic beta cell damage in diabetes mellitus. However, the therapeutic usefulness of IL-1ra in human insulin dependent diabetes mellitus is questionable.

Graft Versus Host Disease

Acute graft versus host disease (GVHD) is initiated by T-cells in the donor graft responding to antigenic differences on recipient cells. Tissue damage in GVHD, however, may be mediated by IL-2 release from activated T-cells leading to the production of pro-inflammatory cytokines by macrophages in the donated marrow.

Other Diseases

A possible role for IL-1ra in the treatment of other disease processes has recently been reviewed in the following diseases:

Ischaemia and scarring of the central nervous system or heart.

Chronic myelogenous leukaemia and asthma.

Crescentic nephritis and pulmonary fibrosis in animal studies.

Active immunity to memory and healing.

REFERENCES

1. Sood S. Cytokines – Guest lecture. Proceedings of CME– PAIN. XVII ISSPCON, Jamnagar, 2002.
2. Cabot PJ. Immune-derived opioids and peripheral antinociception. [Review] Clinical and Experimental Pharmacology and Physiology. 2000, 28(3):230–2;2000; 28(3): 230–2.
3. Clatworthy AL, Grose E, Immune-mediated alterations in nociceptives sensory functions in *Aplysia californica*. Journal of Experimental Biology 1999;202:623–630.

4. DeLeo JA, Rutkowski MD, Stalder AK, Campbell IL. Transgenic expression of TNF by astrocytes increases mechanical allodynis in a mouse neuropathy model. Neuroreport 2000 11(3):599–602; .
5. Hori T, Oka T Hosoi M Abe M Oka K. Hypothalamic mechanisms of pain modulatory actions of cytokines and prostaglandin E2. Annals of the New York Academy of Sciences 2000, 917;106–20; 2000.917:106–20.
6. Joyce A, DeLeo Raymond W, Colburn. Proinflammatory Cytokines and Glial Cells: Their Role in Neuropathic Pain. Neuroreport 2001, 12; 292
7. M. Empl MD, S. Renaud MD, B. Erne, P. Fuhr MD. et al. TNF - alpha expression in painful and non painful neuropathies. Neurology 2001; 56 (10): 22
8. Plata-Salaman CR. Central nervous system mechanism contributing to the cachexia anorexia syndrome. Nutrition 2000;16(10):1009–12.
9. Ramer MS, Thompson SW, McMahon SB. Causes and consequences of sympathetic basket formation in dorsal root ganglia. Pain. 1999 (Supple 6:) S111–20.

•••

OPIATE RECEPTORS : NEWER PERSPECTIVES AND CLINICAL SIGNIFICANCE

5

The prediction and discovery of opioid receptors in 1973 preceded the recognition and documentation of endogenous opiate like compounds. These landmark discoveries introduced an era of prolific research which is going to lead to DNA coding and molecular structure of opiate receptors and will result in definite description of molecular biology of opioids. Cloning of opiate receptors with expression of single receptor types in separate lines will allow their pharmacologic functional and biochemical characteristics to be determined[1]. Opiate receptors differ in their configuration, anatomical distribution and affinity ligands. (Table 5.1)

Table 5.1: Characteristics of Opiate Receptors[3]

	μ	δ	κ
Tissue bioassay	Guinea pig ileus	Mouse vas deferens	Rabbit vas deferens
Endogenous ligands	Encephalin β endorphins	Encephalin	Dynorphin
Exogenous agonist ligand	Morphine Phenylpiperidines DAMGO, DAGO	DPDPE DADLE Deltorphin	μ 50488 Butorphanol Bremazocine
Antagonist	Naloxone Naltroxone	Naloxone Naltrindole	Naloxone N or BNI
Cloned (human)	Yes	Yes	Yes
Subtypes	1, 2, 3	1, 2, cx, ncx	1, 2, 1a, 2a, b
G-protein coupled	Yes	Yes	Yes
Adenylate cyclase	Inhibits	Inhibits	Inhibits
Ca^{++} channels K^{+} channels conductance	Inactivates Increases	Inactivate Increases	Inactivates Increases
Actions	Analgesia, sedation, respiratory depression, miosis, bradycardia, nausea, vomiting and increased GI mobility	Supraspinal analgesia, respiratory depression	Diuresis, spinal analgesia, dysphoria, decreased respiration
Site of action Supraspinal	Periductal grey area, median and Magnus raphe nuclei, giganto-cellular and reticullar	Periductal grey area, pallidus raphe nucleus, gigantocellular reticular	Periductal grey area, caudal, linear, median magnus and reticular
Spinal cord	Yes	Yes	Yes

Opiate receptors belong to the superfamily of G protein coupled receptors constituting 80% of all known receptors *e.g.*, muscarinic, adenylate cyclase, adrenergic, GABA and somatostatin receptors. Direct inhibitory actions of opioids are mediated by receptors coupled to pertussis toxin – sensitive to G_1/G_0 proteins and direct excitatory effects via a cholera toxin – sensitive G_5 like protein. The opioid receptor activated G protein effector system can be divided into – short-term effectors (K^+ and Ca^{++}) and long-term effectors involving cAMP and phosphatidylinositol. Both μ and δ receptors activate inwardly rectifying K^+ channels and all opiate receptor types can inhibit opening of voltage dependent Ca^{++} channels.[2] The K^+ channel effects results in hyper polarization of neuronal membranes, decreasing synaptic transmission while Ca^{++} reduction can decrease neurotransmitter release (Table 5.1).

At periductal grey area, opiate receptor stimulation results in impulses that alter the degree of inhibition of neuronal pods, reducing the transmission of nociceptive information from periphery. At spinal level action is at nerve synapses either presynaptically (as neuromodulators) or postsynaptically as neurotransmitters.[3]

to very high affinity site μ_1 as well as to the high affinity site (*k, d* or *a*) depending upon the ligand used. Naloxazone and naloxonazine were reported to abolish the binding of each ligand to μ_1 site. Furthermore in vivo studies, naloxazone was found to be selectively blocking morphine induced anti-nociception but did not block morphine induced respiratory depression or the induction of morphine dependence.[3]

δ_1 and δ_2 : This subdivision of δ receptor subtypes was proposed on the basis of in vivo pharmacological studies (Table 5.2). In rodents in vivo, the supraspinal antinociceptive activity of DPDPE can be selectively antagonized by BNTX2 or DALCE, whereas deltorpine I and D_3LET activity can be reversed by 5′-NTII.[5]

Best evidence to support subdivision of δ-receptors comes from inhibition of adenylcyclase activity and from δ receptor-mediated elevation of intracellular Ca^{++} in the Ndb-47 cell line where BNTX selectively antagonized DPDPE and naltriben selectively antagonized deltrophin II.

The pharmacological properties of the cloned DOR-1 receptor are between those predicted for either the δ_1 or δ_2 subtypes. DPDPE and deltrophin II are both potent displacers of [3h]- diprenorphine binding to mouse and human receptors which is not consistent with δ_1 or δ_2 classifications the [3h]-diprenorphine binds to the recombinant receptor's displacement by naltriben suggests it to be δ_2 subtype.[5]

Table 5.2 : Delta Receptor Subtypes[5]

Receptors subtypes	Antagonists	
	competitive	Non equilibrium
δ_1	DPDPE/DADLE	BNTX DALCE
δ_2	Deltorpine T1/DSLET	Naltriben 5′-NTII
DOR 1	DPDPE	Naltriben

δcx and δncx : This subdivision was based on the hypothesis that one type of δ-receptor (δcx) was complexed with μ-receptors or perhaps κ receptors, whereas δncx was not found to be associated with an opioid receptor complex.[6] There are in existence subtypes of δncx, *i.e.*, δ (ncx-1) and δ (ncx-2), the δ (ncx-1) receptor may be synonymous with δ_1-receptor while δ cx synonyms with δ_2 receptor.

κ-receptors : The first κ-receptors characterization came from work using [3H] ethylketocylazocine (EKC) in guinea pig brain. This pointed to the existence of a non-homogenous population of high affinity binding sites, thus leading to κ_1- and κ_2- sites sensitive for DADLE.

Newer Advances in Opiate Receptors

Recently it has been reported that heroin and morphine-6-glucuronidase but not morphine, still produce anti-nociception in mice in which MOR-1 gene in opioid receptors was disrupted in exon-1. However, MOR-1 gene disruption in exon-2 all three agonists were not effective antinociceptives. It was concluded that antinociceptive actions of heroin and morphine-6-glucuronide could be through a receptor produced through gene product[4] MOR 1_A, 1_B, 1_C, 1_D, 1_E, 1_F.

Receptor Subtypes – μ_1 and μ_2 Subtypes

This subdivision was proposed by Pasternak et al. to explain their observation in radioligand binding studies that (3P) labelled μ_1 and δ and κ ligands displayed biphasic binding characteristics[4]. Each radioligand binds

The DADLE sensitive κ_2 site bound β_1 endorphin. Labelling with [3H]-etorphines revealed two additional sites *i.e.*, κ_2 that bound [Met] enkephalyl-rg-gly-leu and another κ_3 or "MRF" that bound [Met5] enkephalyl-arg-phe with high affinity.[7]

Table 5.3 : Kappa receptor subtypes[7, 8]

Subtype	Sub-subtype	Ligand binding
κ_1	κ_{1a}	[3h]-U-69593
	κ_{1b}	α-neo-endorphin
κ_2	κ_{2a}	[3h]-bremazocine(κ_{2a1}) nor-BNIenadoline(κ_{2a2})
	κ_{2b}	Endorphin and DADLE (κ_{2B1} and κ_{2B2})
	κ_3(MRF)	DAMGO + enadoline

There were proposed further subdivision of κ_1-site into κ_{1a} and κ_{1b}. There was in existence a third κ_3 subtype insensitive to *m*-50, *m*-88. On the other hand, Rothman (1990)[8] reported subdivision of κ_2 binding of [3H]-Bremazocine into 2a- and 2b- sites which were further subdivided using combination of depletion of (μ and δ sites) and suppression against the binding of (I^{1251}) OXY. So were defined the κ_{2a-1} and κ_{2a-2} sites, having relatively high and low affinities respectively for nor-BNI and enadoline and κ_{2b-1} and κ_{2b-2} sites with a low affinities for DAMGO and α-neo endorphin.

Correlating Genes with μ-, δ- and κ- Receptor Subtypes

Though there is little evidence, yet for different genes encoding the different subtypes of μ, δ and κ-receptors, these subtypes may result from different post transitional modification of the gene product (glycosylation, phosphorylation, etc.) from receptor dimerization to form homomeric and heteromeric complexes or from interaction of the gene product with associated proteins such as RAMPs.[9]

The orphan receptor The ORL_1 bore a high degree of structural homology towards classical receptor type in rat, mouse and man. However, there is no corresponding pharmacological homology as there is no endogenous ligand terming it as an "orphan opioid receptor". A little affinity is possible on the benzomorphan, bremazocine by changing Ala 213 in TM5 to the conserved Lys of μ, κ. and δ, or by changing val-glu-val 267–279 sequence of TM6 to the conserved lie-his-lie motif.[10]

Apart from selective opioid ligands (Table 5.4), there are other less well characterized opioid receptors like ε-receptors specific for β endorphin,[12] τ-receptors with affinity of encephalin, λ-receptors with affinity for 4,5 epoxymorphins and ξ-receptors.

Endogenous ligands : In the mammals endogenous opioid peptides are derived from four precursors: pro-opiomelanocortin, pro-enkephalin, pro-dynorphin and pro-nociceptin. The last one having affinity for ORL_1, receptors only[13] (Table 5.5).

Table 5.4 : Selective Opiate Ligands [10,11]

Receptor type	μ-receptor	δ-receptor	κ-receptor	ORL1
Selective agonists	Endomorphin-1 Endomorphin-2 DAMGO	(D-Ala2) deltorphinT (D-Ala2) deltorphinT1 DPDPE, SNC80	Enadoline μ - 50488 μ - 69593	None
Selective antagonists	CTAP	Natrindole TIPP-ψ ICI-174864	Nor binaltorphimine	None
Radioligand	(3H)-DAMGO	(3H)-natrindole (3H)-PCI-DPDPE (3H)-SNC121	(3H)-enadoline (3H)-46593	(3H)- nociceptin

Table 5.5 : Mammalian Opioid Ligands

Precursor	Endogenous peptide	Amino acid sequence
Pro-opiomelanocortin	β-endorphin	YGGFMYSEKSQTPLVTL FKNAIIKNAYKKGE
Pro-dynorphin	(met) enkephalin (leu) enkephalin	YGGFM,YGGFL,YGGFMKF YGGFMRLG,YGGFMRRV-NH2, YGGFMRRV-NH2
Pro-enkephalin	Dynorphin-A and B Dynorphin -A(1–8) α and β-neoendorphi	YGGFLRRIRPKLKWDNQ YGGFLRRI,YGGFLRKYP YGGFLRRQFKVVT, YGGFLRKYPK
Pro-nociceptin/QFQ Pro-endomorphine	Nociceptin Endomorphine 1 Endomorphine 2	FGGFTGARKSARKLANQ YPWF-NH2 YPFF-NH2

Development and Clinical Application

The exogenous non-peptide ligand *e.g.*, morphine, codeine and thebaine existed even before the discovery of endogenous peptides. The respiratory depression, tolerance, side effects of morphine provided the stimulus to seek analogues with selective analgesic property. The evolution occurred from epoximorphine, morphinans (levorphanol), benzomorphan (pentazocine) to phenyl-piperidine (Pethidine) and 4-amino-piperidine (fentanyl). The morphine structure was simplified in methadone, while thebaine was simplified to oripavine derivatives. The introduction of an additional six membered ring leads to a highly potent etorphine which is a thousand times more potent than morphine. The μ-receptor affinity drugs provide good analgesia alone or with adjuncts. The piperidine related fentanyl is used perioperatively for induction and maintenance of anaesthesia. Benzomorphans (nalorphine) are associated with dysphoric and psychotomimetic effects.[15]

The κ site was associated with ketazocine with a powerful antinociceptive effect. The κ-receptor characterization led to attempted design of compounds like spiradoline (U-62,066) and enadoline (CI-977) with greater selectivity and potency but with CNS mediated sedation and dysphoria.[15] A peripherally mediated effect for inflammatory conditions can be found in asimadoline. The neuroprotective properties of κ-receptors can be advantageous in stroke and head injury.

The discovery of enkephalins and of δ-receptors leads to the synthesis of compounds lacking addictive properties of morphine. Applying the "message-address" concept which produced antagonist naltrindole lead to the discovery of delta selective agonists TAN-67 or SB213698[16] which may have a superior profile as analgesics.

The prospects for clinical utilites of ORL_1 receptor in the brain leads to a motor impairment which may be a disadvantage to the development of ORL_1 agonists.[10]

REFERENCES

1. Reisine T. Review: Neurotransmitter receptors. V. Neuropharmacology, 1995;34:436.
2. Wandless AL, Smart K, Lambert DG. Fentanyl increases intracellular Ca^{++} concentration in SH-5Y5Y cells. Brit. J. Anaesth. 1996;76:461.
3. Bailey PL, Egan TD, Stanley TH. Intravenous opioid anaesthetics. In: Anesthesia Miller RD. 5thEd. Churchill-Livingstone, Philadelphia, 2000;2323–51.
4. Schuller AGP, King MA, Zhang J, et al. Retention of heroin and morphine-6B-glucuronide analgesia in a new line of mice lacking exon 1 of MOR-1. Neuro Science, 1999;21:151–6.
5. Jiang A, Takemore AE, Sultana M et al. Differential antagonism of opioid antinociception by DALCE naltrindole, 5 pr, NTII: Evidence for delta l receptor subtypes. J. Pharmacol: Exp. Ther: 1991;257:1069.
6. Rothman RB. In : Handbook of Exp. Pharmacology. Herz A, Springer verlog. Berlin, 1993;104:1–217.
7. Pick CG, Paul D, Pasternak GW. Nalbupine : a mixed kappa 12 and kappa 3 analgesic in mice. J. Pharmac. Exp. Ther. 1992;262:1044.

8. Rothman RB. Binding surface analgesia of [3H]-U-69593 and [3H]- bremazocine and affinity for β-endorphin and α-neo endorphin in guinea pigs. Peptides, 1990;11:311.
9. McLatchie Lm, Neil JF, Main MJ et al. RAMPs regulate the transport and ligand specificity of calcitonin specific receptors like receptors. Nature, 1998;393:333–39.
10. Mogil JS, Pasternak GW. The molecular and behaviour pharmacology of orphonin FQ nociception peptide and receptor family. Pharmac, Review, 2001;53:281.
11. Reisine T, Pasternak G. Opioid analgesics and antagonists in Goodman-Gillman's. The pharmacological basis of therapeutics. Hardman JG, Limbird L (eds). 9th Ed. McGraw Hill, New York, 1996;521–555.
12. Wuster M, Schulz R, Herz A. Specificity of opioids towards the mew, delta and eita opiate receptors. Neuroscience, 1979;15:193–196.
13. Nakanishi S, Inoue A, Kita T et al. Nucleotide sequence of cloned c DNA for bovine corticotrophin-β-lipoprotein precursor. Nature, 1979;278.423.
14. Teranius L. Families of opioid peptides and classes of opioid receptors In: Adv. in pain research and ther. Fields Hl, Dubnor R, Covero F (Eds). 9th Ed. Raven, New York,1985;463:477.
15. Terman GW, Bonica JJ. Spinal mechanisms and their modulation. In: Bonica's management of pain. Loeser JD. Ed. Lippincotts, Williams and Wilkins, Philadelphia, 2001;72–152.
16. Dondio GC, Geoffrey D, Giardina G et al. The role of "spacer" in the octahydro-isoquinoline series. Discovery of SB213698, a nonpeptidic, potent and selective deltaopioid agonist. Analgesia. Elmsford, NewYork, 1995;1:394–9.

•••

DORSAL HORN RECEPTORS AND DRUGS ACTING ON CHRONIC PAIN

6

A 17-nation survey by Rawal[1] showed Opioids used intrathecally/epidurally in 10% patients as clonidine also was used by most of the respondents. Many neurotransmitters and neuro modulators were involved in the dorsal horn. Excitatory amino acid glutamate acts at N-methyl-D-aspartate (NMDA) and non-NMDA receptors. *e.g.,* AMPA (alpha amino 3-hydroxy 5-methyl 4-isoxazdepropionic acid), kainate and metabotropic glutamate receptors[2].

Table 6.1 : Dorsal Horn Receptor and Peptides

Presynaptic		Post synaptic	Role	Drugs acting
Peptides	Glutamate Substance P	AMPA receptor (Na^+ influx) Neurokinin-1 (IP3, DAG) NMDA(Mg^{++}, Ca^{++}, Na^+ outflow)	Central sensitization Long-term memory(increased)	Ketamine MK-801
Receptors	Opioid (kappa, mu, sigma) GABA B, 5HT 3 alpha 2 adenosine	GABA B, GABA A 5HT 1B alpha 2 adenosine	Decrease nociceptive input Increase noradrenaline	Opioids Benzodia-zepines Clonidine Seratonin

Several peptides released by primary afferents *e.g.,* substance-P and neurokinin A (acting through neurokinin receptors) calcitonin gene related peptide, opioid receptors, GABA, serotonin and adenosine receptors are receptors involved in neurotransmission and neuro modulation[3]. These reduce or modify the nociceptive impulse and offer a multimodal choice for pain relief.

The opioids have been used for postoperative pain mainly, also used in malignant and nonmalignant pain. Intrathecal or epidural drug delivery is dictated by operative procedure and projected duration of the need for analgesia. Epidural route is preferred following withdrawal of subarachnoid microcatheters following risk of post dural puncture headache and CSF leakage. Opioid agonists possess different selectivity against different types of pain *e.g.,* Mu (μ) against thermal pain, kappa (κ) against pressure or visceral pain (Butorphanol, buprenorphine) in case of the later drugs, response difference in sex occurs due to oestrogen-opioid interactions in the dorsal horn.[4] Morphine is used in the range of 1-6 mg and 0.1 mg, fentanyl 0.025-0.1 mg and 0.005-0.01 mg by epidural and intrthecal route respectively. The respiratory depression remains a major side effect with the use of opioids.

Alpha 2 Agonists

Clonidine and adrenaline provide spinal analgesia in acute and chronic patients. It provides dose related anxiolysis, sedation and augments the quality and duration of peripheral nerve block with local anaesthetics. It is taken 2 mg epidurally and 150–450 microgram intrathecally. Side effects include hypotension and bradycardia which is not present with the more potent dexmeditodimine[5]. A dose of 0.35 mg/kg intrathecally provides motor blockade upto 177.2 minutes when used

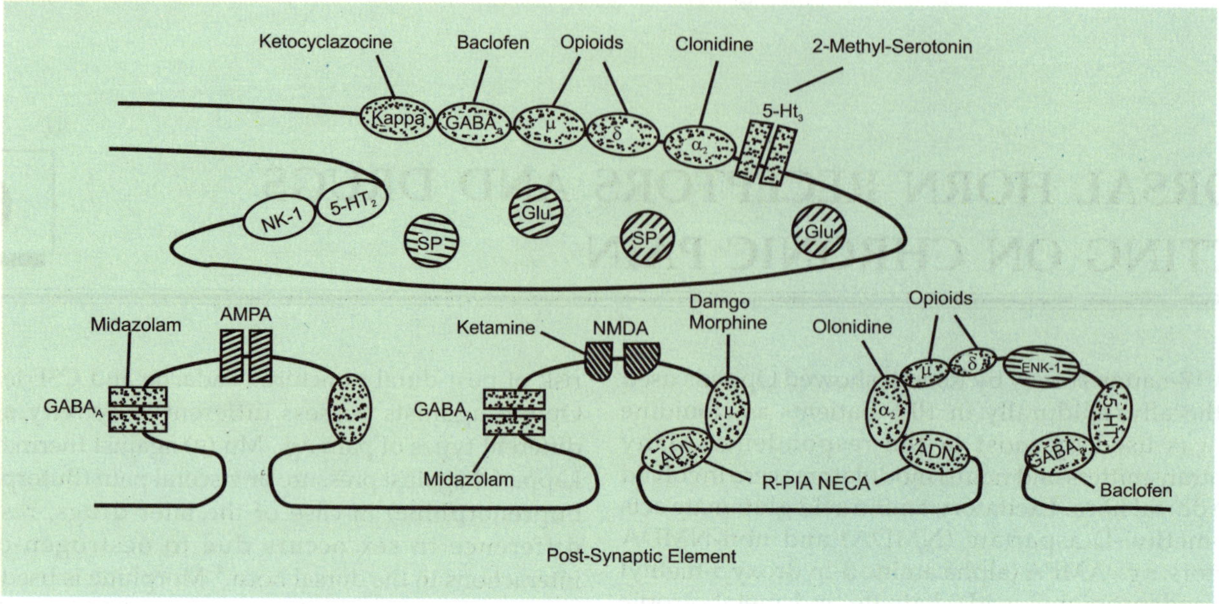

Fig. 6.1 : Dorsal horn receptors and drugs acting on it

along with sensorcaine (Kumar et al.), there was no hemodynamic or other side effects[6].

Cholinomimetics and Cholinesterase Inhibitors

Stimulation of cholinergic receptors is a mechanism of endogenous analgesia. The muscarinic agonists may have a role in producing analgesia *e.g.*, cholinesterase inhibitor neostigmine. However, there is a poor effect to side effect ratio. Intrathecal (100 mg) produced nausea, vomiting and transient lower extremity weakness, which is dose related[7].

Benzodiazepines

Benzodiazepines enhance the effect of GABA upon GABA-A receptors and produce analgesia, which is reversible with benzodiazepine antagonist flumazenil as well as the GABA antagonist bicuculline. Baclofenac used for spasticity acts on GABA-B, while muscimal acts on GABA-A receptors. In animal studies, limited data on intrathecal and epidural midazolam suggests a potential neurotoxicity after a single dose[5].

Ion Channel Blockers

Because spinal nociception depends upon ion flux to trigger postsynaptic depolarization in dorsal horn neurons mu or delta opioid agonist inhibit potassium flux, kappa agonist inhibit calcium flux and local anaesthetics inhibit sodium flux. Calcium influx initiates the intracellular cascade of genetic and biochemical responses to pain. Calcium channel blockade potentiates opioid analgesia while suppressing opioid abstinence syndrome. L type voltage calcium channel block (L-VSCC) may not provide effective analgesia when given alone, but nimodipine potentiates morphine analgesia. However, N type VSCC abound on neurons and its synthetic analogue SNX 11 is a potent analgesic for morphine resistant pain of neuropathic or malignant origin. Side effects are nausea, orthostatic hypotension, headache, constipation and confusion. Preclinical data on potassium channel block also points towards analgesic effects[5].

NMDA agonists

Ketamine block the open calcium channels on NMDA receptor complex. It has been used along with local anaesthetics and opioids to prolong post-operative analgesia without any respiratory depression. However, epidural/spinal Ketamine produces a shorter duration of analgesia with possibility of psychomimetic effects.

Other NMDA open channel blockers *e.g.*, dextromethorphan, phencyclidine and glycine binding drugs have been used in experimental stages. Amitriptyline is found to suppress NMDA induced hyperalgesic states intrathecally in animals. It also enhances analgesia by augmenting the effects of noradrenaline and serotonin[5].

NSAIDs and Nitric Oxide Synthase Inhibitors

These inhibit intracellular enzymes activated by calcium entry into the postsynaptic cell (nitric oxide synthase and phospholipase). These in turn generate nitric oxide and arachidonic acid, the later being a substrate for cyclo-oxygenase isoenzymes, COX-1 and COX-2. Spinal injection of NOS inhibitor L-NAME blocks thermal hyperalgesia as well as NMDA induced hyperalgesia. Lysine salicylate intrathecally provide analgesia for refractory cancer pain. Acetaminophen intrathecally provide analgesia and reversal of hyperalgesia[8].

Adenosine and Non Opioid Peptides

Adenosine receptors A1 and A2 are linked to analgesia, through spinal cord adenosine release, which if blocked by intrathecal theophylline producing hyperalgesia. Opioids and serotonin when used intrathecally release adenosine and produces analgesia[9].

Action: Steroids reduce inflammation by reducing biosynthesis of phospholipase A2 inhibitor, preventing prostaglandin synthesis, thereby preventing hyperalgesia. Complications include dural puncture (1%), headache, abscess, meningitis, and Cushing's syndrome.

Neurolytic Agents[5]

They are important therapeutic analgesic adjuvants, as they don't provide definitive causative relief in chronic pain conditions especially in cancer and trigeminal neuralgia. Their validity is proved by WHO stepladder where 10% of the patients can be provided with these as a multimodal therapy.

Mechanism of action: Neurolytic agents disrupt pain pathways for a long time while sparing other functions.

Table 6.2 : Comparison of Various Studies

Authors	Cause of back pain symptoms	Duration of	Treatment	No. of injections	Success rate Vs control	Follow-up>1 year (% patients)
Beliveau[11]	Disc lesion	Not specified	MP 80 mg in 42 mL 0.5% procaine Vs 42 mL 0.5% procaine caudal	1–2	18/24 (75%Vs 67%)	26%
Cuckler et al.[12]	PID, spinal stenosis, laminectomy	13 weeks– 36 months	MP 8 mg in 5 mL 1% procaine. Lumbar.	1	25/42 (61 Vs 62.5%)	41%
Dike et al.[13]	Degenerated disc	< 1 year	MP 80 mg in 10 mL NS Vs 10 mL NS lumbar	1–2	21/3 60% Vs 31%	14%
Amboff et al.[14]	Laminectomy	1–2 year	Epidural and subarachnoid injections	1	89/151 (59%)	14%
S. Parekh, P.Kumar[15]	PID, laminectomy, disc degeneration, spondylolisthesis	6 months – 1 year	Epidural hydrocortisone 50 mg Vs 1mg morphine with 0.125% 8 mL Bupivacaine		56% Vs 40%	35%Vs 10%

Other peptides are substance P and related tachykinins like somatostatin, produce epidural / spinal analgesia. However, histopathological changes in spinal cord may present which is dose related. A dose of 20 microgram may be neurotoxic in rats, but doses below 15 microgram are not[10]. Its use was abandoned until its stable analogue octreotide produced analgesia in cancer patients by intrathecal infusion[5].

Intrathecal /Epidural Steroids

Indications: Nerve root irritation and inflammation in PID, spondylolisthesis etc.

There may be a selective lysis of unmyelinated Schwann cells by neurolytic agents, while L.A acts on unmyelinated fibres. However, capsaicin and ricin have a selective toxic action on dorsal root ganglion neurons, which can be exploited clinically in chronic patients.

Neurolytic agents
1. Local analgesics in toxic doses.
2. Alcohol 95%, phenol 5–10%, glycerol 50–100%.

3. Physical neurolysis CO_2 laser, cryoanalgesia.
4. Chemoneucleosis–capsaicin, ricin.

Absolute alcohol 95–100% solution (SG 1.0), can be used intrathecally and in peripheral nerves. It produces a characteristic burning sensation for a few minutes leading to a warm numb sensation which can be blunted by L.A. denervation and pain relief comes after a few days. Alcohol acts by dehydrating and precipitating the proteins in neurons. Complications include neuritis after peripheral nerve block.

Phenol: 1–5 mL of 3–10% is used alone or with water, saline, glycerin. Conc. > 6.7% is not stable at room temperature. Glycerin is added for intrathecal injection, there is less burning sensation than with phenol.

Butyl amino benzoate: A lipophyllic ester local anaesthetic is absorbed slowly and prolongs its action. 2.5% to 10% is used for epidural/spinal block in chronic pain requiring repeated injections with few side effects.

Chemoneucleosis: Capsaicin and ricin are used in the disc for intractable pain. This injection is made superior to posterior superior iliac spine and iliac crest and 10 cc lateral to L3 spinous process under fluoroscopic guidance using 4–12 mg in the disc space. There is a failure rate of 7–30% with systemic allergy reaction prevented by anti-histaminics and steroids (16%).

Further scope: Drug delivery by intrathecal and epidural pump placements.

REFERENCES

1. Rawal N, Neuroaxial administration of opioids and non opioids. In Brown DL (ed). Regional anesthesia and analgesia. pp208–231, Philadelphia WB Saunders Co, 1996.
2. Wilcox GL. Excitatory neurotransmitter and pain, In bond MR, Charlton JE and Wool CJ Vol 4, pp 97–117, Amsterdam, Elsevier.
3. Bond MR, Charlton JE and Woolf CJ, (eds). Proceedings of 6th world congress on pain, Pain research and management series, vol 4 pp 97–117, Amsterdam, Elsevier, 1991.
4. Amandusson A, Hermansion O, Blomquist A, : Estrogen receptor like immuno reaction in dorsal spinal horn and medulla of female rat, Neuroscience. lett. 196;25;1995.
5. Cousins MJ, and Bridenbaugh (eds). Neural blockade in clinical anaesthesia and management of pain 3rd edition, p 946. Philadelphia, Lippincott Raven, 1998.
6. Kumar P,Vyas AH. Clonidine with lignocaine or bupivacaine intrathecal in spinal analgesia. Ind. Journal of anaesthesia, 1993;41:240–242.
7. Lauretti GR, Reis, Prado WA, Klampt JG. Dose response study of intrathecal morphine Vs intrathecal neostigmine, their combination or placebo for post op analgesia in patients undergoing anterior and posterior vaginoplasty. Anaesth. Analg. 1996;82:1182.
8. Malmberg AB, Yaksh TL. Antinociceptive actions of spinal NSAIDs on formalin test in rats. J. Pharm. Exp. Therapy, 1992;163:136.
9. Delander GE, Wahl JJ. Behaviour induced by putative nociceptive neurotransmitter is inhibited by adenosine or adenosine analogues co-administered intrathecally. J. Pharm. Exp. Therapy, 1988;246,565.
10. Chrubasik J, Meynadier J, Scherpereli P et al. The effect of epidural somatostatin on post op analgesia, Anaesth. Analg. 1985;4:3085–3985.
11. Brown JH. Pressure caudal anaesthesia and back manipulations – conservative method of treatment of sciatica. Northwest medicine, 1960;59:905–909.
12. Cuckler JM, Bernini PA, Weisel Sm et al. The use of epidural steroids in the treatment of lumbar radicular pain. J. Bone joint surgery, 1985;67:63–66.
13. Dike TFW, Burry HC, Grahma R. Extradural corticosteroids injection in management of lumbar nerve root compression. Brit. Med. J. 1973;2:635–637.
14. Arnhoff FN, Triplet HB, Polcornoy B. Follow up status of patients treated with nerve blocks for low back pain, Anaesthesiology. 1997;46:170–178.
15. Kumar P, Kumar K. Epidural hydrocortisone for the relief of low backache (abstracts) Ind. Pain, 1986;1(1), 68.
16. Raj PP(ed). Practical management of pain, 2nd edition , p 850, 1992. Mosby Year book Inc; St. Louis.
17. Kumar P. Epidural ketamine and morphine in post operative pain.Ind. pain. 1986[1];1:46–49.
18. Kumar P. Postoperative pain relief following intrathecal Ketamine. J.Anaesth. clin. pharmac. 1986;2:99–101.
19. Kumar P. Intrathecal Ketamine for postoperative pain. Ind. pain, 1990;4:21–24.

7

PLACEBO EFFECT

Anzio Effect

What pain signifies makes a big difference in how it is perceived. Fear, anxiety and stress can make pain seem worse than it is. Cancer pain is often magnified because it is interpreted as a signal of disaster. However, hope and encouragement can make pain seem less than it is. During second World War American soldiers wounded during the battle at a place called Anzio needed less morphine than did civilians with similar wounds.[1] The presumed reason now known as anzio effect, was that while for civilians the wounds were a source of anxiety, for soldiers they meant going home.

If a patient is assured that he will recover and is treated with sympathy, his pain will often disappear. In the same way a simple placebo can have a curative effect. The placebo effect is in part due to the stimulation of the body's endorphin system. When endorphin's action is inhibited by a narcotic antagonist, placebos may not work.

Unfortunately, the psychological element in chronic pain has often led physicians to miss patient's complaints. But only very few percentage of chronic pain patients are hypochondriacs or hysterics.[2]

The placebo effect is said to occur when an intervention that is not expected to have an effect, produces one.[3] The effect can be in any realm of biological function. (*e.g.*, sports, learning, anxiety control, wound healing, weight loss or analgesia). In case of analgesia: "sugar pills" are able to produce significant reductions in reported pain intensity in about 30% of the population. Since pain cannot be measured directly, the placebo effect cannot be measured accurately.

Myths Surrounding Placebo Response

Quackery

From 18th century the word placebo became attached to quackery. With the rational medicine development, placebo could be used as a word, empirics and silly chirugeons. As a form of description, placebo was a deception either for diagnostic purposes or to get rid of unwanted or unprofitable patients. This leads to use of more bread pills, drops of coloured water and powders of ashes than of all other medicines put together which can be considered as a pious fraud.

A Tiresome and Expensive Artifact

A considerable cost of clinical trials for new drug resides in legal requirements for a placebo trial. This is assigned to the fault of a meddling bureaucracy but also the existence of some patients showing responses to placebo therapy, which is considered as an intrusion in the search of true mechanisms.

A Question of Logic

The very mention of a placebo trial is likely to be taken as a hostile questioning of the logic on which the therapy is based. To request as investigation of the placebo component, an inevitable part of any therapy, is to invite anger. Further confusing the question of whether something should work with the question of whether it does work.

The Reality of the Senses and Perceptions

Everyone measures his own sanity by cross checking their sensation with objective reality. This may be because of everyone possesses a separate entity, a mind, which can decide whether to ignore the bell or write a poem about it.

Explanation of Placebo Response

Affective

Placebo affects the unpleasantness of pain while leaving the intensity dimensions unaffected. Placebo may operate by decreasing anxiety, however, anxiety reduction is not a component of placebo effect rather than the cause of it.

Cognitive

The commonest accepted explanation of placebo effects is that the placebo effect depends on the expectation of the subject. Placebo reactors can be identified before the trial by simply asking the subject what they expect to be the outcome of the therapy. The doubtful ones don't respond to placebo, while those with high expectations do.

Expectations in a laboratory experiment may be more limited than in a clinical setting explaining the less rates and intensity of placebo effects in the former.

Conditioning

An active powerful drug produces a powerful effective physiological response in the same manner that food produces salivation, the unconditioned stimuli. If placebo is given repeatedly this effect declines. This is a characteristic of the Pavlovian responses, where simple repeated ringing of bells lead to a steady decline of the salivation, unless the conditioning is reinforced by occasional coupling of the bell with the food.

Response Appropriate Sensation

Certain classes of sensations are locked to the response which is appropriate to the situation in contrast to the classical view that sensation is always locked to the situation which provokes it, especially in certain types of body sensations only. In case of pain three characteristics are important.

1. The patient is usually fully aware of the injury and its consequences, but describes the initial sensation in neutral words *e.g.*, bangs, blows, thumps.
2. In hospital analgesia is precisely located near the original injury and does not apply to the subsequent stimuli. *e.g.*, introduction of an intra-venous line.
3. This leads to the expected pain by the next day leading to overall immobilization of the part, avoidance of the contact on the painful area, withdrawal, sleep etc. All three response patterns are observed in animals as well as in humans. There are two sequential uses of the sensory input. The first is used to assign priority and second to guide the motor behaviour. It is proposed that pain only appears as a conscious phenomena in the second epoch of sensory analysis after the first period during which the priority was established and during which consciousness is not altered.

The placebo effect is clearly powerful and infiltrates all aspects of therapy. It represents a practical, ethical and scientific challenge. When a patient approaches a physician, he assumes that the recommended therapy is based on a rational tested scientific scheme, which has been validated and is a part of successful modern medicine. When the physician prescribes a placebo, he is utilizing the patient's expectations created by reputation.

This is the reason for mandatory "double-blind" study designs. Exhaustive studies and large number of subjects are essential in evaluating any intervention *e.g.*, physical (TENS), psychological (biofeedback or pharmacological opioid). Some individuals may be more than others able to modulate processing of nociceptive information. There is no psychological or other test that can predict the existence of placebo effect or its potency in any patient. The presence of placebo analgesia does not mean absence of a nociceptive process[4]. This point is critical and often ignored by some who claim to be able to interrupt "differential" spinal, epidural or peripheral nerve blocks. This is also ignored by those who propagate novel therapies producing 30–40% success[5]. These therapies have no apparent common mechanism, so the published effect must be regarded with more than usual skepticism. The placebo effect is endorphin mediated, has neither been confirmed or refuted.[6]

Nacebo Effect

Just as theoretically ineffective interventionals are beneficial, there are many ineffective interventions producing adverse effects. Such negative placebo effect is known as nacebo effect. All placebo controlled studies produce a significant incidence of adverse effects produced by placebo itself, these effects are same as that of the active agent, specially after the patient is fully informed of potential adverse effects of an active agent. This does not imply any nociceptive or psychogenic process.[4] A diagnostic nerve block can define the structures involved in pain generation but cannot predict the extent, intensity and duration of permanent nerve blocks.

Factors Influencing Nonspecific Effects[7]

1. Patient's positive attitude towards physician.
2. High anxious states show the greatest response.
3. Patient expectations of the treatment effects. Symptoms may occur when an individual becomes aware of symptoms in others *e.g.*, mass hysteria.

4. Treatment adherence has a better response to it. The mortality outcome also depends on treatment adherence.
5. Provider factors *e.g.*, warmth, friendliness, sympathy, prestige and positive attitudes have better outcome with placebos.

Placebo Effect can be Explained[8] on

1. Decreased anxiety levels affect physiological process and increase symptom reporting.
2. Learning experience of the post treatment (conditioned response) *e.g.*, needle phobia, medical equipment and hospitals.
3. Expectations of pain relief with a treatment may result from a prior classic conditioning and may potentiate drug effects. This may lead to behaviour changes *e.g.*, resuming functional activities.
4. Endorphin effects – high doses on naloxone abolished the placebo response. However, there are contradictory results as well.

Harnessing the Placebo Effects[7]

1. Convey warmth, interest and genuine concern.
2. Convey realistic 'optimism' about treatments prescribed.
3. Display qualifications, merits of physician to boost physicians prestige.
4. Convey an air of confidence but not arrogance.
5. Elicit and address patient's worries, concerns and goals.
6. Let the patient know that physician has reviewed his history, medical records and conduct a thorough examination.
7. Provide a diagnosis and realistic prognosis to the extent possible.

REFERENCES

1. Beecher HK. Measurement of subjective response. Oxford University Press, New York, 1999.
2. Kumar P. Progress in pain therapeutics. A review article. Indpain, 1986;1(2):103–108.
3. Fields HL, Levine JD. Biology of placebo analgesia. Am. J. Med. 1981;70:745–746.
4. Raj PP. Practical management of pain II ed. St. Louis. Mosby yearbook, 1992;76.
5. Koob GF, Bloom FE. Cellular and molecular mechanisms of drug dependence Science, 1988;242:715–723.
6. Crevert P, Albert LH, Goldstein A. Partial antagonism of placebo analgesia by naloxone. Pain, 1983;16:129–143.
7. Turner JA. Nonspecific treatment effects. In: Bonica's management of pain. Loeser JD(ed). Philadelphia. Lippincott-Williams and Wilkins, 2001.
8. Gracely RH, Verbal descriptor measures of pain clarify mechanisms of analgesia due to narcotics, brain stimulation and placebo. Anesth. Prog. 1987;34:113–127.

•••

SECTION–III

Assessment of Pain

METHODS OF CLINICAL PAIN ASSESSMENT

8

Clinical pain assessment strategies differ in several important ways from strategies used to assess experimental pain[1]. In experimental pain research, the subject is usually a normal, healthy volunteer and the painful stimulus being judged is of known intensity and duration. In the laboratory settings one can easily use psychophysical techniques ranging from judgements of pain threshold to more advanced cross-modality matching or sensory decision theory methods. Data collection is carried out by trained research assistants using sophisticated, often computerized equipment. In the clinical settings, the patient is asked to make judgements about their own pain experience and to report these impressions to a therapist. The patient is often in distress and the pain may vary in intensity, duration and quality. The clinician rarely has the luxury of research assistants and, therefore, must rely on assessment methods that are practical, inexpensive and well tolerated by the patient. The results of a clinical pain assessment have important implications for the diagnosis and treatment of the patient's pain.

The assessment of pain in clinical settings is based on two major methods: self report of pain and direct observation of pain-related behaviours.

Self Report of Pain

Patients presenting for treatment of pain are routinely asked to describe the intensity, location and quality of their pain. These self-reports of pain are considered to be an important component in history taking and in ongoing evaluation of treatment effectiveness. Clinical researchers have demonstrated that reliable and valid measures of self-reported pain can be obtained using a variety of techniques.

Pain intensity has been assessed using numeric, visual analogue, or verbal category scales. Numeric scales are one of the oldest and most commonly employed methods of assessing pain. Use of these scales involves: (1) presenting the patient with a series of numbers (0-10) that are anchored by descriptors (*e.g.*, 0 = no pain, 10 = intolerable pain), and (2) asking the patient to select a number to rate the intensity of their pain at a particular time (*e.g.*, present pain, most and least pain in past week). The visual analogue scale, developed and popularized in Great Britain has been used to assess pain intensity in many pharmacologic studies.[2] Table 8.1 displays a Visual Analogue Scale (VAS). The scale is a 100 mm line anchored at the endpoints by descriptors such as "no pain" and "pain as bad as it can be." The patient is asked to place a mark on this line indicating the intensity of his pain. The VAS may be presented as a horizontal or vertical line and may have additional descriptors and line demarcations to indicate varied levels of pain. The VAS is scored by measuring the distance in millimeters from the endpoint "no pain" to the patient's mark on the scale. Although these scales have long been thought to have greater sensitivity than numeric scales, recent studies raise questions about the sensitivity of the VAS in detecting changes in pain intensity in chronic pain patients.

Verbal category scales consist of a series of pain intensity descriptors (*e.g.*, none, slight, moderate, intense, very intense). The patient is asked to select the one adjective that best describes his pain. Verbal category scales have a long history of use in pharmacologic studies. Until recently, there has been little standardization in these verbal scales with regard to the number and content of descriptors or scoring methods. Tursky et al.,[3] maintains that psychophysical scaling of verbal pain descriptors can greatly enhance the utility of verbal category scales of practicing clinicians. He has rigorously evaluated pain descriptors that appear capable of measuring the intensity and unpleasantness of pain. The intensity of unpleasantness descriptors tested by Tursky et al.,[3] are displayed in Table 8.1.

Table 8.1 : Self Report assessment of pain using V A S and Pain descriptors

Visual Analogue Scale (10 cm long)		Psychological Word descriptors[3]
Pain as bad as it can be	10	**Unpleasentness**
		Distressing
		Tolerable
	9	Awful
		Unpleasant
	8	Uncomfortable
		Intolerable
		Bearable
	7	Agonizing
		Miserable
	6	Distracting
		Not unpleasant
		Intensity–
	5	Moderate
		Just noticeable
	4	Mild
		Excruciating
		Very strong
	3	Very Intense
		Severe
	2	Intense
		Very weak
		Strong
	1	Weak
		Not noticeable
No Pain	0	

The major advantages of pain intensity measures are their simplicity, low cost and ease of administration for repeated measurements. The one major disadvantage of these measures is that they typically assess only one dimension (intensity) of a complex experience. It is generally agreed that pain intensity measures should be combined with other behavioural indices of pain status such as medication intake, of time spent in bed each day.

Pain location is best assessed by using a body chart or pain map[4]. This consists of an outline of a human form or body area. The patient is asked to shade in those areas in which pain is experienced. Special markings or shadings also may be used to indicate symptoms other than pain, *e.g.*, numbness, tingling. Pain location measures may be scored for anatomical accuracy to asses tendencies toward exaggeration or for extremity of pain complaints (percentage of body area affected). Excellent work has recently been done in developing quantifiable pain location measures for use with cancer patients.

Quality of pain measures were notably lacking until the adjective checklist of the McGill Pain Questionnaire (MPQ) was developed.[5] The MPQ consists of a series of 20 sets of adjective descriptors designed to assess the evaluative, sensory and affective components of the pain experience. The patient is asked to select the one adjective descriptor in each relevant category that best describes his pain. The adjectives are arranged in ascending order of intensity within each category. Scores are computed by adding the rank values of the adjectives. Separate scores can be calculated for the affective, evaluative and sensory dimensions of the MPQ and total scores based on all descriptors also are often computed.

The MPQ is very widely utilized in clinical research studies of chronic pain. The reliability and validity of this measure has been supported by many investigations. The MPQ has been translated from English into many other languages. The major concern about the MPQ is the difficulty level of the words used in the scale. To overcome this problem, clinicians are urged to read the scale to their patients and provide definitions of pain descriptors when needed rather than rely on a written response format.

Direct Observation of Pain Behaviours

Individuals having pain engage in certain behaviours (guarded movement, painful facial expressions) that communicate to others the fact that they are having pain. Fordyce[6] calls these behaviours, pain behaviours and argues that they should be routinely assessed in evaluating pain. Because pain behaviours are overt, they can be directly observed and recorded by a clinician, spouse, or trained observer.

Clinicians often informally monitor pain behaviours such as medication intake, time out of bed (uptime), days missed from work, or number of visits to physicians. Systematic monitoring of these behaviours can be achieved through the use of behavioural diaries[6]. Clinician or spouse pain behaviour checklists also can provide valuable information of patient's pain status.

Recently, observation procedures for recording motor pain behaviours have been developed by several clinical research teams, assessing five pain behaviours commonly displayed by low back pain patients: guarding, bracing, rubbing, grimacing and sighing[7]. Table 8.2 contains definitions of these motor pain behaviours.

Table 8.2 : Pain Behaviour Categories

Guarding: Abnormally stiff, interrupted, or rigid movement while moving from one position to another.

Bracing: A stationary position in which a fully extended limb supports and maintains an abnormal distribution of weight.

Rubbing: Touching, rubbing, or holding the affected area of pain for at least 3 seconds.

Grimacing: An obvious facial expression of pain which includes furrowed brow, narrowed eyes, tightened lips, corners of mouth pulled back, and clenched teeth.

Sighing: An obvious exaggerated exhalation of breath usually accompanied by shoulders first rising and then falling; cheeks may be expanded.

The behaviours coded appeared to be valid indices of pain in that they are correlated with patient ratings of pain intensity, were sensitive to treatment effects and discriminated low back pain patients from pain-free normal and depressed controls.[7]

The primary advantage of direct observation methods is that they are more objective and reliable than self-report measures. These measures, however, are somewhat more expensive, since they often require trained observers. Pain behaviours are not direct reflections of the pain experience and should not be construed as correlating perfectly with reports of pain intensity. They complement but probably should not take the place of other pain measures.

Implications for Management

Clinical pain assessment is a continuing and integral part of the process of treating pain.[1,6] The methods of assessment described above not only evaluate the effectiveness of treatment. The results of pain assessment have important implications for patient management at each of these stages of treatment.

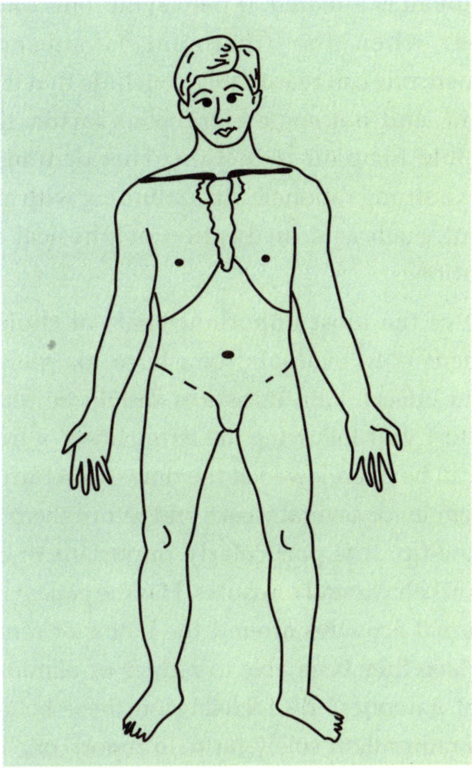

Fig. 8.1 : Pain map for location of pain complaints by patients

Problem Identification

Clinical pain assessment methods yield valuable information about presenting pain complaints. By asking a patient to make several 0–10 ratings daily, frequency, severity and duration of pain intensity can be measured by keeping a diary. Graphing of daily data helps in evaluation of treatment outcomes.

Graphing of daily data on pain or pain behaviour is an excellent method of evaluating treatment outcome for individual patients.

Single case experimental designs[8] provide a rigorous test of the efficacy of pain management methods in individual patients. These designs usually require that a pretreatment base line level of pain and pain behaviour be established over 3 to 14 days. After the baseline period, treatment techniques are introduced and record-keeping continues. By comparing records, kept during treatment to records kept during baseline, one can gauge the effectiveness of treatment. If treatment is effective, a substantial decrease in pain should be achieved after the treatment is initiated. If pain symptoms once again increase, when the treatment is subsequently withdrawn, one can reasonably conclude that it was the treatment, and not some extraneous factor, that was responsible for pain reduction. This demonstration provides a strong rationale for continuing with a specific treatment, such as a medication or physical therapy intervention.

One of the most important goals of clinical pain assessment is to evaluate long-term maintenance of treatment effects. Pain measures should be repeated 6 months to 1 year following the termination of treatment. Patient can be interviewed at the time of a return visit, or to fill them in for several weeks and return them by mail. On follow-up, it is particularly important to examine changes in behavioural measures. Has the patient resumed their normal activities around the house or returned to work? Have they been able to reduce or eliminate their intake of narcotics? By focusing on these behavioural changes rather than solely on pain report, one can best establish the significance of therapeutic change.

Measurement of Pain

The use of radiant heat to obtain psychophysiological standards to pain has been proposed earlier to measure clinical pain[1]. Later it becomes necessary to measure the subjective experience of pain without reference to external causes. The measurement of pain is, therefore, essential to determine the initial intensity, perception qualities and time-course of pain, so as to differentiate among different pain syndromes can be ascertained and investigated and diagnosis is reached.

The importance of pain measurement:

1. To determine pain intensity, quality and duration.
2. To aid in diagnosis.
3. To help decide on the choice of therapy.
4. To evaluate the relative effectiveness of different therapies.

Three dimensions of pain as suggested by Melzack and Casey (1968)[2] were sensory discriminative, motivational affective and cognitive evaluation. These in turn are influenced and subversed by rapid or slow spinal conduction systems and higher central systems. All these three forms of activities then influence motor mechanisms responsible for complex pattern of overt responses that characterize pain.

The Language of Pain

Descriptions of burning quality of pain after peripheral nerve injury or stabbing, cramping quality of visceral pain provides key to diagnosis and treatment. Describing a pain, patient often finds himself at lose of words. This is not due to the paucity of words, they are in the abundance, often seem to be absurd *e.g.*, splitting, shooting, gnawing, wrenching, squeezing or stinging. Sometime patient thinks it is essential to make a statement that someone is skewing red hot poker through his toes and slowly twisting it around.

For a scientific foundation, it is essential to measure it. It is essential to have a number, if efficacy of a drug is to be known. But overall intensity is also important to know if the drug decreased the burning or cramping feeling.

Rating Scales: VAS, McGill Pain Questionnaire, (MPQ), Descriptor Differential Scale (DDS) and behavioural and physiological approaches.

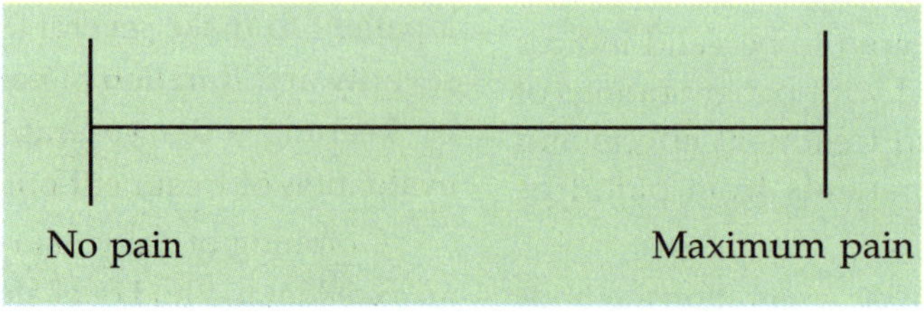

Fig. 8.2 : Visual Analogue Scale

McGill Pain Questionnaire

Patient's Name ———— Date ———— Time ———— am/pm

PRI: S ———— A ———— E ———— M ———— PRI (T) ———— PPI ————
(1 – 10) (11 – 15) (16) (17 – 20) (1 – 20)

1. FLICKERING —
   QUIVERING —
   PULSING —
   THROBBING —
   BEATING —
   POUNDING —
2. JUMPING —
   FLASHING —
   SHOOTING —
3. PRICKING —
   BORING —
   DRILLING —
   STABBING —
   LANCINATING —
4. SHARP —
   CUTTING —
   LACERATING —
5. PINCHING —
   PRESSING —
   GNAWING —
   CRAMPING —
   CRUSHING —
6. TUGGING —
   PULLING —
   WRENCHING —
7. HOT —
   BURNING —
   SCALDING —
   SEARING —
8. TINGLING —
   ITCHY —
   SMARTING —
   STINGING —
9. DULL —
   SORE —
   HURTING —
   ACHING —
   HEAVY —
10. TENDER —
    TAUT —
    RASPING —
    SPLITTING —
11. TIRING —
    EXHAUSTING —
12. SICKENING —
    SUFFOCATING —
13. FEARFUL —
    FRIGHTFUL —
    TERRIFYING —
14. PUNISHING —
    GRUELLING —
    CRUEL —
    VICIOUS —
    KILLING —
15. WRETCHED —
    BLINDING —
16. ANNOYING —
    TROUBLESOME —
    MISERABLE —
    INTENSE —
    UNBEARABLE —
17. SPREADING —
    RADIATING —
    PENETRATING —
    PIERCING —
18. TIGHT —
    NUMB —
    DRAWING —
    SQUEEZING —
    TEARING —
19. COOL —
    COLD —
    FREEZING —
20. NAGGING —
    NAUSEATING —
    AGONIZING —
    DREADFUL —
    TORTURING —

PPI
0 NO PAIN —
1 MILD —
2 DISCOMFORTING —
3 DISTRESSING —
4 HORRIBLE —
5 EXCRUCIATING —

BRIEF —	RHYTHMIC —	CONTINUOUS —
MOMENTARY —	PERIODIC —	STEADY —
TRANSIENT —	INTERMITTENT —	CONSTANT —

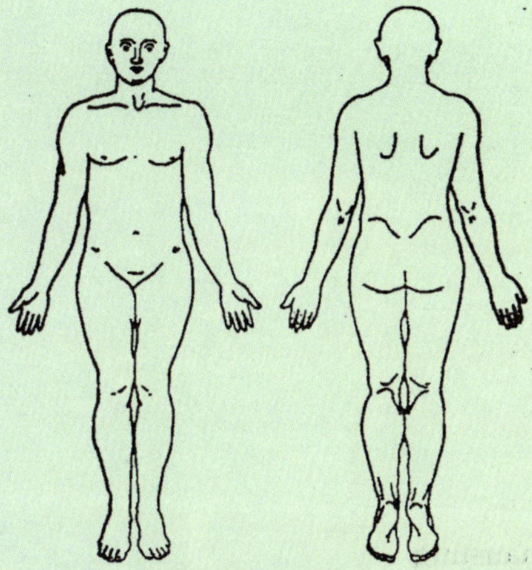

E = EXTERNAL
I = INTERNAL

COMMENTS :

Fig. 8.3 : McGill Pain Questionnaire, Descriptors fall into four major groups: sensory, 1 to 10; affective, 11 to 15; evaluative, 16; and miscellaneous, 17 to 20. The rank value for each descriptor is based on its position in the word set. The sum of the rank values is the "pain rating index" (*PRI*). The "present pain intensity" (*PPI*) is based on a scale of 0 to 5

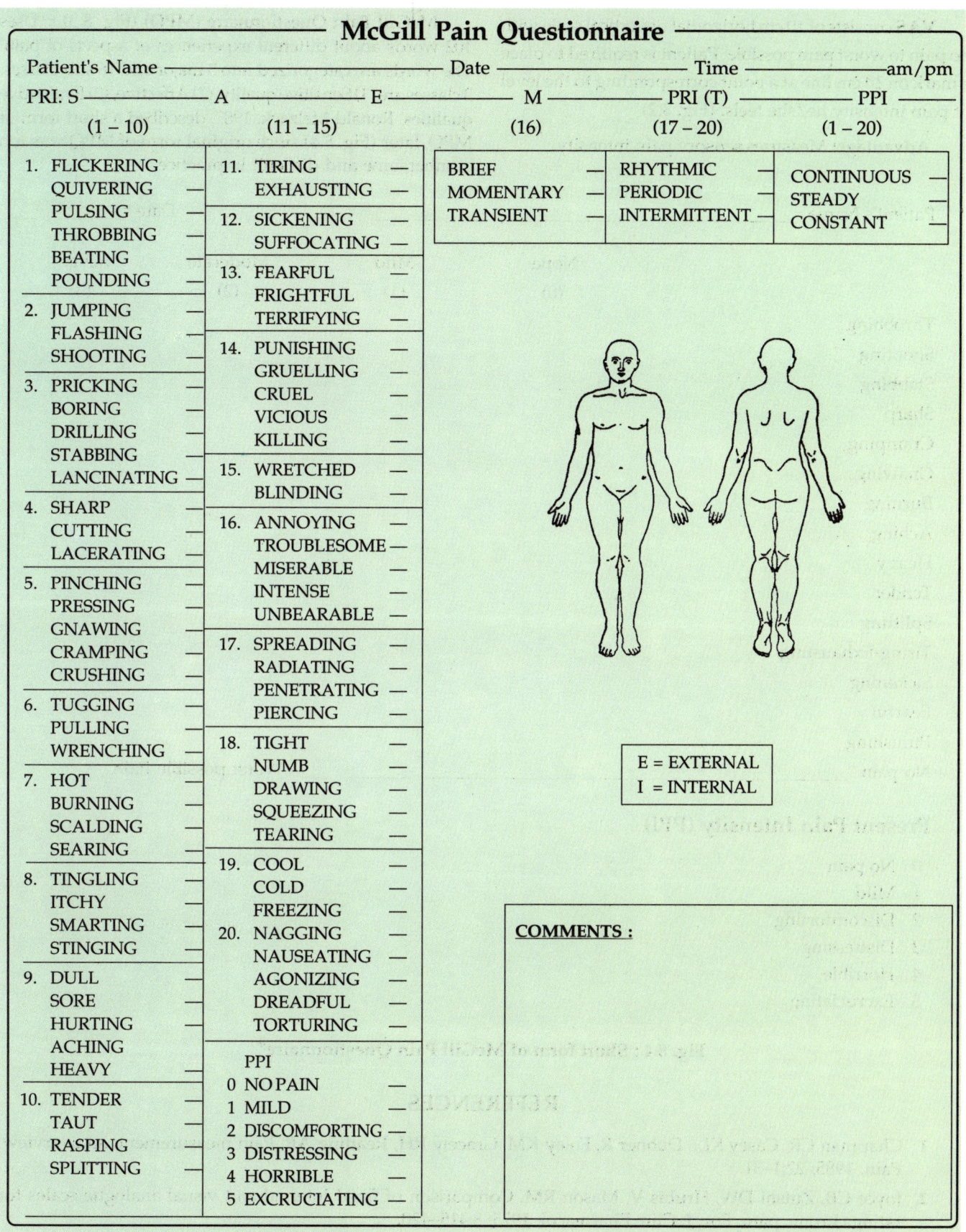

VAS consists of 10 cm horizontal or vertical scale with no pain to worst pain possible. Patient is required to place a mark on 10 cm line at a point corresponding to the level of pain intensity he/she feels. (Fig. 8.2)

Advantage: Measures sensory pain intensity.

McGill Pain Questionnaire (MPQ) (Fig. 8.3) : Uses 102 words about different experiences of aspects of pain. The words are categorized into 3 major and 16 sub-classes. 3 classes are (1) Sensitive quality, (2) Affective, (3) Evaluative qualities. Ronald Melzack, 1987, described a short form of MPQ, later (Fig. 8.4) since original form of MPQ was too cumbersome and difficult in practice.

Patient's Name : ______________________________ Date :__________

	None (0)	Mild (1)	Moderate (2)	Severe (3)
Throbbing				
Shooting				
Stabbing				
Sharp				
Cramping				
Gnawing				
Burning				
Aching				
Heavy				
Tender				
Splitting				
Tiring-Exhausting				
Sickening				
Fearful				
Punishing				

No pain ______________________________ Worst possible Pain

Present Pain Intensity (PPI)

0 No pain
1 Mild
2 Discomforting
3 Distressing
4 Horrible
5 Excruciating

Fig. 8.4 : Short form of McGill Pain Questionnaire[9]

REFERENCES

1. Chapman CR, Casey KL, Dubner R, Foley KM, Gracely RH, Reading AE. Pain measurement: an overview. Pain, 1985; 22:1–31.
2. Joyce CB, Zutshi DW, Hrubis V, Mason RM. Comparison of fixed interval and visual analogue scales for rating chronic pain. Eur. J. Clin. Pharmacol, 1975; 8:415–420.
3. Tursky B, Jamner LD, Friedman R. The pain perception profile: a psychophysical approach to the assessment of pain report. Behav. Ther. 1982;13: 376–394.
4. Keele KD. The pain chart, Lancet, 1948; 2: 6–8.

5. Melzack R. The McGill Pain Questionnaire: Major properties and scoring methods. Pain, 1975; 1: 277–279.

6. Fordyce W.E. Behavioral methods for Chronic Pain and Illness. Mosby, St. Louis, 1976.

7. Keefe FJ, Block AR. Development of an observation method of assessing pain behavior in chronic low back pain patients. Behav. Ther. 1982; 13: 363–375.

8. Hersen M, Barlow DH. Single Case Experimental Designs. Pergamon, New York, 1976.

9. Melzack R. The Short-form McGill Pain Questionnaire. Pain, 1987;30:191–197.

•••

IDENTIFYING PSYCHOLOGICAL INFLUENCES ON CHRONIC PAIN PROBLEMS FOR ASSESSMENT AND TREATMENT

9

The primary purpose of the psychological evaluation of the chronic pain patient is to assess whether psychological and behavioural factors are associated with the patient's pain, suffering and disability, and if so, to delineate these relationships as precisely as possible. A secondary purpose is to determine psychological treatments appropriate for the patient and the conditions necessary for optimal chances of successful treatment. The psychological evaluation cannot be used to determine the aetiology (organic or psychological) of the pain or to predict how an individual patient will respond to surgery for the pain problem.

Patient Preparation for the Psychological Evaluation

Most chronic pain patients believe that a psychological evaluation is not relevant to their pain, and many worry that referral for such an evaluation implies that their pain is viewed as "not real" or "psychological". Patient's guardedness and defensiveness during the evaluation can be reduced and cooperation increased, if the patient understands the purposes of the assessment. It is helpful to prepare the patient by explaining that the evaluation is to be done not because it is believed the pain is "psychological", but because chronic pain usually negatively affects activities, mood, and/or interpersonal relationships, and these changes can in turn make it harder to cope with the pain. The patient can be told that a psychological evaluation can provide information useful in determining factors that may be increasing suffering and disability as well as in planning treatments.

If psychological testing is included in the evaluation, this should be described. Interviewing a spouse or "significant other" (family member, friend) is an essential part of the evaluation, and patients may be told that such interviews can increase the understanding of the patient's pain problem by providing another perspective on pain-related changes that have occurred over time.

Components of the Psychological Evaluation[1]

Table 9.1 shows an outline that can be used for interviewing the patient. Patient guardedness may be reduced by starting the interview with questions about the patient's history and current experience of pain, then proceeding to explore pain-related behaviours, activity changes, and family responses. After some rapport has been established, patients tend to be more comfortable discussing psychological problems. A guide for interviewing significant others is provided in Table 9.2.

Table 9.1. Patient interviewing form

I. **History of the Pain Problem**
   A. Onset, course
   B. Description of present pain
   C. Factors that increase and decrease pain
   D. Time patterns to pain

II. **Previous Treatments and Responses**

III. **Explanatory Model and Treatment Expectations**
   A. Cause of pain
   B. Treatment expectations

IV. **Behavioural Analysis**
   A. Patient activity changes
   B. Spouse activity changes
   C. Pain behaviours
   D. Family responses to pain behaviours
   E. Family responses to well behaviours
   F. Impact of pain on marital, sexual and family relationships
   G. Avoidance learning

V. **Deactivation**

VI. **Drug and Alcohol Use**
   A. Upload and sedative-hypnotic medication use, type and amount
   B. Alcohol use, past and present
   C. History and current use of other psychoactive drugs (*e.g.*, amphetamines, marijuana, cocaine)

VII. **Vocational Assessment and Compensation/Litigation Status**
- A. Educational and work history
- B. Vocational plans
  1. Return to work a realistic goal
  2. Job availability
  3. Retraining needed
- C. Receiving financial compensation
  1. Amount, and amount of former job income
  2. Expected duration of compensation
- D. Any current or planned litigation
- E. Implications of improved health status for litigation, compensation claims

VIII. **Social History**
- A. Family relationships
- B. Family history of pain
- C. Family/subcultural attitudes toward pain, illness, disability
- D. Family history of drug/alcohol abuse
- E. Family history of psychological disorders, treatment
- F. History of abuse, neglect

IX. **Recent Life Stress**
- A. Nature and dates
- B. Association of stressors with pain, activity changes, mood

X. **Psychological Dysfunction**
- A. Screening for depression, anxiety disorders, somatization disorder, dementia
- B. History of psychological disorders and treatment

I. History and Current Subjective Experience of the Pain

It works well to start with the patient's interview by asking about the circumstances surrounding the onset of the pain problem, and about how the pain has changed in severity, location, and frequency over time. Knowledge of systematic diurnal fluctuations in pain and factors associated with increases and reductions in pain, can suggest contributors to pain, suffering, and disability, such as environmental forces and stressors.

II. Responses to Previous Treatment

Information about treatments patients have received previously and their effects is important in planning future treatment. It is necessary to inquire about the nature and extent of previous treatments, in that a particular treatment may be reported to have been unhelpful, when in actuality an adequate trial was not given because of insufficient duration or dose, or inappropriate application.

III. Patient and Spouse Explanatory Model of Pain and Treatment Expectations

It is important to ask both the patient and the spouse what they believe to be the cause of the pain and their expectations and goals regarding further assessment and treatment. If, as is often the case, the patient and/or spouse believe that the medical work-up has been inadequate and that surgery will be necessary to eliminate the cause of the pain, behavioural treatments will not be accepted and will usually not be successful until these views are modified. Likewise, if the patient's goal is to obtain or continue receiving financial compensation for pain, treatment aimed at improved physical functioning and return to work is unlikely to succeed.

IV. Behavioural Analysis[2]

A patient's pain behaviours may be maintained by social or environmental contingencies and a major component of the psychological evaluation is a behavioural analysis to determine whether such processes are present and to identify specific pain behaviour-contingency relationships. Some contingencies include indirect positive reinforcement of pain behaviour by the avoidance of aversive situations or activities, as well as direct positive reinforcement of pain behaviour.

(*a*) To identify positive consequences associated with pain behaviours, it is important to ask the patient and significant other separately what activities the patient is not doing or doing less because of the pain and how frequently each activity is performed now versus before the onset of pain. If the patient is not engaging in activities that were pleasurable and regularly performed before the pain began, this information is useful in planning behavioural goals for treatment. If there are minimal losses or increases, in pleasurable activities, and/or if aversive responsibilities are no longer required because of the pain, it is likely that operant (learning) factors are influencing pain behaviours.

(*b*) Asking how life would be different for the patient and spouse if the pain were decreased also provides information about the "costs" of the pain and potentially meaningful goals. A behavioural treatment programme is unlikely to be successful if realistic goals cannot be identified.

(*c*) Asking both patient and significant others how others know when the patient has increased pain and how others respond at those times, is necessary in order to assess whether there is direct social reinforcement of pain behaviours. If family members frequently respond to the patient's verbal and nonverbal pain behaviours, it is likely that social reinforcers play a role in maintaining pain behaviours.

(*d*) It is also important to inquire about others' responses to "well behaviours"; that is, behaviours inconsistent with the sick role. In some cases, patient activity is followed by spouse's attempts to discourage that activity or to take it over, or in others, with withdrawal of affection and attention or renewed demands. Both responses may lead to increased pain behaviours.

(*e*) The impact of pain on marital, sexual and family relationships should also be explored. Operant factors may be present, for example, if pain has brought the couple closer together or resulted in decreased sexual activity when more frequent sexual activity had been aversive for the patient.

(*f*) An avoidance learning process sometimes leads to consistent avoidance of specific body movements. Certain pain behaviours (*e.g.*, limping) may reduce pain during the acute phase following an injury. Over time, these behaviours become habitual and the patient believes that not engaging in them would result in increased pain. Such patients may be taught that increased pain with movement does not indicate tissue damage and that movement of the painful body part is necessary for rehabilitation and treated with a programme of gradually and systematically increasing active physical therapy.

V. Deactivation

Excessive resting is common in cases of chronic pain and remains in decreased strength, stamina, and flexibility. Such physical changes can then lead to increased pain when activities are attempted; further reinforcing patterns of inactivity and the conviction that activity is harmful. In addition inactivity may result in decreased exposure to pleasurable activities and increased opportunity to focus on the pain, both of which may contribute to depression and further withdrawal, perpetuating a vicious cycle of increasing pain and inactivity. Activity diaries, on which patients record activity and position (reclining, sitting, standing/walking) each hour, are a good source of information about the time spent resting each day. Excessive time spent resting indicates the need for a treatment programme involving gradual systematic increases in duration of daily activities.

VI. Drug and Alcohol Abuse

Chronic pain patients and their significant others should be asked about the patient's amount of alcohol, opioid and sedative-hypnotic medication use, as excessive use of these substances is common. Some patients use pain to obtain drugs or as a rationale for excessive alcohol/drug use, and withdrawal symptoms may be labelled as "pain". Asking about recreational drug use and having kept two-week diaries of medication use can be helpful, although patients may under-report actual use.

VII. Vocational Assessment

Knowledge of the patient's vocational history often is very important in understanding the pain problem and in the treatment planning. If the patient is not currently working, is return to work a desired and realistic goal? If so, what type of work? Patients who receive financial compensation for the pain may fear the loss of this steady income.

The extent to which financial compensation for disability of litigation related to the pain influences the maintenance of a patient's pain behaviours and response to treatment is difficult to determine. Nonetheless, the interviewer should inquire as to the details of compensation and litigation issues, as well as the patient's understanding of the implications of getting better for future financial compensation, so that these factors may be considered in treatment planning and implementation.

VIII. Social History

A brief childhood and family history can yield information concerning patient's learning experiences concerning pain and illness. Questions may also be asked of spouse's about their personal and family history to determine if they may be responding to the patient's pain behaviours in a maladaptive way based on past experiences. A family history of depression or other psychological disorders, familial alcohol or drug abuse, or childhood abuse or neglect can alert the clinician to the potential contribution of such factors to the patient's current situation.

IX. Recent Life Stress

An association between life stress and the onset of and/or maintenance of a chronic pain problem is often seen, although patients may initially deny or minimize this relationship. Often, the interview with the significant other reveals information about significant stresses affecting the patient. Identification of stressors and their effects on pain, suffering, and family functioning frequently indicates directions for treatment, such as relaxation training, stress management training, or marital or family therapy.

X. Psychological Disorders

Depression is a particularly prevalent and treatable disorder in chronic pain populations and, therefore, should be assessed routinely as part of the psychological evaluation. The American Psychiatric Association Diagnostic and Statistical Manual, Third Edition (DSM

III) specifies diagnostic criteria. Chronic pain patients often deny or minimize dysphoria while acknowledging other depressive symptoms such as, persistent irritability, fatigue, insomnia, and suicidal ideation. Accurate diagnosis of depression in this population may be quite difficult because these symptoms may be produced by; excessive alcohol or opioid or sedative-hypnotic medication use. Anxiety and somatization disorders are also seen with some frequency in chronic pain patients, and should be assessed. In older patients, previously undiagnosed dementia is not uncommon.

Table 9.2. Interview form for significant other (Family Member)

I. **Explanatory Model and Treatment Expectations**
   A. Cause of pain
   B. Treatment expectations and goals

II. **Behavioural Analysis**
   A. Patient activity changes
   B. Spouse activity changes
   C. Patient pain behaviours
   D. Family responses to pain behaviours
   E. Family responses to well behaviours
   F. Factors that increase, decrease pain
   G. Time patterns to pain
   H. Impact of pain on marital, sexual, and family relationships

III. **Recent Patient Life Stresses**
   A. Stressors and dates
   B. Association with patient pain behaviour, mood, activity changes

IV. **Patient Medication, Alcohol, Substance of Abuse**
   A. History
   B. Current use

V. **Patient Mood, Cognitive Functioning**
   A. Depression, anxiety symptoms
   B. Cognitive functioning

VI. **Significant Others, Family and Social Background**
   A. Past experience with chronic pain or illness
   B. Family attitudes, responses toward pain and illness

Psychological Scoring Methods[3]

There are many issues to which appropriate use of psychological tests are relevant. Such issues include patients' psychological mindedness, their capacity for insight, their affective responsibility, their selfdestructive tendencies, their motivation for a change and many factors pertaining to their treatment and prognosis. Various such shows are briefed below:

Minnesota Multiphasic Personality Inventory (MMPI)

It is designed to provide an objective assessment of some of the major personality characteristics that affect personal and social adjustment. Hathaway and Mckinely found useful in assessing emotional disorders that occur secondary to pain complaint or pre-existing personality disorders that could potentially affect patient's response to treatment. It contains 550 questions, disadvantage is that it is tedious to administer due to its length. It takes about ninety minutes to do. Difference between functional / psychogenic and organic pain difficult to assess.

Million Behaviour Health Inventory (MBHI)

It is a self report inventory, consists 150, true/false items that measure personality styles and attitudes relevant to specific illnesses. Additionally it contains a prognostic index that attempts to predict ones response to pain treatment. The MBHI, developed for medical patients, serves in both diagnosis and treatment planning, facilitating and when needed, psychotherapeutic intervention.

Symptom Checklist – 90R

An example of self report inventory covering a gamut of symptoms, the SCL - 90R is a checklist composed of 90 items, covering common clinical dimensions, each item is rated for a degree of distress on a 5 point scale, yielding scores for the number of symptoms reported as well as the degree of experienced distress. Nine primary symptom dimensions are tapped; somatisation, observative, compulsive, interpersonal sensitivity, depression, anxiety, hostility, phobic anxiety, paranoid ideation, and psycholocism. The scale has been widely used in for reflecting changes occurring in psychiatric treatment and has proved useful with both inpatient and outpatient population.

Disadvantage : 1. It is more suitable for psychiatric population.

2. It is time consuming.

General Health Questionnaire (GHQ – 28)

This psychological score developed by D. Goldberg is a self administered screening instrument designed to detect current diagnosable changes in the mental health status and to identify causes of potential mental disorders having a detailed diagnosis to a psychiatrics interview.[3]

The General Health Questionnaire was designed for use in primary health care settings, in the general population surveys or in general medical practice.

It consists of four sets of seven questions each. There are four choices to each question. For the first two choices, marks awarded are zero and for last two choices marks awarded is one. Total is done for all 28 questions. Score of 8/9 is the discriminating score, the GHQ yielded a sensitivity of 99%, a specificity of 75%, a positive predictive value of 67%.

Uses:

- It is simple to understand and administer.
- It is useful for non psychiatric patient.

Since it is based on items concerning physical functions in first instance and then, only secondarily does it ask about psychiatric states.

When score is above 9, patient has a probable psychological component and it is an indication for some drug treatment –Tricyclic antidepressant.

GENERAL HEALTH QUESTIONNAIRE GHQ–28 FORM INSTRUCTIONS TO THE PATIENT

Please read this carefully:

We should like to know if you have had any medical complaints; and how your health has been in general, over the past few weeks. Please answer ALL the questions on the following pages simply by underlining the answer which you think most nearly applies to you. Remember that we want to know about present and recent complaints, not those that you had in the past.

It is important that you try to answer ALL the questions.

Table 9.3 : General health questionnaire GHQ–28 form instructions to the patient

HAVE YOU RECENTLY					
A1 -	been feeling perfectly well and in good health?	Better than usual	Same as usual	Worse than usual	Much worse than usual
A2 -	been feeling in need of a good tonic?	Not at all	No more than usual	Rather more than usual	Much more than usual
A3 -	been feeling run down and out of sorts?	Not at all	No more than usual	Rather more than usual	Much more than usual
A4 -	felt that you are ill?	Not at all than usual	No more more than	Rather than usual usual	Much more
A5 -	been getting any pains in your head?	Not at all	No more than usual	Rather more than usual	Much more than usual
A6 -	been getting a feeling of tightness or pressure in your head?	Not at all	No more than usual	Rather more than usual	Much more than usual
A7 -	been having hot or cold spells?	Not at all	No more than usual	Rather more than usual	Much more than usual
B1 -	lost much sleep over worry?	Not at all	No more than usual	Rather more than usual	Much more than usual
B2 -	had difficulty in staying asleep once you are off?	Not at all	No more than usual	Rather more than	Much more than usual
B3 -	felt constantly under strain?	Not at all	No more than usual	Rather more than usual	Much more than usual
B4 -	been getting edgy and bad-tempered?	Not at all	No more than usual	Rather more than usual	Much more than usual
B5 -	been getting scared or panicky for no good reason?	Not at all	No more than usual	Rather more than usual	Much more than usual

B6 -	found everything getting on top of you?	Not at all	No more than usual	Rather more than usual	Much more than usual
B7 -	been feeling nervous and strung-up all the time?	Not at all	No more than usual	Rather more than usual	Much more than usual
C1 -	been managing to keep yourself busy and occupied?	More so than usual	Same as usual	Rather less than usual	Much less than usual
C2 -	been taking longer over the things you do?	Quicker than usual	Same as usual	Longer than usual	Much longer than usual
C3 -	felt on the whole you were doing things well?	Better than usual	About the same	Less well than usual	Much less well
C4 -	been satisfied with the way you've carried out your task?	More satisfied	About same as usual	Less satisfied than usual	Much less satisfied
C5 -	felt that you are playing a useful part in things?	More so than usual	Same as usual	Less useful than usual	Much less useful
C6 -	felt capable of making decisions about things?	More so than usual	Same as usual	Less so than usual	Much less capable
C7 -	been able to enjoy your normal day-to-day activities?	More so than usual	Same as usual	Less so than usual	Much less than usual
D1 -	been thinking of yourself as a worthless person?	Not at all	No more than usual	Rather more than usual	Much more than usual
D2 -	felt that life is entirely hopeless?	Not at all	No more than usual	Rather more than usual	Much more than usual
D3 -	felt that life isn't worth living?	Not at all	No more than usual	Rather more than usual	Much more than usual
D4 -	thought of the possibility that you might make away yourself?	Definitely not	I don't think so	Has crossed my mind	Definitely have
D5 -	found at times you couldn't do anything because your nerves were too bad?	Not at all	No more than usual	Rather more than usual	Much more than usual
D6 -	found yourself wishing you were dead and away from it all?	Not at all	No more than usual	Rather more than usual	Much more than usual
D7 -	found that the idea of taking your own life kept coming into your mind?	Definitely not	I don't think so	Has crossed my mind	Definitely has

A ☐ B ☐ C ☐ D ☐ Total ☐

Short form of the Beck Depression Inventory

Instructions

On the questionnaire are groups of statements. Patient is asked to read the entire group of statements in each category. Then asked pick out the one statement in that group which best describes the way he feels that day, (that is, right now!) He circles the number beside the statement chosen. If several statements in the group seem to apply equally well, is to be circled each one.

Patient is advised to read all the statements in each group before making his choice *e.g.*

A. Sadness

0. I do not feel sad.
1. I feel sad or blue.
2. I am blue or sad all the time and I can't snap out of it.
3. I am so sad or unhappy that I can't stand it.

B. Pessimism

0. I am not particularly pessimistic or discouraged about the future.
1. I feel discouraged about the future.
2. I feel I have nothing to look forward to.
3. I feel that the future is hopelss and that things cannot improve.

C. Sense of Failure

0. I do not feel like a failure
1. I feel I have failed more than the average person.
2. As I look back on my life, all I can see is a lot of failures.
3. I feel I am a complete failure as a person (parent, husband, wife).

REFERENCES

1. American Psychiatric Association, Diagnostic and Statistical Manual of Mental Disorders, Third Edition, American Psychiatric Association, Washington D.C., 1980, pp 494.
2. Fordyce W.E. Behavioural methods for chronic pain and illness, C.V. Mosby, St. Louis, 1976, pp 236.
3. Kumar.P., Vats. A, Chandnani A. Psychosomatic evaluation of patients with cancer and trigeminal neuralgia pain. Ind. J. Pain. 2000;14(2):24–27.

•••

QUANTITATIVE SENSORY TESTING IN CLINICAL TRIALS

10

Spontaneous Pain Versus Evoked Pain

Spontaneous pain is most commonly used as the primary outcome measured in clinical trials of acute and chronic pain. Visual Analogue Scales (VAS), 10-point Numeric Rating Scales (NRS), or 4–5 Point Verbal Rating Scales (VRS) are most commonly used to measure pain[1]. These pain scales allow separate measurement of different dimensions of pain, such as emotional and sensory aspect[2].

However, measurement of spontaneous pain has its limitations[1]. Some pain patients do not suffer from ongoing pain, but rather from pain attacks evoked by certain stimuli. Movements may evoke or increase pain in both acute and chronic pain. Therefore, even when spontaneous pain is successfully treated, increased activity leading to movement-evoked pain may also increase spontaneous pain and obscure the treatment effect. The ability to move, cough, and start exercising is an important goal for treatment of acute pain, and it is

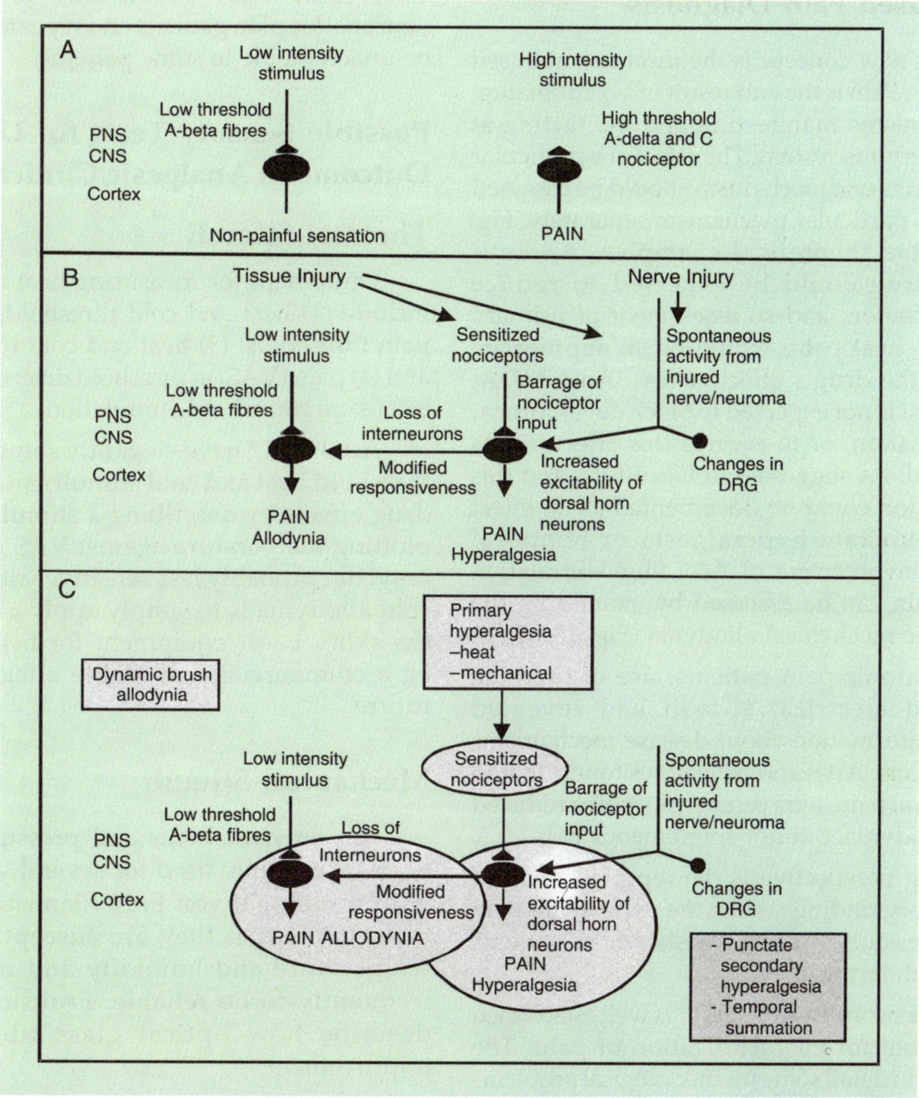

Fig. 10.1 : Modification of noxious stimulation from tissues at dorsal horn

not necessarily measured if we simply assess spontaneous pain at rest. The limitation of using only spontaneous pain as an outcome measure becomes even more evident when the concept of mechanism-based pain classification is addressed.

The Plasticity of the Nervous System

During the last decade, pain research has focused on plasticity in the nervous system after tissue and nerve injury. Tissue injury induces *peripheral sensitization* of nociceptors, and the subsequent afferent barrage induces a hyper-excitable state in the spinal cord dorsal horn, often referred to as *central sensitization*. Nerve injury can produce the same result. These changes explain the increased pain from previously painful stimuli (hyperalgesia) and pain from previously non-painful stimuli (allodynia) experienced after acute injury as well as in chronic pain syndromes. Fig. 10.1B.

Mechanism-Based Pain Diagnosis

An important new concept is the mechanism-based pain classification[3]. Pain is the end result of a combination of several mechanisms manifesting and interacting at several levels of nervous system. The effect of a particular treatment that affects one mechanism should be assessed by measuring this particular mechanism separately. Fig. 10.1C shows some theoretical examples. An anti-inflammatory drug could be expected to reduce peripheral sensitization, and so assessment of primary hyperalgesia (*e.g.*, heat pain) would be an appropriate way to measure the drug's effectiveness. An NMDA-receptor antagonist is not expected to block development of central sensitization, or to reverse this effect, it has already developed. As suggested in Fig. 10.1C, and this mechanism of action could be documented as an effect on secondary punctate hyperalgesia or temporal summation. The involvement of $A\beta$ - fibre stimulation as a source of pain can be assessed by examining the degree of dynamic mechanical allodynia (Fig. 10.1C).

In trials in chronic pain patients, use of thermal, mechanical, and electrical stimuli had revealed interesting new information about disease mechanisms and treatment effects. Attal and colleagues found that in patients with central pain, intravenous morphine reduced brush-evoked allodynia, but not spontaneous pain[4].

An interesting perspective is the reported reversal of abnormal sensory findings when the underlying pain condition is successfully treated, as shown in patients suffering from orthoarthiritis.

Quantitative Sensory Testing (QST) is well established as a diagnostic tool for characterization of pain. The reviews described in detail some methodological problems that must be taken into account[5]. They include ambient temperature, the test algorithm, the slope of the time/stimulus curve, examiner variability, and the importance of testing both affected and corresponding unaffected areas in the same individual.

Suprathreshold Stimuli

For diagnostic purposes, emphasis has been placed on determination of sensory thresholds and pain thresholds. These thresholds describe quantitative aspects of sensory function. In pain patients, qualitative perception at thresholds can be changed as well, as has been shown for cold allodynia: VAS ratings of pain evoked at the cold pain threshold could be reduced by the opioid alfentanil as well as ketamine[5]. However, supra-threshold stimuli seem to be more sensitive measure for assessment of treatment effects[4]. The same has been shown for mechanical stimuli; pain during suprathreshold stimulation is more sensitive. On the other hand, suprathreshold stimulation can impose a burden on patients as it can evoke long-lasting increase in pain. Therefore, it can be difficult to measure in some neuropathic pain patients and repeated measurement can be unacceptable to some patients.

Possible Sensory Tests for Use in Assessing Outcome in Analgesic Clinical Trials

Thermal Stimuli

Equipment for measuring heat and cold thresholds include (1) heat and cold thresholds, (2) heat and cold pain thresholds, (3) heat and cold tolerance thresholds, and (4) pain (VAS) at threshold determination and during brief suprathreshold stimulation.

Attal et al.[4] have elegantly shown how brief supra-threshold heat and cold stimuli can be used to evaluate drug effects by describing a stimulus-response curve, plotting temperature against VAS ratings of pain. An easy, but probably less sensitive, alternative for testing cold allodynia is to simply apply a drop of acetone on the skin[6]. Laser equipment for heat stimulation may be a commercially available alternative in the near future.

Mechanical Stimuli

von Frey filaments and pressure algometry have been successfully used for several years. One problem with traditional von Frey filaments, made of plastic material, is that they are susceptible to changes in temperature and humidity and must be calibrated frequently to be reliable. Fruhstorfer et al. (2001)[7] describe how optical glass fibres represent an improvement.

Hand-held pressure algometers can similarly be better standardized with modern computer techniques[8], although these devices are not yet commercially available Table 10.1. The use of mechanical stimuli is summarized in Table 10.2.

Table 10.1 : Nature of Mechanical Stimulus with corresponding proposed test tool

Nature of Stimulus	Research Tool
Static - Punctate	von Frey filaments
Blunt	Pressure algometer
Dynamic - Spatial distribution	Artist's brush
	Cotton wool Swab.
	Electrical tooth brush
Temporal distribution	Repeated von Frey hair stimulation *e.g.*, 2–3/ sec.

Table 10.2 : Pain Symptoms, mechanisms, and drugs with proposed tests

Pain symptom	Mechanism	Drug	Test
1. Reduced heat pain threshold in primary area	Inflammation: peripheral sensitization	Anti- inflammatory drugs	Heat pain threshold.
2. Tactile dynamic allodynia in non-inflamed tissue (AB - fibre mediated)	Central sensitization	NMDA-receptor antagonists; opoids.	Brush allodynia.
3. Tactile static hyperalgesia in non-inflamed tissue ($A\delta$ - fibre mediated).	Central sensitization	NMDA-receptor antagonists	Punctate hyperalgesia or pain (VAS) evoked by suprathreshold stimuli.
4. Spontaneous burning pain	Spontaneous C-fibre activity	Sodium Channel blockers.	Spontaneous pain.
5. Temporal summation of pain	Central mechanisms	NMDA-receptor antagonists (opioids)	Repeated von Frey Stimulation (2–3/ sec.) electrical stimulation.
6. Cold allodynia	Central sensitization? Reduced inhibition?	Opioids, NMDA-receptor antagonists	Acetone drop; pain due to supra-threshold cold stimuli.

Temporal Summation of Pain

Temporal summation of pain is a physiological mechanism present in healthy individual[2]. However, facilitation of central summation is a common finding in chronic pain. In such patients a single stimulus evokes minor pain, but repeated stimuli at low frequencies (*e.g.*, 2–3/ second) can evoke excruciating pain with long-lasting after sensation and spatial spread of pain. From a mechanism-based view, it would be of great interest to measure drug effects on this particular mechanism. This can be done with repeated von Frey stimulation[1]. Equipment for rapid heat stimulation using heat foils is under development that will allow measurement of temporal summation of heat pain[5].

Spatial Aspects of Abnormal Pain

In the patients with allodynia for thermal or mechanical stimuli, spatial aspects are determined by defining the area of allodynia or hyperalgesia. A number of methods are in use, but these methods are not easily comparable.

Summary

In the era of the mechanism-based pain classification, measurement of spontaneous pain is insufficient for proper characterization of pain syndrome and drug effect. QST has the potential of adding important information critical to correct assessment of the effect of analgesic drugs acting on specific pain mechanisms. However, at present there is no consensus regarding methodology. The methods in current use must be further developed as validated.

REFERENCES

1. Stubhaug A. Clinical trials for acute and chronic pain. In: Rice AS, Warfield C, Justins D, Eccleston C. (Eds). *Clinical pain management.* London : Arnold, 2002.
2. Price DD. Psychophysical measurement of normal and abnormal pain processing. In: Boivie J, Hanson P, Lindblom U, (Eds). *Touch, Temperature, and Pain in Health and Disease: Mechanisms and Assessments,* Progress in Pain Research and Management, Vol. 3. Seattle: IASP Press, 1994; pp 3–25.
3. Woolf CJ, Max MB. Mechanism-based pain diagnosis: issues for analgesic drug development. *Anesthesiology* 2001;95:241–249.
4. Attal N, Gaude V, Brasseur L, et al. Intravenous lidocaine in central pain: a double-blind, placebo-controlled, psychophysical study. *Neurology,* 2000;58:554–563.
5. Jorum E, Arendt-Neilsen L. Sensory testing and clinical neurophysiology. In: Rice AS, Warfield C, Justins D, Eccleston C, (Eds). *Clinical Pain Management.* London: Arnold, 2002, in press.
6. Vestergaard K, Andersen G, Gottrup H, Kristensen BT, Jensen TS. Lamotrigine for central poststroke pain: a randomized controlled trial. *Neurology,* 2001;56:184–190.
7. Fruhstorfer H, Lindblom U, Schmidt WG. Method for quantitative estimation of thermal thresholds in patients. *J. Neurol. Neurosurg. Psychiatry.* 1976;39:1071–1075.
8. Polianskis R, Graven-Nielsen T, Arendt-Nielsen L. Computer-controlled pneumatic pressure algometry—a new technique for quantitative sensory testing. *Eur. J. Pain.* 2001;5:267–277.

•••

PAEDIATRIC PAIN ASSESSMENT

11

Paediatric pain is apparently under-treated. In a hospital unit, at least 20% of ventilated children and 40% of non-ventilated patients may be under-treated for pain.[1] There are two main reasons for this problem. The first is the difficulty inherent in assessing the intensity of children's pain. The second reason is the reluctance on the part of the medical professionals to administer pain medications even after the child is thought to be in pain because of fear of complications. As a result, we do not assess paediatric pain well and when assessed, we do not treat it adequately. Pain assessment in children is complicated. The classic scenario of the non-complaining silent child who lies still and rigid after surgery may seem like an ideal patient to the inexperienced staff, but he may be lying still because of pain. The child may be terrified to move in case it hurts and may not complain for fear of getting an intramuscular injection. Therefore, accurate assessment is necessary to quantify the pain.

To assess pain, a variety of factors, such as the nature of the noxious stimuli; physiological, behavioural, and emotional responses of the child; the patient's self-report; environmental and situational factors; and parental opinions of the child's current pain should be considered. One of the simplest ways to assess pain is to ask the patient. Verbal self-report of pain works well in older children, but it is the younger non-verbal patient who presents the most difficulty for pain assessment and in whom there is the greatest risk of under-treatment.[2] The assessment of pain in children is further complicated because child's pain is rated by a parent, a nurse, and the child from different perspectives.[3] Nurse's rating reflect child's behavioural distress, parent's rating reflects their subjective perception of child's pain and parent's own anxiety and the child's self-report is associated with the child's age.[3] Age of the child influences nurse rating and self-report, but does not affect parent's rating of pain. Chronic pain in children is even more difficult to assess because it is modified by the presence of anxiety, fear and depression in children as young as 2 years of age.[4]

The goal of pain assessment is to collect accurate data to determine which actions should be taken to alleviate or abolish the pain, and to evaluate the effectiveness of these actions. If excellent pain assessment is not followed by rigorous pain management techniques, the effort will not benefit the patient.[5]

Methods of Measuring Pain in Children

The child's response to pain is multidimensional with three clinical components: (1) physiological–increased heart rate, blood pressure, muscle tension, hormonal response etc.; (2) Behavioural–agitated movement, grimacing, crying, avoidance, etc.; (3) Self-report of pain, fear, or anxiety. Besides these clinical parameters, various laboratory and radiological tests aid in the assessment of pain.

Physiologic Measures

In acute pain, it is possible to detect physiologic changes in heart rate, respiration, blood pressure, oxygen saturation, and palmer sweating, skin, blood flow and intracranial pressure.[6] However, adaptation rapidly occurs and autonomic responses return to normal, making it difficult to assess chronic pain by physiological changes alone.

Behavioural Measures

Another method of assessing and measuring children's pain relies on observation of behaviours. Vocal and non-verbal behaviours are used to assess pain in children. **Vocal behaviours** include crying, moaning, screaming and verbal expression of pain, and anxiety. **Non-verbal behaviours** include muscular rigidity, facial expressions, agitation, clinging, flailing and altered sleep patterns. Behaviours should be scored in a checklist format. Inter-rater reliability, in general, is increased when behaviours are scored in a checklist format (namely, as present or absent), in contrast to rating the intensity of the behaviour on a Likert-type scale (that is, 1 to 5).

Self-report Measures

Assessment of children's pain must emphasize the child's perception of the experience because pain is essentially a subjective experience. Patient's self-report is the most accurate and reliable evidence of the existence of pain and its intensity. Belief in the authenticity of a patient's pain perception is central to its effective management.[7] Children are able to indicate the varying levels of their hurt, if the adult can provide an appropriate device for doing this. Most 3-year-old and older children are able to understand the concept of hurt. They can also indicate intensity by choosing a picture, poker chips, or a rung on a ladder.

There are three types of self-report measurements:

(A) **Facial Expressions:** A series of pictures of faces in varying degrees of pain are presented and the child is asked to choose the picture that represents his own pain. The Faces Pain Scale,[8] and Oucher Scale[9] use this technique to measure pain.

(B) **Analogue Scales:** Patients are asked to grade their pain on a straight, horizontal line with a happy, smiling face at one end and a sad, crying face at the other. Measurements such as Visual Analogue Scale and Pain Thermometer[10] are examples of the analogue scales used to assess the degree of pain in older children and adults.

(C) **Other Measurements:** They include a combination of facial and analogue scales, such as Poker Chip tool, picture scale and Smiley Analogue scale.[9]

At this point of time, self-reports are the best indicators of the child's subjective experience. They are readily accessible and easy to administer. When carefully taught to use these instruments, children are able to describe the varying levels and characteristics of their discomfort. Children younger than 5–7 years of age may be limited in their ability to verbally describe pain, and health providers should not rely on "spontaneous, formal complaints". Older children may use any of the modified self-report methods.

Laboratory and Radiological Tests: Various neurophysiological and neurobiological tests, such as Positron Emission Tomography (PET), infrared or microwave thermographic imaging, functional MRI, thermoencephaloscopy, cortical power spectrum analysis, somatosensory evoked potentials or nuclear magnetic resonance spectroscopy have been developed. None of these tests are presently used for clinical evaluation of pain.[11]

Assessment of Pain in Children by Age Groups

Neonates

This group includes full term neonates up to 1 month of age and preterm up to 60 weeks postconceptual age. It was previously thought that newborns do not feel pain because of incomplete myelinization of the sensory nerves. A-delta fibres are not completely myelinated in neonates. They are not efficient in transmitting pain, but the normally unmyelinated C fibres make up for any lack by transmitting noxious stimuli. Because of the newborn's size, the intraneuronal distance is much shorter and, therefore, accommodates for the incomplete myelin sheaths. Pain transmission develops very early in intra-uterine life, Gianna et al. noted that foetal intra-hepatic vein needling produced biochemical stress response as early as 23 weeks post-conceptual age.[12] Anand and his colleagues have demonstrated that infants, even preterms, develop physiologic stress responses and some develop serious complications from inadequate anaesthesia during surgery.[13] In neonates, behavioural and physiological parameters are interpreted together to judge whether the baby is in pain. Premature Infant Pain Profile (PIPP) was developed specifically to assess pain of the premature infants.[14] PIPP measures not only premature baby's behaviour, heart rate, oxygen saturation, and facial expressions, but it also takes into consideration infant's gestational age in assessing pain.

Neonatal Infant Pain Scale (NIPS) was developed for assessing pain in neonates up to 6 weeks after birth.[15] It measures facial expression, cry, breathing pattern, position of arms and legs and the state of arousal.

Krechel and Bildner proposed **CRIES scale** for pain assessment in neonates.[16] It is a modification of the Apgar score. It measures **Crying, Required O_2 for $SaO_2 > 95$, Increased vital signs, Expression, and Sleep patterns (CRIES).[16]** Each of the five categories is scored on a 0 to 2 scale for a maximum score of 10. It is a simple and easy to remember system. However, use of oxygenation as a measure may create an artifact since oxygenation is affected by many factors.

A variety of broad assessment tools of varying complexities such as **OPS (Objective Pain Score),[17] COMFORT score** (to measure distress in the Intensive Care Unit)[18] and **CHEOPS (Children's Hospital of Eastern Ontario Pain Scale)[19]** have been developed for children and full term neonates. The common features of many of these tools include facial expression, body position, mobility, crying, blood pressure, heart rate, oxygen saturation, respiratory rate and sleeplessness.

Currently there is no adequate technology or methods in clinical settings to clearly differentiate neonate's responses to pain from the responses due to hunger, discomfort or anxiety, or to identify variations in the levels of pain.

Infants

Pain in infants is assessed by nurse's observation, parental observation, or by scales such as OPS,[17] COMFORT,[18] and CHEOPS[19]. An infant cries due to hunger, discomfort, pain, fear, or anger. However, the cry because of pain is of greater intensity and frequency. The total crying time due to pain is lower than for those for discomfort or fear. Johnston and Strada[20] used a multidimensional approach to study infant pain. They included observations of cry, body movement, facial expression, and heart rate. Of all the variables measured, they found that facial expression was the most consistent and clear indication of pain.[20] Characteristic changes occurred in three areas of the face: brows furrowed and eyes tightly closed, nasal roots broad and bulged, and mouth angular and open. Other behaviours associated with pain include rigid and withdrawing torso, kicking, thrashing, and protective limbs.

Grunau and Craig analyzed nine specific facial actions in neonates during non-noxious heel rub and presumably noxious heel lance[21], brow bulge, eye squeeze, nasolabial furrow, open lips, vertical stretch mouth, horizontal stretch mouth, lip pursue, taut tongue, and chin quiver. Significantly more facial movement was revealed when the infants experienced heel lance than when they experienced heel rub. Actions 1 to 4 occurred in 99 per cent and action 8 occurred in 70 per cent of the infants soon after heel lance. In addition, infants differed in facial response according to their sleep-awake state; those who were more awake demonstrated a more pronounced response. Differences were also revealed according to the handling by the laboratory technicians performing the heel lances. The progression, frequency, velocity, and timing of infant's withdrawal response to heel sticks derived from sophisticated photogrammetric techniques, and detailed characteristics of infant crying have also been used as indicators of pain-distress behaviour to noxious stimuli in infants.

Some infants are so small or debilitated by their illnesses that they may be unable to respond physiologically to pain. Radioimmunoassay, spectro-graphic cry analysis, and facial-coding systems are techniques that quantify pain but are not yet feasible for pain assessment in routine clinical situations.

Self-Report Measures of Pain

Measure	Type of Measure	Strengths and Limitations
Visual Analogue Scale	Premeasured line with either vertical or horizontal orientation, the length of which is taken to represent the continum of the pain experience with one end defined as "no pain" and the opposite end as "severe pain."	Very simple to use in children at least 5 years old. Children 3 and 4 years old have significant comprehension problems with the measure. Portable, time efficient and inexpensive; a well validated measure, focuses primarily on pain intensity without consideration for the affective, evaluative and motivation components of pain.
Oucher Scale	Numerical VAS (0–100) for children who can count and Photographic Facial Expression Scale for children who cannot count.	Can generally be used in children at least 3 years old. Three multi-ethnic versions are available; cost of scale and large format may be prohibitive. Very good psychometric properties and clinical utility.
Wong-Baker Scale	Faces scale consisting of six cartoon faces ranging from smiling face for "no pain" to tearful face for "worst pain."	Can be used in children at least 3 years old, but some 4–5 years-olds have difficulty. Easy to administer. "Worst pain" face has tears and not all children cry when in pain, so worst pain may be underestimated. Smiling "no pain" face may lead to higher reportd pain scores compared to the neutral face. Well liked by children. Good psychometeric properties and clinical utility.
Bieri Faces Pain Scale	Facial expression scale consisting of seven faces ranging from neutral face for "no pain" to a face with a square open mouth, closed eyes, and furrowed brow for "worst pain."	Similar to other facial expression scales but they have no faces with smiles or tears, so have avoided the problems associated with these expressions, including (*a*) confounding of pain intensity with pain affect, and (*b*) overestimation of pain with "smiling" as compared to neutral faces.

Bieri Faces Pain Scale-Revised	Facial expression scale consisting of six faces ranging from a neutral face for "no pain" to a face with a square open mouth, closed eyes, and furrowed brow for "worst pain".	Appropriate for use in children at least 4–5 years old. Consistent with the most widely used metric for scoring (0–100) and conforms closely to a linear interval scale. Good construct validity.
Coloured Analogue Scale (CAS)	Color analogue scale consisting of a 143-mm tetragon that is white at one end (labelled "no pain") progressing through increasing colour intensity to dark red at the oposite end (labelled "most pain"), scored 0-10 in increments of 0.25.	Appropriate for use in children 5–16 years old. Easy to use and portable. Easy to score with scoring on back of scale. Limited to measurement of pain intensity. Very good psychometric properties. Recommended for use with Facial Affective Scale.
Poker Chip Tool	Concrete ordinal rating tool. Child rates pain intensity by choosing one of four poker chips representing "pieces of hurt where one piece equals "a little hurt" and four pieces equals "the most hurt you could ever have".	Well understood by young children at least 4 years old. Extensively tested reliability and validity. Widely applied across populations and situations. Easy to use and portable.

Pre-schoolers

It is thought that 3 to 7 years old children are cognitively unable to symbolize, abstract, or quantify. Therefore, the pre-schooler may tell us that it hurts, but the process of obtaining pain intensity scores is a challenge. It may also be a challenge to hold the attention of preschool children while teaching them to use the measures. Researchers have devised many creative ways to help these children indicate the degree of their "hurt". Some of these devices include line drawings of faces, a photographic scale of facial expressions (Oucher scale), a Poker Chip Tool, colour scales, a ladder scale, and linear analogue scales.[9] Following are examples of some of the commonly used measurement techniques:

(A) The Oucher scale developed for 3 to 12 years old uses colour photographs of an actual European-American child for pain intensity cues.[8] It consists of two vertical scales – a photographic and a numerical. The photographic scale consists of six different pictures of the face of a child. The child's expressions demonstrate increasing discomfort from "no hurt" to the " biggest hurt" you can ever have. Similarly, on the numerical scale, 0 means no pain and 100 means extreme pain. The photographic scale is useful for 3 to 7 years old children, whereas, 7 to 12 years old children may use the numeric scale. An alternate version of the Oucher scale has been developed using photographs of Hispanic and African-American children for non-Euro-American children.[22]

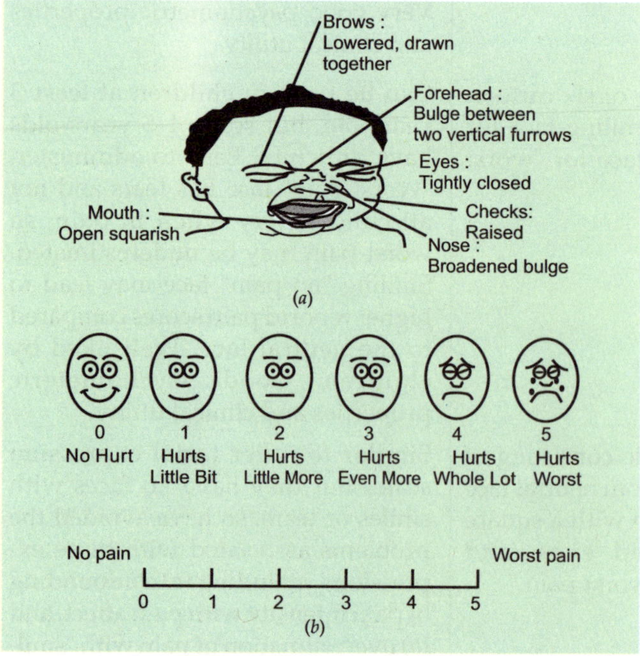

Fig. 11.1. (*a*) : Wong scale (*b*) Faces scale

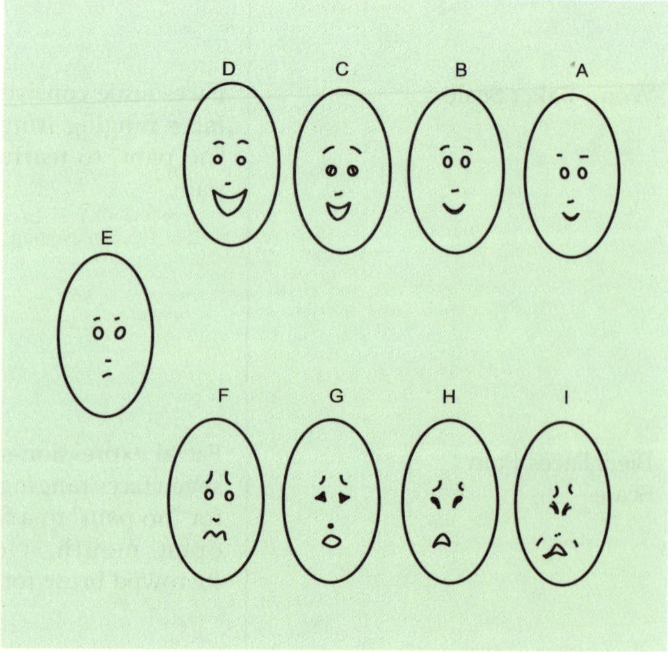

Fig. 11.2 : McGrath's Cheops scale

(B) The Poker Chip Tool allows children to quantify pain when they select one to four poker chips to indicate the level of their discomfort.[10]

(C) Colouring body outlines to express the site and degree of pain has been an effective method of obtaining information from preschool children. Colouring has special appeal for children and provides an appropriate way for pre-schoolers to express themselves about their subjective experiences. They select colours (crayons or markers) to indicate the "worst hurt" the child has ever had, "hurt" and "no hurt at all." They then colour their hurt on a body outline. Such outlines of both boys and girls with front and back views are available.

(D) The Linear Analogue Scale (LAS), which includes facial expressions at each end of a horizontal line, is more abstract and, therefore, requires more advanced cognitive development than is required for the Oucher and other face scales.[23] In its simplest form, the Visual Analogue Scale (VAS) is a 10-cm line with the anchor words "no pain" and "the worst pain possible" at the ends.[23] Another form of the VAS is the **ladder scale**. It is used with both adults and children. Patients are asked to choose the level of their pain from a drawing of a ladder, with higher rungs indicating greater pain.

(E) McGrath et al. developed CHEOPS (Children's Hospital of Eastern Ontario Pain Scale) to measure pain in children age 1 to 7 years during the postoperative period.[19] The types of behaviours noted include verbal expression, cry, facial expression, torso movement, and touch and leg movement. Behaviours are scored for the intensity of pain and related distress reflected. The CHEOPS, however, was developed by observing children who were emerging from anaesthesia. Recent research using the CHEOPS suggests that behaviours alone may not provide valid indicators of pain intensity after discharge from the recovery room. Child's behaviour may also be different from that expected from the self-report scores. Beyer and McGrath compared self-report and behavioural pain measures in 3–7 years old post-surgical children.[24] They noted that many children who reported severe pain manifested few of the behavioural indications of distress used in the CHEOPS. (Fig. 11.2)

(F) Assessment of pain often includes assessment of distress. This is particularly true in the cancer ward and Intensive Care Unit. Children in these settings are distressed because in addition to pain, they have anxiety and depression. Gauvain-Piquard et al., described a 17-item rating scale to measure distress in preschool children with cancer.[4] In addition to pain and anxiety behaviours, behaviours indicative of depression such as social withdrawal are included. It is interesting to note that in this sample, anxiety was negatively correlated with pain.

A second technique of measuring distress in the intensive care unit is the **COMFORT SCALE**. It was developed to assess distress of children in the Intensive Care Unit. It measures alertness, calmness, respiratory response, physical movement, mean arterial pressure, heart rate, muscle tone, and facial expression.[18]

School aged Children

Developmentally, school-aged children are beginning to understand abstract phenomena. As children become more comfortable with numbers and the concept of quantification, graphic and visual analogue scales developed for adults become more appropriate. The analogue scales with happy and sad faces at the anchor points would be appropriate for school aged children, as long as they understand they are rating pain, not happiness. It has been noted that significantly higher pain ratings are given on scales that have a smiling "no pain" faces compared with scales that have neutral "no pain" faces.[25] Variations of the adult scales such as the Coloured Analogue Scale (CAS), Facial Affect Scale (FAS) and Children's Pain Inventory (CPI) score, have been developed for children.[26] Two of the commonly used measurements are OPS and FPS. The Objective Pain Score (OPS) measures crying, complaint of pain, movement, agitation, posture and blood pressure.[17] The Faces Pain Scale (FPS) consists of seven faces increasing in pain intensity and approximating equal intervals as assessed by children.[8]

There are a variety of factors that might affect children's pain scores. Nausea tends to make a child "feel bad all over," and this will probably be reflected in the pain score. Scores should not be obtained until after the child vomits. This may also be true if children are hungry or they have to void or defecate, or if they need repositioning. Similarly, fear and anxiety may also affect the scores children give. Although it is not possible to eliminate all of these extraneous factors, it is possible to reduce their influence by careful explanations to children and appropriate timing of data collection.

If self-reports are used, the child must have the chance to learn how to use them and practice with them. One of the best ways to do this is to get them involved by remembering and rating past pain experiences. Listening to their descriptions and ratings of pain is essential for assessing the face validity of self-reports. If a child reports a 1 (on a 0 to 5 scale) for the hurt he felt when he broke his leg and reports a score of 5 for a stubbed toe, the health provider has cause to believe that the child does not understand the task and is unable to use the instrument. Adults should not judge the child's score; such as to say "Is your hurt REALLY that bad?" If their scores are criticized, children will agree with the adult.

As children mature and experience more types of pain, they use more meaningful words to describe the variation of pain experienced. The McGill Pain Questionnaire has been used extensively in adults, but may be used in older children and adolescents.[27] It includes 78 verbal descriptors of pain and a graphic rating scale. Savedra and colleagues found 9 to 12 years olds were able to select from a list of 24 verbal descriptors from the initial work on the McGill Pain Questionnaire – the words that best described their pain.[28] Tesler, et al., noted that 8 to 17 years olds identified 67 useful words to describe pain and assigned an intensity value to each.[29]

Adolescents

Developmentally, adolescents are able to abstract, quantify, and qualify phenomena, and, therefore, may have little difficulty in using scales developed for adults, such as 0 to 100 numerical scales and visual analogue scales. Practically, all adult scales such as VAS and McGill Questionnaire may be used. Adolescents, in contrast to younger children, may include psychological and emotional factors in descriptions of their pain experiences. Adolescents exhibit fewer types of distress behaviour than younger children in response to pain due to increased behavioural control and more localized response in this age group. Muscle tension is the only behaviour exhibited in adolescents more than in children. When groaning and flinching are included as behaviours, adolescents and children had similar total distress scores. It is important to note that adolescents who are ill may regress to earlier stages of development. Thus, simpler scales may be necessary during acute illness episodes.

Premature infants, neonates and children, all experience pain. It is sometimes difficult to assess the intensity of their pain, but we must be able to judge whether they are in pain or not. Any one or a combination of pain measurement scales may be used to systematically assess pain and to evaluate the effectiveness of the treatment. Whenever possible, analgesics should be given non-invasively. Pain relief should not be administered in a painful way, as this will only add insult to injury and may make subsequent pain measurements difficult. If intramuscular injections are given to relieve pain, children quickly learn to say they do not hurt even when they do. Thus, hurtful pain relief strategies will inhibit children from providing honest and accurate pain assessment data. Although there are always exceptions, oral or intravenous routes seem to be more acceptable to children.

REFERENCES

1. Koehler H, Schulz St., Wiebalk A. Pain management in children: Assessment and documentation in burn units. Eur J Pediatr Surg 11:40–43;2001.
2. Llyod-Thomas A. Assessment and control of pain in children. Anaesthesia 50:753-756;1995.
3. Manue SL, Jacobsen PB, Redd WH. Assessment of acute pediatric pain: Do child self report, parent ratings and nurse ratings measure the same phenomenon? Pain 48:45–52;1992.
4. Gauvain-Piquard A, Rodary C, Rezvani A, et al. Pain in children aged 2–6 years: a new observational rating elaborated in a pediatric oncology unit. Pain 31:177–188;1987.
5. Beyer JE, Wells N. The assessment of pain in children. Pediatric Clin North America 36:837–854;1989.
6. Sweet SD, McGrath PJ. Physiological measures of pain, In Measurement of pain in infants and children ed. Finley GA and McGrath PJ, IASP press, 1998.
7. Hall SJ. Pediatric pain assessment in intensive care units. Intensive and critical care nursing 1:20–25;1995.
8. Bieri D, Reeve R, Champion G. et al. The Faces Pain Scale for the self assessment of the severity of pain experienced by children: development, initial validation and preliminary investigation for ratio scale properties. Pain 41:139–150;1990.
9. Knott C, Beyer J, Villarrmel A et al. Using the Oucher developmental approach to pain assessment in childhood. MCN 19:314–320;1994.
10. Champion GD, Goodenough B, von Baeyer CL, et al. Measurement of pain by self report, techniques. In Measurement of pain in infants and children ed. Finley GA and McGrath PJ, IASP press, 1998.
11. Anand KJS. Neurophysiological and neurobiological correlates of supraspinal pain processing: measurement techniques. In Measurement of pain in infants and children ed. Finley GA and McGrath PJ, IASP press, 1998.
12. Gianna KX, Sepulveda W, Kourtis P et al. Foetal plasma cortisol and B. endorphin response to intrauterine needing . Lancet 344:77–81;1994.
13. Anand KJS, Sippell WG, Aynsley-Green A. Randomized trial of fentanyl anesthesia in pre-term babies undergoing surgery: effects of the stress response. Lancet 1:62–66;1987.
14. Stevens B, Johnson C. Premature infant pain profile. Development and initial validation. Clin J Pain 12:13–22;1996.
15. Lawrence J, Alcock D, McGrath P et al. The development of a tool; to assess neonatal pain. Neonatal Network 12:59–66;1993.

16. Krechel SW, Bildner J. CRIES: A new neonatal postoperative pain measurement score. Initial testing of validity and reliability. Pediatric Anesthesia 5:53–61;1995.
17. Hannallah RS, Broadman LM, Belman BA et al. Comparison of caudal and ilioinguinal/iliohypogastric nerve blocks for control of post-orchidopexy pain in pediatric ambulatory surgery. Anesthesiology 66:832–834;1987.
18. Amuel B, Hamlett KW, Marx CM, et al. Assessing distress in pediatric intensive care environments: the COMFORT scale. J pediatric psychology 17:95–109; 1992.
19. McGrath PJ, Johnson G, Goodman JT. CHEOPS: A behavioural scale for rating postoperative pain in children. Advances Pain Research and Therapy 9:395–402; 1985.
20. Johnston CC, Srada ME. Acute pain response in infants: A multi-dimensional description. Pain 24:373–382; 1986.
21. Granau RVE, Craig KD. Pain expression in neonates: Facial action and cry. Pain 28:395–410; 1987.
22. Villarruel AM, Denyes MJ. Pain assessment in children: Theoretical and empirical validity. Adv Nurs Sci 14:32–41;1991.
23. Johnston CC. Psychometric issues in the measurement of pain. In Measurement of pain in infants and children. Finley GA, McGrath PJ, IASP press, 1998.
24. Beyer JE, McGrath PJ, Berde CB. Discordance between self report and behavioural pain measures in children Aged 3–7 years after surgery. J Pain and Symptoms Manag 5:350–356;1990.
25. Chambers C, Giesbrecht K, Craig KD et al. A comparison of faces pain scales for the measurement of pediatric pain: children's and parents ratings. Pain 83:25–35;1999.
26. McGrath PA, Seifert CE, Speechley KN et al. A new analog scale for assessing children's pain: an initial validation study. Pain: 64:435–443;1996.
27. Melzack R. The McGill pain questionnaire: Major properties and scoring methods. Pain 1:277–299;1975.
28. Sevendra MC, Tesler MD. Assessing children's and adolescents' pain. Pediatrician 16:24–29;1989.
29. Tesler M, Savendra M, Ward J, et al. Children's language of pain. In Pain research and clinical management. Dubner R, Gerhart G, Bond M, Amsterdam, Elsevier,1988 pp 348–352.

•••

SECTION–IV

Pharmacology

CLINICAL PHARMACOLOGY OF OPIOIDS

12

Morphine is still considered to be the opioid drug of choice by many practitioners, a place it has essentially occupied throughout recorded history. However, some of the other potent μ-receptor agonists are gaining popularity for a variety of reasons.

The commonly prescribed opioids (agonists and antagonists) bind preferentially to the μ-receptor, they do associate with all three types. Morphine and normorphine (a minor morphine metabolite) show greatest relative preference for the μ -receptor. Methadone (which also is a potent NMDA-receptor blocker) shows a significant binding to δ-receptors, while buprenorphine, and to a lesser extent naloxone, avidly bind to all three receptor types. In fact, the binding affinity of buprenorphine to the μ -receptor is smaller than that of naloxone, which explains why the latter only partially reverses buprenorphine toxicity.

Codeine and heroin display exceedingly poor binding to opioid receptors, which raises the possibility that both are prodrugs, where the pharmacologically active species are morphine and 6- monoacetyl morphine[1] respectively. In addition, codeine also shows low relative efficacy at the μ-receptor in human neuroblastoma cells.[2] A similar situation probably occurs to oxycodone, where the metabolite oxymorphone may be substantially responsible for the pharmacodynamic effects. Alternatively, the intrinsic nociceptive effects of oxycodone may be mediated via κ-receptors.

While pethidine is considered to be a potent μ -receptor antagonist, its binding to all three opioid receptors is relatively weak. This binding of morphine, methadone, buprenorphine and naloxone, to the cloned human μ -receptors show excellent congruence with the equivalent animal data. Fentanyl shows a similar binding affinity, while codeine demonstrates greater binding affinity to the cloned human receptor.[3] Thus, for these commonly administered compounds, there is not enormous variability in their affinity for the human μ -receptor.

Physicochemical Properties of Opioids

The physicochemical properties of drugs substantially control their passive transfer across biological membranes. Two factors, their relative lipophilicity, low partition coefficient and degree of ionization at physiological pH affect the rate and extent of transmembrane flux and binding to critical receptors. For various opioid drugs, there are small differences in their molecular weights, but greater differences in their pK_a and lipophilicity. The higher the O/W partition coefficient value, the greater is the lipophilicity. In vitro studies using human cadaver meningeal membranes have shown a bell-shaped curve for a plot of meningeal permeation versus O/W partition coefficient, with the optimal permeability occurring around 130 (alfentanil).[4] Thus, more hydrophilic (*e.g.*, morphine) or lipophilic (*e.g.*, sufentanil) opioids have a lower meningeal permeability. This biphasic relationship is hardly surprising when opioid drugs, like all drugs, must traverse multiple aqueous and lipid bilayers (*e.g.*, membranes) to reach their site of action at the opioid receptor. Consequently, drugs with partition coefficients towards the extremes are disadvantaged with respect to transmembrane permeability compared to opioids with a more well-balanced partition coefficient.

Table 12.1 : Binding Affinities of Various Opioids to Guinea Pig and Cloned Human Opioid receptors[3]

Binding affinity				
	Guinea pig			cloned human
Opioid	**Delta**	**Kappa**	**Mu**	**Mu**
Morphine	90	317	1.8	2.0
Normorphine	310	149	4.0	ND
Levorphanol	5.6	9.6	0.6	1.9

Codeine	>10,000	ND	2,700	65
Methadone	15.1	1,628	4.2	4.2
Fentanyl	151	470	7.0	1.9
Pethidine	4,345	5,140	385	ND
Pentazocine	106	22.2	7.0	ND
Buprenorphine	1.3	2.0	0.6	0.5
Naloxone	27	17.2	1.8	1.4

Time curve is to manipulate (*i.e.*, delay) the absorption rate, as in the case of various sustained-release oral morphine, oxycodone, and hydromorphone formulations and transdermal fentanyl. The prolonged analgesia associated with these formulations is achieved by altering the absorption profile of the opioids.

Pharmacokinetic Aspects

The effective option to predictably change the shape of the blood opioid concentration – oral dosage forms.

Immediate Release Formulations

The peak opioid concentration usually occurs within 30–60 minutes (*i.e.*, T_{max} value) following the oral administration of opioid drugs as an immediate-release solution or tablet. The oral bioavailability (*i.e.*, proportion of opioid absorbed following oral administration compared to a standard parenteral [usually intravenous] dose) for opioid drugs displays both significant interpatient and absolute variability.

Food can influence oral morphine absorption, depending on the type of formulation administered. For example, food results in increased Area Under the Curve (AUC) following immediate-release formulations but has more variable effects with modified-release formulations, depending on the formulation.[5]

Sustained or Modified-release Formulations and Bioequivalence

Many of these modified-release morphine formulations are not bioequivalent, which indicates that either the rate and/or the extent of morphine absorption is different between the formulations.[5] The clinical implications of a lack of bioequivalence between formulations is that care should be exercised if physicians change modified-release formulations in individual patients as dosage adjustments may be necessary to reoptimize pain control. Some of the modified release morphine formulations can be administered once every 24 hours. The outcome with respect to analgesia and side effects were equivalent to those seen with morphine formulations administered every 12 hours.[5]

Table 12.2 : Opioid Pharmacokinetics and the Role of Metabolites

Opioid	Terminal half-life (h)	Clearance (L/min)	Equian-algesic Dose (mg) i.v.,/i.m.	Dosing interval (h)	Oral bioavail-ability (%) oral	Active meta-bolities
Morphine	2-4	0.8-1.2	10/30-40	2-4/12,24	10-50	M6G
Pethidine	3-4	0.6-0.8	100/200-300	2-4	30-60	Norpethidine
Methadone	6-150	0.1-0.3	10/2-5	8-24	60-90	No
Fentanyl	3-7	0.7-1.5	0.1/0.025-0.05	3 days	<2/90	No
Codeine	3-4	0.6-0.9	60/120	2-4	60-90	Morphine
Oxycodone	2-6	0.4-1.1	5-10/15	3-4/12	40-130	Oxymorphone
Hydromor-phone	2-4	0.4	2/3-4	4-6	35-80	No phone

Chronopharmacokinetic Variability

Chronopharmacokinetic variability may be defined as differences in the rate and/or extent of absorption or changes in metabolism and excretion with consequential alterations in the blood concentration-time profile for the same dose of drug, depending on the time of day the dose is administered.[5]

Buccal Formulations

Fentanyl has negligible oral bioavailability because the drug undergoes a cytochrome P450 isoform 3A4 catalyzed N-dealkylation to form norfentanyl in both the liver and intestines.[6,7] However, this drug has been successfully administered via the buccal mucosa in a unique formulation (termed a hardened lozenge on a stick or the "fentanyl lollipop" although the latter term is now actively being discouraged) as a non-invasive treatment of acute pain in paediatric patients and also for incident or unpredictable breakthrough pain in adult patients with severe cancer pain.

Other Routes of Administration

Transdermal Formulations

The fentanyl pharmacokinetics from the formulation (Transdermal Therapeutic Systems or TTS-Fentanyl, Duragesic, Janssen-Cilag) are characterized by slow absorption through skin (partially controlled by a rate-control membrane that forms part of the formulation), and by a long duration of effect, upto 3 days. A reservoir in the stratum corneum immediately below the patch is established over 12–16 hours once a system is applied, and then constant blood fentanyl concentrations are maintained for upto 3 days. Desaturation of this depot occurs after system removal and pain relief is maintained while analgesic blood concentrations are being established from newly applied patches. It is serendipitous that the rate of desaturation from the old site (immediately under the patch that has just been removed) is approximately equal to the rate of saturation from the newly applied patch, thereby maintaining constant blood fentanyl concentrations.[7] Studies in cancer pain suggest that TTS-fentanyl has similar pain control to MS Contin (controlled release morphine sulfate); but with a lower incidence of constipation.[7] TTS-fentanyl has also been used to treat noncancer pain and pain related to AIDS.

Spinal Administration

While spinally (*i.e.*, epidural or intrathecal) administered opioids (and other drugs and drug combinations) are primarily considered in the treatment of severe pain in cancer patients when optimized orally administered drugs no longer provide adequate analgesia. This route of administration is increasingly being used in chronic noncancer pain.[9] The spinal route of administration is used because of a perceived more favourable balance between improved pain relief and the incidence and severity of adverse effects compared to oral opioids due to a selective spinal action. The small opioid doses administered intrathecally (in comparison to oral doses of the same opioid) result in negligible and subtherapeutic blood opioid concentrations. In contrast, however, there is rapid and significant vascular absorption following epidural opioid administration, the extent of which varies among opioids.[10] Thus, analgesia observed within 1–2 hours of a bolus epidural opioid probably is a combination of both a spinal and a supraspinal (and perhaps peripheral) action of opioids secondary to significant blood opioid concentration, whereas the analgesia after approximately 2 hours is due to a selective spinal analgesia effect.

Intranasal Administration

The absorption of opioid drugs from the nasal mucosa has been used to treat breakthrough or incident pain and also for preoperative sedation. Nasal spray bottles that deliver an accurate volume of solution (and therefore dose) as a spray per activation are used for this route of administration. Fentanyl[8], oxycodone and sufentanil[9] have been effectively administered in this manner. The intranasal bioavailability for oxycodone and sufentanil was 45% and 78% respectively. Administration of intranasal sufentanil as either drops or a spray had essentially the same effect on the degree of postoperative sedation[10].

Pulmonary Administration Using Aerosol or Nebulizated Solutions

Evidence suggests rapid, extensive but variable absorption of both morphine and fentanyl[10] after inhalation of drug solutions that have been aerosolized. In fact, the mean blood concentration-time profiles, following pulmonary administration were similar to those seen with intravenous administration, which raises the possibility of a non-invasive option for breakthrough or incident pain. While these studies used specialized apparatus to create the small droplets that constitute the aerosol, the absorption of opioid drugs from traditionally nebulized solutions is less efficient and results in lower bioavailability and more variable postoperative analgesia[12].

Parenteral Administration

The absorption of all opioids following either intravenous, intramuscular, or subcutaneous administration has been well characterized over a prolonged period and consequently is not considered in detail here.

Rectal Administration

The rectal route is frequently used in patients who have difficulty in swallowing or have significant vomiting despite optimized antiemetic therapy. The absorption of drugs from the rectum is notoriously variable and depends greatly on the nature of the formulation used. Liquid rectal formulations (solutions or suspensions) frequently have reasonable, rapid and predictable absorption, but meet with generally low patient acceptance, because the solution is difficult to hold in the rectum, particularly in ambulant patients.

While rectal bioavailability of opioids from solid dosage forms can be extensive (greater than oral bioavailability of the same dose), it is highly variable, and the precise anatomical location of the suppository in the rectum is a crucial factor governing the extent of avoidance of hepatic first-pass metabolism and hence rectal bioavailability.[5]

While vaginal pessaries can also be used to administer opioid drugs, this route of administration is not greatly favoured by most female patients.

Metabolism

The liver is the primary site of biotransformation of most drugs, including opioid drugs. Metabolism also occurs to a variable extent (depending on the opioid) in the organs of the body that come into initial contact with the opioid. For example, during absorption from the gastrointestinal tract (following oral administration) and lung (pulmonary administration). Indeed other organs (*e.g.*, kidney and brain) also metabolize opioid drugs. Although the skin has demonstrable capacity to metabolize a range of drugs, fentanyl is not metabolized during Transdermal absorption.[5]

The terminal half-life for most opioids varies between 2 and 7 hours, the notable exception being methadone, where the extremes are as short as 6 hours and as long as 150 hours. Although most patients will be in a range of 12– 60 hours.[13]

Morphine is mainly metabolized by conjugation with glucuronic acid to form the 3- and 6-glucuronides (Phase I reaction), with a minor route being N-demethylation to produce normorphine (Phase II reaction). Codeine and heroin (3,6-diacetylmorphine or diamorphine) are morphine analogues. Codeine is converted to morphine via hepatic metabolism catalyzed by cytochrome P450 isoform 2D6.[14] Thus codeine is considered to be a prodrug for morphine in view of its poor binding to the μ-receptor. However, the major metabolite is codeine-6-glucuronide, which, unlike morphine-6-glucuronide (M6G) would not be expected to have significant analgesic activity as it would require conversion to M6G by O-demethylation.

Fentanyl is metabolized in the liver by N-demethylation catalyzed by the 3A4 isoform of cytochrome P450 to form norfentanyl. There are other minor routes of metabolism including amide hydrolysis and hydroxylation.[6] The metabolites are believed to be inactive. The 3A4 isoform is also the major determinant of both alfentanil and sufentanil metabolism.[15]

Pharmacogenetic Aspects of Cytochrome P450 Metabolism

Cytochrome P450 2D6 is involved in the metabolism of codeine (and its derivatives) to morphine (and corresponding derivative) by O-demethylation. There is a polymorphic distribution of this isoform in Caucasians, such that 8–10% of the population lack the capacity to perform this conversion. This variation results in the subdivision of patients into two groups, either extensive or poor metabolizers. Thus, poor metabolizers will not experience analgesia following codeine administration. Further, codeine metabolism could be inhibited in extensive metabolizers by the concurrent administration of other drugs, also metabolized by this isoform. It has been suggested that it is predominantly codeine and not morphine that is responsible for the side effects observed following codeine administration.[16]

Renal Excretion

Analgesic and toxic effects observed after morphine administration to patients with poor renal function are probably due to M6G rather than morphine. M6G accumulates[17] and it is not uncommon to be unable to detect morphine in blood samples collected a few hours after morphine administration. Similarly, norpethidine accumulates at a greater rate in patients with renal insufficiency, with a corresponding greater potential for neurotoxicity. Therefore, other opioids such as fentanyl, methadone or possibly hydromorphone should be considered in lieu of morphine in chronic noncancer pain patients with significantly reduced renal function.

Metabolite Pharmacodynamic Effects

Some opioid metabolites have pharmacological effects that are either positive (*i.e.*, contribute to analgesia) or negative (*i.e.*, contributes to the adverse events profile). Morphine-6-glucuronide and normorphine have intrinsic analgesic activity, particularly the former. The status of morphine-3-glucuronide (M3G), is still controversial with suggestions ranging from it being inactive[18] to being a functional antagonist at other receptors[19] because it does not bind to opioid receptors.

Opioid Use in Drug Dependent Patients

Increasing attention is being given to the relationship between the long-term prescription of opioids to treat chronic noncancer pain and drug-seeking behaviour or frank opioid addiction.[20] Pain is seen by some patients as the vehicle that may be more likely to convince practitioners to prescribe opioids rather than admitting to a drug dependence problem. However, it is essential to recall that opioid dependent individuals can suffer from chronic pain just like any other member of society. Recent evidence suggests that methadone maintenance patients can demonstrate a hyperalgesic response to experimental pain, depending on the pain stimulus employed.[21] These findings only add an additional layer of complexity as they indicate that acute pain should be taken seriously and treated aggressively in opioid dependent patients.

Sex Difference in Reported Pain and Analgesic Response

While the accusation of sex difference and reported pain is not a new concept, interest in this area has dramatically increased over the last decade. For example, a Special Interest Group of the IASP on Sex, Gender and Pain was established in 1996 at the 8th World Congress on Pain in Vancouver. There are many examples of sex differences; women are more likely than men to report chronic pain conditions, but prevalence rates vary for condition and age[22]. The reasons for this variability are numerous and include hormonal, psychological, neurophysiological, and neuropharmacological factors.

Acute pain studies using various μ-receptor agonists have shown variable results, with some authors indicating that males require more postoperative analgesia than females, but have evidenced no differences in plasma concentrations or minimum effective concentrations of the opioid agonist[23]. Other studies suggest no gender difference in analgesic consumption rates.

A series of studies have shown that κ-receptor agonists result in improved analgesic outcomes for females that are not convincingly explained by sex differences in pharmacokinetics.[24] There is also suggestion of a sex difference in the analgesic response to NSAIDs such that only male volunteers reported pain responses to ibuprofen administration following an experimental stimulus, but there was no difference in pharmacokinetics between males and females.

Tramadol is administered as a racemate and has a dual mechanism of action; the *d*-enantiomer exhibits preferential but weak binding activity at μ-receptors and is a more potent inhibitor of serotonin reuptake, while the *l*-enantiomer is more efficient in blocking norepinephrine uptake.[25]

The combination of morphine and ketamine may result in improved analgesia in patients with neuropathic pain compared with morphine alone. Ketamine is also an NMDA-receptor blocker and acts at a site different from the NMDA recognition site. However, the *d*-enantiomer has more potent blocking action at the NMDA-receptor than does the *l*-enantiomer.[26]

Morphine, hydromorphone, fentanyl, codeine and naltrexone are devoid of NMDA-receptor antagonist activity, while levorphanol has very weak blocking action compared to dextromethorphan.

REFERENCES

1. Inturrisi CE, Shultz M, Shin S, et al. Evidence from opiate binding studies that heroin acts through its metabolites. Life Sci 1983;33:773–776.
2. Traynor JR. The μ-opioid receptor. Pain Rev. 1996;3:221–248.
3. Gourlay GK. Chronic pain, clinical pharmacology of the treatment of acute and chronic pain. In: Max M (Ed). Pain 1999-an updated review: refresher course syllabus. Seattle: IASP press, 1999, pp 433–442.
4. Bernard CM. Epidural and intrathecal drug movement. In: Yaksh TL (Ed). Spinal drug delivery, Amsterdam: Elsevier, 1999, pp 239–252.
5. Gourlay GK. Sustained relief of chronic pain: pharmacokinetics of SR morphine. Clin Pharmacokin 1998;35:173-190.
6. Labroo RB, Paine MF, Thummel KE, et al. Fentanyl metabolism by human hepatic and intestinal cytochrome P450 3AS: implications for inter individual variability in disposition, efficacy, and drug interactions. Drug metab dispos 1997;25:1072–1080.
7. Gourlay GK. Treatment of cancer pain with Transdermal fentanyl. Lancet 2001; 2:165–172.
8. Zeppetella G. An assessment of the safety, efficacy and acceptability of intranasal fentanyl citrate in the management of cancer related breakthrough pain: a pilot study. J pain symptom manage 2000;20:253–258.
9. Takala A, Kaasalainen V, Seppala T, et al. Identification of human cytochrome P450 3A4 as the enzyme responsible for fentanyl and sufentanil N-dealkylation. Anesth Analg 1996;82:167–172.
10. Vercauteren M, Boeckx E, Hangreefs G, Noorduin H, van den Bussche G. Intranasal sufentanil for perioperative sedation. Anaesthesia 1988;43:270–273.
11. Mather LE, Woodhouse A, Ward ME, et al. Pulmonary administration of aerosolized fentanyl: pharmacokinetic analysis of systemic delivery. Br J clin pharmacol 1998;46:37–43.
12. Higgins MJ, Asbury AJ, Brodie MJ. Inhaled nebulised fentanyl for postoperative analgesia. Anaesthesia 1991;46:973–976.

13. Plummer JL, Cherry DA, Cousins MJ. Estimation of methadone clearance: application in the management of cancer pain. Pain 1998;33:313–322.
14. Eckhardt K, Li S, Ammon S, et al. Same incidence of adverse drug events after codeine administration irrespective of the genetically determined differences in morphine formation. Pain 1998;76:27–33.
15. Tateishi T, Krivoruk Y, Ueng YF, et al. Pharmacokinetic comparison of intravenous and intranasal administration of oxycodone. Acta anaesthesiol Scand 1997;41309–41312.
16. Desmeules J, Gascon MP, Dayer P. Magistris M. Impact of environmental and genetic factors on codeine analgesia. Eur J Clin Pharmacol 1991;41:23–26.
17. Portenoy RK, Foley KM, Stulman J, et al. Plasma morphine and morphine-6-glucuronide during chronic morphine therapy for cancer pain: plasma profiles, steady state concentrations and the consequences of renal failure. Pain 1998;41:13–19.
18. Hewett K, Dickenson AH, Mcquay HJ. Lack of effect of morphine-3-glucuronide on the spinal antinociceptive actions of morphine in the rat: an electrophysiological study. Pain 1993;53:59–63.
19. Gong QI, Hedner J, Bjorkman R, Hedner T. Morphine-3-glucuronide may functionally antagonize morphine-6-glucuronide induced antinociception and ventilatory depression in the rat. Pain 1992;48:249–255.
20. Goldman B. Diagnosing addiction and drug seeking behavior in chronic pain patients. In: max m (Ed). Pain 1999- an updated review: refresher course syllabus. Seattle: ASP Press, 1999; pp 1–20.
21. Doverty M, White JM, Somogyi AA, et al. Hyperalgesic responses in methadone maintenance patients. Pain 2001a; 90:91–96.
22. Fillingim RB (Ed). Sex, gender, and pain, progress in pain research and management. Vol. 17. Seattle: IASP Press, 2000.
23. Gourlay GK, Kowalski SR, Plummer JL. Cousins MJ, Armstrong PJ. Fentanyl blood concentration–analgesic response relationship in the treatment of postoperative pain. Anesth Analg 1988;67:329–337.
24. Miaskowski C, Gear RW, Levine RD. Sex-related differences in analgesic responses. In: Fillingim RB(Ed). Sex, gender, and pain, progress in pain research and management. Vol. 17. Seattle: IASP Press, 2000, pp 209–230.
25. Kieslowski CJ, Raffa RB, Porreca F. Tramadol and its enantiomers differentially suppress C-fos-like immunoreactivity in rat brain and spinal cord following acute noxious stimulus. Eur J Pain 1998;2:211–219.
26. Lodge D, Jones M, Fletcher E. Non-competitive antagonists of N-methyl-D-aspartate. In: collingridge GL, Watkins JC, (Eds). The NMDA receptor, Oxford: Oxford University Press, 1994; pp 104–131.
27. Gorman AL, Elliott KJ, Inturrisi CE. The *d*- and *l*- isomers of methadone bind to the non-competitive site on the N-methyl-D-aspartate (NMDA) receptor in rat forebrain and spinal cord. Neurosci lett 1997;223:5–8.

•••

NEWER METHODS OF OPIOID DRUG DELIVERY

13

Current interest in improving the management of pain by the use of opioid analgesics has led to the search for newer methods of opioid drug delivery. Opioids can be given by (1) sublingual, (2) continuous subcutaneous infusion, (3) transdermal, (4) continuous spinal opioid infusion and (5) intraventricular injection. Each of these modes of administration shares the advantage that they can be used for continuous or repeated administration of an opioid analgesic when injections and oral dosing are to be avoided (Table 13.1). In addition, each of these methods may have advantages in certain therapeutic situations and each mode of administration requires consideration of pharmacological and pharmacokinetics factors.

Table 13.1 : Comparison of New Methods of Opioid Delivery[2,3,4]

Consideration	Continuous Spinal	Continuous Subcutaneous	Continuous Transdermal	Continuous Intraventricular	Continuous Sublingual
Avoids im/sc injections	Yes	Yes	Yes	Yes	Yes
Avoids need for iv access	Yes	Yes	Yes	Yes	Yes
Circumvents oral absorption	Yes	Yes	Yes	Yes	Yes
Use by ambulatory	Yes	Yes	Yes	Yes	Yes
Ease of management	Responsible specialist needed	Responsible specialist needed	Self-administered	Responsible specialist needed	Self-administered
Complications	Infrequent but potentially serious	Infrequent, mild	Unknown serious	Potentially serious	Mild

Sublingual Administration

Although the sublingual route is not a common route of administration for opioid analgesics, it offers a number of potential advantages over injections or the oral route (Table 13.1). The total sublingual and buccal area is small compared to the gastrointestinal tract.

However, the potential exists for a rapid absorption of drugs in this area which are rich in blood and lymphatic vessels. In selecting the opioid that might be suitable for use by the sublingual route, consideration must be given to the principles governing absorption through the oral mucosa and to the physiochemical properties of the opioids (Table 13.2). If the drug is administered in a solid dosage form, then the first step is the dissolution of the dosage form in the tissue fluids (Fig. 13.1).

Table 13.2 : Physicochemical Properties of Opioids

Drug	Partition coefficient *	pK_a
Morphine	0.00001	7.9
Hydromorphine	0.0001	
6-Acetylmorphine	0.0012	
Levorphanol	0.01	9.4
Heroin	0.043	

Meperidine	1.7	8.5
Fentanyl	19.6	8.4
Methadone	44.6	9.3
Buprenorphine	60.3	

* Heptane and Phosphate buffer at pH 7.4

The opioids are weak bases and can exist in two forms, an ionized and a unionized form. It is the unionized form that passes rapidly through lipid membranes into the systemic circulation. The more lipid soluble is the unionized form of the opioid, the faster it will be absorbed. As shown in Table 13.2, there are large differences among the opioids in their Partition Coefficient (PC), an experimentally determined constant that is a measure of lipid solubility. For example, the PCs of methadone and buprenorphine are 6 orders of magnitude larger than the PC for morphine. Indeed morphine is the least lipid soluble of all the clinically used opioids. The order of increasing lipid solubility of opioids (Table 13.2) predicted quite well the order of increasing sublingual absorption. The second important factor is the ionization constant or pK_a of the opioid, for it determines the relative amount of ionized and unionized species at a particular pH. The opioids have pK_a that vary from 7.9 to 9.4 (Table 13.2), so that by raising the pH of the dosing solution, we can increase the proportion of unionized species of opioid in the sublingual cavity. By control of pH and selection of a lipid soluble opioid, it should be possible to develop opioids, in addition to buprenorphine, that are suitable for sublingual administration.

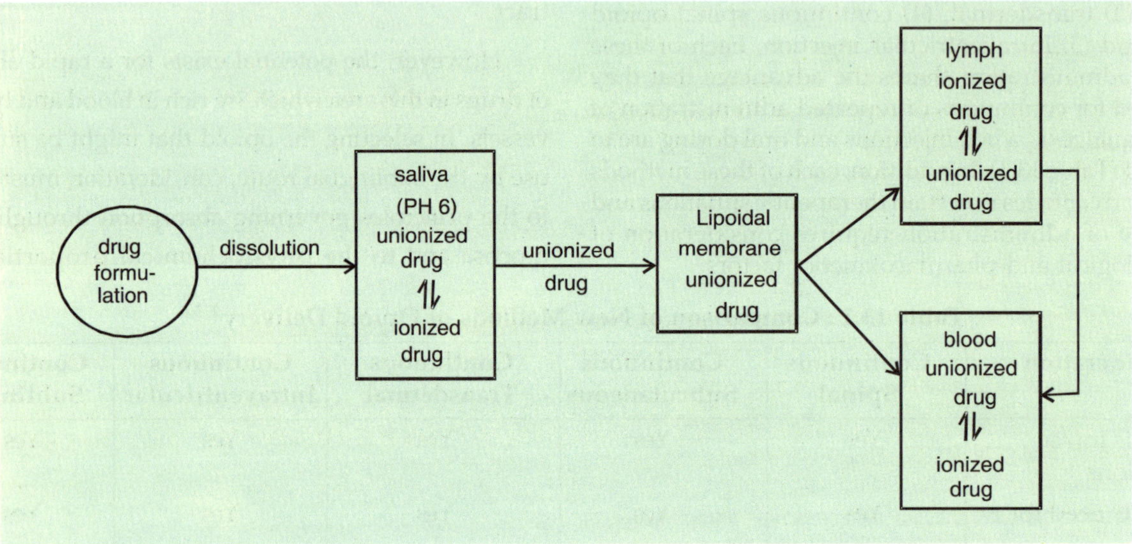

Fig. 13.1 : A schematic representation of the sublingual absorption of a drug that is ionized at physiological pH

Continuous Subcutaneous Infusion (CSCI)

Opioids injected subcutaneously in aqueous solution are generally rapidly absorbed with time to reach the maximum concentration in plasma from 10 to 30 min. Faster or slower absorption is possible depending on the vascular of the site, the ionization and the lipid solubility of the opioid, the volume of the solution. Opioids, being relatively small molecules, are absorbed directly into the capillaries and the absorption process appears to be limited by blood flow. A prime determinant of the absorption rate from a subcutaneous site is the total surface area over which absorption can occur. Although the subcutaneous tissues are somewhat loose, and moderate amounts of fluid can be administered, the normal connective tissue matrix prevents indefinite lateral spread of the injected solution. The properties shown to be important for the absorption of opioids from the sublingual cavity will also influence subcutaneous absorption.

Table 13.3 : Guidelines for Continuous Subcutaneous Infusion (CSCI)

1. Most opioid analgesics available for parenteral use can be administered by CSCI (meperidine [pethidine] and pentazocine are irritating to tissues).
2. May initiate CSCI with the same opioid analgesic that patient has been receiving by the alternate route.
3. Starting dose is calculated using equianalgesic conversing tables (see Table 13.5) with use of rescue doses and titration to effect.
4. Equipment: a portable infusion pump, drug delivery bags, and a 27-gauge paediatric butterfly needle.
5. Home management requires instruction of patient and family.

Coyle et al.[5] have evaluated continuous subcutaneous infusion of opioids using a portable infusion pump attached to a 27-gauge butterfly needle in the management of pain in cancer patients. Based on these observations, guidelines for the selection of the opioid and starting dose for CSCI are given in (Table 13.3).

The appropriate management of patients by the use of CSCI requires special considerations as outlined in Table 13.4 and equianalgesic starting doses for some opioid administered by CSCI are given in Table 13.5. These workers found that the steady state plasma morphine concentration varied from 13 to 24 mg/mL during CSCI with a dosage of 2 mg per hour for 12 days in a 22 year old cancer patient.[5]

CSCI has been demonstrated to be a relatively simple, safe and effective method for opioid administration to adults and children in pain. Additional studies are required to continue the development of guidelines of CSCI and determine whether any currently available opioids may possess pharmacokinetic or other properties that make them particularly useful for CSCI.

Table 13.4 : Special Considerations with Continuous Subcutaneous Infusion (CSCI)

1. Local irritation at the site of administration (usually when volume exceeds 1 mL per hour)—more frequent rotation of site infusion.
2. Pain breakthrough due to poor absorption from a particular site — change infusion site.
3. Rapidly escalating pain in terminal patients may necessitate the discontinuation of CSCI.
4. Availability of a clinical nurse specialist to assist in home management.

Table 13.5 : Equianalgesic Conversion Ratios[6]

Opioid	**Equianalgesic Doses (mg)**	
Analgesic	PO	IM/SC
Morphine	30.0	10.0*
Hydromorphone (Dilaudid)	7.5	1.5
Levorphanol (Levo-Dromoran)	4.0	2.0
Methadone	20.0	10.0

* A 1:3 ratio has been used because of repetitive administration

Continuous Transdermal Delivery

The newest and perhaps most challenging method of opioid drug delivery involves the development of a transdermal drug delivery system (Fig. 13.2).

A continuous transdermal delivery system for opioid administration offers a number of potential advantages including ease of self-administration (Table 13.1). A critical consideration in the absorption of drugs applied to the skin surface is the properties of the epidermis. This is because despite its thinness the epidermis is a formidable barrier to the absorption of most drugs. Most of the resistance to drug diffusion encountered in the epidermis results from the ultra thin, outermost layer of dead cells called the stratum corneum, the intracellular space of the corneum contains a unique protein called keratin. Together with a lipid rich medium comprising 15% to 20% of the total stratum corneum, the overall organization is designed to minimize water loss at the body surface. This organization also confers a high resistance to the diffusion of most chemicals. The physiochemical properties of a drug that make it suitable for transdermal delivery are:

1. Sufficient lipid solubility to penetrate tissue to the capillaries.
2. Adequate water solubility to allow fairly concentrated solutions (>1.0 mg/mL) to be incorporated into the drug reservoir.
3. High relative analgesic potency since it reduces the bulk of the reservoir system.

These considerations have led to the use of the potent, highly lipid soluble opioid, fentanyl in a transdermal delivery system currently under development. Preliminary results indicate that after a lag period of 2–3 hours, fentanyl appears in plasma and 12 hours are required for steady state plasma fentanyl levels to be achieved. Additional pharmacokinetic and analgesic studies are required before this potentially useful drug delivery system can be adequately evaluated.

Continuous Spinal Opioid Infusion (CSOI)

Continuos spinal infusions of opioids represent relatively a new development in spinal opioid analgesia. Therefore, it is worthwhile to first review the principles and considerations in the spinal opioid analgesia. Spinal opioid analgesia is defined as the introduction of opioids into the epidural or subarachnoid space for the management of acute and chronic pain. Since its introduction in the late 1970s, it has been used for the management of acute pain in the intra and postoperative period, for obstetrical analgesia and for chronic pain due to cancer and of non-malignant origin (Table 13.6)[4].

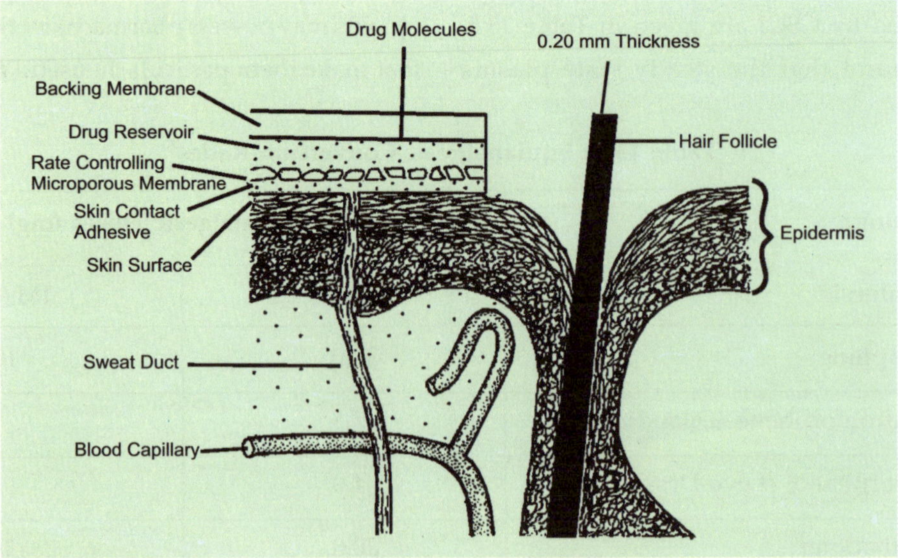

Fig. 13.2 : A schematic representation of the flow of drug from a transdermal delivery system through skin into the systemic circulation

Table 13.6 : Equianalgesic Conversion Ratio's[6]

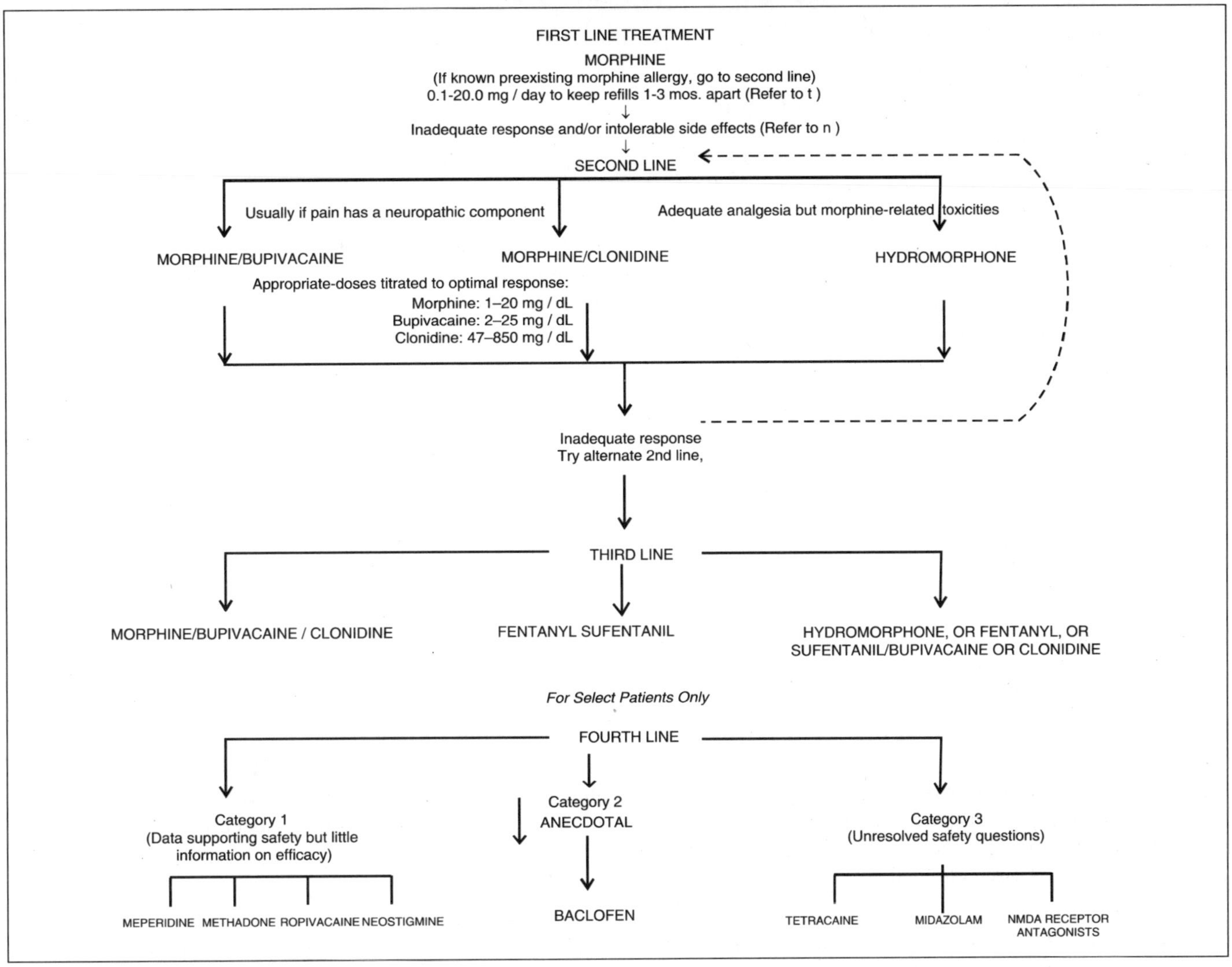

Spinal opioids offer potential advantages over systemic opioid administration including a substantially longer duration of analgesia at much lower dose. Furthermore, if the opioid remains localized to the site of administration then selective activation of spinal cord opioid receptors could provide segmental analgesia without supraspinally mediated adverse affects. Opioid analgesia is free of the sympathetic, motor and proprioceptive adverse effects produced by local anaesthetics. However, adverse effects occur with spinal opioids including sedation, nausea and vomiting, respiratory depression, urinary retention and pruritis[4]. The most feared adverse effect, respiratory depression, occurs as a consequence of rostral redistribution of opioid to supraspinal brainstem sites by movement in the CSF or systemic uptake into the circulation.

Considerable anatomic and pharmacological evidence has accumulated to support the mechanism and site of action of spinal opioids at the dorsal horn of the spinal cord. Opioid receptor densities are the highest in the marginal zone and in the substantia gelatinosa of the dorsal horn. These areas of spinal cord receive primary nociceptive afferent terminals of A delta and C fibres and microinjection of opioids suppress noxious evoked activity of lamina V neurons. In addition the analgesic effects of intrathecal opioids are dose dependent, stereo specific, antagonized by naloxone and subject to the development of tolerance.[7]

Table 13.7 lists some of the factors that determine the response to spinal opioids. Because of the difficulties involved, if any, controlled studies have compared graded doses of spinal opioids to obtain relative potency estimates. These values are critical for the appropriate comparison among spinal opioids of analgesic time action characteristics and the incidence and severity of adverse effects. It is well established that there are multiple opioid receptor types and that the μ, κ and δ-receptor types are to be found in the spinal cord. Currently we lack opioids for use in humans that are highly selective for each of these receptors. However, animal studies have been encouraging[8] and the use of selective opioids and opioid peptides will no doubt improve the specificity of this mode of administration and may overcome the limitations imposed by tolerance.

Table 13.7 : Factors Determining the Response to Spinal Opioids

1. Relative analgesic potency
2. Receptor selectivity
3. Pharmacokinetics in CSF and spinal cord
4. Tolerance to opioids

Calculations by Bullingham et al.[2] predict relatively little uptake of morphine from CSF into the spinal cord at equilibrium (Table 13.8). The persistent CSF morphine levels favour redistribution to supraspinal sites. Thus the **low lipid solubility and limited uptake into spinal cord of morphine results in a slow onset of action while the slow egress from CSF and spinal cord results in a relatively long duration of action.**[4] Furthermore, the supraspinal redistribution of morphine in CSF predisposes to effects mediated cephalad, while respiratory movements may enhance the spread of morphine from spinal to supraspinal CSF with pharmacological consequences.

In contrast to morphine, methadone is very lipid soluble (Table 13.2) and is rapidly taken up from the lumbar CSF into the spinal cord (Table 13.8). Rapid egress occurs from CSF leaving a very little methadone available in CSF to move supraspinally. **Thus lipid soluble opioids such as methadone and fentanyl are characterized by a more rapid onset but a shorter duration of action than morphine.** The opioid lofentanil presents a third pharmacokinetic profile. Its lipid solubility is similar to that of methadone resulting in rapid onset, but it appears to possess high affinity at μ-receptors, resulting in a longer duration of action. Increased information on these pharmacokinetic factors will improve our ability to select the most appropriate opioid for each patient.

Table 13.8 : Distribution of Opioids from CSF to Spinal Cord

Opioid	Brain: plasma ratio	Cord: CSF ratio	Initial Dose in Cord (%)
Morphine	0.046	0.06	3.8
Methadone	1.23	3.1	67.0
Fentanyl	10.58	34.7	95.8

Note : Calculated assuming a cord volume = 10 mL, CSF volume = 15mL, and assuming cord concentration = brain concentration.

Respiratory depression is less common in patients who have developed some degree of opioid tolerance due to prior systemic administration of opioids. Unfortunately the development of tolerance can also significantly reduce the therapeutic efficacy of spinal opioids. Thus, the best time to initiate spinal opioids in patients with

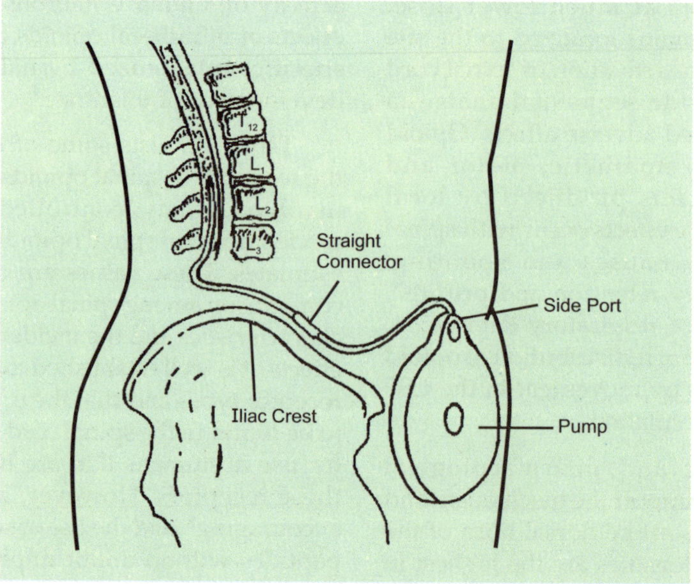

Fig. 13.3 : A schematic representation of infusaid pump with catheter in the epidural space at L1-L2

chronic pain due to cancer is not yet clear. The difficulties posed by the tolerance development suggest that the chronic use of spinal opioids requires different approaches. Yaksh et al.[8] found that in morphine related tolerance, rats very little cross tolerance, occurs to the delta opioid receptor agonist, DADL, administered intrathecally. Moulin et al.[10] found that intrathecal DADL produced safe and effective analgesia in cancer patients with some degree of tolerance to systemic opioids.

Patients with cancer pain require individualization of dose regardless of the route of administration. Cousins and Mather[4] have reviewed the use of long-term epidural catheters to administer opioids. Another innovation is a totally implanted system for continuous spinal opioid infusion. In addition to the advantages indicated in Table 13.1 CSOI avoids the use of neurolytic agents or neurosurgical procedures for pain control and allows preoperative assessment of the patient's response to spinal opioids.

A schematic of the Infusaid model pump 400 is shown in Fig. 13.4. The pump includes a 47 mL drug chamber, which is under compression from a temperature sensitive bellows. The pump delivers opioid at a constant low rate (2 to 4 mL/day) for 14 to 21 days into a silastic catheter, which is implanted under local, regional and general anaesthesia into the epidural or subarachnoid space. The pump model also has an auxiliary side port (Fig. 13.4), completely bypassing the pump mechanisms by implanting the pump in a subcutaneous pocket in the abdomen or chest (Fig. 13.3).

However, tolerance appears to develop rapidly in some patients and more slowly in others. Tolerance development with or without escalation in pain due to disease progression results in failures after 2–6 months of CSOI. To date, mechanical problems associated with the catheter system and CSF hyromas have been reported. No evidence of catheter induced spinal cord pathology or epidural abscess or meningitis was found in the series.[3,7]

Intraventricular Injection

Intraventricular injection of opioid has been reported to be of value in the management of chronic cancer pain. The procedure requires the implantation of an Ommaya reservoir to allow IVT opioid administration. The selection of patients and guidelines for the use of IVT are discussed by Lobato et al.[11] Table 13.1 compares IVT administration with the other methods. The only opioid used in these reports was morphine in doses that ranged from a starting dose of 0.25 to 1 mg given 1 or 2 times a day[12], to a maximum dose of 1 to 15 mg given 1 to 3 times per day. Nausea and vomiting occurred in 20% to 60% patients, and other opioid effects including drowsiness and disorientation were reported. The patients developed respiratory depression 4 to 9 hours after the initial morphine dose. Complications included catheter obstruction and a meningitis, treated successfully with antibiotics. The development of tolerance required a progressive increase in dose. Pharmacokinetic studies confirm very high ventricular CSF levels of morphine, which decay within at 1/2 to 7 hours.[8] IVT morphine is distributed to cisternal and lumbar CSF[8]. Since opioids can act at spinal and supraspinal sites to produce analgesia, the mechanisms of IVT analgesia may involve multiple sites. It can be assumed that IVT administration of opioids mediate adverse effects, such as nausea and vomiting and sedation. It is unlikely that these limitations to the selectivity of IVT administration can be circumvented with available opioids.

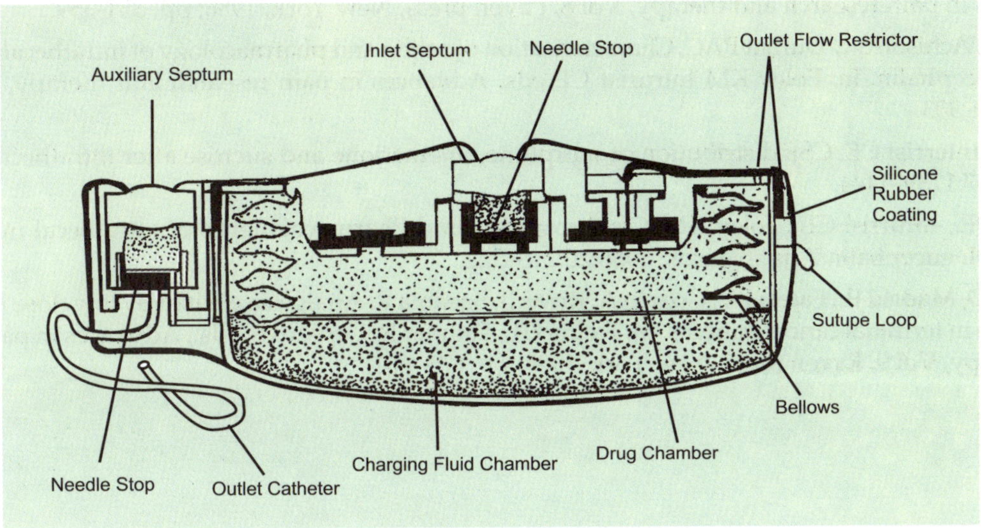

Fig. 13.4 : A schematic cross section of the model 400 Infusaid implantable drug delivery system[7]

REFERENCES

1. Beckett AH., Hossie RD. Buccal absorption of drugs. In: Brodie BB.,Gillette J.R, eds.Handbook of experimental pharmacology, vol 28, Springer-Verlag, New York, 1971; pp. 2–46.
2. Bullingham RES, McQuay HJ, Moore RA. Extradural and intrathecal narcotics. In: Atkinson RS, Hewer CL, eds., Recent advances in anaesthesia and analgesia, vol 14, Churchill Livingstone, New York, 1982; pp. 141–156.
3. Coombs, DW, Maurer LH, Saunders RL, Gaylor M. Outcomes and complications of continuous intraspinal narcotic analgesia for cancer control pain, J. Clin. Oncol, 1984; 1414–1420.
4. Cousins M.J., Mather L.E. Intrathecal and epidural administration of opioids, Anaesthesiology, 1984; 276-310.
5. Coyle N., Mauskop A., Maggard J., Foley K.M. Continuous subcutaneous infusions of opiates in cancer patients with pain, Oncol. Nur. For., 1986;53–57.
6. Foley KM The treatment of cancer pain, N. Engl. J. Med., 1985; 213:84–95.
7. Greenberg HS. Continuous spinal opioid infusion for intractable cancer pain. In: Foley KM, Inturrisi CE, eds., Advances in pain research and therapy, Vol 8, Paven press, New York, 1986; pp. 351-359.
8. Yaksh TL, Achison SR, Durant PAC, Characterisation of action and pharmacology of intrathecally administered DADL encephalin. In: Foley KM Intrurist CE eds. Advances in pain research and therapy, 8, Raven, New York, 1986;303.
9. Payna R, Interrisi CE. CSF distribution of morphine, methadone and sucrose after intrathecal injection. Life Sci 1986;37:1139–1144.
10. Moulin DE., Inturrisi CE., Foley KM. Cerebrospinal fluid Pharmacokinetics of intrathecal morphine sulfate and DADL encephalin Ann. Neurol., 1986;20:218–222.
11. Lobato RD, Madrid JL, Fatela LV, Gozalo A, Rivas JJ, Saeabia R. Analgesia elicited by low dose intraventricular morphine in terminal cancer patients. In: Fields HL, Dubner R, Cervero F, eds., Advances in pain and research and therapy, Vol 9, Raven press, New York, 1985; pp. 673–681.

•••

NON STEROIDAL ANTI-INFLAMMATORY DRUGS (NSAIDs)

14

For more than 100 years little was known about the mode of action of NSAIDs, the predominant group of drugs, used to reduce pain and inflammation. This group has been enlarged recently by the introduction of selective cyclooxygenase-2 compounds. Within last 50 years a coherent pharmacological picture has been created. The discovery of prostaglandins synthesis does not explain as to why aspirin and (acidic) NSAIDs exert anti-inflammatory and analgesic effects, while non-acidic pyhenazone and acetaminophen are analgesic only.[1] All acidic antiinflammatory are highly bound to plasma proteins with pK_a between 3.5–5.5. A high protein binding and an open endothelial layer of vasculature, there is a high concentration in the inflamed tissue, GIT, kidney and block the COX-2 locally. By contrast neutral pK_a value drugs like phenazone are evenly distributed throughout the body. These acidic NSAIDs cause acute side effects in GIT (ulcer), blood stream (inhibition of platelet aggregation), kidney, (fluid and K^+ retention) and respiratory mucosa (asthma) (Fig. 14.1).

Table 14.1 : Acidic NSAIDs (Brune and Lanz, 1985)[3]

Sub class	pK_a (protein) binding)	Time to peak plasma concentration	Elimination half-life	Single dose range (max. daily dose)
Low potency				
➢ Aspirin	3.5	-0.25 h	20 min	0.05–0.1 g (6 g)
➢ Salicylic acid	2.9	0.5–2 h	2.5–7 h	0.5–1 g (6 g)
➢ Ibuprofen	4.4	0.5–2 h	2–4 h	0.15–100 g (300 g)
High potency				
➢ Acetyl proprionic acids (ketoprofen, blurbiprofen)	4.2	0.5–2 h	1.1–4 h	15–100 mg (300 mg)
➢ Arylacetic acids (diclofenac)	4	0.5–24 h	1–2 h	25–75 mg (200 mg)
➢ Indomethacin, ketorolac	4.5	0.5–2 h	2.6–11.2 h	25–75 mg (200 mg)
➢ Oxicams	4.9	0.5–2 h	4–10 h	4–12 mg (16 mg)
Intermediate potency				
➢ Salicylates diflunisal	3.8	2–3 h	8–12 h	250–500 mg (1g)
➢ Arylproprionic acid	4.15	2–4 h	13–15 h	0.5–1 g (2 g)
➢ Arylacetic acids 6MNA	2.4	3–6 h	20–24 h	0.5–1 g (1.5 g)
Highpotency (slow elimination)				
➢ Oxicams	5.1	3–5 h	14–160 h	20–40 mg (initially 40 mg)
➢ Tenoxicam	5.0	3–5 h	25–175 h	20–40 mg

CYCLOOXYGENASES

In 1991 two different genes code for cyclooxygenases COX-1 and COX-2 were discovered, cloned, sequenced and characterised[4]. These enzymes form a hydrophobic groove or channel opening through the membrane, the substrate (arachidonic acid) or an inhibitor inserts into this groove. The COX-2 proteins display a larger channel than COX-1.[5]

Physiopathology of COX-1 and COX-2: The COX-1 isoenzyme is present in most tissues and produces prostaglandins. The COX-2 is an inducible isoenzyme, which acts in inflammatory cells (*e.g.*, macrophages and synoviocytes) after exposure to proinflammatory cytokines and is down regulated by glucocorticoids. In the kidney (macula densa) and other areas of the urogenital tract and in the CNS, COX-2 is significantly present, over in the absence of inflammation. Induction of COX-2 beyond base line levels in the peripheral nervous system and spinal cord is prominent in connection with inflammatory painful reactions. Both these enzymes are blocked by NSAIDs.

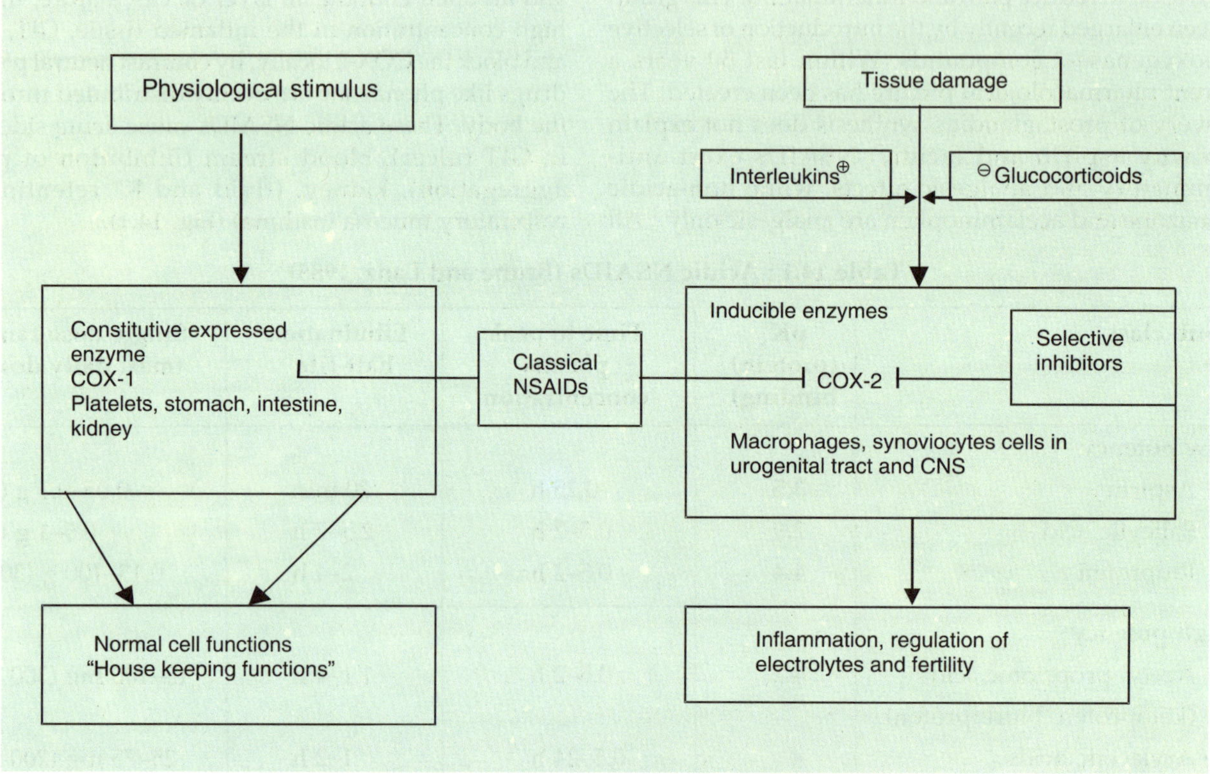

Fig. 14.1 : physio-pathogenesis of COX-1 and COX-2 (Kay Bruce)[6]

Table 14.2 : Indications for NSAIDs

Indications	High dose	Middle dose	Low dose
Acidic NSAIDs			
➤ Spondylitis, gout, arthritis	Diclofenac, indomethacin, piroxicam, ibuprofen	Diclofenac, indomethacin, piroxicam	No
➤ Cancer pain (bone)	Diclofenac, ibuprofen, piroxicam, indomethacin	Diclofenac, ibuprofen, piroxicam, indomethacin	Acetyl salicylic acid, ibuprofen
➤ Active arthrosis (inflammation)	No	Diclofenac, ibuprofen, piroxicam, indomethacin	Ibuprofen ketoprofen
➤ Myofascial pain	No	Diclofenac, ibuprofen, piroxicam, indomethacin	Ibuprofen ketoprofen
➤ Trauma (swelling)	No	Diclofenac, ibuprofen, piroxicam, indomethacin	Ibuprofen ketoprofen

➢ Post operative pain	No	Diclofenac, ibuprofen, piroxicam, indomethacin	Ibuprofen ketoprofen
Nonacid NSAIDs			
➢ Acute pain and fever	Coxibs	Pyrozolinones	Anilines
➢ Spastic pain (colic)	?	Yes	No
➢ Associated with fever	?	Yes	No
➢ Cancer pain	?	Yes	Yes
➢ Headache, migraine	Yes	Yes	Yes
➢ Associated viral infections	?	Yes	Yes

Nonacidic NSAIDs

Anilines

Most widely used drug of this group, acetaminophen (paracetamol) was discovered at the same time as aspirin. They are weak and possibly indirect inhibitor of cyclooxygenases. Specially at COX-2. upto 1g/kg/ b.w. doses, it has few side effects except liver toxicity. Acetaminophen is metabolized to toxic nucleophilic benzoquinones that bind to DNA and structural proteins in parenchymal cells in liver and kidney. Glutathione or N-acetyl cystine administration in early stages can prevent the liver necrosis. Indications are fever, mild pain in viral infections, recurrent headache and can be used in children. Acetaminophen can be used in combination with aspirin and caffeine but can cause nephropathy[8].

Phenazones (depyrone and propyphenazone)

Used as antipyretic and analgesics. They can lead to agranulocytosis. All antipyretics can cause Stevens-Johnson syndrome, Lyell's syndrome and shock reactions. All nonacid NSAIDs are devoid of GIT and renal toxicity.

Prostaglandins and Hyperalgesia

The analgesic action of NSAIDs is due to inhibition of the production of prostaglandins at the site of inflammation and in the CNS. Prostaglandins sensitize primary afferent nerve C-fibres and thereby activate the silent nociceptors causing primary hyperalgesia by targeting at the tetrodotoxin resistant Na^+ channels. A peripheral inflammation stimulates prostaglandin in the dorsal horn of spinal cord leading to secondary hyperalgesia and allodynia[9]. The prostaglandin interferes with glycinergic inhibition in the spinal cord.

Table 14.3 : Nonacid NSAIDs

Pharmacological subdivision	Plasma protein binding	Time to peak concentration	Elimination half-life	Single dose (daily dose)
Acetaminophen paracetamol	5–50%	0.5–1.5 hr	1.5–2.5 hr	0.5–1 g (1-6 g)
Phenazone (antipyrine)	<10%	0.5–2 hr	5–24 hr	0.5–2 g (1-6 g)
Propylphenazone	10%	0.5–1.5 hr	1–2.5 hr	0.5–2 g (1-6 g)
Metamizole (depyrone)	20–50%	1–2 hr	2–4 hr	0.5–2 g (1-6 g)
Selective COX inhibitors				
Celecoxib	>90%	2–4 hr	9–15 hr	40–200 mg (400 mg)
Rofecoxib	>80%	2–4 hr	12 hr	12–25 mg (25 mg)

Inhibition of COX-2 Activity by NSAIDs

The NSAIDs act at the COX active site which is at the end of a hydrophobic channel that runs from the membrane binding surface of the enzyme into the interior of the molecule.

- ➢ Aspirin irreversibly inactivates both COX-1 and -2 by acetylating an active site and thereby interfering with the binding of arachidonic acid in the active site.
- ➢ However, ibuprofen competes with arachidonic acid for COX active site.

While flurbiprofen and indomethacin cause a slow, time-dependent, reversible inhibition of COX-1 and -2 by formation of a salt bridge between carboxylate of the drug.

Clinical Use of Acidic NSAIDs

Acidic NSAID compounds (aspirin) at high doses (>3g/day) inhibits not only pain and fever but also inflammation *i.e.*, swelling, redness and warming. These compounds differ in their potency, with single doses ranging between a few mg (ornoxicam) to about 0.8 g (ibuprofen) and also differ in their pharmacokinetic characteristics (time to peak action and oral bioavailability). However, these drugs lack a relevant degree of COX-2 selectivity (inhibitors of COX-2 at concentrations that does not block COX-1. That is why these drugs are classified according to their potency and elimination of half-life.

Selective COX-2 Inhibitors

The slow absorption and elimination of Coxibs make them poor candidates for acute pain. However, they are effective for osteoarthritis and rheumatoid arthritis. Both of them show analgesic potency comparable to that of traditional NSAIDs.[9]

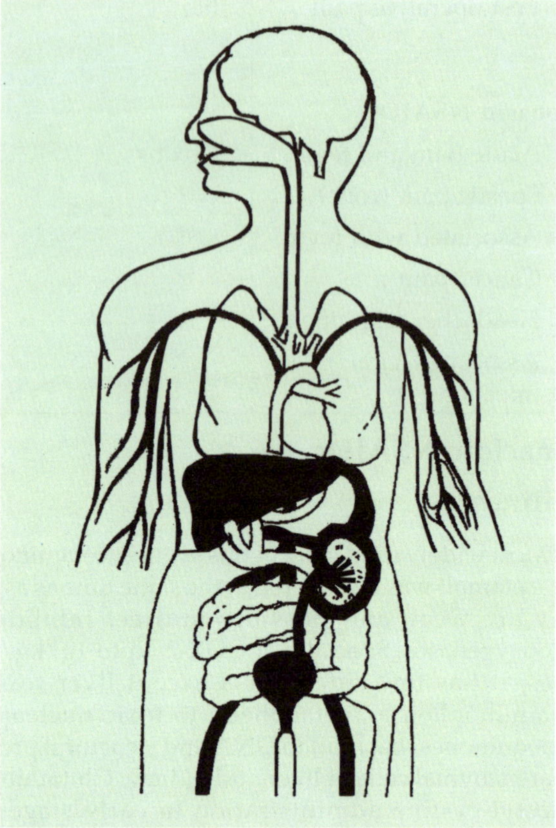

Fig. 14.2 : Distribution of acidic antipyretic analgesics in the human body (dark) areas shows increased concentrations)

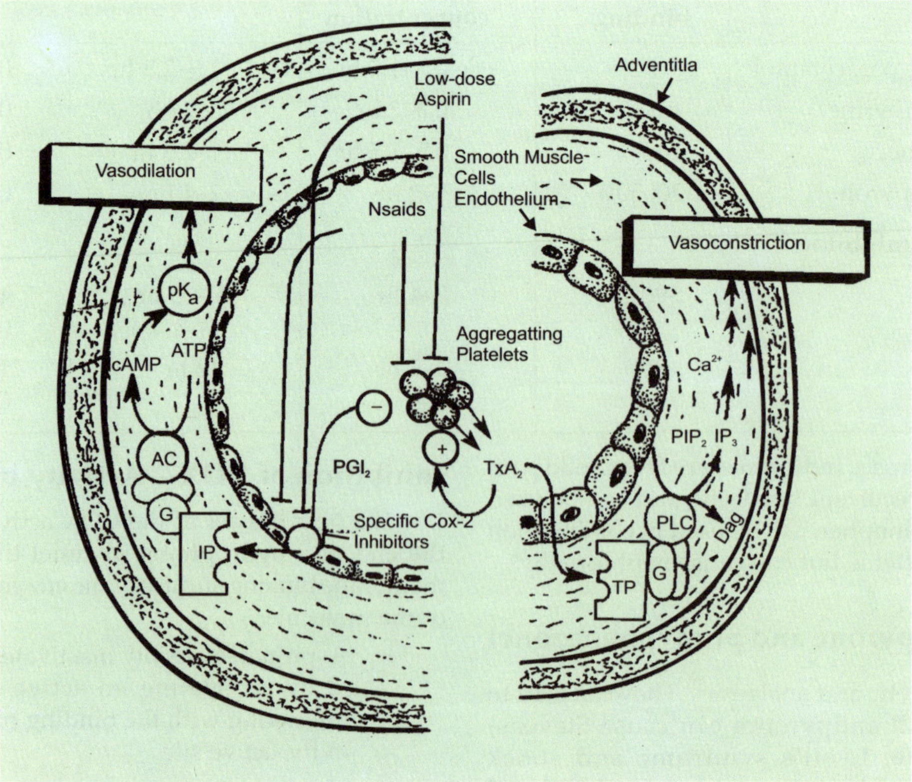

Fig. 14.3 : Regulation of periheral vascular tone by prostacyclins and thromboxane A2

COX-2 and GIT

Even in double clinical doses celecoxib and rofecoxib cause a significantly lower incidence of upper GIT due to the protective action of the prostaglandins secreted from COX-1. However, there is some dyspepsia with an incidence lower than that seen with NSAIDs, but higher than with placebo.[10] These drugs may influence ulcer healing by interfering with associated angiogenesis. The rofecoxib has been recently withdrawn from the Indian and US market due to GI actions.

COX-2 and Kidney Functions

COX-2 immunoreactivity was detected in renal vasculature, medullary interstitial cells and macula densa, whereas COX-1 was detected in the collecting ducts, loop of Henle and renal vasculature. This can offend renin-angiotensin system. Therefore, COX-2 inhibitors can cause peripheral oedema, hypertension and exacerbation of pre-existing hypertension by inhibiting salt and water excretion by kidney. The prostacylin reduction can lead to reduced Na^+ excretion comparable to other NSAIDs. So it is advisable to use them with caution in patients with fluid retention, hypertension and heart failure.

COX-2 and Cardiovascular System

COX-2 inhibitors can alter the thromboxane-prostacyclin balance by inhibiting the vasoprotective prostacyclin in endothelial cells. This can lead to hyper-coagulability. However, these complications are comparable to other NSAIDs. However, VIGOR study showed four fold increases in the incidence of myocardial infractions as compared to naproxen[11] in patients with rheumatoid arthritis.

So COX-2 inhibitors may provide a significantly improved risk benefit ratio in terms of GIT safety especially in old age patients and in patients receiving glucocorticoids and anticoagulants. However, available COX-2 inhibitors do not compare favourably with the old nonacidic antipyretic analgesics *e.g.*, acetaminophen and propylphenazines.

REFERENCES

1. Graf P, Glatt M, Brune K. Acidic nonsteroid anti-inflammatory drugs accumulating in inflammed tissue. Experientia, 1975;31:951–954.
2. Day RO, Francis H, Vial J, Geisslinger G, Williams KM. Naproxen concentrations in plasma and synovial fluid and effects on prostanoid concentrations. J. Rheumatol.1995; 22:2295–2303.
3. Brune K, Lanz R. Pharmacokinetics of non-steroidal anti-inflammatory drugs. In: Bonta II, Bray MA, Parnham MJ(eds). The pharmacology of inflammation, handbook of inflammation, Vol. 5. Amsterdam: Elsevier, 1985; p 413–449.
4. O. Banion MK, Sadowki HB, Ninn V, Young DA. A serum and glucocorticoids regulated 4-kilohase m-RNA encodes a cyclo-oxygenase related protein. J. Biol. Chem 1991;266:23261–23267.
5. Kurumball RG, Steven Sam, Gierse JK. Structural basis for the selective inhibition of cyclooxygenase – 2 by anti-inflammatory agents. Nature 1996;384:644–648.
6. Kaybrun E. Non opioid (antipyretic) analgesics. In; Pain 2002 an update review. Refresher course syllabus. Maria Adele, Ed. Giamberdiko, IASP press, Seattle, 2002; 365–379.
7. Samad TA, Moore KA, Sapirstein A. Interleukin 1 beta-medicated inductin of COX-2 in the CNS contributes to inflammatory pain hypersensitivity. Nature 2001;410:471–475.
8. Porter GA. Acetaminophen/ aspirin mixtures : experimental data Am. J. Kidney Dis. 1996; 28(supp):30–33.
9. Fitzgerald GA, Patroro C. The coxibs selective inhibitors of cyclooxygenases 2. N. Engl. J. Med 2001;345–346.
10. Langman MJ, Jensen DM, Watson DJ. Adverse upper gastrointestinal effects of rofecoxib compared with NSAIDs. JAMA, 1999;282:1929–1933.
11. Bombardier C, Laine L, Reicin A. Comparison of upper gastrointestinal toxicity of rofecoxib and naproxen in patients with rheumatoid arthritis. VIGOR study group. N. Engl J Med 2000;343:1520–1528.

•••

15

PSYCHOTROPIC DRUGS AS ANALGESICS

Both the non-psychiatrist and the psychiatrist can find it hard to disentangle the way in which psychotropic drugs promote pain.

The diagram, given below indicates how to begin with the causes of pain and recognize that the causes may be multiple, whilst the final experience is unitary. Pain is not to be understood as a psychological experience at one time and a physical experience at another. It always is just one experience. However, it can have many different causes grouped either as physical or psychological. Thus there is duality of causes, but monism of the final phenomenon. The final experience is always a psychological event.

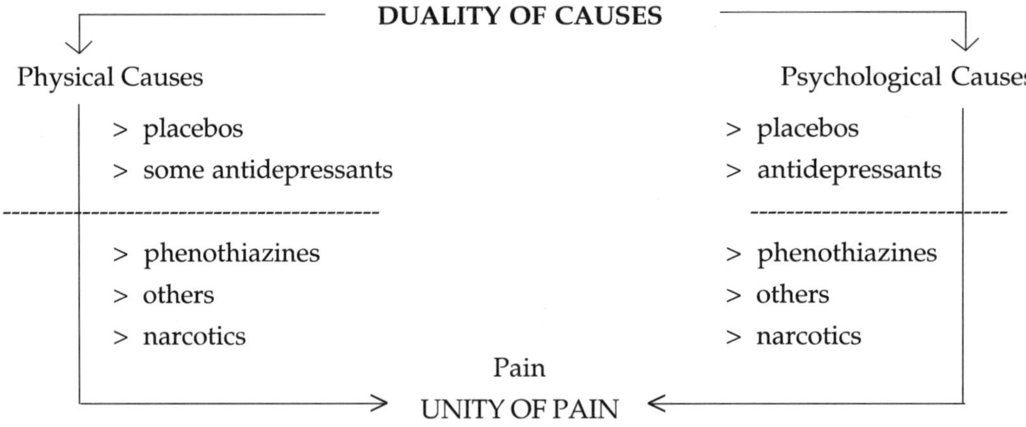

Many different drugs may affect physical causes or psychological causes of pain[1,2]. For example, pain even when it is due to lesions, may be relieved by placebos, perhaps sometimes more than when it is due to hypochondriasis. Some antidepressants relieve pain, of course by relieving depression, which produces it. But other antidepressants may relieve pain because they have analgesic effects, even when there is no depression.

A few patients have no organic cause which can be recognized for pain. At the same time they have pain and they are not depressed. That is to say, they do not meet the criteria for a sad mood, low spirits, and associated phenomena. Magni et al.[3] collected a group of patients who had such a pattern of pain and examined them systematically for other phenomena which are associated with depression like a family history of depressive spectrum disorders. They found that imipramine binding was reduced in patients with this pattern of illness in the same direction as patients with depression but not to the same extent. In an additional study these authors demonstrated that there was a response of the pain to antidepressants, particularly in those patients who had a reduced number of imipramine binding sites and who had a family history of depressive disorders[4]. This suggests that there are sometimes patients whose cerebral pathophysiology is such that they will respond to antidepressants, in the same way as patients with depression, but who lack the evidence of a depressed mood.

1. Deafferentation pain *e.g.*, Causalgia, phantom pain, and thalamic pain.
2. Pain from carcinoma.
3. Pain from major lesions *e.g.*, Rheumatoid arthritis or osteoarthritis.
4. Pain from minor lesions with concomitant psychological change.
5. Pain from musculoskeletal disturbances *e.g.*, Fibrositis syndrome or mechanical back pain.

Several drugs overlap in their functions. Carbamazepine is an anticonvulsant and was first used in neurology. It is now well and widely established for the relief of trigeminal neuralgia. For more than 20 years it has been suggested that it will ameliorate the mood, especially of epileptic patients, but more recently of others. It is now used to relieve manic-depressive illness and depression.

It prevents manic-depressive illness in some patients and perhaps depression as well and may even antidepressant.

It is a drug, which overlaps, in its neurological and psychiatric effects. It is commonly used for other pains besides trigeminal neuralgia. It should be considered particularly

1. There is recognizable nerve damage.
2. There are sharp or stabbing or jabbing pains.

Drug	First Use	Second Use
Carbamazepine	Epilepsy, trigeminal neuralgia	Manic-depressive illness
Lithium	Manic-depressive illness	Chronic cluster headache
Diazepam	Anxiety	Muscle relaxant

By contrast, lithium carbonate is used primarily in psychiatry and has been spread to neurology. Its first use is for manic-depressive illness. It is known that in relatively small doses it is helpful for a number of cases of chronic cluster headache. The latter is an organic disease probably related to sympathetic dysfunction.

Another drug used first in psychiatry and then on physical grounds is diazepam, which is used for anxiety and also for muscle relaxation. At present, clonazepam appears to be coming to the fore as a potential drug for the relief of pain. Formerly, it was mostly considered to be a benzodiazepine, which happened to be useful for epilepsy, myoclonic jerks and perhaps rare dystonic disorders.

Phenothiazines

Phenothiazines are widely used for pain[6]. The rationale for their use is that they have numerous central and peripheral effects including a local anaesthetic action in the laboratory.[7,8] There is also laboratory evidence of analgesia being induced by them. *e.g.*, in mice.

Possible Uses

They have been put forward or recommended for use with thalamic or central pain and other deafferentation pain *e.g.*, causalgia, neuralgias, neuropathy, and phantom pain, disc lesions. They are also potentially helpful with carcinoma. Sometimes they are used for pain, which causes insomnia, or for persistent troublesome pain for which no other control is available *e.g.*, cluster headache.

Evidence

The evidence in favour of the use of these drugs is limited. Intravenous methotrimeprazine has been shown to be comparable with morphine.[2] Two single dose trials of phenothiazines compared with narcotics, have shown them to be comparable with each other.[1,7] However, longer trials do not support case reports which have suggested the benefit of phenothiazines.

Disadvantages

These include the production of depression. This is perhaps a controversial statement, but anyone who has seen a patient control pain by raising the dose of methotrimeprazine, develop depression which was removed by an increased dose of antidepressant and then reduce both phenothiazines and antidepressant simultaneously without a recurrence of the depression, until the next time the phenothiazines was raised, is unlikely to feel that there is nothing in the statement. Further, a number of patients regularly complain of dysphoria or unpleasant subjective feelings when they are given phenothiazines. Thus many will not take them and it is unwise to persuade a patient to feel wretched one way in order to cure the wretchedness of pain with a given drug. If patients reject phenothiazines for pain because of dysphoria, never urge them further upon these drugs.

Sedation is both an advantage and a disadvantage of phenothiazines. Anticholinergic effects are common and well recognized and include hypotension, constipation and retention of urine. Tardive dyskinesia and parkinsonism are important side effects for which care must be taken. They lead to a simple precaution. If phenothiazines are used, monitor the patient regularly for tardive dyskinesia. Warn the relatives of the patient that this may emerge. Undertake liver function tests and blood dyscrasias occasionally.

Favoured phenothiazines

These are methotrimeprazine, fluphenazine, pericyazine and chlorpromazine.

Recommendation :

Try amitryptyline first. Use only phenothiazines with antidepressants.

Antidepressants

Antidepressants are probably the most widely used psychotropic medication for pain.

Rationale

1. Serotoninergic drugs promote antinociceptive effects via the peri aqueductal grey matter. They promote stimulation-produced analgesia. Many antidepressants are serotoninergic. Hence, it is often thought that serotoninergic antidepressants will be the most effective analgesics.
2. Tricyclic antidepressants and monoamine oxidase inhibitors potentiate opiate analgesia.
3. The mouse writhing test is positive for amytriptyline at least.

Objections

1. The rat hot plate tail flick test is negative for most or all antidepressants.
2. Non depressed patients did not respond in at least one trial to the use of amitriptyline.
3. Zimelidine is more serotoninergic than amitriptyline but less analgesic.[10]
4. Maprotiline is reportedly effective in tension, headache and is highly catecholinergic. But tension headache depends upon a psychological mechanism as well as a physical one.

Evidence

There are a number of adequate positive control trials of antidepressants compared with placebo in the treatment of organic conditions causing pain *e.g.*

Condition	Drug (No. of Trials) [1, 2]
Arthritis	Imipramine
Arthritis	Dibenzepin
Diabetic neuropathy	Amitriptyline
Diabetic neuropathy	Imipramine
Low back pain	Clomipramine
Migraine	Amitriptyline
Neoplasm	Imipramine
Post-herpetic neuralgia	Amitriptyline

The key test of antidepressants as an analgesic without depression being present was undertaken by Watson et al.[11] In this study using amitryptyline double blind vs. placebo, 24 patients with post-herpetic neuralgia were studied, of whom only one showed a worthwhile response to placebo, whilst 16 showed a good or excellent response to amitryptyline. The Beck depression inventory scores indicated that 14 out of the 23 patients were not depressed. 11 of these 14 had good to excellent pain relief. In the whole study, using amytryptiline and placebo, only 1 patient responded to placebo. The response to amitryptyline in the nondepressed patients compared with the placebo is significant at the level< 0.01.

Perhaps other antidepressants besides amitryptyline are analgesic, but the evidence has not been brought forward. Likely candidates include imipramine and perhaps doxepin. As already mentioned, zimelidine is not particularly analgesic. One controlled trial does support it, but did not distinguish well between depressed and nondepressed patients. Another trial, open and comparative between amitriptyline and zimelidine showed amitriptyline to be much better[10].

It is unlikely that the serotoninergic effects of amitriptyline account for its special antidepressant benefits, in relation to migraine, it is said that it may have some calcium channel blocking effects which might account for its analgesia, but this does not appear to be the favoured explanation in relation to other types of pain, such as post-herpetic neuralgia. Salter and Henry[9] have produced evidence that adenosine may be related to the modulation of pain. Their evidence is based on the fact that adenosine mediates the depression of spinal dorsal horn neurons, which is induced by the peripheral vibration in the cat. In other words, adenosine mediates the depression of spinal. It might be the case that the analgesic effect of antidepressants is related to some other feature than their serotoninergic characteristic, perhaps their adenosinergic than zimelidine. Dipyridamole is adenosinergic and some initial open observations suggest that it has analgesic qualities.

Disadvantages

They have numerous anticholinergic effects particularly in the case of the most effective one, amitryptyline. Weight gain is a problem as well as dry mouth, constipation and sometimes retention of urine, hypotension, cardiac arrhythmias and very rarely glaucoma. If antidepressants are combined with phenothiazines as is sometimes advantageous for the control of pain, these effects are increased.

Other Psychotropic Drugs

Benzodiazepines are sometimes used for pain. They relieve anxiety and may act upon the muscle contraction effect. An increasing role has been suggested for clonazepam. Narcotics of course also have psychotropic effects but are mainly considered to be analgesics.

Nonsteroidal antiinflammatory drugs may work psychologically but presumably only through a placebo action. The following table summarizes the relative strength of some of these effects.

Drug	Physical causes	Psychological causes
	Effects	
Placebo	+/–	+/–
Some or all antidepressants	+++	
Phenothiazines	+	+/–
Benzodiazepines	+	+
Lithium carbonate	+/–	+/–
Carbamazepine	++	+/–
Narcotics	++++	+
NSAIDs	++	+/–

Some or all antidepressants are highly effective as analgesics in certain circumstances. Narcotics are the most effective analgesics in physical circumstances but less so in psychiatric illness. Phenothiazines are of less use as a rule for pain from psychological causes than they are for pain from physical causes. For carbamazepine the same is true. Lithium carbonate is useful for very specific cases of either physical or psychological illness and the same may be true for benzodiazepines.

REFERENCES

1. Bloomfield S, Simard-Savoie S, Bernier J, Tetreault L. Comparative analgesic activity of lovomepromazine and morphine in patients with chronic pain, Can. Med. Assoc. J., 1964; 90: 1156–1159.
2. Lasagna RG, DeKornfeldt TJ. Methotrimeprazine: a new phenothiazine derivative with analgesic properties Am. Med. Assoc., 1961; 178-887–890.
3. Magni G, Andreoli F, Arduino C, et al. 3-H Imipramine binding sites are decreased in platelets of chronic pain patients Acta Psychiat. Scand.,1987.
4. Magni G, Andreoli F, Arduino C, et al. 3-H Imipramine binding sites in chronic pain patients treated with mianserin. Acta Psychiat. Scand,1987.
5. Melzack R, Wall PD. Pain mechanisms: a new theory, Science, 1965; 150: 971–979.
6. Monks R, Merskey H. Psychotropic drugs. In: Wall P.D. Melzack R, eds., Textbook of Pain, Churchill Livingstone, Edinburgh, 1984;526–637.
7. Montilla E, Fredrik WS, Cass LJ. Analgesic effect of methotrimeprazine and morphine, Arch. Intern. Med., 1963;111:91–94.
8. Ncordenbos W. Pain, Elseiver, Amsterdem, 1959.
9. Salter MW, Henry JL. Evidence that adenosine mediates the depression of spinal dorsal horn neurons induced by peripheral vibration in the cat, Neuroscience, 1987.
10. Watson CPN, Evans RJ. A comparative trial of amitryptyline and zimelidine in post herpetic neuralgia, Pain, 23, 1985; 387–394.
11. Watson CPN, Evans RJ, Reed K, Merskey H, Golsmith L, Warsh J. Amitryptyline versus placebo in post herpetic neuralgia. Neurology, 1982; 32:671–673.

•••

PSYCHIATRIC DRUGS AND MANAGEMENT OF CHRONIC PAIN

16

The role of psychiatry in management of patients with chronic pain can be divided into three major areas:

1. Psychiatric consultation.
2. Psychiatric liaison to a multidisciplinary team.
3. Psychiatric therapy per se.

Evaluation of Patients with Chronic Pain

Prior to working with patients with chronic pain, a comprehensive general medical evaluation, followed by pertinent subspeciality medical/surgical assessment is necessary. Many of the psychiatric diagnoses remain tentative until the contribution of organic pathologies are clarified.

Pain history

Regardless of the role assigned to a psychiatrist, the first order practice is to evaluate the patient by obtaining an accurate pain history. In most cases, the conclusions of the medical and surgical evaluation are expressed as being negative or as containing findings inadequate to explain the pain on an organic basis. However, this is not sufficient cause to justify the diagnosis of psychogenic pain. Positive findings are necessary for a psychiatric diagnosis.

To start with, a first-hand description of circumstances surrounding the onset of pain is important. Accumulated evidence of repeated negative examination, unsuccessful surgical procedures, or treatment failure increase the chances that now a psychological component is playing a significant role. In checking for associated complaints, vegetative symptoms of depression are most important. Their presence is notable even though the patient, who has chronic pain, typically attributes them to the discouragement of living with pain, and thus denies depression.

History of drug use is another important area. Drug dependency is usually well disguised, both from the physician and the patient. To clarify this issue, one must not be distracted by the relative need for medication, the seemingly unquestioned right of the patient with pain to whatever medication will help, or the opinion of previous physicians.

If the patient has a history of a chronic or recurrent medical problem in childhood, the response pattern may be repeated when problem with pain develops in adulthood. A variation of this theme is the existence of a parent or sibling who has chronic pain problems and perhaps serves a model for the patient's pattern of morbidity.

Complicating Factors

Socioeconomic Factors: In our culture, the individual who complains of pain is usually accorded respectful attention by family, friends, and employer — particularly if medical evaluation produces some diagnostic label for it. Being in pain may offer gratifications that even an adequately adjusted person find appealing; more so the deprived or stressed person or the one with psychological impairment.

Financial compensation is the most tangible reward of all. Many patients disavow and relationship between their pain and money; they profess a wish to return to work if the pain is removed, and this is seemingly their genuine, conscious intention. As a matter of fact, most chronic pain patients have an adequate work record before the onset of present illness, as they often emphasize. Nevertheless, potential financial reward and security profoundly increase attention to the painful area. Whether to work in the presence of distress or to accept a declared disabled state with steady financial reward is a difficult dilemma for anyone.

Legal factors: The contribution of legal factors overlaps with these economic issues. This is an area in which the physician finds it most difficult to function objectively and to assure that the patient's best interests are served.

When injury is done, the victim has a right to compensation. Deprivation of some bodily capabilities or impairment of well being generally entitles the patient to some sort of allowance from an adversary or from society in general. The means to obtain this is through the legal system; however, the adversary system promotes an emotion-laden interaction involving the patient. Under these circumstances, even the most independent and well motivated person becomes focused on his or her pain. Morbidity is often increased and effective treatment may have to be set aside until litigation is resolved.

Family issues: While pain is a sense of hurt, a subjective phenomenon is known only to the afflicted person, it does serve a communicative role between the patient and people around him, family members in particular. This pain communication does not always work to the patient's advantage. A high degree of mutuality is usually associated with the pain problem that has itself become important in the family dynamics. The pain complaint and reaction to it becomes a method of communicating concern, affection, demand and hostility. These issues necessitate that family members participate in the treatment of chronic pain.

Chemical dependency: The typical chronic pain patient is using two or three analgesic and /or sedative/ hypnotics, and sometimes alcohol. For this type of patient, chemical dependency is a major risk. About one-half of these patients abuse medications or are frankly dependent upon them. Polypharmacy is a typical pattern.

Naturally, the pain patient seeks pharmacologic relief; it is prompt, simple, and advocated by physicians. Unfortunately, chronic pain and its associated insomnia, tension, and fatigue do not respond satisfactorily to current analgesics and sedatives which are useful in managing acute pain. Soon the chronic pain is complicated by medication, side effects and psychologic and /or physical dependency. The psychologic presentation of patients with chronic pain typically involves the following drug effect: subtly impaired cognitive functions, drug-seeking behaviours, diminished motivation, social withdrawal, and amplification of pain.

Depression: The relationship between chronic pain and depression is of particular clinical importance. The reported incidence of depression in patients with chronic pain varies widely from 25% to 87%.[1,2] The causal relationship between chronic pain and depression is unclear. Is a pain a depressive symptom or is depression a result of chronic pain? Is there a shared mechanism involved? While the answer is unclear, the depressive component of chronic pain requires clinical attention which should include the consideration of an antidepressant.

Mental Behavioural Status Examination

The behavioural examination begins while the psychiatrist is taking the pain history (Table 16.1). The patient's description of the painful area and of changes he has seen, felt or heard, for which there are no significant objective findings, are good indications of central amplification factors.

Table 16.1 : Mental and Behavioural Status Examination

Pain Behaviour:

* ✶ Description of pain (quality, change)
* ✶ Verbal and non-verbal pain behaviour
* ✶ Subjective pain level (scale of 0–10)

Attitude:

* ✶ Distortion of medical opinion
* ✶ Distortion of past treatment
* ✶ Acceptance of psychiatric help

Nursing or Family Observations:

* ✶ Demand for continuous care
* ✶ Drug-seeking behaviour
* ✶ Conflicts with paramedical staff
* ✶ Rejection of encouragement and help
* ✶ Withdrawal

It is useful to have the patient estimate the severity of pain. This can be done on a 0–10 scale, 0 being no pain and 10 the maximum pain, one can imagine experiencing. This subjective estimation of the pain level by the patient allows comparison of the observed features of pain and a specific subjective determination by the patient.

The patient's understanding of other medical opinions should be examined. This often indicates unrealistic expectations, selective denial, or psychotic distortions. The individual's description of past treatment also may reveal fixed and unrealistic beliefs about "inadequate care." These patients are often chronically dissatisfied and do not respond to any treatment.

Working Diagnosis: Finally, a working diagnosis is in order. In practice, a complex mixture of structural-psychologic-social factor is the rule and it is difficult, if not impossible, to confirm the priority and aetiology of pain, *i.e.*, organic peripheral pathology v/s psychiatric disorder. DSM-III-Revised proposes changing the designation of psychogenic pain disorder to "idiopathic pain disorder" which does not imply psychological factors causing the pain, but rather that the pain stems from multiple factors.

A more practical designation is "chronic pain disorder" to which can be added further description, *e.g.*, including components of chronic radioculopathy, depression, central pain amplification, and medication dependency, etc. Of course, these components could also be listed as separate diagnoses.

Psychiatric Therapies / Management

Prior to considering management of chronic pain, every patient deserves consideration of curative treatment, such as surgery, anaesthetic block, electro stimulation, analgesic agents, acupuncture, or any psychiatric treatment modalities that might produce pain relief.

Electroconvulsive Therapy (ECT): Even though depressed patients are more analgesic than normal subject to experimental stimuli, pain is not an uncommon accompanying symptom of depression. Case reports of successful ECT in patients with chronic pain and suicidal depression or pain as a component of a delusional system have been documented. However, early relapse into pain and depression is common. Instances of chronic pain, the use of ECT can be justified only if the pain has delusional quality or is associated with other major psychiatric symptoms.

Psychotherapy: Before the advent of the concept of management of chronic pain, psychodynamic psychotherapy was the main psychiatric approach to patients with chronic pain. Unfortunately, theoretical reconstructions of the nature of chronic pain did not have direct impact on the treatment outcome in most cases; psychodynamic, psychotherapy of patients with chronic pain has been frustrating, at best for both parties concerned.

Time limited cognitive or supportive therapies, in the context of a multidisciplinary approach, or in combination with physical therapy and/or a trial of and maintenance on some medications, seem to be more productive. Supportive psychotherapy usually involves helping patients to clarify their problems, reviewing the options available to them occasionally giving advice and also supplying the type of concern and regard which boosts self-esteem. In contrast, cognitive therapy focuses upon cognitive strategies such as, attention focusing, imagery production, and thought management.

Apart from individual therapy, conjoint marital therapy, family therapy and group therapy also play a role in pain management. Conjoint therapy is almost always indicated in chronic illness, since there is often the development of dependence on the spouse, who may unwittingly reinforce the patient's invalidism.

Pharmacotherapy

Analgesics: Narcotic analgesics are treatment of choice for acute pain and progressive pain associated with malignancy. As noted previously, prolonged use of analgesics in general, narcotics in particular, produce more complications than therapeutic effects in the case of patients with chronic pain. Some researchers claim, however, a certain group of patients can be successfully maintained on a small dose of narcotic analgesics without developing dependency.

Anxiolytic: In clinical settings, anxiety is often associated with the acute pain accompanying MI, trauma, infection, and surgery. In such situations, minor tranquilizers are a useful adjunct to analgesics. This also applies to anxiety accompanying the pain of progressive disease such as cancer. In the case of patients with chronic pain, however, the use of anxiolytic is limited.

Antidepressants: Since chronic non progressive pain is often accompanied by depressive symptoms, a consideration of an antidepressant is often indicated. The mode of action is unclear. However, there are evidences that the Tricyclic antidepressants do have an analgesic function separate from their antidepressant effect. They also facilitate sleep and allow discontinuation of sedative hypnotics which may be contributing to the patient's morbidity. Most investigators report some response in patients with chronic pain to the antidepressants, with suggestion that those substances blocking serotonin uptake are preferable.

Tricyclic antidepressants and phenothiazines in combination are reportedly effective in chronic pain problems. Specific indications are in post-herpetic neuralgia, diabetic neuropathy, and in other central pain states involving deafferentation. Again, the mechanism is unclear and often the pain returns when the medication is stopped. Amitriptyline and fluphenazine are a combination often used.

Biofeedback and Self Regulation Techniques

Biofeedback techniques use instrumentation to provide the patient with information about changes in bodily functions of which the person is usually unaware. Self regulation techniques (*e.g.*, hypnosis, autogenic training and meditation) are used to help the patient control internal physiological states.

In pain states, anxiety and attention variables affect reported pain. It is possible to modify these factors with EMG and skin temperature, biofeedback training and through the use of relaxation techniques. In some patients, these adjuncts facilitate pain reduction and promote sleep. They are self-help techniques that encourage the patient in dealing with persistent pain.

Pain Management Programme

Comprehensive pain programmes have as their goals the intention to help the patient cope with pain more effectively, to reduce the intake of medication, to teach self-help methods and if possible to reduce nociceptive pain. A psychiatrist could be the director or a member of a multidisciplinary programme working in an outpatient setting.

In most psychologically oriented programmes, treatment consists of the following components: behaviour modification, physical rehabilitation, medication managements, education-cognitive therapies, group discussion, biofeedback-relaxation techniques, family member participation and supportive psychological treatment.

Usually the behaviour modification techniques are the most crucial components of such treatment programmes and require the most experience to have them applied in an affective way. Such techniques typically include:

1. Approaching pain behaviours, both physically and verbally, with a neutral response. In response to defined chronic pain complaints, the staff members say nothing, change the subject or leave the room briefly. Obviously, this approach must be carefully explained to the patient and his or her family before admission. Subtle, adversive responses, behaviours are pain-reinforcing.
2. Reinforcement of increased physical activity, independent functioning and social interaction.
3. Further reinforcement by graphing techniques of the patient's physical achievement.
4. Reinforcement of improved functioning by the patient's review of videotape.
5. Provision of pain related medications on an as-needed basis during the evaluation phase and fixed times thereafter. This eliminated the p.r.m. patient-staff interaction which is felt to be a pain reinforcer.[2] Administration of pain-related medications in a vehicle which makes the patient unaware of the dose. This again requires careful explanation of type of drugs to be used and the reduction schedule followed, emphasizing that prevention of physical complications is assured.

Such a treatment programme involves a multidisciplinary approach. Specialized psychological training must be provided to nurses, physical therapists, and occupational-vocational therapists. Physician's colleagues also require explanation to avoid misunderstanding about treatment goals.

Family participation is a vital part of the programme. The family needs to know what the patient has gone through and learn how to respond neutrally to pain behaviour with positive regard toward healthy behaviours.

REFERENCES

1. Kramlinger KG, et al. Are patients with chronic pain depressed? Am. J Psychiatry, (1983);140: 747–749.
2. Large RG. The psychiatrist and the chronic pain patient: 172 anecdotes, Pain, (1980); 9: 253–263.
3. Swanson DW. Results of behaviour modification in the treatment of chronic pain Psychosomatic Med.,(1979); 41:,55–61.

•••

ANTIEPILEPTIC AND MEMBRANE STABILISING DRUGS AS ANALGESICS

17

The capacity of the neuron to generate and conduct action potentials is the essential element that enables it to fulfill its role of transferring information. Drugs that have the capacity to interfere with impulse generation have the potentiality, therefore, to switch off excitable cells. If the drugs affected some neurons more than other neurons, then the possibility arises that certain specific circuits could be silenced. The excitability of the neuron resides in its sodium channels. These are discrete aqueous pores that span the membrane and exist in an open and closed state. At resting membrane potentials the sodium channel has a closed molecular configuration. When the membrane is progressively depolarized, an increasing number of sodium channels change from the closed resting form to an open active form. This voltage dependent increase in sodium conductance results in an inrush of sodium ions generating the depolarizing phase of the action potential. The action potential is terminated because the sodium channel can exist in the open state only for a short self limited period; it rapidly decays to a closed state *i.e.*, however, different from the closed resting state. The difference is that this closed form of the channel cannot be opened by depolarization of the membrane, it is effectively inactivated (Fig. 17.1). The inactivated form of the channel can be converted to the resting closed form. It is the proportion of sodium channel at the resting membrane potential that are in the inactivated or resting state that determines the excitability of the neuron.[1]

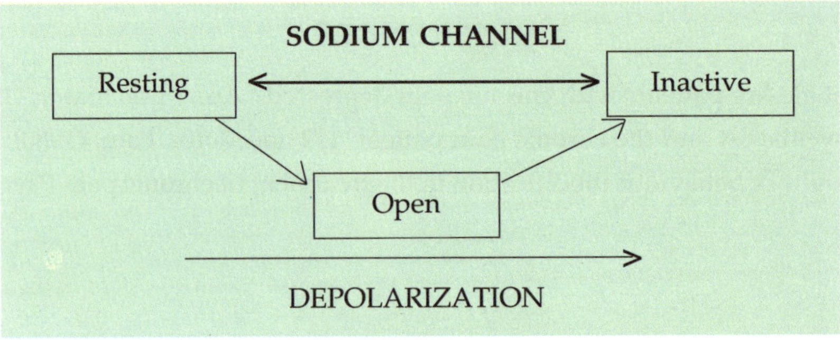

Fig. 17.1 : The sodium channel is a voltage-dependent protein that spans the neuronal membrane. At resting membrane potentials the channel is closed, but can be activated by depolarisation to the open form. The active form rapidly decays to a closed inactive form

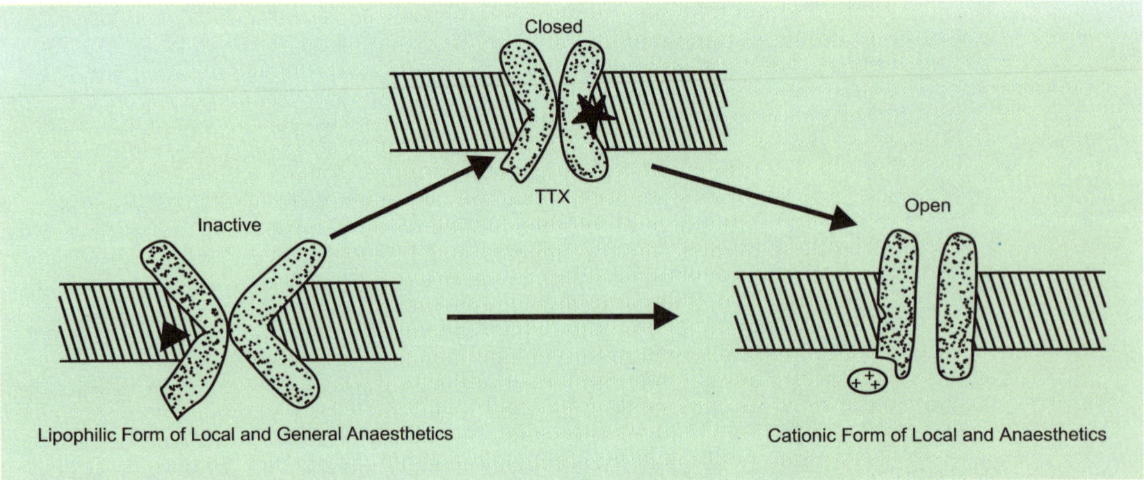

Fig 17.2 : A representation of the three different ways that drugs can interact with the sodium channel. Only membrane stabilising drugs such as lignocaine or procaine and antiepileptics, such as carbamazepine or diphenyl hydantoin interact with the receptor in a voltage-dependent way

Three classes of drugs have the capacity to interact with the sodium channel (Fig. 17.2). The first is that class of which tetrodotoxin TTX is the best example. This toxin, produced by the puffer fish, binds to sodium channels in a non-voltage dependent way and prevents the channel from opening. The second class is exemplified by the aromatic linked tertiary amines[2] and the antiepileptics diphenylhydantoin and carbamazepine.[3] These drugs, when they are in the cationic form appear to bind specifically in a classic manner to a voltage dependent receptor on the inner surface of the molecule that is only exposed when the membrane is depolarized. Having bound to the receptor, these drugs alter the distribution of the sodium channel, so that most of the channels are maintained in the inactive form. The third class of drugs are the uncharged or lipophillic form of the local anaesthetics and the general anaesthetics which interact with the sodium channel in a non-receptor mediated way to alter macroscopic permeability *i.e.*, membrane in inactive state.

Two factors could be involved in the antinociceptive or analgesic actions of membrane stabilizing drugs. The first relates to the concept of conduction safety and the second to use or frequency dependent block.

Conduction Safety

Under normal circumstances, depolarization activates sufficient sodium channels to generate more inward current than is required to produce a full overshooting action potential. The margin of safety is of the order of seven. Conduction will fail, if either the threshold rises high enough or the amplitude of the spike decreases, reducing the safety factor below 1. The conduction safety of the neuron is not distributed homogenously along its surface. Branch points, where impedance mismatches can occur, area of lower density of sodium channels, variations in transition kinetics, Schwann or glial cell influences, ionic concentration gradients, all can influence conduction safety. It is possible that certain neurons have a lower conduction safety than others and, therefore, would be more sensitive to membrane stabilizing drugs. If C primary afferent neurons were particularly sensitive, because for *e.g.*, of the small size of their terminal branches, then systemic administration of sodium channel blockers could produce a greater effect on these than on other neurons.

Frequency or Use Dependence

The major effect of membrane stabilizing drugs or the antiepileptic drugs diphenylhydantoin and carbamazepine is to bind to the sodium channel once it has been activated.

The interaction of these drugs with the channel is, therefore, voltage dependent. Consequently cells which fire at high frequencies with repetitive bursts or show sustained depolarization will be more susceptible to the actions of the drugs than those cells which fire infrequently. If certain particular types of afferent input produce a prolonged depolarization or elicit high frequency discharges, then this input would be more susceptible to blockade by the membrane stabilizing drugs than inputs that did not have these effects. C afferent fibres do have the capacity to produce prolonged depolarization of dorsal horn neurons. This may partly explain the more selective action of lignocaine or tocainide on C than on A afferent fibre evoked activity[4].

In clinical conditions, the membrane stabilizing drugs could be effective either on those sensory conditions resulting from C inputs or those conditions associated with abnormal paroxysmal activity in primary afferent or second order neurons, such as trigeminal neuralgia. Development of safe, effective sodium channel blocking drugs that can be administered orally would appear to be a priority for the future treatment of many intractable pain conditions.

REFERENCES

1. Strichartz GR. ed. Local anaesthetics. Handbook of experimental pharmacology. Vol. 81, Springer-Verlag, Berlin, 1987.
2. Wiesenfield-Hallin Z, Lindblom U. The effect of systemic tocainide, lidocaine and bupivacaine on nociception in the rat. Pain, 23, 1985;357–360.
3. Wilbur M. Pharmacology of diphenylhydantoin and carbamazepine action and voltage sensitive sodium channels, Trends Neurosci. April 1986;147–151.
4. Woolf CJ, Wiesenfield-Hallin Z. The systemic administration of local anaesthetics produces a selective depression of C afferent fibre evoked activity in the spinal cord, Pain, 1985; 23: 361–374.

•••

PAEDIATRIC ANALGESIC PHARMACOLOGY

18

Paediatric analgesic dosing guidelines are continually modified based on new clinical research information. Dosing guidelines are approximate and should be modified according to clinical conditions.

Acetaminophen

Acetaminophen (paracetamol) is now the most widely used analgesic for children in most countries. Overall, it shows excellent safety, even in infants.[1] Recent studies have concluded that: (*a*) Rectal dosing is relatively inefficient and delayed. Initial doses of 30-40 mg/kg in infants and children, and doses of 20 mg/kg in preterm neonates are safe and yield therapeutic concentrations. (*b*) Daily maximum oral or rectal dosing guidelines have been recommended in the following ranges: children, 90–100 mg/kg/day: infants, 80–90 mg/kg/day; term neonates, 60–75 mg/kg/day; preterm neonates > 32 weeks, 45–55 mg/kg/day. (c) Toxicity may be increased by fever, dehydration or concurrent hepatic impairment.

NSAIDs appear to increase the risk of bleeding following tonsillectomy in some studies, but not in others.[2] While it is difficult to identify controlled analgesic trials for NSAIDs in neonates several recent studies have examined the safety and effectiveness of ibuprofen, compared to the previous standard, indomethacin, for closure of a patent ductus arteriosus in preterm neonates. Preliminary evidence suggests that ibuprofen may offer a better safety profile, in terms of less detrimental effects on cerebral, renal and mesenteric blood flow and blood flow velocity.

COX-2 Inhibitors

An abstract of a pharmacokinetic trial of rofecoxib in 2–5 year old children was presented at the American College of Rheumatology in November 2001. This study recommended daily dosing of 0.6 mg/kg to achieve plasma concentrations similar to a 25 mg tablet in adults. Higher doses of 1 mg/kg/day may be appropriate for a full antiinflammatory effect in children. However, in view of its withdrawl from Indian market, it is not used now in children.

Opioids

Recent studies of opioids have predominantly been conducted in the perioperative setting, in intensive care, and in the management of cancer pain.

Infusions in Non-intubated Patients

Opioid infusions show generally good analgesia, relatively infrequent episodes of hypoventilation[3] and a high frequency of peripheral opioid side effects,[4] continuous electronic monitoring, especially oximetry is generally recommended for infusions in infants; this recommendation is especially strong for infants under 6 months of age. One study found no difference in stress responses between infants receiving intermittent morphine compared with those receiving continuous morphine infusion.[5]

Nurse- and Parent-controlled Analgesia [6]

Nurse-controlled analgesia is used widely at major paediatric centres worldwide, and appears to be generally safe and convenient as a method for titrated dosing of opioids in infants and younger children, or among children with developmental disabilities.

Parent-controlled analgesia is widely accepted in palliative care. Its use in opioid-naive children in the postoperative setting remains controversial. While many parents develop very sophisticated skills in pain assessment and an understanding of potential respiratory depressant effects of opioids, others may not, particularly if the hospital does not provide a formal programme for parent education. If parent-controlled analgesia is to be considered, education standards and patient monitoring standards must be regarded as necessary preconditions.

Table 18.1 : Oral dosing guidelines for commonly used non-opioids analgesia

Drugs	Dose (mg/kg) (<60 kg)	Dose (mg) (<60 kg)	Interval	Daily max Dose (mg/kg) (<60 kg)	Daily max Dose (mg/ (> 60 kg)
Acetaminophen	10–15	650–1000	4	100	4000
Ibuprofen	6–10	400–600	6	40	2400
Naproxen	5–6	250–375	12	24	1000
Aspirin	10–15	650–100	4	80	3600
Rofecoxib	0.6	25	24	0.6	50

Local anaesthetics and regional anesthesia and analgesia.

Several topical anaesthetics are in widespread use, including EMLA cream (Lidocaine and Prilocaine; Astra pharmaceuticals) and Ametop (tetracaine). EMLA has previously appeared more effective than placebo and less effective than dorsal penile block for newborn circumcision. Ropivacaine appears safe and effective for epidural infusions in infants and children. Adult humans and animal studies suggest that it may have a slightly greater therapeutic index compared to bupivacaine. Levo-bupivacaine may provide a similar increase in therapeutic index.[7]

Table 18.2 : Opioid analgesic initial dosage guidelines

Drug	Equianalgesic Doses		Usual Starting i.v. or s.c. Dose and Intervals		Parenteral Oral Dose Ratio	Usual Starting Oral Doses and Intervals	
	Parenteral	Oral	Child < 50 kg	Child >50 kg		Child <50 kg	Child >50 kg
Codeine	120 mg	200 mg	—	—	1:2	0.5–1 mg/kg every 3–4 h	30-60 mg every 3–4 h
Morphine	10 mg	30 mg (chronic) 60 mg (single dose) kg/h	Bolus: 0.1 mg/kg every 2–4 h; infusion : 0.03 mg/ 1.5 mg/h	Bolus: 5–8 mg every 2–4 h; infusion:	1:3 (chronic); 1:6 (single dose) release :	Immediate release : 0.3 mg/kg every 3–4 h; sustained release 20–35 kg; 10–15 mg every 8–12 h, 35–50kg; 15–30 mg every 8–12 h	Immediate release 15–20 mg every 3–4h; sustained 30–45 mg every 8–12h
Oxycodon	—	15–20 mg	—	—	—	0.1– 0.2 mg/ kg every 3–4 h	5–10 mg every 3–4 h
Metha-done	10 mg	10–20 mg	0.1 mg/ kg every 4–8 h	5 mg every 4–8 h	1:1–2	0.1–0.2 mg/ kg every 4–8 h	5–10 mg every 4–8 h
Fentanyl	100 µg (0.1 mg)	—	Bolus : 0.5–1 µg/kg every 1–2 h; infusion: 0.5–2 µg/kg/h	Bolus: 25–50 µg every 1–2 h; infusion: 25–100 µg/hr	—	—	—

Hydromorphone	1.5–2 mg	6–8 mg	Bolus : 0.02 mg every 2–4h; infusion: 0.006 mg/kg/h	Bolus: 1 mg every 2–4 h; infusion: 0.3 mg/h	1:4	0.04–0.08 mg/kg every 3–4 h	2–4 mg every 3–4 h
Meperidine (Pethidine)	75–100 mg	300 mg	Bolus : 0.8–1 mg/kg every 2–3 h	Bolus : 50–75 mg every 2–3 h	1:4	2–3 mg/kg every 3–4 h	100–150 mg every 3–4 h

Epidural infusions of local anaesthetics, particularly in combination with Clonidine or opioids can provide outstanding analgesia when employed in a setting of advanced expertise in both technical aspects and postoperative management. Epidural analgesia is labour intensive.

Anticonvulsants

Anticonvulsants are used widely for neuropathic pain in children. Gabapentin has become the most widely prescribed anticonvulsant, because of its apparent safety and efficacy profile compared with many of the older anticonvulsants. There are insufficient data at present (either based on adult use for pain or paediatric use for epilepsy) for recommending some of the newer anticonvulsants, such as topiramate,[8] pregabalin, or lamotrigine, for treatment of neuropathic pain in children.

Antidepressants

Antidepressants are also widely used for neuropathic pain in children, as well as for migraine prophylaxis and for treatment of sleep disturbances among patients with many forms of chronic pain as with adults, Selective Serotonin Uptake Inhibitors (SSUIs) have become more widely prescribed as first-line agents for mood disorders. Tricyclic are more commonly chosen for neuropathic pain, migraine prophylaxis, or enuresis, or as second line therapy for treatment of depression or attention-deficit hyperactivity disorder with hyperactivity.

A considerable number of paediatric analgesic safety and efficacy studies have been conducted in recent years. There is a need for further improvements in study design, and for better methods of assessing a variety of outcomes, including non painful symptoms and side effects. Multicentre efforts may facilitate studies of analgesics in the treatment of chronic pain in children.

REFERENCES

1. Lesko SM, Mitchell AA. The safety of acetaminophen and ibuprofen among children younger than two years old. *Paediatrics;* 1999;104:39.
2. Romsing J, Ostergard D, Drozdziewicz D, Schultz P, Ravn G. Diclofenac or acetaminophen for analgesia in paediatric tonsillectomy outpatients. Acta Anaesthesiol Scan 2000;44:291–295.
3. Lynn AM, Nespeca MK, Bratton SL, Shen DD. Intravenous morphine in postoperative infants: intermittent bolus dosing versus targeted continuous infusions. Pain 2000;88:89–95.
4. Esmail Z, Montgomery C, Courtrn C, Hamilton D, Kestle C. Efficacy and complications of morphine infusions in postoperative paediatric patients. Paediatr Anaesth 1998;8:145–148.
5. Bouwmeester NJ, Anand KJ, van Dijk M, et al. Hormonal and metabolic stress responses after major surgery in children aged 0-3 years: a doube-blind, randomized trial comparing the effects of continuous versus intermittent morphine. Br. J Anaesth 2001;87:390–399.
6. Monitto CL, Greenberg RS, Kost-Byerly S, et al. The safety and efficacy of parent-/nurse-controlled analgesia in patients less than six years of age. Anesth Analg 2000;91:573–579.
7. Kothane DS, Sankar WS, Shubina M, et al. Sciatic nerve blockade in infant, adolescent, and adult rats: a comparison of ropivacaine with bupivacaine. Anesthesiology 1998;89:1199–1208.
8. Gilron I, Booher SL, Rowan JS, Max MB. Topiramate in trigeminal neuralgia; a randomized placebo controlled multiple crossover pilot study. Clin Neuropharmacol 2001;245:109–112.

•••

SECTION–V

Cancer Pain

MAGNITUDE OF CANCER PAIN AND RELATED SYMPTOMS

19

Of the more than 9 million patients in the world, half of them occur in developing countries. As majority of these present in advanced stage, the only realistic options are pain and palliative care.

The cancer patient faces a wide range of psychological and physical problems. There is a fear of death, physical disability and dependence on others. But the most feared consequence of cancer, however, is pain. Moderate to severe pain is experienced by 30 to 60 % of cancer patients during active therapy and in 90% of patient with advanced disease. Pain is often a remainder of an impending death and has profound impact on the patient's emotions, mood and distress. Thus the cancer patients with pain are more likely to develop psychological disorders than those without pain.[1]

Pain also heightens the burden on the patient's family, in terms of financial difficulty due to the cost of patient's care and treatment. There are associated emotional burden and physical strain on the attending relatives. Similar problems are faced by staff nurses and physicians who face complex diagnostic and therapeutic challenges, inability to cope with treatment failures. Cancer patients need more nursing care with the aim of improving the quality of life of the patients.[2]

The management of associated problems like poor nutrition, problems related to urogenital, renal and CNS and CVS also need a multidisciplinary approach by a specialized team consisting of an oncologist, surgeons, psychiatrist, anaesthesiologist, radiotherapist and trained nurses. This has lead to specialized cancer wards in major hospitals. The challenges posed during terminal stage of cancer needs special care homes called hospices where care, rehabilitation and treatment are provided by a dedicated team. In spite of technological advances, made in last 50 years, the physician's attitude towards the cancer patient is of resignation, relegating him to doom. Most of the terminal patients are sent back home to die. The physicians and care givers lack knowledge of the pain and other related symptoms. The attitude of care givers should be changed from treatment of malignancy only, to the specialized care, rehabilitation and quality of life especially in the end stage. The non availability of morphine which is due to government restrictions is another hurdle in our country which incidentally is the highest producer of opium in the world. There is a baseless fear of addiction in the cancer patients which is basically a drug dependence and not drug abuse. The WHO and Indian Society for Study of Pain have been guiding the physicians and imparting technological know how with a little success. It is heartening to note that there are opening more and more pain clinic services at district level every year.

World Health Organization has documented following reasons for inadequate cancer pain control[2].

1. Absence of national policies on cancer pain relief and palliative care.
2. Lack of awareness on the part of health care providers, policy makers, administrators and the public that most cancer pain can be relieved.
3. Shortage of finances, limitation of health delivery systems and personnel.
4. Concern that medical use of opioids will produce psychological dependence and drug abuse.
5. Legal restrictions on the use and availability of opioids.

Following factors contribute to under treat-ment of cancer pain:

(A) **Patient related : Pain under-reporting**

1. Fear of disease progression.
2. Perceived lack of time or inadequate time spent with physician.
3. Poor compliance with prescribed medications.

(B) **Physician related**

1. Legal issues – opioid prescriptions.
2. Difficulty assessing pain complaints.
3. Lack of information, expertise on cancer pain management.
4. Desire to provide untried, latest pain management techniques.

This can be dealt with by :

1. Education of patients and health care providers.

2. Establishment of pain management practice/ programmes.

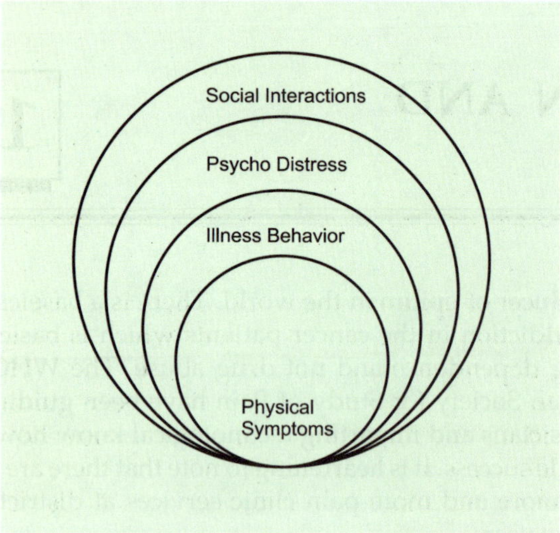

Fig. 19.1 : Biopsychosocial phenomenon

3. State cancer pain initiative, parallel to advanced cardiac life support and advanced trauma life support programmes.

Paradigm of Pain

A joint report of the College of Anaesthetists and The Royal College of Surgeons highlighted the need to treat acute pain. The acute pain later becomes chronic following tissue damage and which becomes a complex biopsychosocial phenomenon. The Fig. 19.1 shows an illustration of pain in cancer management[3] involving complex psychosocio-behavioural phenonenon.

The Fig. 19.2 shows the author's conception of the patient's suffering from pain. The centre of the diagram

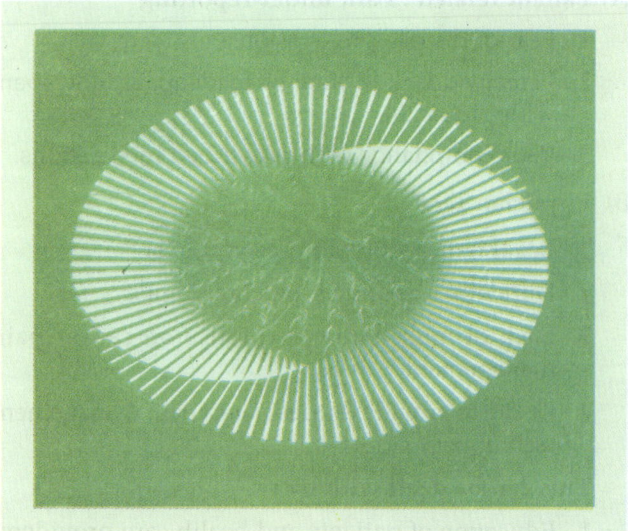

Fig. 19.2 : Whirlpool of pain

shows electric shock like sensation represented by electric ray fish sending electrical shocks, which in turn leads to somatic and psychological changes in the body and its surroundings as well, thus causing a whirlpool in the surrounding waters.[4]

Prevalence and Magnitude of Cancer Pain in India[5]

At any given time there are about 1.5 million people suffering from cancer in India. As cancer detection facilities are poor, most of the patients are already in an advanced stage of the disease and need palliation for cancer-related and other symptoms.

As accurate statistics are not available, it is difficult to say how many of these patients are having pain and the degree of severity of their pain. Based on figures from some more affluent developed nations it may be estimated that about 70% (1.05 million) of the victims of cancer are in pain at some stage or the other of their disease and require relief by effective intervention by pain clinicians.

Of the various possible interventions, neurolytic nerve blocks, continuous patient-controlled analgesic administering devices and use of skin patches of narcotic and other analgesic are beyond the reach of a majority of these patients, either because of the non-availability of experts or because of high costs.

Oral morphine and adjuvants, therefore, remains the only universally applicable intervention for relief of pain in these patients. All palliative care centres should ensure continued availability of oral morphine and adjuvant drugs.

There is almost a total lack of awareness amongst our people on how cancer presents and progresses. The facilities for early detection and so-called early curative interventions are also few and far between. As a matter of fact, medical facilities in general are still beyond the reach of the common man, both logistically and financially.

As a result of this, patients with cancer when they present for medical consultation have already reached a stage when their disease is beyond any curative intervention. Palliative care remains the only choice in these circumstances.

Pain: The Most Important Symptom in Cancer, Requiring Relief

As conscientious members of the society in general and as physicians serving the patients, we have to endeavour to chalk out plans for relief of pain, in not only in cancer patients, but also in patients with pain of other categories, whose number may run into millions at any given time.

Patients are suffering unnecessary pain, according to a survey in USA. More than three-quarters of patients questioned said, they had experienced pain as a result of drugs or surgery either for cancer or for other diseases.[5] However, fewer than half had been told to expect this by a caregiver, and only one in ten had been given any written material on techniques for pain control. Adequate pain relief is generally thought to be possible in nine out of ten cancer cases, but most patients were unaware of any methods of doing this including pain-relieving skin patches, and suppositories containing pain-relieving drugs, which could be within the reach of some of such patients.[5]

The Suffering Resulting from Pain

Pain is subjective and unpleasant feeling and results in psychological, behavioural, and even physical changes. Pain can be a destructive disease as well. Persistent pain, when the threat of injury has passed and the wound has healed, no longer serves its useful protective purpose. Persistent chronic pain can be as disruptive as the original injury with far reaching consequences that impact on every aspect of human existence. These physiological and psychosocial consequences result in decreased mobility, anger, depression (incidence 30–100%) disrupted family life, loss of earning power and significant cost to society.

This multidimensional nature of chronic pain entitles it to be considered as a disease entity in and of itself. Pain is a universal experience that a staggering number of people live with everyday. Estimates of the number of chronic pain sufferers vary and have grown significantly in the last ten years. In 1983, it was estimated that more than 75–80 million people in America alone suffered chronic pain. In 1966 more than 120 million Americans suffered from chronic pain. A few other current estimates from varying sources include arthritis pain – 16 million, low back pain – 19 million of which 11.7 million are impaired and 2.6 million are permanently disabled, headache – over three million, chronic neuralgia – eight million, cancer pain – 2.5 to 3 million, and post-herpetic neuralgia 28,000. Although estimates vary, it is obvious that pain is a very prevalent health problem in India also, in fact, it may be the greatest health care problem in India. A study in 1999 for the American Pain Society estimated that nine per cent of U.S. adult population are suffering from moderate to severe non-cancer related chronic pain.[2]

Categories of Pain

The three major categories of pain are:

1. Cancer pain.
2. Non-malignant pain.
3. Psychogenic pain.

Cancer patients may be classified into five groups :

1. Patients with acute cancer related pain.
2. Patients with chronic cancer related pain due to either progression or therapy.
3. Patients with pre-existing chronic benign non-malignant pain and cancer related pain.
4. Patients with chemical dependency history and cancer related pain.
5. Dying patient who must be provided comfort.

Problems of Managment

Management to be effective has to be preceded by an accurate assessment of the type and severity of pain and the impact of pain on the life of the pain sufferer. When the assessment is complete, ancillary testing performed, and a diagnosis is reached, a plan for managing the pain must be formed.

The treatement will depend on the aetiology of the pain. However, there are some basic principles for managing pain. The most important principle is that pain is a multidimensional problem that impacts all aspects of the patient. All of the physiologic effects of pain must be treated but equally important are the psychological, social, spiritual, and economic components. No practitioner is adequately prepared to manage all of the aspects. A multidisciplinary approach draws together specialists from many specialties to work collaboratively to develop and implement a treatment plan. An interdisciplinary team composed of pain practitioners, medical, nursing, rehabilitation and psychosocial specialists and clergy co-ordinated by a case manager has the best chance of improving the quality of the chronic pain sufferer's life. Not all patients will need all specialties but the programme can be tailored to meet each patient's needs. The goals are to identify and treat aetiologies that can be managed medically or surgically, provide physical, occupational and recreational rehabilitation to maximize the level of acitivity, identify and treat psychosocial problems and maladaptive behaviours, and give the patient the necessary education and tools to take control of the pain and his life.

Table 19.1 : Characteristics of pain[6]

1. Number of pains		
(*a*) Single site of pain	–	46
(*b*) Multiple sites of pain	–	68
2. Duration of worst pain		
(*a*) 1 month	–	46
(*b*) 1 - 3 months	–	31
(*c*) > 3 months	–	37
3. Intensity of pain		
(*a*) No pain	–	0
(*b*) Mild pain	–	4

(*c*) Moderate pain	–	38
(*d*) Severe pain	–	62
(*e*) Excruciating pain	–	10
4. Temporal pattern		
(*a*) Continuous	–	64
(*b*) Intermittent	–	48
5. Radiation of pain		
(*a*) Present	–	67
(*b*) Absent	–	47
6. Palliative factors		
(*a*) Lying down	–	2
(*b*) Rest	–	10
(*c*) Fomentation	–	8
(*d*) Others – Massage rubefacient	–	1
7. Provoking factors		
(*a*) Eating food	–	48
(*b*) Coughing	–	25
(*c*) Ambulation	–	23
(*d*) Change of position	–	8

Table 19.2. Distressing and annoying symptoms other than pain[6]

1. General symptoms		
(*a*) Fatigue	–	86
(*b*) Fever	–	20
(*c*) Breathlessness	–	22
(*d*) Sleep disturbance	–	94
• Due to pain	–	84
• Due to anxiety	–	3
• Due to both	–	9
2. GI symptoms		
(*a*) Hiccups	–	3
(*b*) Fullness after meals	–	10
(*c*) Anorexia	–	35
(*d*) Nausea	–	16
(*e*) Vomiting	–	9
(*f*) Constipation	–	37

Table 19.3. Number of patients with various mechanisms and various causes of pain[5]

1. Mechanism of pain		
(*a*) Somatic nociceptive	–	23
(*b*) Visceral nociceptive	–	0
(*c*) Neuropathic	–	19
(*d*) Somatic and neuropathic	–	62
(*e*) Somatic and visceral	–	4
(*f*) Visceral and neuropathic	–	3
(*g*) Somatic,. visceral and neuropathic	–	3
2. Cause of Pain		
(*a*) Tumour related	–	97
(*b*) Treatment related	–	1
(*c*) Related to both (*a* and *b*)	–	14

Medical, surgical, and anaesthetic treatment will be diagnosis-specific. Pain can be managed medically with both non-opiate and opiate analgesics. Specific pain syndromes or aspects of pain may respond to antidepressants, antiolytics, anticonvulsants, hormones, psychoactive agents, cardiovascular agents, and radiopharmaceuticals to name a few. Transcutaneous electrical stimulation may provide non-pharmacological pain control. Surgical procedures may correct a pain producing aetiology, correct a complication of chronic pain, or may be aimed at interrupting a nerve pathway. Anaesthetic nerve blocks can help diagnose or treat pain. Implantation of local anaesthetics or opiates via drug implants have been used in the west. Spinal cord stimulators that can control pain without drugs may be appropriate for some patients.

Rehabilitation is aimed at improving the patient's overall level of function. Physical medicine may be specifically indicated for some pain syndromes, but all chronic pain patients can benefit. Chronic pain patients tend to be deconditioned from restricted activity. Physical medicine (Physiotherapy) can improve strength, flexibility, and cardiovascular condition. Occupational therapy can help get the patient back to work, either in the home or in a paying job, improving the sense of self-esteem and easing finanical strain.

Recreational therapy improves physical and mental well-being and helps the patient develop activities that divert attention away from pain. The psychosocial team is a very important component of pain management. Psychological testing can help diagnose pain and its effects. It can then help the patient deal with anxiety, anger, depression, and stress associated with chronic pain. Behaviour modification techniques are crucial to gaining control and keeping control of chronic pain. Patients can be taught self relaxation, guided imagery, distraction, and biofeedback to gain control of pain. Since chronic pain impacts the family as well as the patient, attention to family can be provided. Social services can help the patient take full advantage of resources available in the community.

Nurses are often the health care professionals that spend the most time with the patients. They are an invaluable resource for assessing pain and implementing therapy. **Nurses may act as case managers or patient advocates.** Clinical specialists and nurse practitioners may provide services in many disciplines.

Poor diet and weight gain or loss may often be side effects of chronic pain or its treatment. Opiates may suppress appetite and cause constipation. The inactivity resulting from pain contributes to obesity. A dietician can work with patients to correct these problems.

Alternative therapies can be useful for some patients. Yoga, acupuncture, massage therapy, chiropractic treatment, therapeutic touch, and meditation, to name a few have all been found to help some patients and should be utilized.[1]

Team Leadership

With multiple disciplines involved, good communication, integration, and co-ordination are of paramount importance to good management. One person, usually the pain specialist, should act as the team leader. The leader brings the specialities together to formulate a management plan and then on a regular basis as indicated to evaluate and reformulate the management plan. The leader facilitates communication between specialists and assures that treatment progress according to the plan. The leader is the patient's primary contact for questions, concerns, and problems.

Conclusions

Cancer pain is an unsolved problem in India. The number of patients is overwhelming. The available resources are limited and there is hardly any awareness on the part of patients of their right to seek and obtain relief from pain. The physician owes it to the millions of victims of pain to evolve ways and means for an effective pain relief in the cancer patients.

REFERENCES

1. Firzgbon DR and Chapman. Cancer pain In: Bonica's Management of Pain, Loeser (Ed), Lippincott Williams and Wilkins, Philadelphia, 2001;623–703.
2. World Health Organization. Cancer pain relief and palliative care. Technical report series, 804, Geneva, Switzerland, 1990.
3. Aitkenhead AR, Rowtham DJ and Smith G. Textbook of Anaesthesia. 5th Ed. Churchill-Livingstone, Edinburgh;2000.
4. Kumar P. Souveneir (cover page) Proceedings of XVII National ISSPCON, Jamnagar;2002.
5. K.Pandey. Prevalence and magnitude of cancer pain.Proceedings of XVII ISSPCON, Jamnagar; 2002.
6. Joad AK, Gupta P. Pain profile in patients of advanced Head and neck cancer seen at a pain a clinic at Jaipur. INDPAIN, 2001;15(2):18–27.

•••

20

MANAGEMENT OF CANCER PAIN

Three Dimentions of Cancer Pain

Pain is an unpleasant sensory and emotional experience associated with actual or potential tissue damage or described in terms of such damage.[1] There are three components or dimentions of pain on the basis of physiology.

1. **Sensory :** Tumour associated pain including a nociceptive, somatic or visceral or neuropathic.

   Somatic pain is further subdivided into (*a*) well localized **cutaneous**, (*b*) diffused dull **deep tissue** pain and (*c*) a sickening **visceral pain**. The **neuropathic component** arises due to tumour compression and invasion of nerves. This pain is associated with loss of motor and sensory functions and is characterized as a burning pain *e.g.,* brachial and lumbosacral plexus.

   The somatic pain can be treated by analgesics and neurosurgical techniques, while neuropathic pain responds to these partly, making pain management in some patients very difficult.

2. **Emotions and suffering :** A sustained nociception and other problems lead to suffering due to negative emotional arousal and elicit associated stress responses.

   There is a perceived threat to the self, leading to perceived helplessness in the face of threat and exhaustion of psychological and personal resources for coping with that threat[2]. This suffering is different from pain by affecting ability to cope, depletion of physical, psychological and social resources.

3. **Psychological factors :** Psychological factors enhance pain severity. Thus the relation between pain severity and disease pathology is not in a linear fashion. The cancer related pain has higher level of perceived disability and fear responses, reducing their activity and leading to hopelessness and depression.

Consequences of Pain and Depression in Cancer Patients

1. Suffering : significant contribution in major organic disease.
2. Medical evaluation and disease can be complicated.
3. Outcome and severity are adversely affected.
4. Recovery and compliance is delayed.
5. Suicidal tendency due to undetected depression.
6. Pain when poorly managed leads to reactive depression in life threatening disease.

Approach to the Patient

1. Knowledge of the temporal aspects of pain – Acute, chronic or incidental.
2. Understanding of the physiological mechanism – Somatic, visceral and neuropathic.
3. Identifying the types of patients with pain.
4. Diagnosis of cancer pain syndrome.

Assessment Approach in Cancer Pain Management[1]

1. Believe the patient's complaint of pain.
2. Take a careful history of pain complaint.
3. Assess the characteristics, site, pattern, aggravating and relieving factors of pain.
4. Clarify the temporal aspects of pain, acute, sub–acute, chronic, and intermittent.
5. Assess type of patient – Psychological state and degree of suffering.
6. Careful medical and neurological examination and monitoring.
7. Performing and reviewing the diagnostic procedures, knowledge of their limitations.
8. Evaluation of extent of disease – Site, metastasis, stages periodically.

9. Defining and treating specific pain syndromes.
10. Treat the pain to facilitate necessary work up.
11. Provide continuity of care from evaluation to treatment to ensure patient's compliance and to reduce anxiety, using single prescribers.
12. Individualize the management approach to the needs of the patient.
13. Informed consent explaining the risks of treatment including opioids, neurolysis, etc.

Pain Management Options

1. WHO 3 – Step ladder for pain relief is the most commonly used method of starting simple analgesics at first, than switching over to opioids and adjuvant in moderate pain.
2. The severe pain needs neurosurgical interventions *e.g.*, Patient Controlled Analgesia (PCA).

   The PCA offers patients a sense of control over their pain and is preferred over by most patients as compared to intermittent injections.
3. Spinal analgesia using epidural opioid or analgesic adjuvant, injected intermittently or infused continuous through a catheter or implantable infusion pump device.
4. Intermittent continuous local neural blockade *e.g.*, intercostal, deep cervical, stellate, intrapleural, brachial and peripheral nerve blocks using analgesic adjuvants or neurolytics.
5. Physical agents *e.g.*, massage application of hot or cold, TENS and others.
6. Cognitive behavioural interventions *e.g.*, relaxation, distraction biofeedback pain imagery. These methods reduce pain and anxiety, but do not substitute pharmacological management.

Table 20.1 : Pain-relieving modalities for localized malignancy pain

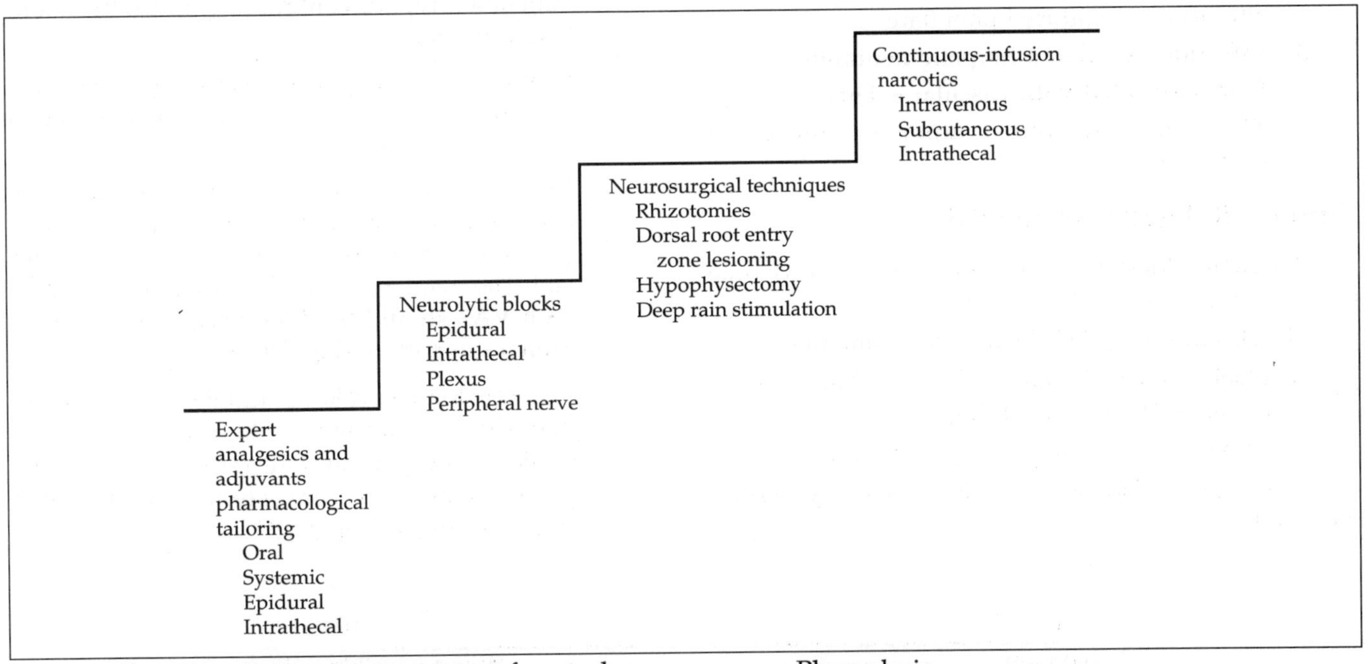

Pain Syndromes in Cancer

Acute pain is related to diagnostic and therapeutic interventions, while chronic pain is caused by direct tumour infiltration.[2]

1. **Acute pain associated with diagnostic interventions:**

   Lumbar puncture headache

   Transthorasic needle biopsy

   Arterial and venous blood sampling

   Bone marrow biopsy, percutaneous biopsy

   Colonoscopy

   Myelography

   Thoracocentesis.
2. **Acute post-operative pain** after

   Myelography

   Pleurodesis

   Tumour embolisation

   Suprapubic catheterization

   Intercostal catheter

   Nephrostomy insertion.
3. **Acute pain associated with analgesic technique:**

   Local anaesthetic infiltration

   Opioid injections

   Opioid headache

   Spinal opioid hyperalgesia syndrome

   Strontium – 89 induced pain flare.
4. **Pain associated with chemotherapy:**

   Intravenous infusion pain due to venospasm, phlebitis

Hepatic artery infusion, intrathecal methotrexate meningitis

Intraperitoneal chemotherapy pain, Bone pain, colony induced chest, palmer, gynaecomastia, digital ischaemia pain, mucositis, perineal discomfort, peripheral neuropathy, joint pain.

5. **Pain associated with hormonal therapy:**

   Leutinising hormone releasing factor tumour flares in prostate cancer

   Hormone induced pain flare in breast cancer.

6. **Immunotherapy:** Interferon-induced acute pain.
7. **Radiotherapy induced pain:**

   Incident pains associated with positioning

   Oesophageal mucositis

   Acute radiation enteritis and proctocolitis

   Early onset brachial plexopathy

   Radiation myelopathy

   Strontium-89 induced pain flare.

8. **Infection associated herpetic neuralgia.**
9. **Pain associated with vascular events:**

   Thrombosis in limbs, superior vena caval obstruction.

Tumour Related Chronic Pain

Bone pain – Metastasis, marrow expansion, vertebrae C_7-T_1, T_{12}-L_1, sacrum, joints.

Muscle cramps and skeletal muscle tumours.

Headache and facial pain – Intracerebral, base of skull metastasis, IX nerve neuralgia.

Ear and eye syndromes – Otalgia, eye pain.

Peripheral nervous system – Radioculopathy, herpes, plexopathy.

Cancer Therapy Associated Chronic Pain

Post chemotherapy – Peripheral neuropathy, avascular necrosis of femur and humerus.

Post surgical – After mastectomy, radical neck dissection, thoracotomy, phantom stump pain, pelvic floor myalgia and frozen shoulder.

Chronic Post Radiation Pain

Plexopathy – Brachial, lumbosacral, peripheral nerve tumour induced by radiation.

Chronic radiation myelopathies.

Chronic radiation induced enteritis and proctitis.

Burning perineum, bone necrosis.

Pain Intensity Scores[1]

1. Patient self-reports continuously in adults should take precedence.
2. Simple descriptive pain intensity scale of no pain, mild, moderate and severe, worst possible (verbal descriptor scale).
3. Visual analogue scale – A graphic rating scale using a ten centimetre base–line with no pain at one end (0) to worst possible pain on the other end. The frequency and evaluation of self-report with VAS should be done in any new pain or changes in pattern (Fig. 20.1).
4. Numeric Rating Scale – A number is assigned to intensity of pain on a scale of 0 to 10; with 0 reflecting no pain and 10 reflecting the worst possible pain. This score is easy to work with in clinical settings. (Fig. 20.2)

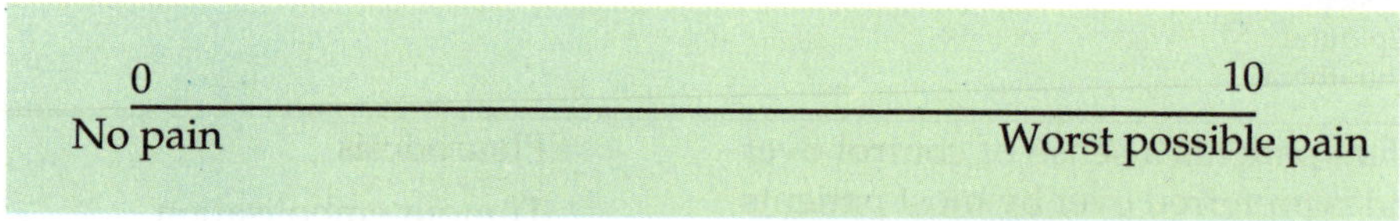

Fig. 20.1 : Visual Analogue Scale (VAS)

Visceral pain – Hepatic, retroperitoneal, intestinal obstruction, peritoneal.

Perineal pelvic floor neuralgia – Adrenal, ureteric, ovarian and lung cancer pain.

Tumour related gynaecomastia.

Radiological Investigations

1. Plain film radiography *e.g.*, for breast cancer and skeletal metastasis, in later scintigraphy, bone scan with tracer isotope may be better with SPECT.

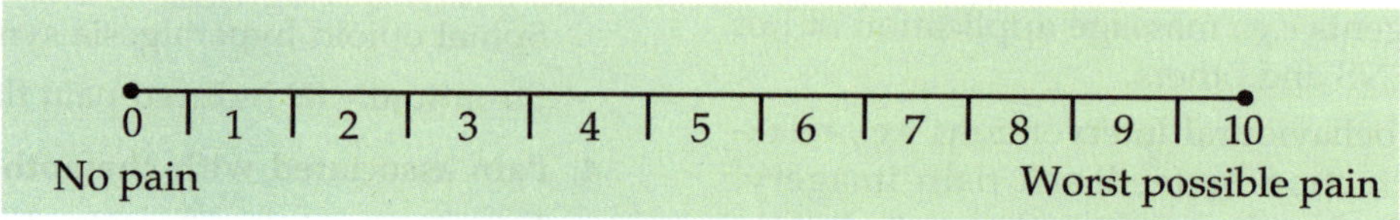

Fig. 20.2 : Numeric Rating Scale

2. CT scan–more sensitive for detection of destructive bone lesions.
3. MRI – is highly sensitive to skeletal metastasis especially in bone marrow, MRI differentiates between traumatic and pathological compressions and delineates the whole spine.
4. FDG - PET scanning is an area of current research.

REFERENCES

1. American Society of Anaesthesiologist's Task force on pain management. Cancer pain section. Anaesthesiology. 1996;84:1243–1257.

2. Wall PD and Melzack R. Textbook of pain. 5th edition. Churchill-Livingstone, Edinburgh, 2001;1018–1019.

•••

21

TREATMENT OF CANCER PAIN

Pain is not a simple sensation, but a complex physiological and emotional experience. The many reasons for failure to relieve pain have been well described.

Table 21.1 : Consequences of untreated pain

Causes of failure to relieve pain	Consequences
Belief that pain is inevitable	Failure to treat
Inaccurate diagnosis of the cause	Inappropriate treatment
Lack of understanding of analgesics	Prescribing of inappropriate, Insufficient or infrequent analgesics
Unrealistic objectives	Dissatisfaction with treatment
Infrequent review	Rejection of treatment by patient
Insufficient attention to mood and morale	Lowered pain threshold

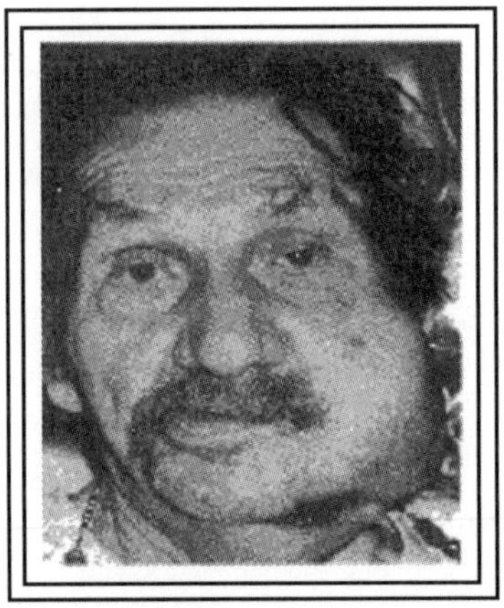

Fig. 21.1 : Facial expressions of patient with squamous cell carcinoma of mandible

Table 21.2 : Acute and chronic pain

Acute pain (*e.g.*, fracture)	**Chronic pain** (*e.g.*, cancer)
Patient : obviously in pain	May only seem depressed
Complains loudly of pain	May only complain of discomfort
Understands pain	Sees pain as unending and meaningless
Primarily affects the patients	Pain overflows to affect family
Doctor : Treatment straight forward.	Treatment may be complex
Parenteral analgesics acceptable	Oral analgesics preferable
Effects acceptable	Side effects unacceptable

Causes of Pain

Table 21.3 : Treatment of pain depending on cause

Cause of pain	First line treatment	Second line	To consider
Visceral: from involvement of abdominal, pelvic or intrathoracic organs	Analgesics	Steroids may help, if compression by tumour is implicated	Nerve blocks–celiac plexus for retroperitoneal pain, spinal for pelvic pain
Bone pain Direct spread or distant metastases	1. Palliative radiotherapy 2. Analgesics 3. NSAIDs	Immobilization (*e.g.*, orthopedic-pinning long bone) (NSAID)	Nerve blocks
Colic –constipation –obstruction	Clear lower bowel Faecal softeners Antispasmodics	Laxatives Analgesics	Enema Celiac plexus block
Soft tissue infiltration	1. Analgesics 2. NSAIDs	Steroids may be helpful	Nerve block
Nerve pain –compression –dysaesthetic –stabbing	Analgesics Amitriptyline Valproate Carbamazepine	Radiotherapy Steroids Nerve block Nerveblock	Nerve block transcutaneous nerve stimulation
Infection- deep –Superficial without cellulitis	Systemic antibiotics Local disinfectants with debridement	Analgesics Analgesics	Nerve block local surgery topical local anaesthetics
Pleural pain Lymphoedema	Antibiotics 1. Gentle massage 2. Exercises 3. Compression hosiery 4. Elevation	Intercostal block if localized, analgesic if extensive 1. Intermittent positive pressure bandaging 2. Analgesics	NSAIDs Steroids if due to recurrence Diuretics don't help
Headaches from raised intracranial pressure	Steroids	Analgesics	
Gastric –irritation –distension	Stop irritants Antacids Asilon	H_2 blockers, Metoclopramide, domperidone	
Rectal –tenesemoid	Chlorpromazine	Diazepam	Nerve block
Pain in paralyzed limbs	Physiotherapy, passive movements	NSAIDs	Muscle relaxants, nerve block

1. Visceral pain may result from hepatic metastasis, lung tumours, pancreatic carcinoma with retroperitoneal involvement and peritoneal involvement by tumour. Pain is often a continuous dull ache but may be interrupted by sharp pains, if an organ moves when the patient changes the position.
2. Bone pain may cause local tenderness, or dull ache worsened by movement. Increasing pain on movement with time suggests an impending fracture.
3. Nerve pain will usually be within the distribution of one or more nerves. Compression produced by variable qualities of pain, with or without motor and sensory changes. Nerves destruction may produce dysaesthetic (hypersensitivity, pins and needles, burning pain) or a stabbing pain.

Principles of Pain Control

1. DO NOT WAIT FOR A PATIENT TO COMPLAIN – ASK AND OBSERVE. Patients with chronic pain do not always look in pain. Clues lie in what drugs have failed. Whether sleep is disturbed and if the activity is limited. Some patients prefer to be asked about "discomfort" rather than "pain". The family's comments are often helpful.
2. ACCURATELY DIAGNOSE THE CAUSE OF PAIN. 80% of the patients have more than one site of pain, 34% have more than four separate pain.
3. USE REGULAR ANAESTHESIA, IN DOSES TITRATED TO EACH INDIVIDUAL SUCH THAT PAIN IS PREVENTED FROM RETURNING. If a drug is known to give effective relief for 4 hours, then it needs to be prescribed 4 hourly. CONTINUOUS PAIN WILL NOT BE CONTROLLED BY "AS REQUIRED" OR "PRN"PRESCRIBING.
4. SET REALISTIC GOALS. Initially a pain free. Full-night's sleep should be the aim, followed by relief during the day, freedom from pain on movement is more difficult to achieve in nerve compression and bone pain.
5. REASSESS REPEATEDLY AND REGULARLY. Accurate analgesic titration demands reassessment. This is an essential requirement for effective care.
6. EMPATHY, UNDERSTANDING, DIVERSION AND ELEVATION OF MOOD ARE ESSENTIAL ADJUNCTS TO ANALGESICS. Drugs are only part of overall management.

Table 21.4 : Analgesic classification

Non Opioids	Aspirin and others non-steroidal anti-inflammatory drugs Paracetamol
Opioids	
Opioids agonists	**Opioids Agonist/Antagonists**
1. Weak codeine dihydrocodeine dextropropoxyphene	**Weak** (pentazocine)
2. Strong morphine dextromoramide diamorphine (Pethidine) phenazocine (dipipanone) Oxycodone	**Strong** buprenorphine (meptazinol) (nalbuphine)

Table 21.5 : Comparison of Analgesics

Mild analgesic	Opiates
1. Less effective in large doses–ceiling	1. Dose related analgesia
2. Used orally– less effective, no dependence	2. IV., I.M, S.C., epidural, intrathecal
3. Used in chronic low grade pain in OPD	3. Used in acute pain
4. Diverse mechanism of action, treats cause	4. Opiate receptor, nonspecific
5. Fewer side effects – gastric	5. More side effects– n/v
6. Used in combination	6. Administered individually
7. Aspirin, NSAIDs, paracetamol	7. Morphine, buprenorphine, fentanyl

OPIOIDS – any chemical capable of stimulating opioid receptor.

1. Opiates – Analgesics derived from opium (*e.g.*, morphine).
2. Agonists – Analgesics with morphine like effects only.
3. Agonist/antagonists–Analgesics with effects similar to morphine but which may antagonize the effects of an agonist analgesic; if both are given together.

The Analgesic Staircase

Choosing an analgesic solely on the basis of pain severity often fails since clinical estimates of pain severity are highly subjective. A choice based on analgesic response tailors the analgesic to the patient, if pain fails to respond to a non opioid, then a weak opioid is the next step. If a weak opioid fails then a strong opioid is the next logical step.

1. Changing from one weak opioid to another will not achieve better pain control.

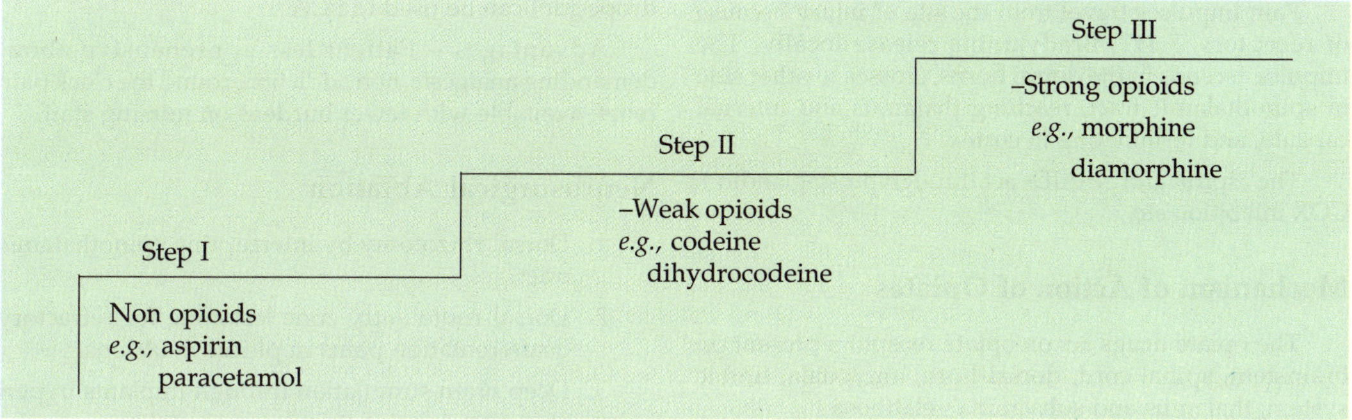

Fig. 21.2 : The analgesic staircase

4. Narcotics – Now obsolete as a term to describe strong opioids.
5. Analgesics in (brackets) in this classification are not recommended for routine use in cancer pain.

2. The decision to start a strong opioid is made by a logical series of decisions not as a last resort.
3. Patients with cancer do not automatically need strong opioids.

Table 21.6 : Stepwise use of NSAID analgesics in cancer pain

First step: THE NON OPIOID

Non Opioid Analgesics			
Drugs	**strength**	**dose**	**comments**
Aspirin	300 mg	300–600 mg	useful adjuncts in bone pain
Dispersible BP		4–6 hourly	gastric irritant
Paracetamol	500 mg	0.5–1 g 4 hourly	lack of gastrointestinal effects
Ibuprofen	400 mg	400 mg 4 hourly	gastritis
Diclofenac	50 mg	50–75 mg 8 hourly	gastritis, renal dysfunctions
Naproxen	250 mg	250–500 mg 8 hourly	gastritis, renal dysfunctions

Second step: THE WEAK OPIOIDS

Weak opioids			
Codeine phosphate			
Tablets BP	15/30/60 mg	15–60 mg	Approximately 1/12th as
Syrup BP	25 mg/mL	4 hourly	potent as morphine
Dihydrocodiene			Approximately 1/10th
Tablets	30 mg	30–60 mg	as potent as morphine
Elixir	10 mg/mL	4 hourly	
Dextropropoxyphene	Equivalent of	One capsule	Accumulation occurs,
Capsules BP	65 mg HCl salt	4–8 hourly	especially with poor renal function

Dextropropoxyphene and paracetamol (co-proxamol)	(32.5 mg) each tablet	2 tablets 4–8 hourly	Dose interval may have to be increased in the elderly

Third step: THE STRONG OPIOIDS

The strong opioids are often necessary to treat cancer pain adequately. They are not euphoriants or sedatives.

Mechanism of Pain

Pain impulses travel from the site of injury because of receptors, 5 HT, Bradykinins release locally. The impulse ascends in the dorsal horns, crosses to other side in spinothalamic tract, reaching thalamus and internal capsule, and terminating in cortex.

The aspirin and NSAIDs act through prostaglandin / COX inhibition etc.

Mechanism of Action of Opiates

The opiate drugs act on opiate receptors present on brainstem, spinal cord, dorsal horn, amygdala, limbic system, thalamus and substanitia gelatinosa.

Types of Opiate Receptors

The μ-receptors produce supraspinal analgesia, γ-produce dysphoria and κ-receptors produce spinal receptors analgesia and sedation. δ-receptors act selectively on leu encephalin. There are further subdivisions of above receptors depending upon the ligand blocking their action. This has lead to cloning of various receptor types with the aim to produce an ideal opiate without any side effects.

Endogenous Opioids

Body produces endogenous opioids like substance which control the nociception most of the times. This works in the pain relief due to various non-conventional methods. Can be released by stimulating the sites given below.

1. Endorphins – in hypothalamus, IIIrd ventricle
2. Leuenkephalin – brainstem and spinal cord
3. Metenkephalin – dorsal horn, morphine like.

The actions of all these can be reversed by naloxone.

Patient Controlled Analgesia (PCA)

Self administration of a small dose of analgesic drug according to patient's own experience of pain. PCA is available for I.V., epidural, or subcutaneous route. PCA is better liked by patients providing better satisfaction, relieving coughing and overall morbidity, as compared to I.M. route. A watch on instrument malfunction, careful planning of doses by physicians, loading a requisite dose of analgesic with a periodic review of pain, lockout interval and costs, are to be effectively worked out.

Opioids like morphine, fentanyl, and butorphanol alone or with additives like ketamine, ketorolac, droperidol can be used in PCA.

Advantages – Patient less apprehensive about demanding analgesic, non addiction, round the clock pain relief, available with fewer burdens on nursing staff.

Neurosurgical Ablation

1. Dorsal rhizotomy by interrupting spinothalamic tract.
2. Dorsal route entry zone lesioning for refractory deafferentation pains in plexus avulsions.
3. Deep brain stimulation through implants in peri aqueductal, peiventricular grey matter.
4. Cryo or thermal lesioning of gasserian ganglion and pituitary (75% success).

Dependence

PSYCHOLOGICAL DEPENDENCE IS NOT OBSERVED IN ADVANCED CANCER ON OPIOIDS[1]

Patients treated with infrequent or insufficient analgesics will ask for more, but this is not dependence, simply an appropriate demand for adequate pain relief. Physical dependence does occur, but clinical experience shows that when pain is relieved by other means such as nerve blocks, opioid dose can be reduced without precipitating withdrawal symptoms.

Tolerance

TOLERANCE TO OPIOID ANALGESIA IS SLOW TO DEVELOP. Tolerance to analgesia is easily matched by small dose increases. After three months a plateau is reached whereby effective analgesia can be maintained for long periods at fixed doses.[2] Respiratory tolerance is very rapid and respiratory depression is not a problem in patients on long time oral morphine.[3] The only exception is when pain (a stimulus to respiration) is suddenly relieved by other means (*e.g.*, a nerve block), when respiratory depression can occur, if the dose has not been reduced beforehand. Most patients on a fixed dose of opioids can be reassured that any residual drowsiness will disappear within 3–5 days. Tolerance to nausea and vomiting takes longer, but prophylactic antiemetics such as haloperidol can usually be stopped after 10 days. In contrast there is no observable tolerance to constipation and regular laxatives must be prescribed with opioids.

If the initial dose of opioid is low enough not to cause side effects, the dose can be increased until pain control is achieved, knowing that the patient is becoming tolerant to most of the side effects, but not to the analgesia.

Which opioid?

Oral morphine or diamorphine are the strong opioids of choice. They are of equal efficacy and there is no evidence that regular oral medication with one has any advantages over the other. This is not surprising since diamorphine is rapidly metabolized to 6-mono acetyl morphine and morphine[4].Their differing rates of absorption result in different potencies, but a higher potency does not implicate increased efficacy, simply less drug can be given to have the same effect.

Morphine sulfate is chemically stable in water and its shelf life is determined by microbial contamination. The addition of 0.25% v/v chloroform prevents microbial contamination upto 3 weeks. Sodium metabisulphate 200 ppm may be a more effective antimicrobial for long time[5].

Initial dose

Opioid requirements depend on previous analgesic requirements and age, weight, height and surface area correlate poorly with the amount of opioid needed. Patients with poor hepatic function appear to metabolize morphine normally and there is now some evidence that the kidney has an important role in eliminating opioids such as morphine.[6]

The initial dose should be chosen as follows:

1. Previously on non-opioid: Dihydrocodiene 30 mg 4 hourly.
2. Previously on weak opioid: 10 mg oral morphine 4 hourly.

3 mg **2 mg**

ORAL MORPHINE = ORAL DIAMORPHINE

3. Previously on strong opioids: equivalent dose of morphine. Calculate the 4 hourly doses and increase this by 50% if the patient was not pain controlled.

These rules can be safely followed for those with poor hepatic function. For the elderly, frail or those with poor renal function, these rules still apply but the doses may have to be increased more slowly.

Conversion to Controlled - release Morphine

60 mg diamorphine or morphine solution per 24 hours (*i.e.* 10 mg 4 hourly) is approximately equivalent to 60 mg controlled - release morphine per 24 hours (*i.e.* 30 mg –12 hours)

The last dose of morphine or diamorphine solution and the first dose of controlled-release morphine should be given together.

Controlled trials have shown formulation to be equivalent, mg for mg with oral morphine sulphate solution. However, two observational studies suggest that it was also

Table 21.7 : Oral strong opioids of choice

Drug	Typical starting dose	Equivalent doses of oral morphine	Dose interval	Comments
Morphine hydrochloride or sulphate solution	10 mg	10 mg	4 hourly	Titrate dose of the individual patient
Diamorphine hydrochloride –solution –tabs (10 mg)	7.5 mg	10 mg	4 hourly	Interchangeable with morphine as long as potency difference is taken into account
Controlled-released morphine sulphate (MST continuous) tabs	30 mg	See notes below	12 hourly	Effective over 12 hours. Unnecessary to prescribe more often than 8 hourly. Do not use for breakthrough pain, since it takes 4 hours before effective blood levels are reached. Do not crush or cut the tablets

equivalent, mg for mg, with diamorphine. This disparity may be due to the 22% greater bioavailability of controlled–release morphine compared with morphine sulphate solution. This would suggest that in practice patients can be transferred from either morphine or diamorphine solution with little or no adjustment of the controlled-release morphine needed.[2]

Night Time Doses

On a four-hourly regimen for oral morphine, it is possible to avoid giving in the middle of the night by increasing the bedtime dose by 50–100%. This gives sufficient analgesia over the following 8 hours; possibly reduced renal function overnight, keeps plasma morphine levels elevated. There is no evidence that higher bedtime doses increase night-time mortality in advanced cancer patients, even when these patients are receiving a hypnotic. Patients on more than 100 mg oral morphine for hourly are likely to need a 2 a.m. dose, although the reason for this is not clear. An alternative is then to transfer the patient completely to controlled-release morphine. There is no logic in using controlled-release morphine at night and four hourly morphine solution at daytime.

Dose Increases

Doses should be titrated to the patient's pain. Effective doses range from 5 mg or less of oral morphine 4-hourly to more than 500 mg 4-hourly. Recommended maximum dose has no relevance to the control of cancer pain.

Doses are increased in 30–50% steps. A typical sequence of increases of 4 hourly morphine sulphate solution would be 5 mg/10 mg/15 mg/20 mg/45 mg/ 60 mg/90 mg. For pain that needs rapid control two or more steps can be taken each day. Elderly patients or those with poor renal function may only need increases every 3–5 days because of morphine accumulation.

Table 21.8 : Approximate oral opioid equivalents

Opioid	Conversion factor to oral morphine	Opioid	Conversion factor to oral morphine
dextropropoxyphene	× 1/10	diamorphine	× 1.5
dihydrocodeine	× 1/10	dextromoramide	×2
		morphine Parenteral	×2
pethidine oral	× 1/8	diamorphine Parenteral	×3
dipipanone	× 1/2	phenazocine	×3
papaveratum	× 2/3	levorphanol	×5
oxycodone	× 1	hydromorphone	× 6
methadone	× 1	buprenorphine	× 50

Other Strong Opioids

Table 21.9 : Alternative opioids to morphine and diamorphine

Opioid	Typical starting dose	Equivalent dose of morphine	Route	Dose interval	Comments
Phenazocine 5 mg tablets	2.5 mg	7.5 mg	Oral sublingual	6–8 hourly	Possibly causes less nausea when given sublingually
Levorphanol 1.5 mg tablets	1.5 mg	7.5 mg	Oral	6–8 hourly	May be less well tolerated at higher doses
Dextromoramide 5/10 mg tablets 10 mg suppos.	5 mg	10 mg (po) 5 mg (pr)	Oral / sublingual / PR	3 hourly	Little evidence that it is effective for more than three hours in cancer pain

Pentazocine	20 mg	10 mg	I.M. /I.V.	4–6 hourly	Limited use in cancer
Butorphanol	2 mg, 0.5 mg	15 mg	I.M Epidural	6 hourly	Psychomimetic sedation
Buprenorphine	0.3 mg, 0.1 mg	10 mg	I.M. Epidural	6 hourly 6–20 hourly	Withdrawal symptoms

The following strong opioids have few or no advantages over those already described. They are discussed in alphabetical order:

Buprenorphine: Side effects are similar to morphine and although, it is said to have little action on bowel cancer patients. Buprenorphine require laxatives.[7] It is a partial agonist and shows a ceiling effect to analgesia. It has a high affinity for morphine receptors.

Dipipanone with cyclizine. Dose increases are limited due to sedation caused by the 30 mg cyclizine in each tablet.

Nefopam: A non opioid analgesic that can be given orally or sublingually. It appears to be approximately 1/3 as potent as oral morphine. There is a ceiling effect to analgesia. It may induce convulsions and should be avoided in the presence of cerebral metastases. It has no place in advanced cancer pain.

Pethidine: Its short duration of action of 2–3 hours makes it impractical for use in cancer pain.

Phenazocine: It commonly causes dysphoria and hallucinations.

Sublingual only: Buprenorphine.

Sublingual buccal or oral: dextromoramide, diamorphine, morphine nefopam, phenazocine.

The sublingual route is usually unacceptable in very ill patient with little saliva.

Rectal Route

This route may be the route of choice when the oral route is no longer practical. Injections, however, can be easier to give, cause no great discomfort and may be better tolerated.

Spinal Routes

Extradural or intrathecal routes may have a place in treating some patients, but these routes are not free of side effects, including delayed respiratory depression and itching[8]. The method needs practitioners skilled in this technique.

Intrathecal injections – Opioids neurolytics used for accurate placement of neurolytic agents in indoor patients:

Table 21.10 : Rectal Analgesics

Suppository and strength	Typical starting dose	Equivalent dose of morphine	Route	Dose interval	Comments
Oxycodone pectinate Suppose:10 mg	30 mg	30 mg	PR	6-8th hourly	Sedative and long acting, useful over-night
Morphine (as hcl or sulphate) Suppose.10/15 /30/60 mg	10 mg	10 mg	PR	4th hourly	Can be made upto any dose upto 150 mg
Dextromoramide Suppose.10 mg	10 mg	10 mg .	PR	3 hourly	Short duration limits its use

Alternative Routes of Administration

THE ORAL ROUTE IS ALWAYS PREFERABLE AND USUALLY POSSIBLE.

Sublingual or Buccal Route

This route may be useful in patient with vomiting or dysphagia. The following analgesics can be used in this way.

Indications – Carcinoma of cervix, rectum, pelvis

Agents used – Absolute alcohol (95%) hypobaric, diffuses fast, relief shorter, inflammation, burning at site

Phenol – 5% hyperbaric, local analgesic. Used aqueous or in glycerol, effective diffusion

Chloroceresol – 5% in glycerol, hyperbaric, effective diffusion

Complications – Patchy degeneration, arachnoiditis, retention of urine, paresis, headache, nausea and vomiting

Drug Delivery Implants by Spinal Routes

Type I – Simple epidural, intrathecal catheter. Analgesia for few days provided.

Type II – Tunnelled catheters, for pain relief for a few weeks.

Type III – Reservoir port, provides analgesia for a few months.

Type IV – Continuous infusion; provide analgesia for more than six months.

Type V – Programmed infusion, analgesia for more than a year.

Epidural – Opioids, neurolytics.

Indications – Same as intrathecal catheter and infusion pumps.

Diagnosis and therapy – Vascular phenomenon, visceral pain.

Agents – 3–5 mL of 3–10% phenol.

Advantage – Easy injection, no complication due to dural puncture, position.

Disadvantages – Less precise, dural puncture, neurological complications.

Table 21.11 : Drug delivery systems

Type I	Type II	Type III	Type IV	Type V	Type VI
Simple Epi, S.A.Catheter	Tunnelled Catheter	Reservoir port	Manually activated	Continuous infusion	Programmed infusion
Days	Weeks	Months	Years	Years	

Parenteral Route

There are few indications for Parental Analgesics in cancer patients.

1. In the last few hours, or occasionally days of life.
2. Vomiting while antiemetic treatment is effective.
3. Acute pain for rapid effect (although rectal or sublingual route can be almost as rapid).
4. Dysphagia.

Small volume injections are kinder in thin patients and the high solubility of diamorphine hydrochloride is a useful advantage. Morphine sulphate is less soluble but suitable alternatives are morphine acetate and hydromorphine. Subcutaneous injections through 25G needles is kinder and as effective as intramuscular injections.Continuous subcutaneous infusions can be given by using small battery driven pumps. When changing from the oral to parenteral routes the following dose equivalents apply.

Table 21.12 : Opioid Conversion

3 mg	=	**2 mg**	=	**1 mg**	=	**1.5 mg**
oral morphine		oral diamorphine		inj. diamorphine SC/IM		inj. morphine SC/IM

CONTINUOUS INTRAVENOUS OPIOIDS ARE UNNECESSARY. There is no evidence in chronic cancer pain. The intravenous route provided more analgesia than regular subcutaneous, sublingual or rectal administration. Few very ill patients with cancer either need or want an intravenous infusion. Continuous subcutaneous administration is an alternative.

Painful Procedures

There are occasions when procedures such as dressing changes or manual evacuation of faecal impaction produce pain, which is not covered by regular prophylactic analgesia. It makes little sense to increase this background analgesia.

Nitrous oxide and oxygen: In equal parts (Entonox) inhaled from premixed cylinders is useful when a rapid onset of analgesia is needed, but the effect only lasts a few minutes. Ideally the patients should self administer the gases under supervision, in this way titrating the correct dose for themselves.

Diazepam: It is rapidly effective given intravenously (absorption from the intramuscular route is unreliable). It must be given in a titrated dose no faster than 2.5 mg / minute, until the patients eyes droop and speech becomes slurred. The aim is to stop short of patient losing consciousness. The patient, may still feel some pain during the procedure but will have no memory of the event later. Diazepam emulsion (diazemules) is expensive, but causes less local pain and thrombosis. The rectal route can be used but titration is more difficult and less accurate.

Extra dose of morphine can be given by repeating the normal; oral 4 hourly dose 1 hour before the procedure, or giving the equivalent dose of diamorphine parenterally. The effect will last upto 4 hours. The next 4 hourly doses should be given on time.

Coanalgesics: These are drugs other than analgesics which indirectly relieve pain; they include corticosteroids antibiotics, and antispasmodics. They may be effective without concurrent analgesics.

NSAIDs: These are mild analgesics, but their ability to inhibit prostaglandin synthesis makes them of particular value in bone pain, when prescribed with a strong opioid.

The logic is that prostaglandins may contribute to the osteolysis in bone metastases and to the resulting pain. Radiotherapy is the treatment of choice in the pain of bone metastases, but NSAIDs can be used while the effect of radiotherapy is developing, or if it is impractical such as with multiple rib metastases. The combination of cutaneous pain pruritis and erythema in breast carcinoma ('Cupitch' syndrome) may also be caused by local prostaglandin production and response to NSAIDs.[9] The choice of NSAID depends mainly on cost and patient acceptability.

Aspirin : It is cheap and often effective in a dose of 3 g daily.

Side effects are less common at this dose, but the full anti-inflammatory action doses of 4 g or more are needed which may not be tolerated. Patients who are hypoproteinemic may not tolerate even the lower doses. Flurbiprofen is a potent inhibitor of PGE_2 synthesis and clinically effective at doses of 50–100 mg 12 hourly. An alternative is the salicylates diflunisal in doses of 250–500 mg 12 hourly.

Corticosteroids: Corticosteroids have wide application in advanced cancer. They can reduce the oedema and inflammation that surrounds the tumour and, therefore, ease the pressure on surrounding structures. Although they have anti-inflammatory action, they have a less specific effect on synthesis of prostaglandins and less effective than NSAIDs in bone pain. They can improve appetite and occasionally produce a useful sense of well-being. Side effects are not often troublesome.

Approximately 2% of patients on corticosteroids develop peptic ulcer disease, while upto 5% of patients with advanced cancer may develop complicated ulcer disease. In view of the benefits they bring such risks which are accepted by most physicians.

Dexamethasone is the corticosteroid of choice. It is more potent than prednisolone (2 mg dexamethasone = approx.15 mg prednisolone), resulting in fewer tablets for the patients. Low doses should be taken once in the morning, higher doses can be taken in divided doses, but no later than 6 p.m. to avoid insomnia. High doses should be reduced gradually over 10 days to the lowest dose that controls symptoms. For those unable to swallow tablets, dexamethasone suspension (4 mg/5 mL) is easily made up by pharmacists and is significantly cheaper than soluble prednisolone or betamethasone.

Muscle relaxants : Skeletal muscles spasm may be due to nerve involvement or direct irritation by tumour. Local heat, massage and relaxation techniques may help. The following drugs may be useful[10].

Diazepam : Tablets 2/5/10 mg, syrup 2 mg /5mL,

Table 21.13 : Side effects of analgesic treatment

Side effects	Incidence	Comments
Oral candidiasis	31%	Treatment is simple and effective
Peripheral oedema	20%	Usually mild
Moon face	18%	An advantage in thin patients
Dyspepsia	7%	Usually mild
Hyperactivity	4%	Do not prescribe corticosteroids later than 6 pm

Table 21.14 : Corticosteroids in advanced cancer

Low dose (*e.g.*, 2–4 mg dexamethasone daily) Nonspecific uses Improved appetite Advanced well-being Improve strength	Specific uses Haemoptysis
High dose (*e.g.* 16–24 mg dexamethasone daily) Coanalgesic Raised intracranial pressure Nerve compression Head and neck tumour Pelvic tumour Metastatic joint involvement Malignant pleural pain	Specific uses Cold compression Superior vena caval compression Air ways obstruction Carcinomatous lymphangitis Leucoerythroblastic anaemia Cough due to malignancy

suppositories 5/10 mg. Effective, but at the expense of drowsiness. It has a prolonged half-life so that a single bedtime dose of 5–20 mg is usually sufficient.

Baclofen : Tablets 10 mg, the dose needs to be gradually increased from 5 mg 8 hourly to a maximum of 30 mg 8 hourly. It should be taken with food. Nausea, vomiting, drowsiness and confusion limit its use.

Dantrolene : Capsules 25/100 mg. The dose is slowly increased over several weeks from 25 mg daily up to 100 mg 6 hourly. Drowsiness and weakness are problems, especially in the first weeks of treatment. The therapeutic effect may take several weeks to develop.

Psychotropic Drugs

Phenothiazines : There is no clear evidence that drugs such as chlorpromazine or methotrimeprazine potentiates morphine or diamorphine. There is no place for routinely combining an opioid and phenothiazines.

Butyrophenones and benzodiazepines : Pain in an anxious or agitated patient is likely to improve with counselling and the judicious use of psychotropics such as haloperidol or diazepam.

Antidepressants can be effective in nerve destruction pain which is characterized by a burning sensation and local hypersensitivity. Amitriptyline or dothiepine can be used at a dose of 25 mg increasing every few days until the pain eases or side effects arise.

Anticonvulsants : These can be useful in stabbing pain that can accompany nerve compression. Sodium valproate starting at 200 mg 12 hourly upto 400 mg 6 hourly can be used.

Coanalgesic Therapy

These modes of therapy are adequately covered elsewhere and include radiotherapy, nerve blocks, neurosurgical procedures including pituitary alcohol block, transcutaneous nerve stimulation hypnosis, and acupuncture.

Persistent Pain

If after multiple increases of a strong opioid the pain is still not adequately controlled, a complete reassessment is necessary.

- has the cause of pain correctly diagnosed?
- are analgesics appropriate? Has a new pain developed that needs different treatment?
- have basic principles been followed?
- have the analgesic staircase been followed?
- have appropriate strong opioids been used?
- have coanalgesic drugs been considered?
- is the patient lonely, frightened, anxious or depressed?

REFERENCES

1. Twycross RG. Principles and practice of pain relief in terminal cancer. Update 1972;5(2/115–121).
2. Twycross RG. Clinical experience with diamorphine in advanced malignant disease. International journal of pharmaocology.1974; 9(3)184–198.
3. Walsh TD. Opioids and respiratory functions in advanced cancer. Recent results in cancer research 1984; 89:115–117.
4. Locktidge. Hydrolysis of diacetylmorphine by cholinesterase. Journal of pharmacology 1980; 21(1)1–8.
5. Regnard CFB, Edward S. Chloroform in morphine soln. Pharmaceutical journal 1984; 233:745–746.
6. Mcquay AJ. High systemic relative bio availability of oral morphine, Royal society of medicine. Int. Cong. series. 1984; 64:149–154.
7. Twycross RJ. Narcotic agonist antagonism symptom control in advanced cancer pain relief.1983; 253–269.
8. Yaksh TL. Spinal opioid analgesia. 1981; 293–346.
9. Twycross RJ. Pruritis and pain in encuirass breast cancer. Lancet. 1981; 696.
10. Consumers association. Drugs to relieve plasticity. Drugs and therapeutic bulletin. 1983; 21(1:1–3).
11. Doyle D. Nerve blocks in advanced cancer. Practitioner. 1982; 226:539–544.
12. Myles J. Chemical hyphophysectomy. Advances in pain research, 1979; 373–400.

•••

MORPHINE AVAILABILITY IN INDIA

22

Morphine Availability[1]

1. The problem

Cancer and Pain

- Approximately 1.05 million people experience cancer pain in India every year.
- Cancer pain is often severe and can sometimes be excruciating.
- Severe pain can make activities of daily living impossible.
- Unrelieved pain not only affects the patients, but also the family and the community.

Morphine

- Morphine is an essential drug for cancer pain management.
- Despite India's heavy cancer burden, it consumes far less morphine than most countries.
- India supplies much of the opium to make morphine for increasing use in the rest of the world, but it produces very little for domestic use due to lack of demand.

Access to Morphine

- Institutions that use morphine have problems obtaining a continuous supply of morphine.
- The state licensing system for morphine is so complex that it is nearly impossible to have all the licenses valid at the same time.
- The 1985 antinarcotics law established tough new penalties for violation involving narcotic drugs.
- Morphine consumption is increasing in most of the world. Morphine consumption in India decreased by over 90% from 1985 to 1998.

2. Steps taken : 1992 – 1994[2]

1. Government of India sponsored workshops to discuss the problem of morphine unavailability.
2. The WHO provided free morphine for regional cancer centers: some of which was never used and had to be disposed.

1995

1. The ministry of health, department of revenue and WHO collaborating centre participated in a workshop in New Delhi to review the complexities of morphine regulation.
2. The WHOCC made a systematic study of the federal and state regulatory requirements for obtaining morphine.
3. The Indian association of palliative care (IAPC) established the committee on morphine availability and control to work with the WHOCC and the government of India to improve availability of morphine.
4. WHOCC designated the pain and palliative care society (PPCS) as a WHO demonstration project for studying how to ensure morphine availability.

1996

1. WHOCC prepared guidelines for physicians to obtain morphine under existing regulations; the guidelines were published by the IAPC in the Indian journal of palliative care.
2. At the international level, WHO published a guide to opioid availability and the INCB published the recommendations that national governments throughout the world should identify and remove regulatory barriers to the availability and use of morphine for cancer pain relief.

1997

1. The IAPC and WHOCC submitted to the government of India a proposal to simplify the regulation of morphine.
2. The government of India accepted the proposal, adapted it, and sent it to all state government with instructions to adopt a new regulation to amend state rules to simplify licensing and access to morphine and, therefore, pain relief.

1998

1. The WHOCC, the US cancer pain relief committee and the PPCS conducted the first state level morphine availability workshop at Trivandrum. (Kerala, 24th June 1998) to focus attention on the need to amend state rules.
2. A task force was appointed by the health department to prepare a draft regulation for official submission to the government of Kerala.

1999

1. The government of Kerala adopted the regulation submitted to simplify licensing for morphine.
2. The IAPC , WHOCC and USCPRC sponsored three more morphine availability workshops in Orissa (Cuttack 8th Oct.1999), Maharashtra (Mumbai 4th Oct.1999) and Karnataka (Bangalore 26th Feb.1999). The states of Sikkim and Madhya Pradesh also adopted new regulation to simplify morphine availability.

2000

1. The IAPC, WHOCC, USCPRC sponsored two more workshops on morphine availability during February in Ahmedabad (Gujarat) and Gwalior (Madhya Pradesh).
2. The IAPC and its commitee on morphine availability and control will meet with the WHOCC in Bangalore to assess the progress to improve morphine availability and consider the next steps.
3. The IAPC and WHOCC will meet with the officials of government of India to assess progress and consider next steps.

Special Provisions Relating to Use etc. of Morphine by Recognized Medical Institution

1. Notwithstanding any provision to the contrary in these rules, possession, transport, purchase, sell, import interstate, export-interstate or use of morphine or any preparation containing morphine in respect of recognized medical institution shall be as per the following provisions :
2. **Definition :** in this chapter unless the context otherwise required :
   I. 'Morphine' includes any preparation containing morphine.
   II. 'Recognized' medical institution means a hospital or medical institution recognized for the purpose under this chapter. It is the responsibility of the institution so recognized to ensure that morphine obtained by them is used for medical purpose only.
3. **Recognition of medical institution:**
   I. Every medical institution which intends to be recognized for the purpose under this chapter shall apply to the drug controller appointed by the state government who shall convey his decision within three months of reciept of application.
   II. If it comes to the notice of the drug controller that morphine obtained by recognized institution was supplied for non-medical use or that any of the rules under this chapter is not complied with, for reasons to be recovered in writing, the drug controller may revoke the recognition accorded under these rules.
4. **Duties of recognized medical institution :**
   Every recognized medical institution shall:
   I. Designate one or more qualified medical practitioner who may prescribe morphine. When more than one qualified medical practitioner has been designated, one of them shall be designated as overall in charge.
   II. The designated medical practitioner or the incharge, as the case may be, shall (*a*) endeavour to ensure that the stock of morphine is adequate for patient needs. (*b*) maintain adequate security over stock of morphine, (*c*) maintain a record of all receipts and disbursements of morphine in the format enclosed and (*d*) ensure that estimates, and other relevant information required to be sent by the recognized medical institution under this chapter are sent to the authorities concerned.
5. **Sending of estimates of requirements of morphine by the recognized medical institution :** Every recognized medical institution shall send their annual requirement of morphine by 30th November of the preceding year along with the name and address of the superior from whom they intend to buy it to the drug controller.
6. **Approval of estimates by the drug controller :** The drug controller who received the annual requirement shall consider it, which may if necessary call for necessary clarification. A reply on approved estimates or not accepting the estimates shall be sent before 21st of December of the preceding year. A copy of the communication

shall be sent each to the superior, whose name has been given in the estimate, if the supplier is located in another state, the drug controller of that state, the Drug Controller General of India and the Narcotics Commissioner of India.

7. **Supplementary estimates :** If the requirement of the recognized medical institution exceeds the annual estimate approved by the drug controller, the recognized medical institution may send supplementary estimates at any time to the drug controller, which shall be considered and dealt with by the drug controller in the same manner as the annual estimates.

8. The provision of these rules in other chapters in respect of possession, transport, purchase, sale, import interstate, export interstate or use of manufactured drug shall not apply in respect of a recognized medical institution shall be in accordance with the following provisions applicable till recently.

   (*a*) The recognized medical institution shall place orders for purchase to a manufacturer/ supplier along with a photocopy of the communication of the district drug controller vide which the institution was recognized for the purposes of this chapter and a copy of the communication of the drug controller vide which the approved estimates were conveyed. A copy of the order for purchase shall be sent to the Drug Controller and the Narcotics Commissioner of India by District Drug Controller.

   (*b*) Any manufacturing company shall send morphine to the recognized medical institution under this chapter only on the basis of an order for purchase received along with copies of recognition granted by the drug controller and the approved estimates communicated by drug controller. The manufacturer /supplier shall dispatch the morphine consignment along with a consignment note in quintuplicate. Copies of the consignment note shall be sent by the manufacturer/supplier to the drug controller of the state in which the manufacturer / supplier is located, the drug controller of the state in which the recognized medical institution is located and the Narcotic Commissioner of India. He shall also keep a copy of the consignment note. (c) On receipt of the consignment, the recognized medical institution shall enter the quantity received with date in all the copies of the consignment note, retain the original consignment note, send the duplicate to the supplier, triplicate to the drug controller, the quadruplicate to the drug controller of the state (in cases in which the consignment originated outside the state) in which the supplier is located and the quintuplicate to the Narcotics Commissioner of India.

9. **Maintenance of records :** All records generated under this chapter shall be kept for a period of two years from the date of transaction which shall be open for inspection by the officers empowered by the state government under sections 41 and 42 of the Narcotics Commissioner of India.

10. **Inspection of stocks of morphine :** The stocks of morphine under the custody of a recognized medical institution shall be open for inspection by the drug controller or any other officer subordinate to him or the officers of other departments of the state government empowered under sections 41 and 42 of the Narcotic Drugs and Psychotropic Substances Act 1985.

11. **Appeals :** Any institution aggrieved by any decision of or order passed by the drug controller relating to recognition of any institution, revocation of recognition of any institution or estimates may appeal to the secretary, department of health of the state government within ninety days from the date of communication of such decision or order.

REFERENCES

1. Kumar P. Management of cancer pain and related symptoms. New Delhi, Samvedna, 2003.
2. Proceedings of WHO workshop on Morphine Availability. Ahmedabad, Feb. 2000.

•••

GASTROINTESTINAL SYMPTOMS

23

Constipation

CONSTIPATION CAN MIMIC SOME FEATURES OF CANCER, particularly abdominal masses, nausea, vomiting, pain confusion and diarrhoea. Colic combined with fixed abdominal masses can be easily mistaken for tumour, resulting in inappropriate use of analgesics. If the facility is readily available suppository can be invaluable in this situation. Constipation should be anticipated in all patients on opioids or drugs with anticholinergic actions and in patients who are immobile and with reduced fluid intake or on low fibre diet.

Table 23.1 : The treatment of constipation

Clear lower bowel:	**Start laxative:**
High arachis oil retention enema overnight.	Contact laxative: Isabgul
In the morning:	With danthron: Co danthramer
If rectum full–glycerol suppository	Co danthrusate.
If rectum empty–high phosphate enema	With sennoside:senna
If no success:	
Repeat enema after 24 hours, if faeces are palpable in descending colon. Start laxative.	Upto 20 mL bd Co danthromer forte.
If rectum is impacted:	**If colic precipitated:**
Soft faeces: biscodyl suppository or tablet.	–reduce dose of contact laxative
Hard faeces: manual evacuation.	–add osmotic agent *e.g.*, lactulose.

Table 23.2 : Contact laxative equivalents

6 Co danthromer capsules = 30 mL of Co danthromer syrup	= 10 mL senna syrup
= 3 Co danthrusate capsules	= 2 senna tablets
= 10 mL Co danthromer syrup.	

Nausea and Vomiting

ANTIEMETIC CHOICE DEPENDS UPON CAUSE: Commonly overlooked causes of nausea and vomiting in advanced cancer are constipation, hypercalcemia, pharyngeal stimulation by copious sputum, gastric stasis and drugs, such as metronidazole. Tolerance to opioid induced nausea and vomiting occurs in 7–10 days. Patients transferred from strong opioids to weak opioids are already tolerant, so that an antiemetic is not needed. A single antiemetic is usually sufficient.

In some situations such as bowel obstruction, second antiemetics may be needed but should have a different but appropriate site of action. During the initial period of control of nausea and vomiting the oral route may not be practical. All the antiemetics given below are available in injectable form, but only cyclizine, prochlorperazine, domperidone and chlorpromazine are available in suppository form. In the subcutaneous infusion pump only haloperidol, cyclizine, metoclopramide should be used.

Table 23.3 : The treatment of nausea and vomiting

Stimulation of vomiting centre	First line treatment	Second line treatment
Higher centres – Anxiety, fear	Counselling	Add diazepam 5–10 mg or chlorpromazine 25–100 mg 8 hourly
Directly – DXT to head and neck? – Raised ICP	Cyclizine 50 mg 8 hourly Corticosteroids Cyclizine 50 mg 8 hourly	Chlorpromazine 25–100 mg 8 hourly
Via vagal and sympathetic afferents – Cough	Simple linctus PRN	Add morphine solution 5–10 mg 4 hourly
– Bronchial secretions	Hyoscine hydrobromide 0.3 - 0.8 mg 6 - 8 hourly	Add gentle chest physiotherapy.
– Stretched liver capsule	Corticosteroids	Add Cyclizine 50 mg 8 hourly
– Gastricstasis	Metoclopramide 10 mg 8 hourly Or domperidone 10 mg 8 hourly.	Add dimethicone 10 mL 4 hourly
– Constipation	Clear constipation	Add Cyclizine 50 mg 8 hourly
– Bowel obstruction	Cyclizine 50 mg 8 hourly	Add haloperidol 3–5 mg
Via Chemoreceptor trigger zone – Drugs opioids, Hypercalcaemia,uremia	Haloperidol 1.5–3 mg	Chlorpromazine 25–100 mg 8 hourly
Via vestibular nerve	Add Cyclizine 50 mg 8 hourly	Chlorpromazine 25–100 mg 8 hourly

Antiemetics

Haloperidol preparations: Tablets 0.5, 1.5,5,10, 20 mg.Inj:5/10 mg/mL. Routes: PO/IM/SC. Antiemetic of choice on ctz. Reduced risk of extra pyramidal effects at low doses.

Cyclizine preparations: Tablets 50 mg suppository 50 mg in 50 mg/mL, dose: 50–100 mg 4 – 8 hourly. Routes: PO/PR/SC/IM. Antiemetic of choice acting directly in vomiting centre, anticholinergic side effects at higher doses. Occasionally local irritation when injected subcutaneously.

Metoclopramide preparations: Tablets 10 mg, elixir 5 mg/mL, Inj 5 mg/mL dose: 10-20 mg 8 hourly dose 10–20 mg 8 hourly. Routes PO/SC/IM. Antiemetics of choice to speed gastric emptying. May cause extra pyramidal effects at large doses. Can be given subcutaneously.

Alternatives to the above antiemetics

Prochlorperazine preparations: Tablets 5, 25 mg.syrup 5 mg/mL, and suppositories 5, 25 mg.

Inj 12.5 mg/mL., dose:5–10 mg 8 hourly routes: PO/IM/PR. More sedative and likely to cause dry mouth than haloperidol. Shorter half-life than haloperidol. Too irritant to use subcutaneously. Suppository can be useful.

Domperidone preparations: Tablets 10 mg, susp 5 mg/mL, suppository 30 mg, doses: oral 10 mg 8 hourly. Alternative to metoclopramide especially if extra pyramidal reactions are a risk and rectal route is required.

Chlorpromazine preparations tablets 10, 25, 50, 100 mg, elixir 25 mg/mL, suppository 100 mg.Inj 25 mg/mL, dose:10 – 100 mg 8 hourly. Routes: PO/IM/PR. Comments: Too sedative for routine use. Too irritant for subcutaneous use.

Anorexia

IT IS NORMAL FOR LESS ACTIVITY TO REDUCE ENERGY INTAKE and this should be explained to the patient. It need not be treated. Underlying causes which can be treated include pain, constipation, nausea and vomiting, gastric distension, oral problems, body odours, anxiety and depression, drugs, unappetizing food and food odours. Patients may develop taste abnormalities and may prefer sweeter, colder and spicier foods. So all, attractively presented meals are more likely to be eaten.

If the cause of anorexia is unclear, or difficult to treat, corticosteroids can be effective. Dexamethsone 4 mg may be reduced to 2 mg after one week, can improve appetite and taste. Side effects are unlikely at this dose, but dexamethasone should be stopped if there is no improvement after two weeks.

NASOGASTRIC SUCTION AND INTRAVENOUS HYDRATION ARE RARELY NECESSARY:

1. Contact laxatives are withheld to avoid colic, osmotic laxatives to avoid bowel distension and metoclopramide or domperidone to avoid the upper gut trying to contract against high obstruction.
2. Hyoscine butyl bromide (buscopan) is an alternative to hyoscine hydrobromides and may have less peripheral anti cholinergic effects, such as dry mouth. The dose is 10–20 mg 4–6 hourly PO/SC.

Causes of Obstruction

Recurrent abdominal pelvic cancer can often cause multiple malignant blockages; usually in the small bowel.

Table 23.4 : The Medical Management of Bowel Obstruction

Explanation	Eliminate nausea and reduce vomiting
Dietary advice No fluid/food restriction – Small meals earlier in the day. **Reduce colic** Stop osmotic or contact laxatives. Hyoscine hydro bromide 0.3 mg sublingually 4–8 hourly – if no success, increase hyoscine to 0.8 mg subcutaneously 4–8 hourly	AVOID Metoclopramide or domperidone START Cyclizine 50 mg 6–8 hourly (PO/SC/PR/IM) – if no success ADD haloperidol 3–5 mg nocte – if no success REPLACE Cyclizine and haloperidol with Hyoscine hydrobromide. 0.4 mg SC. 8 hourly.
Reduce background pain	**Soften bowel contents**
Opioids (oral route often possible)	Docussate tablets or syrup 100–200 mg 8 hourly
– Codeine phosphate 30–60 mg 4 hourly.	**Reverse obstruction**
– Morphine sulphate (titrate dose).	Clear constipation Consider dexamethasone 12 mg daily for 1 week. (only occasionally successful)

Intestinal Obstruction

OBSTRUCTION CAN BE MANAGED AT HOME. The traditional preoperative "drip and suck" is successful in controlling the symptoms of obstruction in less than 15% of patients unfit for surgery.[3] These patients can be managed medically without "drip and suck"; free of nausea and pain. An outline of management is given below:

Patients are little troubled by short episodes of vomiting provided that the most distressing symptom, nausea, is controlled by antiemetics. Obstructions distal to the upper small bowel will allow sufficient fluid to be absorbed to prevent significant dehydration. Patients with complete small bowel obstruction have been managed in this way for several weeks before succumbing to the cancer. It is possible to achieve a peaceful phase without the need for nasogastric suction or intravenous hydration which is rarely justified in the last days or weeks of life.

Metastatic obstruction from outside the abdomen is most commonly due to melanoma or due to primaries of breasts or lung. **Constipation** can cause distension, nausea, vomiting and abdominal masses that may not change position far a week or more. A supine abdominal X-ray will differentiate constipation from other causes of obstruction. **Benign adhesions** may occur in upto 20% of patients with recurrent abdominal cancer. Adhesions are more likely if the ileum is obstructed and if the abdomen is previously irradiated[4].

Surgery: The possibility of benign adhesions or a single site of obstruction means that surgery can be considered. Relative simple surgery is often all that is required, such as forming a loop colostomy or dividing adhesions. An understanding surgical opinion can be helpful; although radiology may be needed to show a single level obstruction that is amenable to surgery.

There will be many patients, however, whose tumour is too extensive, who have had previous surgery for obstruction, who are too ill or frail, or who have no wish for further intervention. These should be managed medically as described before.

Proximal obstructions: duodenal or pyloric obstructions are more likely to cause vomiting, but less likely to cause distension. They cause gastric stasis with features of the "squashed stomach syndrome" and must be differentiated from other causes of this syndrome which may respond to metoclopramide or domperidone. Use of these drugs in intraluminal obstructions are likely to cause increased discomfort and colic, the nausea can be treated with cyclizine, but vomiting may still occur several times. These patients may need gastric aspiration to reduce vomiting and IV hydration to prevent thirst.

Oesophageal obstructions present special problems with regurgitation of swallowed saliva, painful dysphagia and epigastric pain. Gastric acid causes precipitation of protein from the tumour producing tenacious material, which is difficult to bring up. Antacids or H_2-receptor blockers can help. Hyoscine hydrobromide 0.3–0.6 mg SC 8 hourly, will reduce saliva production at the expense of the dry mouth which can be treated with local measures. Painful dysphagia can be helped with mucaine and tumour pain with opioids. Consideration should always be given to insertation of an oesophageal tube or to **radiotherapy.**

Feeding and hydration: Some patients will absorb sufficient fluids from their upper gut to prevent significant dehydration. As patient deteriorates and eventually become comatose, their fluid intake reduces, but contrary to common belief, the resultant dehydration need not be distressing.

Ascites

The commonest causes for malignant ascites are primary tumour of the breast, ovary, colon, stomach, pancreas and bronchus. Nearly one third of the primary tumours lie outside the abdomen. Symptoms include abdominal distension or pain, a squashed stomach syndrome, leg lymph oedema and dyspnoea due to diaphragmatic splinting.Treatment plan is outlined below:

Diuretics: The finding of increased renin and sodium retention in malignant ascites has prompted the successful use of spironolactone. The addition of a oral loop diuretic increases the diuresis, although the reduction of the ascites is as much due to redistribution of fluids as by diuresis[5].

Paracentesis: This is best carried out using a peritoneal dialysis, catheter connected to a urinary drainage bag via a urinary catheter with the balloon and tip cut off. The use of 0.5% bupivacaine as local anaesthetic for the puncture site allows pain free drainage for upto 8 hours, if necessary. Puncture sites should be away from scars and the inferior epigastric artery which runs 3–5 cm from the midline in the abdominal wall. Ideal sites are in the left iliac fossa (atleast 10 cm from the midline) and in the midline suprapubically (the bladder should be empty). A lateral approach is advisable in patients with distended bowel–marked distension is a contraindication to paracentesis. If diuretics have been unsuccessful, or the prognosis is short, the slow drainage of 5 litres or more of fluid may be indicated. Contrary to popular belief, there is no evidence that the patient deteriorates rapidly after such a large paracentesis as long as it is done slowly over 8–12 hours.

Peritoneo venous shunt: Insertion of a shunt can be done under a short general anaesthetic and causes fewer problems than for ascites due to benign liver disease. There is no evidence that increased metastatic disease occurs after such a procedure, a tense ascites is preferred prior to insertion, since this encourages drainage. Thereafter inspiratory exercises are used to further encourage drainage.

Diarrhoea

Table 23.5 : Treatment of diarrhoea in advanced cancer

Cause	1st line treatment	2nd line treatment
Infection **Drugs** (*e.g.*, antibiotics, laxatives)	Loperamide–4 mg tabs/syp with each loose stool.	
Constipation	Clear rectal impaction	Treat constipation
Obstruction	Manage obstruction	
Pancreatic steatorrhoea (reduced lipases and bicarbonates)	Pancreatic enzymes	Cimetidine 400 mg at least 30 min before a meal (a night time dose is not necessary) pancrex gelatin capsules (5–10) or granules 93–6 5 mL tspns should be used if cimetidine is prescribed.

Post gastrectomy	Loperamide 2–4 mg tabs / syrup with each loose stool then 12 hourly. If bacterial overgrowth suspected : oxytetracycline 250 mg 6 hourly for 2–4 weeks	Pancreatic enzymes
Post radiotherapy	Low residue diet loperamide–4 mg tabs/syp with each loose stool then 12 hourly	NSAIDs Consider cholestyramine 4 g in water 6 hourly
Bile salt irritation (*e.g.*, ileal resection)	Loperamide–4 mg tabs/syp with each loose stool then 12 hourly	Cholestyramine 4 g in water 6 hourly
Rectal discharge	Predsol enema Metronidazole 400 mg 8 hourly. If anaerobic infection present	Local cryotherapy or diathermy Radiotherapy

Table 23.6 : Other problems and management

Problem	Causes	Features	Treatment
Dry mouth	Dehydration, Phenothiazines, Tricyclic, Hyoscine	Dry tongue thick saliva, difficulty in speaking	Oral hydration if possible, sucking: crushed ice, butter, frozen tonic water. Chewing: pineapple chunks Change drugs *e.g.*, amitriptyline to mianserin, prochlorperazine to haloperidol
Coated tongue	Debility, poor oral hygiene, dehydration, Candida	White/brown or black tongue, reduced taste, halitosis	Cleansing: 2% soda bicarb or 6% H_2O_2 Dissolving: 1 g effervescent ascorbic acid on tongue Brushing:gently with tooth brush Chewing: pineapple chunks
Candidiasis (thrush)	Debility, cross infection, poor oral hygiene	White adherent patches, coated tongue, dryness, redness, soreness or dryness, cheilitis only ulceration only	Ketoconazole 200 mg for 1 week Soak dentures Mouthwash: betadiene
Ulceration	Apthous ulcers Radiotherapy Chemotherapy Dentures Poor oral hygiene	White depressions in mucosa with surrounding inflammation Painful	Tetracycline syrup 10 mL (250 mg mouth wash for 2 min then swallowed) Triamcinolone in oro base Betamethasone 1 mg dissolved in water as a mouth wash
Herpes simplex zoster		Pale vesicles with surrounding redness. Painful, unilateral in zoster	Treat as for painful mouth Consider: acyclovir 200 mg 4 hourly for 5 days

Painful mouth	Ulceration, candidiasis, poor oral hygiene, oral cancer, oral sepsis	Soreness talking, eating and swallowing	Benzydamine as mouth wash 1–2 hourly Choline salicylates to local lesions Consider: local anaesthetic prior to cleansing mouth

Candida: Normally inhabitant of mouths of many patients with cancer, especially of irradiation of head and neck. Most overt candidiasis is the result of over growth of Candida following reduction of host immunity. Fungicidal disinfectants such as betadiene should be used for hand washing in units treating patients with candidiasis.[6]

Ketoconazole vs. nystatin: Ketoconazole 200 mg once daily for one week is at least as effective, more convenient and its cost is similar to one weeks treatment with 2 mL nystatin 4 hourly. Gynaecomastia and hepatic toxicity have been reported with ketoconazole. The incidence of serious hepatic injury is very low and should not preclude its use in advanced cancer.[7]

Oral analgesia: Benzydamine hydrochloride mouth wash provides local anti-inflammatory action and analgesia for 1–2 hours with minimal numbness. Choline salicylates is also effective but can cause pain on application.

Oesophageal tube (Celestin tube), it can be inserted using an endoscope under light anaesthesia.

Hydration and feeding. There are special situations in which it is worth considering hydration and feeding.

Oesophageal gastric and intestinal candidiasis:[8] Radiological appearance in a Barium swallow is characteristic in case of oesophageal candidiasis. Gastric and intestinal candidiasis may present with abdominal pain and watery diarrhoea. Treatment of both is ketoconazole.

Table 23.7 : Dysphagia

Cause	Features	Treatment
Obstruction Eoesophageal tumours	Painful dysphagia with patient describing level of obstruction	Celestin tube Bouginage Radiotherapy Corticosteroids and lasers
Extrinsic compression	As above	Radiotherapy corticosteroids
Neurological Neuromuscular	*e.g.*, brainstem tumour Muscular weakness disorganized swallowing	Hyoscine hydrobromide 0.3–0.8 mg 8 hourly to reduce choking Physical help with swallowing
Perineural spread of tumour(5th,9th and 10th)	Disorganized swallowing Altered sensation in throat and face	Corticosteroids
Mucosal Candidiasis	Painful swallowing, back or retrosternal pain	Ketoconazole 200 mg for 1 week
Radiotherapy	As above	Mucaine 10 mL 2–4 hourly Diflunisal 250 mg bd

Table 23. 8 : Squashed stomach syndrome

Cause	Features	Treatment
Drugs (opioids, anti-depressants), ascites, hepatomegaly.	Nausea-vomiting, epigastric pain, regurgitation, hiccups, early satiation, heart burn	Metoclopramide 10–20 mg 8 hourly PO/SC/IM.
Obstruction	As above	Treat as per obstruction

REFERENCES

1. Hanks GW. Antiemetics for terminal cancer patients. Lancet. 1982; 1410.
2. Dew YS. Changes in taste sensation and feeding behavior in cancer patients. Journal of Human Nutrition, 1978; 32:447–453.
3. Glass RL, Le Duc RJ. Small intestinal obstruction from peritoneal carcinamatosis. The American Journal of Surgery, 1973; 125:316.
4. Walsh HPJ. Is laparatomy for small bowel obstruction justified in patients previously treated malignancy? British Journal of Surgery,1984; 71:933–935.
5. Amiel SA, Blackbuin AM and Rubers RD. Intravenous infusion of furosemide as treatment of ascites in malignant disease. Brit. Medical Journal, 1984; 288:1041.
6. Burnie JP., Lee W, Williams JD et al. Control of an outbreak of systemic Candida albicans. British Medical Journal 1985; 291:1092–1093.
7. Lewis JH, Zimmerman HJ, Benson GD et al. Hepatic injury associated with ketaconazole: injury analysis of 33 cases. Gastroenterology,1984; 503–513.
8. Trier JS and Bjorkman DJ. Esophageal, gastric candidiasis. American Journal of Medicine, 1984; 77(4d): 39–43.

ADVANCED MALIGNANCY–URINARY CARDIORESPIRATORY AND OTHER SYMPTOMS

24

Haematuria

It is unusual for blood loss to be severe, so that iron supplementation may be sufficient to prevent anaemia. Infections should always be excluded both by clinical and urine culture.

Palliative radiotherapy may cause troublesome haematuria arising from bleeding from a malignant lesion in urinary tract.

Bleeding can be minimized by 1% alum irrigation solution. It acts by precipitating proteins in mucosal surface. It is given by continuous bladder irrigation; it is not absorbed, and has no systemic toxicity.

Urinary Incontinence

Investigation of incontinence is rarely appropriate in patients with advanced cancer, and a clinical diagnosis must be made although surgical repair is also inappropriate, the advice of an urologist can be invaluable.Drugs are often the first line of treatment.[1]

Table 24.1 : Urinary retention

Cause	First line	Consider
Constipation	Laxatives	
Drugs (anti-cholinergic)	Reduce dose	Change drug
Tumour obstruction	Phenoxybenzamine or dexamethasone	Catheterization or suprapubic catheter
Naturopathic bladder		
Spastic	Phenoxybenzamine	Intermittent self Catheterization
Flaccid	Phenoxybenzamine	Distigmine 5 mg on alternate days; intermittent self Catheterization

Table 24.2 : Urinary incontinence

Cause	First line	Second line	Consider
Post prostatectomy	Propanthiline, 15 mg before meal +30 mg nocte (upto 90 mg daily)	Imipramine 50–100 mg nocte	Condom, urethral catheter or bag decompression nasally may help
Stress continence	Ring pessary	Ephedrine 30 mg BD, last dose not later than 6 pm	Absorbant pads, tampons, surgery
Urge incontinence	Propantheline 15 mg before meal= 30 mg nocte (upto 90 mg daily)	Imipramine 50–100 mg nocte	NSAID (flurbiprofen), pads, condom,urethral catheter or bag

Neuropathic Bladder • spastic • flaccid	 Large capacity: manual stimulation to void, small capacity: intermittent catheterization regular voiding	 Permanent condom, uretheral catheter or bag Intermittent catheterisation	 Desmopressin nocte may help
Bypassing catheter	Exclude infection or bladder spasm	Have balloon volume	Change to smaller size catheter
Vesico-vaginal fistula	Absorbant pads or tampons	Desmopressin nocte may help	
Overflow	Catheter	Phenoxybenzamine	Distigmine

1. Desmopressin: This synthetic analogue of vasopressin (anti-diuretic hormone) will reduce urinary output overnight and is occasionally helpful in otherwise intractable nocturnal incontinence. A fluid intake /output chart should be started, and no fluids given after 6 pm. Usually 20 microgram of desmopressin is given nasally at 10 pm. It is important the patient produces a daytime output of at least 500 mL, otherwise water intoxication can occur.
2. Intermittent self catheterization is an alternative at home to a permanent catheter. The technique is usually only suitable for women. Catheterization is done at least four times a day. The catheters can be washed after use then boiled or kept in sodium hypochlorite solution.
3. Condom catheters for men are an alternative to a permanent indwelling catheter, but have the disadvantage of leaking, if not carefully fitted. An alternative is a urostomy bag fitted over the penis and adherent to the pubic skin.
4. Sex and the catheter : Some patients and their partners are still able and willing to consider intercourse, but frightened to the catheter. Many women are able to have satisfactory intercourse with an indwelling catheter, although intermittent self catheterization is a better alternative. Men who are able to achieve an erection can do so with a catheter present. Gentle intercourse is possible with a disconnected catheter (after draining the bladder), and placing a condom over penis and catheter. If the ejaculatory mechanism has not been damaged this can still occur with a catheter, but may be painful. Self re-catheterization or a condom catheter is better alternative.

Table 24.3 : Bladder pain or spasm

Cause	First line	Second line	Consider
Infection	Appropriate antibiotic	Bladder washout if catheter present	Phenazopyridine 100–200 mg 8 hourly
Irritation – catheter – tumour	 Remove half water from balloon radiotherapy	 Phenazopyridine Phenazopyridine	 Exclusion of bladder calculus Analgesics
Neuropathic bladder spasm Anxiety	Propantheline 15 mg before meal +30 mg nocte (upto 90 mg daily) Empathetic listening	Hyoscine hydrobromide 0.3–0.6 mg SL/SC PM Propantheline 15 mg before meals 30 mg nocte (upto 90 mg daily)	 Diazepam 5–10 mg

Radiotherapy can occasionally cause bladder pain and spasm. Try phenazopyridine which is a topical analgesic. It colours the urine orange/red.

Cardiovascular Symptoms

Vena caval obstruction: This needs urgent treatment. Superior vena caval obstruction may cause distressing and painful swelling of the head, neck and arms. Inferior vena caval obstruction has a similar effect on the lower half of the body.

Initial treatment consists of high doses dexamethasone 8 mg IV stat, followed by 24 mg daily in divided doses, the last dose no later than dose required to control symptoms. If possible the patient should be urgently referred for radiotherapy.

Anaemia : Anaemia in advanced cancer does not always require treatment. It is usually an anaemia of chronic diseases and does not respond to iron or other supplements. Consequently transfusion is often considered, if the anaemia is profound. This needs careful consideration. If the anaemia is causing postural dizziness or weakness, and the patient is likely to remain active then a transfusion may help. Transfusions are not helpful in controlling drowsiness or dyspnoea and are contraindicated when the prognosis is a few weeks or less. Transfusions are not without risk and repeated transfusions do little to improve a patient's comfort and quality of life.

Leucoerythroblastic anaemia due to marrow infiltration may respond to hormone therapy (*e.g.* Tamoxifen in breast cancer) or appropriate chemotherapy. If these have been tried already, consider high dose dexamethasone.

Respiratory Symptoms

Dyspnoea is subjective and unrelated to the severity of the pathology. The fear of suffocation and anxiety from any cause will make the situation worse. Consequently simple measure, such as cooling fan, opening a window and the security of someone's presence will do much to ease the sensation of dyspnoea. Causes of dyspnoea such as bronchospasm or pulmonary oedema are treated conventionally.

Pleural effusion If symptomatic, this should be drained almost to dryness, not taking more than 1–1.5 liters at a time. It is a common fallacy that fluid will re-cumulate within days of tapping several weeks is more usual and this may be sufficient in an ill patient. Occasionally more rapid accumulation occurs, or the patient's prognosis such that a regular tapping is impracticable. In these cases it is worth instilling a fibrotic agent to prevent re-accumulation. Tetracycline 500 mg is the choice, and is dissolved in 20 mL 0.25% bupivacaine just before use. It is instilled after tapping and the patient is asked to lie on each side, front and back for two to three minutes each way. Mild, temporary, pleuritic pain is usually the only problem.

Lobar collapse which is recent and due to bronchial carcinoma may respond to radiotherapy.

Lymphangitis Carcinomatosa may be helped by dexamethasone, 16 mg daily in divided doses (the last dose not later that 6 pm) reducing to 2–6 mg once daily over the following week. Inhalation of bupivacaine 0.25% using ultrasound nebulizer produces 2 Å size particles which will reach the alveoli and may ease dyspnoea, but the inhalations are not always tolerated.[2]

Opioids are effective at reducing the demand for ventilation without causing clinically significant respiratory depression. Even in the presence of chronic bronchitis or bronchial carcinoma, carbon dioxide retention is unusual. Patient not previously on opioid should be started on 5 mg oral morphine 4 hourly, titrating the dose upward to the response.

Midazolam (1–2 mg) and diazepam has a place in a very anxious, dyspnoeic patient, 5–10 mg stat (po or pr) followed by 5–10 mg nocte.

Respiratory infection : Whether or not to treat a chest infection in a patient with advanced cancer often cause great concern. First it must be remembered that cancer will progress despite antibiotic. Secondly what matters is whether the patient is distressed by infection (*e.g.*, fever, purulent sputum, pruritis, chest pain). In such situation there is a duty to treat in order to preserve right to comfort. Whether to control symptoms with antibiotic or other methods (*e.g.*, cooling for fever, hyoscine for secretion, analgesic for pain) must depend on the prognosis. If this is likely to be weeks or months then antibiotics should be considered. If the prognosis is likely to be hours or days, however, there is no time to wait for antibiotic to work and the other treatment should be used for the patient's comfort.

Cough: Cough may be dry (*e.g.*, mechanical irritation of the pharynx, trachea, bronchial tree, pleura, pericardium or diaphragm) or moist (*e.g.*, infection, chronic obstructive disease, asthma or heart failure). It is not always possible to treat the cause.

Peripheral suppression: Simple linctus or humidified air are soothing preparation which can be repeated as often as required. Bupivacaine 0.25% (maximum 30 mL per day) in 2 –10 Å size particles (via a bird nebulae) is helpful to suppress cough arising anywhere down to the larger bronchi. It is not always tolerated and the larger particles may cause numbness of mouth and throat, preventing safe eating and drinking for several hours. High dose dexamethasone may reduce pleural, pericardial or diaphragmatic irritation by tumour.

Central suppression: Oral morphine sulphate 3–10 mg 4 hourly in a dose that is titrated to the cough.

Methadone should not be used since its long half-life results in sedation.

Haemoptysis: Slight blood stained sputum in bronchial carcinoma is a normal part of the disease. Infection can be simply treated with appropriate antibiotics. Haemoptysis from a pulmonary infarct will settle and needs no treatment. A major haemoptysis is very rarely present.

Frequent haemoptysis due to bronchial carcinoma can be treated with radiotherapy to the mediastinum or low dose dexamethasone. In the rare event of a major haemorrhage and if the patient remains conscious then diamorphine 5–10 mg stat IV and diazepam 5–10 mg IV will ease the fear and distress.

Noisy breathing: Bronchial secretion can produce a "death rattle" which is distressing to relatives and staff, although rarely to the patient who is usually comatose. A few very debilitated but conscious patients are troubled with secretion but are too weak to cough. Treatment is with hyoscine hydrobromide 300–800 micrograms 2–4 hourly. It is sedative but preferable to atropine which can cause CNS stimulation. If high doses are used repeatedly paradoxical agitation can occasionally occur. Frusemide 40 mg IM/IV has been used in resistant cases.

Grunting respiration is occasionally seen in comatose patient. Repositioning often helps. If the patient is breathing rapidly, diamorphine 5–10 mg SC 2–4 hourly will reduce the respiratory rate to normal level and ease the grunting. High dose of diamorphine may be needed, if the patient is already receiving an opioid for pain relief. If the respiratory rate is normal then diazepam 5–10 mg rectally 2–4 hourly can help.

Hiccups

Exclude a squashed stomach syndrome. Diaphragmatic or phrenic nerve irritation from tumour may respond to high dose dexamethasone. If simple remedies fail (*e.g.*, swallowing granulated sugar) and the hiccups are persistent, try chlorpromazine 25–50 mg as a slow IV injection, oral or in routes being less effective.[3]

Dermatological Symptoms

Ulcers

Many unrelated treatments have been proposed for the management of decubitus and malignant ulcers, which reflect the low success rate of any one method. The simplest methods are the best.

1. **Debridement** to remove slough requires the active removal of all dead tissue with forceps and curette. In some areas of established pressure damage access to the underlying dead tissue may be prevented by a hard, dark eschar of dead skin. Wet dressings (gauze with normal saline) will soften the eschar sufficiently to allow debridement.
2. **Cleansing** does not imply sterilization, since ulcers are invariably colonized by bacteria. Antiseptics such as povidone-iodine (Betadine solution) will control overt infection and allow healing to take place. Topical antibiotics in powders, sprays or tulles should not be used since they result in the selection of resistant organisms and can cause local sensitivity which may lead to systemic hypersensitivity. Systemic antibiotics will not reach dead tissue which must be removed by debridement. They should only be used if cellulities is present (after sensitivity tests), or in controlling odours. Chlorine releasing solutions may damage viable tissue and are best avoided.
3. **Radiotherapy** should be considered for all fungating tumours. Bleeding can be a problem from superficial vessels that are damaged during debridement or dressing changes. Gauze soaked in 1 in 1000 adrenaline solution usually stops oozing after a few minutes application. More persistently bleeding vessels can be sealed by applying absorbable gelatin sponge.
4. **Dressing** : Dressings should provide a moist environment and the simplest and cheapest is gauze soaked in normal saline or Ringer's solution. Granuflex is suitable after debridement and can be left for one week between dressing changes. Op-site can protect superficial ulcers in areas subject to repeated trauma (*e.g.*, sacrum). It is semi-permeable and should be left in place until it peels away naturally. Exudate accumulation can be removed with needle and syringe, the puncture hole being sealed with a small square of Op-site. Silastic foam[4] can be useful in deep ulcers where a comfortable dressing is needed, or in facial ulcers.

Generalized Pruritis

An attempt to diagnose the cause should always be made, since specific treatments may then be indicated. In particular drugs, eczema, infestations, contact dermatitis, iron deficiency and uraemia should be excluded. In advanced cancer, however, diagnosis is often difficult and treatments have to be non-specific.

General measures: Patients should avoid heat, hot baths, rough underclothing and rough drying after bath. Preventing a dry skin is essential and measures include; adding oil to the bath, aqueous creams or crotamiton. Calamine is too drying and should be avoided.

Cupitch syndrome (cutaneous pain and itch): This is occasionally seen in patients with en cuirass breast cancer. The skin surrounding the tumour is often red, painful and itchy and may be due to local prostaglandin production. Both pain and itch may respond to an anti-prostaglandin *e.g.*, flurbiprofen or diflunisal.

Jaundice: Pruritis is not always to the severity of the jaundice, probably because the balance of dihydroxy salts seems more important than the total amount of bile salts present. Cholestyramine, 4G, 6 hourly preferentially binds dihydroxy salts in the bowel, but the granules are unpleasant to take. Cholestyramine will be ineffective in total biliary obstruction, since there are no bile salts in the bowel to be absorbed. Methyltestosterone, 10–25 mg 8 hourly, has been used successfully in ill patients with severe pruritis, despite occasionally increasing the jaundice due to cholestasis.

Topical drugs: Corticosteroids can be effective when appropriately applied to inflammatory skin disorders. They tend to be ineffective if applied to itchy skin without lesions. Topical anaesthetics and antihistamines are best avoided.

Systemic drugs: Antihistamines are often used with no evidence of histamine release and any positive effect is probably due to a central sedative effect. Morphine is a rare cause of histamine release, but should be considered with itching starting soon after commencing an opioid. Cimetidine has occasionally been used in itching due to various causes and specifically in Hodgkin's disease[5].

Sweating: Some patients suffer from profuse sweating, particularly at night. It is difficult to treat. It may be due to fear or anxiety. Occasionally the malignancy itself will produce a fever with sweating. Simple measures such as cooling with a fan or sponge are effective. Naproxen has been shown to relieve the fever due to cancers of the breast, lung, and bowel and to Hodgkin's. The usual dose is 250–500 mg bd.

Odours and Discharges

Odours

Most odours are the result of infection and foul-smelling odours are associated with anaerobic bacteria. Attempts to mask a smell with other odours will fail (*e.g.*, air freshners, perfumes). The patient comes to associate the new odour with the unpleasant one and soon it too becomes intolerable.

1. **Reducing Infection.** For anaerobic infections metronidazole (Flagyl) 200–400 mg 8 hourly is the drug of choice. Suppositories (500 mg or 1G) and a suspension (200 mg/mL) are available. There is little evidence that topical metronidazole is effective[4]. Other methods aimed directly at the tumour should be considered, such as radiotherapy or cryotherapy with liquid nitrogen since these may reduce tumour bulk and so reduce the amount of dying tumour tissue that predisposes to infection and odour.
2. **Isolating the odour** may be possible using adsorbants such as charcoal dressings or appliances such as colostomy bags for fistulae. Oxychlorodene has no inherent odour and is effective in removing unpleasant odours. It cannot be applied directly to tissues but can be sprinkled between dressings or into colostomy bags. Granuflex (hydrocolloid) and Sorbsen (calcium alginate) are expensive dressings which can slightly reduce odour.

Discharges

Discharges may occur from fistulae, colostomies and the vagina or rectum. Impacted faeces should always be excluded in rectal discharges.

Fistulae: It may be possible to fit colostomy bags over the fistula. The Paediatric types are easier to fit because of a softer flange. Odour can still pass through "odour-proof" bags and oxychlorodene can then be used. Silastic foam can be used when it is desirable to reduce the amount of discharge as in external fistulae connecting with the oral cavity. The dressing forms a close fitting, comfortable and washable dressing which reduces fluid loss. The foam dressing formed can be washed and re-used frequently.

Vaginal and rectal discharges due to local carcinomas can be helped with antiseptic douches/lavage *e.g.*, povidone-iodine (Betadine vaginal gel or douche). Corticosteroids (given rectally or vaginally) can help. A recto-vaginal fistula may cause stool to be passed vaginally which can be reduced by allowing the stool to become firmer (reduce the laxative or give a low dose of Loperamide). Vaginal discharges from a recto-vaginal fistula can also be reduced with regularly changed tampons. Perineal and perianal skin often need protection from the continual moisture with barrier creams *e.g.* zinc oxide paste. Referral for radiotherapy, diathermy, and cryotherapy or laser treatment should be considered.

Hypercalcaemia

Malignancy is the most common cause of hypercalcaemia, occurring in nearly 10% of patients with advanced cancer. Primaries of the breast and bronchus are the commonest causes. There is no clear relationship with bone metastases and their absence should never preclude a search for hypercalcaemia. The mechanism appears to be increased bone and renal, resorption of calcium due to a parathyroid-like hormone produced by the tumour.

Drowsiness occurs in over half of patients.[2] Other symptoms include thirst, polyuria, nausea, vomiting, anorexia, constipation and a confusional state. It is all too easy to attribute many of these to the cancer or the analgesia, although a combination of drowsiness, thirst and polyuria should always lead to a check of serum calcium. The calcium level should be corrected according to Me albumin (true calcium approximately equals measured calcium + 0.02 × 140 – albumin).

The intensity of treatment will depend on the severity of symptoms and the advanced stage of the cancer.

Severe symptoms require intravenous rehydration with 0.9% saline (4–6 litres in 24 hours may be required), together with parenteral Frusemide to promote calcium excretion. Mithramycin is a cytotoxic agent which in single doses of 25 micrograms/kg has a delayed but sustained effect which may last several weeks.

Repeated doses increase the risk of side effects, particularly bone-marrow depression.

Moderate symptoms will respond to intravenous hydration and parenteral Frusemide.

Mild symptoms may respond to oral rehydration and maintenance therapy alone.

Maintenance therapy: Keeping the calcium within normal limits can be achieved with oral phosphate. Diarrhoea is a common side effect, which may be minimized by loperamide 2–4 mg daily and by increasing the phosphate dose gradually. Reduced renal function due to renal calcification is a long term risk. Patients not tolerating or responding to phosphate may be controlled on the expensive etidronate, a diphosphonate which has a slow onset of action, but a more sustained effect than mithramycin. Corticosteroids are not helpful in hypercalcaemia due to solid tumours (breast, bronchus) but can be useful in myeloma. Hormones should always be considered in primaries of breast (tamoxifen, medroxyprogesterone, aminoglutethemide) and prostate (stilboestrol).

REFERENCES

1. West Moore. Urinary incontinence drugs.1979; 17:418–422.
2. Heyse Moore. Respiratory symptoms in the management of terminal diseases,1984; 113–119.
3. Williamson BWA. Management of intractable hiccup. British Medical Journal, 1977; 2: 501–503.
4. Warrender TS. Op-site and the dhss. British Medical Journal, 1982; 285:378–9.
5. Imard JOP. Cimetidine for pruritis. British Medical Journal, 1980;280:151–2.
6. Stevenson JC. Malignant hypocalcaemia. British Medical Journal, 1985; 291: 421–2.

NEUROPSYCHOLOGICAL SYMPTOMS IN CANCER

25

Cerebral Tumours

Features vary from subtle mood changes to confusional states, with focal signs such as dysphasia, ataxia, or hemiparesis. As intracranial pressure rises there may be headache, nausea and vomiting. Dexamethasone in high doses reduces oedema around a primary or secondary tumour. The daily dose is reduced over 2–3 weeks to the lowest dose that will control symptoms. This dose should continue until there are clear signs that symptoms are progressing. It is then sometimes possible to increase the dose again with good effect, but it is often necessary to remain at this dose to control symptoms. If it is clear that the patient is deteriorating rapidly despite dexamethasone, the dose can be reduced and stopped. Focal neurological signs may respond to radiotherapy. Side effects of whole brain irradiation are alopecia, and occasionally nausea. Increased survival is not claimed when treating metastases. It is less effective than corticosteroids in reducing oedema and these should be given concurrently. Cyclizine is the antiemetic of choice for nausea and vomiting due to raised intracranial pressure. Opioids may be required to control headache. Since respiratory depression is rare with oral opioids, there is little risk of carbon dioxide retention raising intracranial pressure still further.

Spinal Cord Compression

This neurological emergency requires an early diagnosis. Pain with local spinal tenderness is early sign, and subsequent leg weakness or sensory changes strongly suggest compression. Sensory changes can be varied and non-specific. Altered reflexes are useful localizing signs. Sphincter disturbance is a late sign. Metastases from primaries of breast, lung or prostate are the commonest malignant cause.

On suspicion of cord compression dexamethasone should be started, 8 mg IV stat, followed by 24 mg daily in divided doses. This should be followed immediately by radiotherapy. Laminectomy alone appears to be less effective with more complications. The best results are obtained in slowly developing lesions. Acute compression is usually the consequence of local cord ischaemia and, therefore, irreversible.

Lumbosacral Plexopathy

Pelvic tumours may involve the lumbosacral plexus on the posterior wall of the pelvis. Features of a pelvic tumour include leg or perineal pain, leg weakness and sensory loss, sphincter disturbance, tenesmus or bladder irritability and leg oedema. These symptoms may respond to high dose dexamethasone. Symptoms of nerve destruction (stabbing or burning pains, hypersensitivity) may respond to antidepressants or anticonvulsants. Tenesmus may respond to chlorpromazine 25–50 mg 8 hourly.

Anxiety

Drugs can never be a substitute for empathy. True Anxiolytics that are capable of 'Iysing' anxiety do not exist, at best such drugs suppress anxiety. But this can be very helpful in allowing patients to express their fears, an essential first step in treatment.

Haloperidol is relatively non-sedating and can be given in doses of 5–10 mg nocte 12 hourly. Extrapyramidal symptoms occasionally occur at higher doses (restlessness, dystonia, parkinsonian features).

Diazepam can be effective in a single night-time dose of 2–10 mg at the expense of some daytime sedation. A half-life of up to a week makes divided doses unnecessary, but accumulation can occur, which may be mistaken for deterioration due to the cancer. A short course (4–6 weeks) should be planned. Longer courses can result in rebound anxiety starting within 2 weeks of stopping diazepam[2] and this withdrawal syndrome can last several weeks. Doses should be reduced gradually. Midazolam provides better and reliable anxiolysis.

Hypnotics *e.g.*, nitrazepam (half-life 30 hours), temazepam (half-life 8 hours) can be useful in elderly patients to reduce the risk of accumulation. Treatment should be short and the dosage reduced gradually.

Agitation

An agitated patient is frightened and treatment needs to be rapid. Agitation may stem from anxiety alone, or be the result of an acute confusional state. Pain, constipation or urinary retention can also be precipitating factors and must be excluded.

Haloperidol 10 mg, patient is given hourly until the patient settles. It can be given intravenously. Diazepam is useful, if a greater sedative effect is required in a dose of 10 mg PO or PR repeated hourly until the patient settles. Up to 50 mg may be required. Rectally, the injection solution is absorbed faster than the suppository form. Repeated use of the injection solution may cause local irritation. Diazepam can be given intravenously. If a patient becomes increasingly agitated on diazepam, this is an indication to change to chlorpromazine. Initially give 50 mg PO or 100 mg PR, repeating hourly until the patient settles. Titrate the dose to an 8-hourly regimen. Midazolam 1–2 mg. IV can be better than diazepam.

Depression

Depression can be mistaken for sadness, which is a natural emotion felt by most patients. Indicators of depression are early morning wakening and feelings of guilt or worthlessness. Suicidal ideas may reflect a wish to retain control over life or a wish to be less of a burden, and are not always a consequence of depression.[3] Somatic symptoms (*e.g.*, weight loss, anorexia, insomnia) cannot be used as markers of depression. A skilled counsellor is invaluable for depressed patients, in addition to a course of antidepressant. Amitriptyline is the first choice, starting at 25 mg and increasing every few days up to 150 mg.

Confusional States

Confusion in cancer is not inevitable and can often be treated or made tolerable. It may present as disorientation, misinterpretation, short term memory loss include drugs (sedative, opioids, corticosteroids) infection, metabolic disturbances, cardiac or respiratory failure, and in susceptible patients, a full bladder or bowel.

When trying to understand confused patient, a useful concept is that confusion reduces the number of messages from the environment and increases those from the body and memory stores, while making it difficult to differentiate the source of the messages.[4]

The implication is that self awareness is at least partly intact. While this may cause some patient to be very frightened by the confusion it does provide a means of managing confusion. A further implication is that sedative drugs should not be used routinely in order to preserve awareness.

Differentiate between Misinterpretation and Hallucinations.

Psychotropic drugs may be required, if a patient is too agitated to be helped.

Haloperidol 10 mg PO/SC should be given hourly until the agitation settles. If more sedation is required use a short acting sedative such as chlorpromazine 50 mg PO/IM or 100 mg PR, repeated hourly until the agitation settles.

Guidelines for Managing Confusion

Hallucinations arise without an outside stimulus and may need treatment

Diagnose cause : (always suspect drugs)	**Treat, if possible**
Provide	A company (family or friends) A constant routine Light, quite environment
Listen for clues	To understand confusion (ask the attendant)
Explain the cause	It may make the confusion less frightening
Reassure	The patient is still sane
Reorientate	Provide hooks onto which they can hang their reality

Anticholinergic side effects occur (dry mouth, constipation, blurred vision, difficulty in micturition). Dothiepine can be tried in the same doses, or Mianserin 30–90 mg. In general agitated and anxious patients respond to sedative drugs such as amitriptyline and dothiepine, whereas withdrawn and apathetic patients will require less sedative drugs such as imipramine 25–150 mg. It may take a month or more to see a response, after which the doses can be reduced gradually to half of the highest daily dose.

Refusal of medication should be respected unless a patient is likely to injure himself or others.

Listening for clues may uncover a fear of dying, guilt or anger which at least will allow an understanding of the patient's behaviour.

Misinterpretation results from garbled environmental messages poorly interpreted. They can be made worse by droperidol 5–10 mg nocte.

REFERENCES

1. Gilbert RW. Epidural spinal cord compression from metastatic tumor. Annals of Neurology, 1978; 3(1): 40–51.
2. Power KG. Controlled study of withdrawal symptom and rebound anxiety after diazepam, BMJ, 1985; 290: 1246–1248.
3. Stedford A. In: Facing death Patient's family and professionals, 1984; 109–121.

•••

ADVANCED MALIGNANCY: SPECIAL PROBLEMS

26

Hydration and Feeding

There is sometimes an overwhelming need for relatives and staff to give patient water and food. This natural feeling should not be allowed to override the patient's need for comfort. There is no evidence that symptoms of experimental water deprivation or hyponatremia are seen in patient's with advanced cancer.[1] Indeed, intravenous hydration can be distressing and in a very ill patient some dehydration can actually improve comfort. Urinary output drops, so reducing the need for catheterization, and troublesome bronchial secretion lessens. In bowel obstruction, gastric secretions are less, so reducing both vomiting frequency and the need for nasogastric suction. Energy requirements are usually so low and anorexia so complete that feeding is unnecessary.

There are special circumstances, however, when hydration and feeding are both possible and reasonable. There are usually patients with the neurological problems with swallowing. Some of these patients may still have many months of life that they wish to live to the full. In contrast, by the time patients with oesophageal or gastric tumours have completely obstructed they are usually far too ill for feeding or hydration to be justified.

Assistance with feeding : In patients with neuromuscular dysphagia, it is possible with practice and patience to help some patients to swallow by positioning, manual pressure at specific points and the gentle use of droppers to deliver fluids.

Clinifeed tube : This is a fine bore; soft and self lubricating nasogastric tube which is usually well tolerated by patients. The tube is too soft to allow aspiration of the gastric contents and needs a wire introducer to stiffen it sufficiently to allow easy passage. It can pass into the trachea during insertion and gastric placement should be confirmed by:

1. A chest X-ray (when the tip should be below the diaphragm).
2. Injecting 20 mL air into the tube (when bubbling should be heard over the stomach with a stethoscope).

Of the two methods chest X-ray is preferable.

Pharyngostomy may be useful in the very few patients requiring lengthy nasogastric feeding because of swallowing or feeding difficulties. It can be performed under a short GA and results in a small permanent fistula below the jaw angle into which a fine bore feeding tube can be easily inserted.

Diabetes in Advanced Cancer

Drug requirements

The need for hypoglycaemic agents usually reduces as the disease progresses. Reduced food intake and weight loss are major factors. The aim of treatment changed from preventing future complication to preventing symptomatic hypoglycaemia or hyperglycaemia. Acceptable blood glucose ranges are wider, 6–12 millimole /litre fasting and 8–20 mmol/L non-fasting.

Noninsulin dependent diabetics can usually reduce and even stop their oral hypoglycaemic drugs without symptomatic hyperglycaemia occurring.

Insulin dependent diabetics may wish to simplify bd or tds regimens to long acting once daily insulin, such as ultratard. Postprandial blood glucose peaks of up to 20 mmol/L may be well tolerated. This is preferable to distressing symptoms of repeated hypoglycaemia and insulin requirement can often be halved. As the disease progresses insulin requirement will drop further. It is not necessary to continue insulin in comatosed patient because of their cancer.

Diabetes and Corticosteroids

Corticosteroid induced diabetes: Latent diabetes may become hyperglycaemic on corticosteroid but are usually asymptomatic. Thirst and polyurea can be treated with diet, if the patient still has an adequate intake. A short acting oral hypoglycaemic such as tolbutamide bd may be needed.

Non-insulin dependent diabetics already on an oral hypoglycaemic may do better. Once daily insulin if the hyperglycaemia is symptomatic. The simplest regimen is as follows:

Day 1	Insulin 20 units
Day 2	Insulin + stop oral hypoglycaemic
Day 3	Insulin + check fasting glucose

Thereafter, adjust insulin dose according to the fasting glucose (6–12 mmol/L).

Insulin dependant diabetics may need more insulin, but at the same time insulin requirements are reducing because of reduced intake and weight loss. Consequently it is often possible to leave insulin dose unchanged.

Head and Neck Cancer

Pain is the commonest complaint, followed by dysphagia (38%), airway obstruction (28%), fungating ulcer (14%) and mucosal dryness with major bleeding occurring in less than 1 %.[2]

Pain

Co-analgesics are often required. Tumour expansion with small fascial compartment and nerve compression by perineural spread of tumour will respond to high dose dexamethasone. Pain from local bone invasion is treated in the same way as bone metastasis with a combination of analgesic and NSAIDs. Infection is often present and the resulting pain may respond to antibiotic. Nerve destruction is likely in locally invasive lesions and may respond to amitriptyline. Nerve blocks can be of help, especially in brachial plexus involvement. Radiotherapy should always be considered.

Dysphagia

This may be due to tumour obstruction, neuromuscular incardination due to perineural spread of tumour, or splinting of the pharynx by fibrosis and local tumour. Short-term relief can be achieved from high dose dexamethasone and radiotherapy. Dysphagia due to oesophageal candidiasis is easily treated. It is now always helpful to feed or hydrate very ill patient, but when this is appropriate fine bore tube feeding system or even a pharyngostomy are well tolerated.

Airway Obstruction

Strider due to tracheal obstruction by tumour is frightening to the patient and needs urgent treatment. High dose dexamethasone starting with 8 mg IV stat, followed by radiotherapy is the treatment of choice. Fortunately obstruction usually develops over several days, making urgent tracheostomy unnecessary. Referral for excision /vaporizations by carbon dioxide laser should be considered, if this is available.

Fungating Ulcers

Once the area is cleaner and has less odour, there may be a large fascial defect or an orocutaneous fistula which leaks saliva, water and food needing frequent dressing changes. Silastic foam comes as a liquid which is mixed with a catalyst (0.2 mL catalyst to every 10 mL silastic foam) and poured into cavity. A soft, well fitted sponge formed which is comfortable, cosmetically preferable to bulky dressings, and easily washed. To prevent the liquid from the pharynx before it has set, "cling film" can be fitted in and around the fistula, allowing the foam to be poured in with complete safety. The film peels easily away from the set sponge.

Mucosal Dryness

Excessive crusting within the nose following radiotherapy can be softening with 25% glucose in glycerol drop 8 hourly. Secretion and crust can then be loosened with steam inhalation and removed by regular normal saline douches.

Lymphoedema

Oedema due to fluid retention or a low albumin will usually respond to simple measures such as elevation and mild compression. In cancer patient's lymphoedema is due to blockade of lymphatics by malignancy or fibrosis consequent on previous radiotherapy or surgery. It can cause severe swelling, pain and loss of mobility and often needs more intensive treatment. It is a condition that can be treated.

Initial treatment consists of doing the following daily elevation of the arm or leg when sitting or resting. Gentle exercises morning and evening, elastic sleeves and stocking to be worn all day, but which can be taken off at night, and massage. More intensive treatment consists of a compression pump which gently squeezes fluid out of the arm with an inflatable sleeve or, in some centres, a combination of bandaging and massage.

The swelling may resolve in days. However, it can take a year to reduce swelling especially if the lymphoedema has been present for many years. Even if the swelling has not gone down by much, the limb is often more comfortable and easier to move. Most people find they have to continue indefinitely with some treatment such as gentle exercise or wearing a sleeve or stockings. The fluid removed finds its way into general circulation and excreted by kidneys.

Swollen arms and legs are more likely to become infected and dry, cracked skin provides an entry for infection. Careful and thorough skin care is, therefore, essential to keep the skin supple.

Elevation

Arms: When resting in chair or bed during the day arm should be raised to shoulder height by using pillows on the arm rest or small table next to the chair. A sling can worsen the lymphoedema.

Legs: The leg should be up when sitting, at least level with the hips. The foot of the bed can be raised at night by 2–3 inches.

Exercise : This should be gentle, each being done 5–10 times twice a day.

Compression stocking and sleeves : Stocking and sleeves prevent fluid accumulating and give firm support; they must provide enough pressure which should be graduated, being highest at the hand or foot. Some sleeves are made to measure by fitter (in the hospital for shock). "Off the shelf" sleeves are usually cheaper and as effective. Some firms make half and full gloves for those patients with finger or hand swelling. Most leg stocking will take care of foot swelling.

When fitting ensures that there are no crease or wrinkles, and never roll the tops over since this area will act like elastic bands. Initially it is best to wear the stocking / sleeves all days, but taking it off at nights. After a few months it may be possible to leave them off for a few hours. If a separate mitten is used it should never be taken off while the sleeve is still on.

Massage : Massage stimulates the lymphatics near the skin to drain fluid more efficiently and helps to relieve discomfort. The simplest method is to use a hand held electric body massager, the massager comes with an assortment of detachable heads, but the smooth, rounded head need to be used. No lubricant should be applied. Switch to the lowest setting, the massager is rested on the skin with gentle pressure and moved in a circular motion. Massage should start on the unaffected side, front and back, moving across to affected side and down to the affected fingers or toes, concentrating on the root of a limb.

Compression Pumps

These are only needed for swelling that is resolving slowly. They are powered from the mains and intermittently pump up an inflatable sleeve into which the limb has been placed. In the first week the pressure is gradually built up from 30 mm of Hg for 30 minutes once daily to 60 mm Hg 60 minutes twice daily. When using pump, keep the limb elevated and support it on pillow. It is best to remove a compression sleeve or stocking when using a pump, but if they are left the pump pressure should be reduced to 40 mm Hg. Larger pumps with sequentially inflated sleeves can be used in resistant cases.

Cellulitis

This should be suspected in a limb which is red, feels hotter or if the patients complain of acute pain, a burning sensation and feel unwell. Phenoxymethyl penicillin (penicillin V) 500 mg 6 hourly (or erythromycin 500 mg 6 hourly) should be started immediately, continuing on half this dose after one week for at least 6 weeks.

Skin Care and General Advise

The patient should be advised that careful skin care is essential to prevent an entry of an infection, with consequent risk of cellulites. Care includes protection with gloves in garden or kitchen, prompt antiseptic care of cuts and scratches, avoiding direct sunlight or heat, care when manicuring nails, using moisturizing cream at night, avoid shaving with wet razors, and wearing a thimble when sewing. The limb should be used as normally as possible but the patient should not carry heavy shopping with an affected arm or do any exercise actively that makes the limb tired or uncomfortable. Restrictive clothing is best avoided. Finally injections, blood pressure reading or blood samples should not be taken from the affected limb.

REFERENCES

1. Billings JA. Comfort measures for the terminally ill. Is hydration painful? American Geriatrics Journal, 1985; 33(11): 808 - 810.
2. Aird DW. Clinical care in head and neck cancer patients, ENT Journal 1983; 62: 10–30.

CANCER : CHILDREN AND ELDERLY PATIENTS

27

Symptom Control in Children with Cancer

As with the adults, a trusting relationship, together with the maintenance of a reassuring environment is the keystone to effective symptom control in children. This section, however, deals only with the physical control of the commoner symptoms.

Pain

An understanding of child development is essential, particularly when confirming the presence of pain in the pre-school child. It is necessary to look for secondary effects such as the different quality of a cry, irritability, anorexia, insomnia or anxiety. Patients are usually the best judges. Diagnosing the cause of the pain will depend on skillful interpretation of the previous history, symptoms and signs.

Analgesics choice and dose: The principle of the analgesic staircase should be used. Starting doses are shown below. It should be noted that children aged 0–1 years are more sensitive to morphine than older children aged 7–15.[1] It is not unusual for children aged 6 and above to require 'adult 'doses of 5–30 mg or more 4 hourly.

1. The starting doses for strong opioids – Assume the child was previously on a weak opioid.
2. Increased bedtime doses will usually avoid the need for 2 am doses.
3. Laxative should always be prescribed prophylactically.
4. A routine antiemetic is not needed. If nausea or vomiting occurs on an opioid use haloperidol.
5. Controlled release morphine (MST) 5 mg tablets are available on a named patient basis.
6. There can be no indications for using other opioids.
7. Children aged year 0–1 who are inadequately controlled on paracetamol can be switched directly to oral morphine at the doses shown.

Table 27.1 : Starting doses for analgesics in children

Drug Non-opioids	Frequency	0–1	2–5	6–12	13–16
Aspirin (dispersible) Paracetamol (tabs, elixir)	4 hourly 4 hourly	 60 mg	75 mg 120 mg	150 mg 250 mg	300 mg 500 mg
Weak opioids Codeine (tabs, syrup) Dihydrocodiene (elixir)	 4 hourly 4 hourly		 0.2 mg/kg	 0.5 mg/kg 0.5 mg/kg	 15 mg 30 mg/kg
Strong opioids Morphine sulphate (soln) Diamorphine HCl (soln, tabs)	 4 hourly 4 hourly	 0.15 mg/kg 0.1 mg/kg	 3 mg 2 mg	 5 mg 3 mg	 10 mg 5 mg
Controlled released morphine sulphate (MST tabs)	12 hourly		10 mg	20 mg	30 mg

Drug Presentation and Routes of Administration

Constant care and a little imagination are essential when selecting appropriate routes of administration. Contrary to manufacture's belief, children often prefer tablet's to sickly-sweat syrups and elixirs. The taste of solutions and soluble tablets can be improved, if mixed with a fizzy drink or fruit juice. Sublingual preparations are not usually well tolerated and are impractical for young children. The rectal route provides effective and rapid absorption. Subcutaneous infusions using portable, infusion pumps is very simple and effective.

Co-analgesic

NSAIDs and corticosteroids have the indications for pain relief as in adults. Typical doses are shown in Table 27.2.

Table 27.2 : Co-analgesia in children

Drugs	Frequency	0–1	2–5	6–12	13–16
NSAIDs					
Aspirin	4 hourly	–	75 mg	150 mg	300 mg
Naproxen	12 hourly	–	–	10 mg/kg	250 mg
Corticosteroids					
Dexamethasone (low dose)	8 hourly		0.5–1 mg	1–2 mg	2–4 mg
Dexamethasone (high dose)	8 hourly and lunch time	2 mg	3 mg	4–16 mg	

Steroid-induced Cushing's can be severe in children and doses must be reduced to the minimum, required to control symptoms. Battery-driven pump can also be used.

Constipation

Co-danthramer can be made more palatable in a milk shake or by adding fizzy fruit juice. Alternatives are mixing the contents of a co-danthramer capsule with ice-cream, or fruit flavored co-danthramer ice-lollies. Co-danthrusate capsules or senna are solid alternatives, but their relative potencies must be taken into account. Docusate (tablets or syrup) is a weak contact laxative which offers a milder alternative in children.

Bronchial Secretions

As in adults this can be eased with hyoscine hydrobromide (Table 27.3).

Table 27.3 : Hyoscine hydrobromide in children

Drugs	Frequency	0–1	2–5	6–12	13–16
Hyoscine hydro-bromide	2 hourly PRN	15 mcg/kg	150 mcg	300 mcg	30–600 mcg

Nausea and Vomiting

Nausea and vomiting may be due to the tumour, radiotherapy or chomotherapy (Table 27.4).

Table 27.4 : Antiemetics choices and doses

Drugs	Frequency	0–1	2–5	6 –12	13–16
Acting on CTZ					
Haloperidol (tabs, elixir)	12 hourly	25 mcg/kg	200 mcg	400 mcg	1.5 mg
Acting on vomiting centre					
Cyclizine (tabs, inj, suppository)	8 hourly	1 mg/kg	12.5 mg	25 mg	50 mg
Acting on upper gut					
Domperidone (tabs, susp)	8 hourly	0.1 mg/kg	1 mg	5 mg	10 mg
Domperidone (suppos)	8 hourly	0.2 mg/kg	3 mg	15 mg	30 mg

It must be noted that:

1. Low doses of Cyclizine need to be given parenterally. The via a continuous SC infusion pump.
2. Chlorpromazine is an alternative, if greater sedation is required.
3. Metoclopramide is not recommended because of increased risk of extra pyramidal side effects in children.

Agitation

When a calm reassuring environment is insufficient to settle a child, psychotropic drugs, may be necessary. Physical causes of agitation, such as pain must be excluded, if possible. Drug choices and doses are as follows:

Initial doses may have to be repeated until the child settles.

Haloperidol is the least sedative of choice.

Diazepam, if given rectally, the sodium solution is absorbed more rapidly than the suppositories. Repeated use of this injection locally may cause rectal irritation. Diazepam can accumulate and the consequent drowsiness can be mistakenly attributed to cancer.

Midazolan can be used in 1–2 mg doses 1M/1V allowing immediate and reliable action.

4. Age need not alter pain thresholds or tolerance. The similarities of pain experience between elderly and younger patients are far more common than are the differences.
5. Cognitive impairment, delirium and dementia are serious barriers to assess pain in the elderly. Sensory problems such as visual and hearing changes may also interfere with the use of some of the pain assessment scales. However, the clinicians should be able to obtain an accurate self-report of pain from most patients.
6. NSAIDs can be used safely in elderly patients, but their use requires vigilance for side effects, especially gastric and renal toxicity. Opioids are safe and effective when used appropriately in elderly patients; however, elderly patients are more sensitive to analgesic effects of opiate drugs, experience higher peak effect and longer duration of pain relief. (Acute pain management. Operative procedures, USA).

Analgesics may be given safely to geriatric patients, although adjustments of doses are usually required *e.g.*, plasma levels of tricyclic antidepressants are usually higher for a given dose in older as compared to younger patients. I.M. morphine produces longer duration of analgesia in older patients, in part related to prolonged elimination from blood in the elderly[3]. In addition, elderly as well as younger patients with central nervous system disease may be more sensitive to opioids. So the titration of analgesic dose to a given response is even more critical in such patients.

Table 27.5 : Drug choices and doses

Drugs	Frequency	0–1	2–5	6–12	13–16
haloperidol (tabs, inj, elixir)	12 hourly	25 mcg/kg	200 mcg	400 mcg	1.5 mg
diazepam (tabs, elixir, suppos, inj)	nocte	0.2 mg/kg	2–4 mg	5–10 mg	5–40 mg
chlorpromazine (tabs, syrup, suppos)	8 hourly	0.5 mg/kg	5–10 mg	10–25 mg	25–100 mg

Elderly Cancer Patients

Pain considerations in elderly patients can be as follows.[2]

1. Elderly patients often suffer multiple chronic, painful illness and take multiple medications *e.g.* for ischaemic heart disease, diabetes, etc. They are at greater risk for drug-drug and drug-disease interactions.
2. Pain assessment presents unique problems in elderly, since these patients may exhibit physiological, psychological and cultural changes associated with pain.
3. Physicians and elderly patients consider pain to be a normal part of aging. There is a belief that pain cannot be relieved and elderly patients are stoic in reporting.

- ★ The age does not decrease pain perception and sensitivity in the elderly, although emotional suffering related to pain may be less in older patients. The psychosocial factors affecting pain treatment are fairly common.
- ★ Dementia or memory impairment in the elderly leads to cognitive impairment, are unable to attend OPD alone and require special considerations for assessment and treatment.
- ★ There is a significant social, psychological and physical activity limitation in the old patients.

The rule for pharmacological interventions in the elderly is to start low and go slow in view of various diseases existing, or drug interactions. A nurse assisted PCA is effective with none cognitively impaired patients.

Involvement of family and friends in the treatment of old patients helps in treatment compliance and psychosocial problems, especially when there are cognitive impairment and daily activity limitations.

REFERENCES

1. Dahlstorm, Dohle B. Morphine kinetics in children. Clinical Pharm. and Therapeutics.1979; 26(3):354–365.
2. Harkins SW, Price D et al. Geriatric pain. In: Textbook of pain. Wall PD& Melzack R (Eds), 3rd Edition, Churchill Livingstone, Edinburgh, 1994; 769–783.
3. Kaiko RF, Wallelnstein SZ, Rogers AG et al. Narcotics in the elderly. Med. Clinic North America 1982; 66: 1079–1089.

●●●

PSYCHOLOGICAL ASPECTS OF CANCER PAIN PATIENTS

28

Cancer patient faces various stresses like fear of death, physical disability, disfigurement and growing dependency on others. These fears may vary between individuals depending upon patient personality, coping abilities, social support and medical factors. Pain has a profound impact on mood, anxiety, along with complex diagnostic and therapeutic challenges. A multi-disciplinary approach, recognizing the importance of psychological symptoms and psychiatric complications (anxiety, depression, delirium)[1] are presently the best option.

Psychological Impact of Cancer

After an initial period of shock, denial and disbelief, follows a period of anxiety and depression leading to disturbed sleep, diminished appetite, irritability and pervasive thoughts about cancer. These stress responses generally occur temporarily for a few weeks at specific points in the course of cancer *e.g.,* after diagnosis, with relapse, prior to diagnostic tests, surgery, radio and chemotherapy. Psychiatric intervention is not necessary, although anxiolytic sedation and relaxation techniques along with support of family, social workers and hospital staff helps the patient.[1]

Pain is the most feared consequence of cancer. Pain is a psychological process involving nociception, perception and expression and requires addressing both physical and psychological issues, requires services of neurology, neurosurgery, anaesthesiology, rehabilitation medicine, in addition to psychiatrists. Unfortunately psychological variables which are consequences of pain often propose to be the sole cause of pain without addressing to medical factors.

Psychiatric Disorders in Cancer

After an adequate control of pain, it is imperative to reassess the patient's mental state for psychiatric disorders which may increase mood disturbances and thus morbidity and mortality. After a thorough assessment and accurate diagnosis, the treatment of depression, delirium needs behavioural and psychopharmacology.

Depression

Depression occurs roughly in 20–25% of all cancer patients and prevalence increases with higher levels of disability, advanced illness and pain.[2]

The somatic symptoms of depression (*e.g.,* anorexia, insomnia, fatigue, weight loss) are unreliable and lack specificity. Thus psychological symptoms of depression *e.g.,* hopelessness, guilt, suicidal tendency are of greater diagnostic value.[3] A family history of past episodes and organic causes like corticosteroids, chemotherapy, amphotericin, whole brain radiation, etc., further supports the diagnosis of depression. Carcinoma of pancreas patients are associated with higher rate of depression than that of other intra-abdominal malignancies.

Treatment – Depressed cancer pain patients are treated with a combination of antidepressant medication, psychotherapy and cognitive, behavioural techniques.[2] Psychopharmacological treatment is the mainstay of symptom management.

Table 28.1 : Tricyclic antidepressants

Drugs	Doses (mg/day)
Amitriptyline	25-125
Doxepin	25-125
Imipramine	25-125
Decipramine	25-125
Nortryptiline	25-125
Clomipramine	25-125
Second generation	
Bupreprion	200-450
Trazodone	150-300

Serotonin specific re-uptake inhibitors

Fluoxetine Sertraline	20-60 50-200

Heterocyclic antidepressants

Maprotiline Amoxapine	50-75 100-150

MAO inhibitors

Isocarboxazid Phenalazine Tranylcypromine	20-40 30-60 20-40

Psychostimulants

Dexamphetamine Methylphenidate Pemoline	5-30 5-30 37.5-150

Neuroleptics

Haloperidol	20-100

Benzodiazepines

Alprazolam	0.75-6

Others

Lithium carbonate Buspirone	600-1200 15-60

ECT for severely depressed patients, or when antidepressants pose unacceptable side effects.

Anxiety in Cancer Pain Patients

Anxiety syndromes in cancer patients are due to:

1. Reactive anxiety related to the stresses of cancer and its treatment.
2. Manifestation of a medical or physiological problem *e.g.,* uncontrolled pain (organic anxiety disorder).
3. Phobias, panic and chronic anxiety disorders

Reactive Anxiety

Anxiety at critical moments (*i.e.,* waiting for diagnosis, surgery, procedures) can disrupt ability to function normally, interfere with relationships and ability to understand/comply cancer treatments. Benzodiazepines, behavioural techniques, relaxation can reduce the distress.

Organic anxiety

Uncontrolled pain, infection, metabolic derangements can be treated with analgesics, oxygen, antibiotics and antihistamines, steroids related anxiety can be treated with benzodiazepines or low dose antipsychotics.[4] Encephalopathy, hyperthyroidism, carcinoid, primary and metastatic brain tumour also leads to anxiety.

Phobias and Panic

Panic attacks, needle phobia or claustrophobia follow a critical moment and can complicate treatment of cancer. Relaxation training, systematic desensitization and antipsychotic drugs often help control the patient's fear.

Organic disorders – Delirium and dementia incidence may vary from 15–75% depending upon the progress of disease. Other organic disorders are dementia, amnesia, delusion, hallucinations, intoxications, personality and withdrawal disorders.

Delirium is a global cerebral dysfunction characterized by concurrent disturbance of consciousness level, attention, thinking, perception, emotion, memory and sleep awake cycle. Aetiology of delirium is unknown and there is a waxing and waning of above symptoms, often reversible except in terminal multiple organ failure. Haloperidol can control delirium, but produces extrapyramidal symptoms, dystonia, hyperthermia, confusion and high CPK level. Later can be treated by dantrolene sodium. In the last days of patient, methrimeprazine, or midazolam can be used as an alternative to neuroleptics.

Confusional states[6] in cancer is not inevitable and can often be treated or made tolerable. It may present as disorientation, misinterpretation, short-term memory loss and include drugs (sedative, opioids, steroids), infection, metabolic disturbances, cardiac or respiratory failure and susceptible patients – a full bladder or bowel.

When trying to understand a confused patient, a useful concept is that confusion reduces the number of messages from the environment and increase those from the body and memory stores, while making difficult to differentiate the source of the messages. The implication is that self awareness is at least partly intact. While this may cause some patients to be very frightened by the confusion, it does provide a means of managing confusion. A further implication is that sedative drugs should not be used routinely in order to preserve awareness. Haloperidol 10 mg per hour until agitation settles.

Guidelines for Managing Confusion[6]

Diagnose cause : drugs ?	—	treat if possible
Provide	—	accompany, constant routine
Listen for clues	—	to understand confusion (ask relatives)
Explain the cause	—	makes confusion less frightening
Reassure	—	the patient is still sane
Reorientate	—	provide hooks on to which they can hang their reality

Cancer Pain and Suicide

Inadequately controlled pain or poorly tolerated pain can cause suicidal tendency. In addition mood disturbances, hopelessness, depression, delirium in advanced stage of cancer, pre-existing psycopathology, suicide history and inadequate social support.

Euthanasia persistent pain and terminal illness are the primary reasons for those who request for physician-assisted suicide. From a medical perspective, uses of suicide as manifestation of psychiatric disturbance to be prevented. However, philosophically, many in our society view suicide in those who face the distress of a fatal and painful disease like cancer as 'rational' and a means to regain control and maintain a 'dignified' death. This subject is often debatable by physicians (active euthanasia) and public (passive euthanasia).

Active euthanasia is often tolerated under condition that (*i*) the patient's consent is free, conscious explicit and persistent (*ii*) the patient and physician agree that suffering is intolerable (*iii*) other measures of relief have been exhausted (*iv*) second physician must concur (*v*) these facts must be documented. Incidence is 1.8% of deaths in Netherlands. Common reasons for requesting euthanasia[6] loss of dignity–57%, pain–46%, unworthy dying–46%, dependence on others 33%, tired of life 23%.

Cancer Pain and Family (Second Order Patients)

Family members are called upon to provide emotional support, basic care taking, share responsibility for medical decision making,weathering financial and social cost. A programme for family members should include in pain management issues like assessment, administration of medicines, addict emotional support and stress management. In addition to family the staff nurses are also intensively involved in the palliative care and face treatment failures and psychological burnouts.

Cognitive – Behavioural Interventions in Cancer Pain

Hypnosis, biofeed face and multifunctional behavioural interventions are used as adjuncts in cancer pain management. Behavioural includes self monitoring, anticipating anxiety and avoiding it.

Relaxation Technique – Achieve a physical and mental state of relaxation. This includes (1) Passive relaxation (2) Progressive muscle relaxation (3) Medication (4) Focused breathing. Once relaxed patient can use imagination to manipulate or distract pain. Patient imagery includes (1) Pleasant distraction (2) Transformational (3) Dissociative imagery. The patient can imagine pleasant pain free experience, a pain free walk and breaking pain cycle.

Hypnosis – A stage of heightened focus concentration can manipulate pain perception. Three principles of hypnosis are self hypnosis, relax, not fighting the pain and use a mental filter to ease the hurt in pain.

Biofeedback – Includes electromyographic and electroencephalographic assisted relaxation. However, analgesia is not maintained after treatment stops.

Music Therapy – Can capture focus of attention away from pain while aroma therapy can have relaxing and stimulating qualities.

In the end it can be concluded that cancer pain patients are most vulnerable to psychiatric complications needing proper management with antipsychotic drugs along with psychotherapy and cognitive behavioural therapy.

REFERENCES

1. Massive MJ, Holland JC.The Cancer patients with pain; Psychiatric complications and their management. Medical Clinics of North America 1987;71:243–258.
2. Massive MJ, Holland JC. Depression and the cancer patient. Jour Clin. Psychiatry,1990;51:12–17.
3. Plumb MM, Holland JC. Comparative studies of psychological function in patients with advanced cancer. Psychosomatic Medicine,1977;39:264–276.
4. Stiefel FC, Breitbart W, Holland JC. Corticosteroids in cancer : Neuropsychiatric complications. Cancer Investigation,1984,7:479–491.
5. Helig S. The San Francisco Medical Society euthanasia survey, Results and Analysis, San Fransisco Medicine,1988; 61: 24–34.
6. Kumar P. A Hand book of Management of pain and related symptoms. Samvedna, New Delhi, Reprint 2004,29.

•••

29

CANCER THERAPEUTICS

As a patient becomes semiconscious due to the cancer, prescribing requirements will change. The oral route becomes impractical and the need for some drugs will change or cease.[1]

Table 29.1 : Prescribing the drugs in the last hours or days

Drug	Suggested change	Consider
Analgesics		
Paracetamol, aspirin,	Stop	Diamorphine SC 2.5 mg PRN.
Weak opioids	Diamorphine SC 5–10 mg 4 hourly	
Strong opioids	Diamorphine SC 4 hourly at equivalent do dose	SC infusion of Diamorphine
NSAIDs		
e.g., flurbiprofen	Stop	Diamorphine SC 2.5 mg PRN
Corticosteroids		
e.g., dexamethasone	Stop	–
Laxatives		
e.g., co-danthramer	Stop	–
Antiemetics		
Haloperidol	Continue by SC	Prochlorperazine PR
Cyclizine	Injection or infusion	Cyclizine PR
Metoclopramide	-do-	Chlorpromazine PR
	-do-	Domperidone PR
Psychotropic drugs		
Temazepam, Nitrazepam, Diazepam	Diazepam PR	Chlorpromazine PR
Haloperidol	Cont. by SC injection or infusion.	Diazepam PR
Chlorpromazine	Chlorpromazine PR	-do-
Antidepressants	Stop	–
Anticonvulsants	Diazepam PR 5–10 Mg 4–8 hrly.	–
Anti infective	Stop	Alternative treatment For bronchial secretion
Cardiovascular		
Anti arrhythmic	Stop	–
Diuretics	Stop	–

Other drugs		
Bronchodilators	Stop	Hyoscine SC 0.4–0.8 mg 8th hourly
Insulin	Stop	
Hypoglycaemics Iron and vitamins	Stop	

Subcutaneous Infusion Pumps

Should parenteral administration be necessary, repeated injections can be distressing to the patient, nurse and family, and difficult to organize in the home. Continuous SC infusion is a suitable alternative.

Drugs: Diamorphine, morphine sulfate, hyoscine and metoclopramide can be used safely. Cyclizine and methotrimeperazine occasionally cause local irritation. Chlorpromezine prochlorperazine and diazepam are too irritant and should never be used in a SC infusion pump.

Drug Interactions

There are many such drug interactions, but those below are probably of most importance to patients with advanced cancer.

Table 29.2 : Interaction of drugs used in cancer patients.

Drug affected	Interacting drug (s)	Effect
Analgesics		
paracetamol aspirin	metoclopramide	Raised peak blood levels
diamorphine	pentazocine CNS sedatives	Reduced analgesia Increased risk of sedation.
Steroids		
corticosteroids	Loop diuretics, thiazides, phenytoin, carbamazepine aminoglutethemide	Hypokalemia Decreased effect of steroids Decreased effect
dexamethasone		
Antiemetics		
chlorpromazine	propranolol	Increased blood levels
cyclizine	antacids	Decreased Absorption
phenothiazines	phenothiazines	Increased anti-cholinergic tricyclic side effects
metoclopramide	Anti-cholinergic Drugs with anti-cholinergic effects (tricyclics, cpz) opioids haloperidol	Antagonism of metoclopramide Stimulation of upper gut increase in peak blood level of opioids Extra pyramidal side effects
Anticonvulsants		
carbamazepine	dextro-propozyphene, cimetidine	Potentiation
phenytoin	cimetidine, co–trimoxazole, diazepam	Potentiation
CNS sedatives		
diazepam	cimetidine	Increased blood levels
chlormethiazole	cimetidine	Potentiation

Cardiovascular Drugs		
digoxin	bumetanide, furosemide, thiazides cholestyramine	Increased toxicity Due to potassium depletion Decreased absorption
bumetanide	corticosteroids	Antagonism due to Fluid retention
furosemide	indomethacin corticosteroids beta blockers	Hypokalaemia Reduced anti-hypertensive effects NSAIDs
Blood iron (oral)	Antacids, tetracycline	Decreased absorption
Anti-infective ketoconazole	Antacids, anticholinergic, Cimetidine	Decreased absorption
Metronidazole	Alcohol	Disulfiram reaction

Table 29.3 : Common drug doses and side effects

Drug	Dosage	Side effects
acyclovir	P.O. 200 mg 6 hourly (for 5 days)	Rashes, transient rise in urea/ creat
amitriptyline	P.O. 50 – 50 mg nocte	Sedation, dry mouth, constipation
aspirin	P.O. 600 mg 4 hourly	GI irritation, hypersensitivity
baclofen	P.O. 5–30 mg 8 hourly	Drowsiness, fatigue, confusion hypotension, nausea
benzydamine	As a rinse or gargle 15 mL 2 hourly	Local numbness
bethanechol	10–30 mg 8th hourly	Nausea, vomiting, sweating, blurred vision, colic, bradycardia
bisacodyl	P.O./P.R.10 mg after food	Colic, local rectal irritation
bumetanide	P.O. 1 mg daily in morning	Polyurea + loss
buprenorphine	S.L. 1–2 tablets 6–8 hourly	Nausea, vomiting
chlorpromazine	P.O. 25–100 mg 4–8 hourly P.R. 100 mg 6th hourly	Extra pyramidal symptoms, anti-cholinergic effects, hypotension (rarely jaundice)
cholestyramine	P.O. 4 g in water 6th hourly	Constipation, anorexia, nausea, Colic rashes
cimetidine	P.O. 400 mg bd or 800 mg nocte	Confusion, reduced hepatic metabolism
co danthromer	P.O. 10 mL syrup- 10 mL forte syrup bd	Colic perianal rash
co danthrusate cyclizine	P.O. 1 nocte to 3–8th hourly P.O. 50 mg 4–8 hourly	Colic perianal rash Dry mouth, drowsiness, headache
dantrolene	P.O. 25 mg daily upto 100 mg 6th hourly	Weakness, fatigue, nausea, vomiting, drowsiness

dexamethasone	Low dose P.O. 2–4 mg daily (low dose 12–15 mg) not later than 6 pm	Obesity, moonface, candidiasis
diazepam	P.O. 5–20 mg at night	Drowsiness confusion, poor co-ordination, subjective change in voice
diflunisal	250–500 mg bd with food	Nausea, constipation, colic, diarrhoea
dihydrocodiene	30–60 mg 4–6 hourly	Constipation, vomiting
dimethicone	As asilone 10 mL 4–6 hourly	–
distigmine	5–20 mg before break fast	GI irritation, salivation
docusate sodium	100–200 mg 8 hourly	Diarrhoea, colic
domperidone	P.O. 10 mg 8 hourly/Pr 60 mg 8 hourly	Galactorrhoea, gynaecomastia (long-term)
flurbiprofen	P.O. 50–100 mg bd	GI irritation, hypersensitivity
frusemide	P.O. 50–80 mg mane	Polyurea, K^+ loss, rashes
haloperidol	P.O. 1.5 –10 mg nocte	Extra pyramidal symptoms
hyoscine hydro-bromide	S.L/P.O. 0.3–0.8 mg 6-8 hourly	Drowsiness, dry mouth, blurred vision, ileus, constipation, difficulty micturating
ketoconazole	P.O. 200 mg mane For 1 week	Nausea, constipation, rashes, itching
loperamide	2–4 mg PRN (max 16 mg daily)	Nausea, dizziness, dry mouth
metoclopramide	S.C/P.O. 10 mg 4–8 hourly	Extra pyramidal effects, sedation, diarrhoea, dizziness
mianserin	P.O. 30–90 mg nocte	Mild anticholinergic effects
morphine	Median = 20 mg 4 hourly	Nausea, vomiting, constipation
nystatin	P.O. 100,000 units 4 hourly	–
paracetamol	P.O. 0.5–1gm 4–6 hourly	Rare–skin rashes
phenoxybenzamine	P.O. 10 mg nocte	Tachycardia, postural hypotension, dizziness, lassitude
prochlorperazine	P.O. 5–10 mg 8 hourly/im 12.5 mg 6 hourly	Drowsiness, dry mouth
propantheline	P.O. 15–30 mg 8 hourly	Anticholinergic effects
spironolactone	100–200 mg	GI irritation, high K^+, gynaeco-mastia
temazepam	P.O. 10–60 mg nocte	Morning drowsiness
tetracycline (intrapleural)	500 mg in 20 mL 0.5% bupivacaine	Transient local pain, pyrexia

REFERENCES

1. Kumar P. Management of cancer pain and related symptoms. New Delhi, Samvedna, Reprint 2004.

•••

HOSPICE CARE IN CANCER PATIENTS

30

In medieval period in Europe hospices were shelters for the pilgrims. Hospice programmes take bedside care of the dying by ensuring continuity of care across home and inpatient settings. The programmes address needs of patient's pain which left unattended can lead to hopelessness and disability along with patient's family who are emotionally and physically depleted. Palliative and supportire care for terminally ill patients and family can be provided by director on consultation.

Aims of Intractable Cancer Pain in Hospice[1]

1. Identify cause to better treat.
2. Prevent pain – anticipate and prevent rather than treat.
3. Erase pain memory – thus decrease the dosage.
4. An unclouded sensorium.
5. Normal effect relate to environment.
6. Decrease of suffering, increase function and setting therapeutic goals with the help of family.

The hospice model of pain management is as per WHO three step ladder using following methods by a physician, nurse, family and social workers:

1. Drugs
2. Neural blockade
3. Neuroaugmentive – TENS
4. Physical/occupational therapy – exercise, hot/ cold applications.
5. Behavioural: Hypnosis, imagery, relaxation, prayer.
6. Symptom treatment – constipation, vomiting, diarrhoea, bedsores.

Central place of family : In 80% of patient days of care, family members are involved. The family members are helped by nurses, counsellors, social workers. There should be one or more people on call for emergencies 24 hours a day.

The terminally ill patient relies heavily on family members for toilet, bath, medications and the fear of being alone. Adult sons, daughters, relatives, neighbours all are expected to play particular role depending on their jobs and personal ties with the family.

Psychological and spiritual support: The social workers, priests can listen to fears, worries, help clear planning and control the fear, anger, forgiveness to the patient and the family members. They provide bereavement services and transport, cremation for the dead patient.

The palliative care in the hospice enhances comfort and improves the quality of the patient's life. The disease has taken over and the goal of controlling its spread is no longer realistic.

Protocol of Hospice Programme

1. Support staff members of the team meet the patient and his family.
2. Proper authorization by physicians for treatment of pain and related symptoms.
3. Informed consent about protocols of hospice management.
4. Radiotherapy – No active treatment, only conservative radiotherapy on and as need basis for pain and disease control.
5. Chemotherapy, IV antibiotics, blood transfusions, hyperalimentation.
6. Intravenous hydration, if tube feeding fails.
7. Minor colostomy can be performed for relief of symptoms.
8. Oxygen can be used as a comfort measure.

Reasons for Hospice Care

1. A perception of physicians and patients that technology would overcome disease and death always leads to disappointment in terminally ill.
2. Health profession not geared to deal with treatment failure.
3. Obligation to dying patient and family not fulfilled by therapy.
4. Care during active treatment re-emphasized.

Types of hospice programmes

1. Acute hospital care–oncology unit, medical - surgical departments.
2. Inpatient hospice programme–licenced home health agencies.
3. Community Home Health agency–licenced home-health agencies.
4. Long-term facilities – nursing and intermediate care facilities, and 1–3 beded.
5. Case management programme–Spiritual, social, volunteer and bereavement.
6. Volunteer hospice programmes–physician, nurses, social worker follows upto hospital mission.

Admission policy:

1. Diagnosis of cancer.
2. Life expectancy less than 5 months.
3. Referral from family physician.

   It should be made clear to the family and the patient that these services are not curative but palliative only.

Home Care Services:

1. There should be a need of the skilled service.
2. An evidence of family or caregiver should be present before allowing home care.
3. Communication with nearby hospice shall be maintained.

Principles and planning of hospice:

1. Inpatient and his family are treated as a unit of hospital care.
2. Neighbours, friends and others can be primary caregivers.
3. Values, preferences and outlook on life of the patient and his family to be considered.
4. Physiological, medical appliances, drugs, psychological, social, spiritual, economic problems of the patient and family must be fully understood and taken care of.
5. Multidisciplinary medical service team consists of a physician, nurses, social, spiritual volunteer, psychological and bereavement services.
6. Palliative treatment of pain and other physical symptoms, psychological problems.
7. Round the clock services to the patients dying at home, facility for inpatients.
8. Continuous medical care to reduce the feelings of isolation and abandonment.

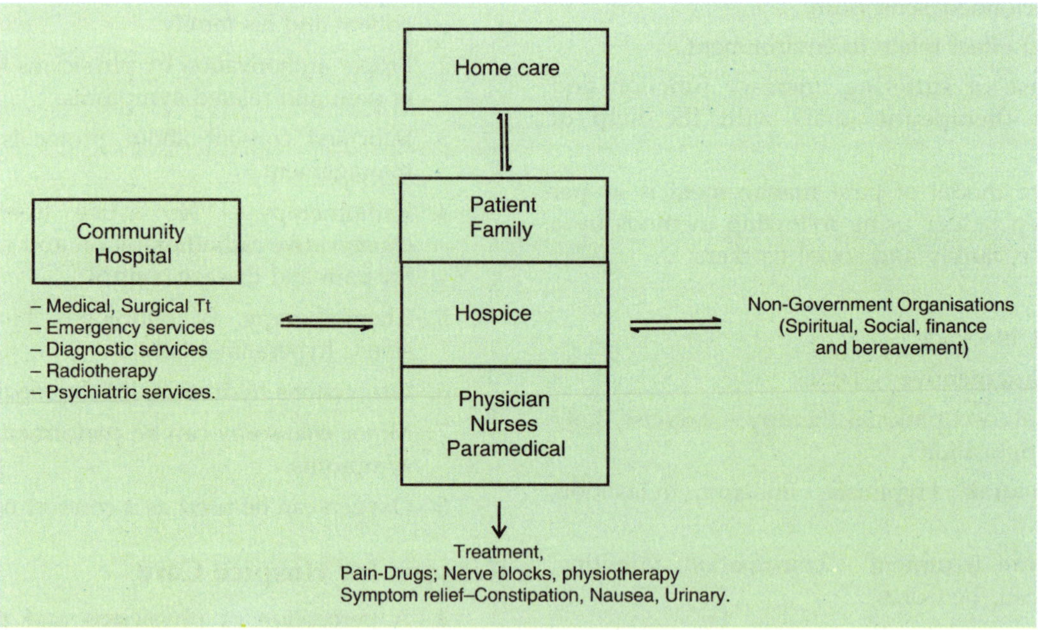

Fig. 30.1 : A flow diagram of hospice care

Hospice ownership

Hospital owned – 46%,
Independent – 35%,
Community – 25%.

Types of Hospice care

Home care – 56%

Inpatient+home care – 31%

REFERENCES

1. Burchman, SL and Ewen, JM. Hospice care–critical issues for the future. In Practical Management of Pain. Raj, PP(Ed). Mosby year book. St. Louis. 1992; 491–504.

•••

PROTOCOL FOR MALIGNANT PAIN THERAPY

31

Treatment of Cancer Pain

Unrelieved pain causes suffering, anger, anxiety, fear, depression and suicidal tendencies. Relief ensures good quality of life.

Basic Principles and Approach to Cancer Pain Management

By modifying the source of pain by treating the cancer: surgery, radiation, bone metastases, chemotherapy.

By altering the central perception of pain: analgesics, antidepressants, anxiolytics.

By interfering with nociceptive transmission within the CNS, Neuraxial analgesia.

Neuroablation.

Psychological care.

Alternative pain management strategies: Acupuncture, TENS.

Immobilization: Rest, cervical collar.

Assessment of cancer pain

Comprehensive assessment is required.

- Type.
- Intensity.
- Pain source.
- Psychological factors.
- Assessment of treatment/pain relief.

WHO analgesic ladder. (Revised in 1996)

Simple and effective method for controlling cancer pain by oral administration of analgesics including oral morphine.

Effective pain relief is achieved in 75–90% of patients.

Ist Step– (Mild Pain)

NSAIDs.

2nd Step–(Moderate Pain)

Mild opioids

NSAIDs

Adjvuvants.

3rd Step–(Severe Pain)

Alternative methods

Nerve blocks,

Continuous infusions,

Strong opioids.

Oral Opioid Therapy

First line approach for patients with moderate to severe pain

Principles of drug therapy for cancer pain

By the mouth

By the clock

By the ladder

For the individual

Attention to detail is vital.

Dose titration = right dose = adequate pain relief with minimal side effects.

Transdermal fentanyl (Duragesic patch) provides continuous transdermal delivery pf fentanyl for 72 hours.

First line modality for moderate to severe pain.

Adjuvant drugs – Tricyclics, steroids (plexopathy pain) , anxiolytics

Laxatives are almost always necessary with opioids. More than 50% need antiemetics

Home Care Services

Terminal patients

Predominant complain pain

Oral NSAIDs, tramadol.

Oral morphine

- Usual dose 50–100 mg per day.
- Rare cases 250 mg per day.
- Nutritional supplementation.
- Psychological support.

Drawbacks

– Retrospective assessment of pain and pain relief according to pain score is not available.

– Accessible only to patients residing in Metros.

Direct drug delivery systems

– Neuraxial drug delivery.

– Intraspinal opioid therapy.

Contraindications

– Thrombocytopenia.

– Coagulopathy.

If these are present, PCA with IV or SC morphine is used.

Numbing the nerves in cancer patients–peripheral nerve blocks

When the drugs are ineffective, nerve blocks provide effective pain relief.

Experts in nerve blocks are few and far between.

Aids – X-ray, imaging aids, CT scan.

– Nerve stimulators, special electrodes, needles.

– Requires hospital admission.

Training needs

– Convince medical authorities.

– Provide adequate facility for training.

– Provides platform for interaction.

– Knowledge database.

Advantages

– Effective and long lasting.

– Reduces frequent visits to doctors.

– Good quality of pain relief.

– 50 – 80% patients may benefit.

Nerve blocks

1. L.A. – lignocaine, bupivacaine.

   Reduced concentrations – lignocaine 0.5%, bupivacaine 0.25%.

2. Diagnostic – somatic or visceral, autonomic block.
3. Side effects assessment – fall in blood pressure, reduced sensation.
4. To determine efficacy of neurolytic blocks.
5. Pain relief outlasts its pharmacologic action.
6. Disadvantages – pneumothorax, haemorrhage, infections.
7. Use of steroid along with L.A. reduces swelling around tumour for weeks.
8. Catheters – spinal, epidural produce symptom relief for weeks.

Neurolytic blocks

Useful in terminal cancer patients.

Advantage for Indian patients (rural areas).

Economically poor background.

Cost effective.

Longer duration of pain relief (4–6 weeks).

Stay at home.

e.g., subarachnoid chemical neurolysis for gynaecological and rectal malignancies.

Success rate 80%.

Neurolytic agents used

– *Absolute alcohol*–painful, intense, recurrence

– *Phenol* 5–10%, biphasic, painless

– *Chlorocresol*

– *Ammonium sulphate*

Neurolytic blockade of peripheral nerves

Used when other therapies:

– fail

– ineffective

– poorly tolerated

– clinically inappropriate

Side effects

– Neuritis

– Recurrence – of pain within a few months *e.g.*, with alcohol.

– In partial/complete denervation further chemical damage to nerve possible.

– Dysaesthetic (neuropathic pain).

Peripheral nerve blocks

– Trigeminal

– Stellate

– Glossopharyngeal

– Intercostal

– Celiac plexus

– Hypogastric plexus.

Regional neurolytic blocks

1. No neuropathic pain
2. When more extensive block needed
   – extensive growth of tumour
   – Increase in pain.
3. Easy access of spinal, epidural routes

Subarachnoid neurolytic blocks

Indications – cancer of cranial nerves
– tumour involves somatic nerves (Breast, abdominal wall, abdominal viscera, pelvis)

Hypobaric absolute alcohol

- patient positioned with involved dermatomes in upper portions
- proper positioning of operative table
- appropriate padding
- stability of patient position
- needles inserted at appropriate level
- 0.10 to 0.25 mL injected at appropriate level

Leave patients for 20 minutes to consolidate block.

Hyperbaric subarachnoid neurolytic block

- Phenol in 10% glycerine, prepared fresh
- Wide bored 18–21 G needles used for phenol
- Patient position–affected position downwards
- 0.5 mL aliquots of phenol for each segment.

Benzocaine

- highly lipid soluble local analgesic
- satisfactory analgesia
- motor blockade, bladder/bowel dysfunction.

Epidural neurolytic block

- 5–10% phenol in saline
- used in bilateral pain
- no motor blockade
- useful for limb plexus block
- slight nerve deficits
- side effects – neuritis
  - excessive spread
  - accidental subarachnoid injection.

Complication of S.A and epidural neurolysis

- less pain, relief after satisfactory block
- unplanned sensory motor deficit
- weakness, numbness, incontinence, neuropathic pain.

Celiac plexus block

Indications – pain due to carcinoma of pancreas, and gastrointestinal tract.

Disadvantages

Blocks may have to be repeated after 6–8 weeks.

Possibility of muscle paresis.

Need of CT scans or C arm image intensifier.

Trained personel to perform the block.

Neuroxial administration of narcotics and NSAIDs

- Using catheter delivery systems.
- Home care possible.

1. **Morphine**–Side effects: pruritis, urinary retention, Respiratory depression, nausea, vomiting, delirium.
2. **L.A.**–Side effects: weakness, numbness, fall in B.P.
3. **Steroids** In inflammatory neuropathy in epidural space.
4. **Clonidine** – $\alpha 2$ adrenergic agonist
5. **Benzodiazepine**
6. NMDA antagonists.
7. Ion channel blocks.
8. NSAIDs.
9. Cholinesterase inhibitors.

Neurosurgical ablation:

- In terminal cancer with short life expectancy.
- Dorsal rhizotomy– No long-term effect.
- Interrupt lateral spinothalamic tract of spinal chord.
- 95% success rate initially,>1year – 25%.
- No analgesia in cervical, upper thoracic.
- Mortality 1% unilateral, 10% bilateral.

Dorsal route entry zone lesioning:

- For refractory deafferentation pain *e.g.*, nerve plexus avulsion.

Deep brain stimulation

- Neurosurgical implantation of electrodes.
- Pain relief–30%–60%.
- In peri aqueductal, peri ventricular grey matter.
- Sensory thalamus in deafferentiation pain.

Radio frequency ablation

First line of treatment in chronic malignant pain syndrome.

Expensive equipment required.

Skilled radiologist required.

Effective method of pain relief, lesion is selective, controllable.

Low incidence of morbidity and mortality.

Neurolytic surgical procedures

- Cryo lesioning.
- Thermo coagulation of Gasserian ganglion.
- Low complication, better pain relief.
- >75% success rate > 9 months.
- Pituitary ablation (side effect – diabetes insipidus).

•••

ROLE OF NON-GOVERNMENT ORGANIZATIONS IN RELIEF OF CANCER PAIN

32

Introduction

Population of India has exceeded 100 crores. At least 0.6% of this population needs palliative care for incurable diseases like cancer and AIDS. Upto 78% of such patients live in rural areas of India. Most of cancer treating centres are situated in urban areas of India. Government run rural primary health centres are overburdened with infective diseases patients. Emphasis of government is to use Rural Primary Health Centres for immunisation and family planning programmes. Resources available can provide palliative care only to the limited number of patients even in crowded urban and Cancer hospitals of India.

Hospital Care

Hospice type of complete palliative care though considered ideal in western countries, have only a limited role in India. Due to financial constraints, only limited number of patients can be treated in these centres. Unfortunately most of these hospice care units are also situated in urban hospitals or semi urban hospices around cities.

Home Care

Cancer pain relief by providing free oral morphine tablets and training centre for cancer patients and their relatives is working at Rajasthan Hospital, Ahmedabad, since last five years[1]. Treatment at this centre has following advantages.

1. This non-government institute runs palliative care programme, encourages home care of terminal cancer patients in their homes in urban as well as rural areas of Gujarat, Rajasthan and Madhya Pradesh.
2. Oral morphine tablets (Plain as well as SR) are provided free for Control of Cancer Pain with support from Global Cancer Concern India.
3. Patient or their relatives are encouraged to visit this centre every two weeks or every month to collect free oral morphine tablets and seek guidance for their symptom control.
4. A trained staff nurse and a computer expert works under guidance of a doctor in this centre.
5. Patients and their relatives are provided free guidance of symptom control with Audio-visual Computer Video Programmes. Printed data and instructions are provided to the relatives for home care of the terminal cancer patients.
6. A trained nurse is employed to guide and training of patients and their relatives at their homes.
7. Strong family support available in India is utilized for success of this home care programme.
8. Control of cancer pain is achieved in practically all patients. Symptom control is discussed in four enclosed charts.

Clinical Report

312 patients (Table 32.1) were treated during 12 months period of November 2000 to December 2001. 67% patients were male, 33% patients were females. 66 patients received 10 mg oral morphine tablets. 62 patients received 30 mg SR oral morphine tablets. 26 patients received 30 mg plain oral morphine tablets. 158 patients were treated as 'Demonstration Patients'. (As per enclosed tables)

Table 32.1 : Patients treated during November 2000 to December 2001

S. No.	Diagnosis	Male	Female	Patient	%
1.	Ca Breast	0	40	40	12
2.	Ca Lung Mets	95	19	114	37
3.	Ca Osteosarcoma	5	02	07	2

4.	Ca Rectum	12	05	17	5
5.	Ca Pelvis	18	07	25	9
6.	Ca Mouth Care	47	15	62	20
7.	Ca Abdomen	33	14	47	15
8.	Total patient	210	102	312	100

- 158 patients (Fig. 32.2) were given demonstration on audio-visual computer video programmes. 96 (64%) patients were males and 62 (36%) patients were females. 158 demonstration patients had main symptoms as follows:
- Constipation patients – 13, Dressing patients – 30, Guidance patients – 85, colostomy and catheter care patients – 30.
- 85 (54%) patients required guidance of Medial and Surgery treatment.
- 30 (19%) patients required training of colostomy and urinary catheter care.
- 30 (19%) patients were trained to undertake dressing of wounds at home.
- 13 (8%) patients were taught home care of constipation including enema at home.
- Demonstration and training of following procedures is undertaken on the patient as well as on computer as required. Training on computer is repeated for illiterate and less educated patients or relatives.
- The computer training course contents are:
  - (*a*) Soap water enema for chronic constipation.
  - (*b*) Glycerine syringe for daily bowl movement.
  - (*c*) Diet control including oral esabgul to control constipation.
  - (*d*) Dressing of open wounds and ulcers in cancer patients.
  - (*e*) Taking care of mouth, teeth and gums and mouth wash in oral cancer patients.
  - (*f*) Bedsore dressing and care of the skin in bed-ridden patients.
  - (*g*) Ryle's tube feeding in oral and oesophageal cancer patients.
  - (*h*) Gastrostomy tube feeding and dressing.
  - (*i*) Prosthesis implantation in breast cancer patients.
  - (*j*) Tracheostomy wound and tube's care and suction of trachea.
  - (*k*) Colostomy tube and wound care.
  - (*l*) Sponging and shampoo and skin care.
  - (*m*) Urinary catheter care.
  - (*n*) Health education on use of Morphine Tablets.
  - (*o*) Psychotherapy is also given.
  - (*p*) Yoga, physiotherapy and breathing exercises.

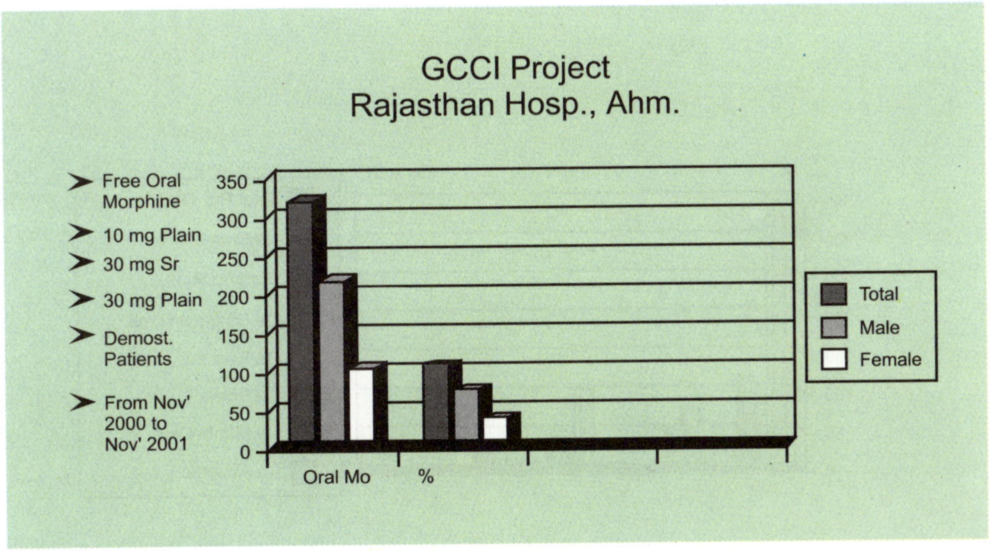

Fig. 32.1 : GCCI Project

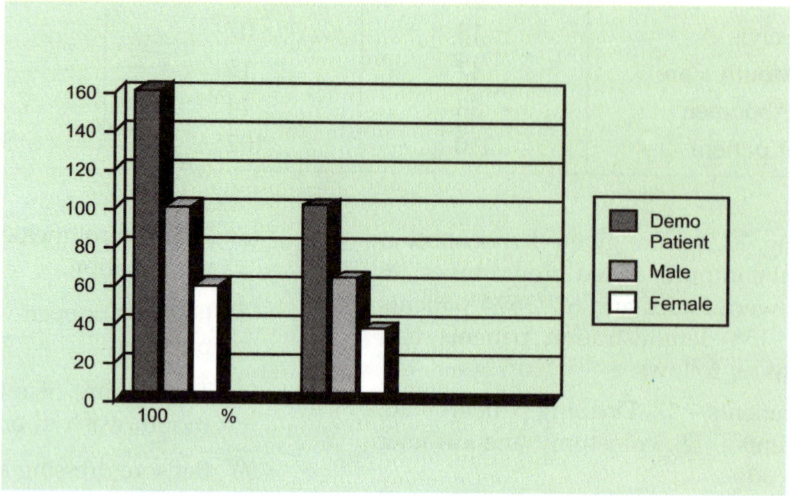

Fig. 32.2 : Demonstration on audio-visual computer video programme

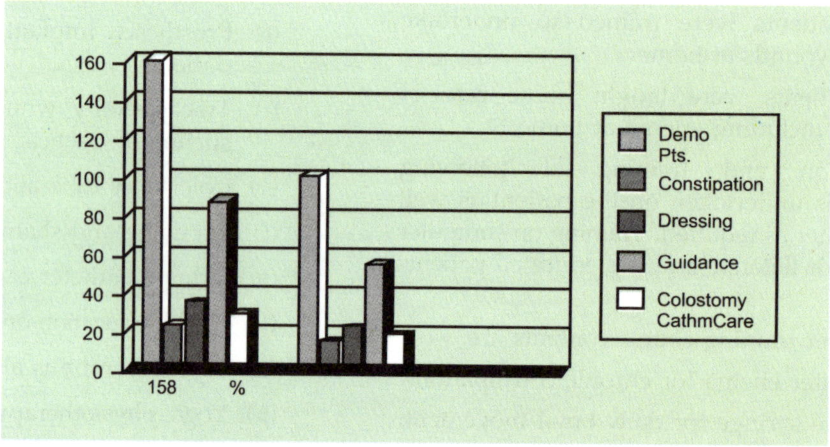

Fig. 32.3 : Symptomatic care

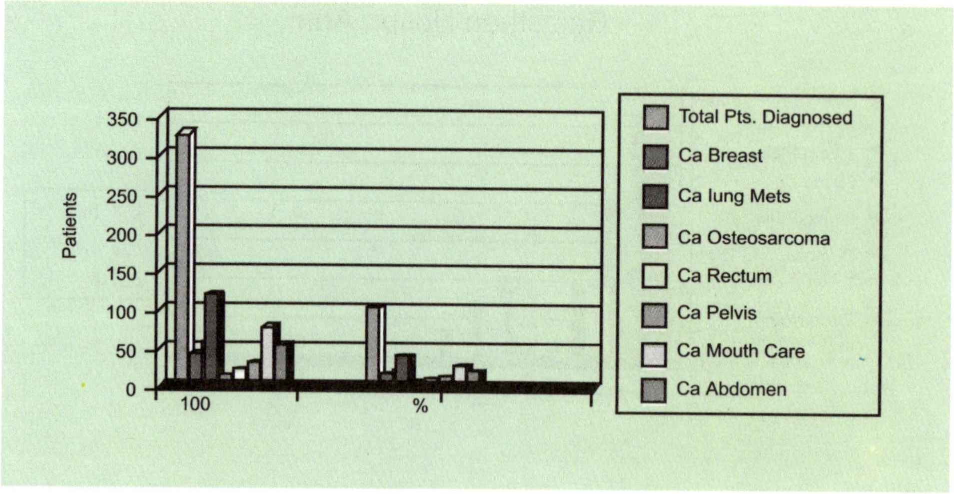

Fig. 32.4 : Cancer patients at pain OPD

Available List of NGOs Working on Cancer Pain in India

1. Indian Society for Study of Pain:

   Over 1300 life members from various specialties working on pain. Established in 1984 at Varanasi under Dr. K. Pandey's guidance with Dr. A. Lal, V. Rastogi, secretary and Dr. Pramod Kumar as treasurer. It is Indian Chapter of International Association for Study of Pain. Official Organization Indian Journal of Pain; present address Dr. R. P. Gehdoo, Secretary, Deptt. of anesthesiology, Tata Memorial Centre and Hospital, Parel, E. B. Marg, Mumbai. Email: rpgk@rediffmail.com.

2. International Association for Study of Pain. IASP with 63 National and Regional Chapters throughout the world. Official Organization– Pain Journal, IASP newsletter, Cancer Pain. Address:IASP Executive Officer, Louisa E Jones, 909, ME, 43rd St., suite 306, Seattle, WA-98105-6020., USA. E-mail: iaspdesk@juno.com, website: www.iasp-pain.org.

3. World Health Organization – cancer pain section.

   WHO, 20, Avenue Appra, Geneva, CH 1211.

4. Samvedna Pain Hospital, NOIDA, Gautam Budh Nagar, UP. It is the only pain hospital in India and anywhere in the world. Official publication. A Handbook on Cancer Pain and related symptoms by Dr. P. Kumar. Website http:/samvednahosp.org

5. South Asian Regional Pain Society– founded 2003 at Dhaka- address: Dr. AKM Akhtharuzzaman, Secretary General, SARPS. Bangbandha Medical College, Deptt. of Anesthesiology, Dhaka, Bangladesh. Email: pain@bd.online.com

6. Pain Clinic OPD. Dr. M. T. Bhatia. Rajasthan hospital, Shahibaug, Ahemdabad, Gujarat.

7. Dr. Rajgopal, Prof and HOD, Deptt. of Anesthesiology and Palliative Care. Medical College. Cochin- Kerala.

8. The information about the cancer pain NGO can be available with the following:

   (*i*) World Health Organization, South Asian Office, Indraprasth Estate-New Delhi.

   (*ii*) Or Geneva, office of WHO.

   (*iii*) Regional Cancer Institutes.

   (*iv*) Medical college pain clinic OPD in all medical colleges and institutes.

   (*v*) Indian Society for Study of Pain.

   (*vi*) Anandlok Hospital, Kolkata.

REFERENCE

1. Dr. Bhatia MT. The role of Non Governmental organizations in cancer pain.Oration Lecture. Proceedings of XVII ISSPCON, 2002.

•••

SECTION–VI

Pain Relief in Specialities

SEDATION AND PAIN RELIEF IN INTENSIVE CARE UNIT

33

The stress response to critical illness can have many deleterious effects. Appropriate use of sedation and analgesia can attenuate the stress, alleviate pain and anxiety, and improve compliance with care. Agitation responds best to anxiolytic drugs; pain is best relieved by analgesics. A combination of these drugs can act synergistically, because most analgesics provide some degree of sedation. In select cases, neuromuscular blocking agents are required, but they should not be used without concomitant sedation and analgesia. Use of agents needs to be tailored to the needs of individual patients; indication, anticipated length of need and underlying organ system derangements are important considerations.

Sedation

Sedation is a general term that refers to the calming of an ICU patient with the use of medications.

Due to a critical illness or injury, an ICU patient may experience unpleasant feelings, agitation, fear or pain. In addition, some of the procedures and supportive care such as, mechanical ventilation may make a patient feel uncomfortable. The ICU staff will attempt to comfort patients by speaking to them and by reassuring them. Often these efforts are not enough to comfort patients and sedation is required.

There are many different medications used for sedation. The selection of a specific medication for a patient depends upon many factors that the doctor must consider. Once selected, the medication may be given to a patient orally, intravenously or intramuscularly. Some medications are given only as needed and the others are given continuously.

Many ICU patients receive sedation because they are agitated. Rarely, patients may have worsening agitation with certain medications used for sedation. This is called a paradoxical reaction to the medication in view of multiple organ dysfunction.[1] Stopping the medication or switching to a different medication usually helps. Sedation is used as long as the patient remains uncomfortable, agitated, anxious, fearful, or in pain. The ICU staff will regularly decrease the medication to see if the patient still needs it.

Potential Complications Associated with the use of Sedation

Each specific medication used for sedation has its own set of side effects and complications. In general, the two most common complications of the sedative medications are depressed breathing and decreased blood pressure. The ICU staff will monitor a patient's breathing and blood pressure during sedation. Many sedative medications cause temporary amnesia and the patient may not clearly remember the events during the period of sedation. If sedation is needed for a long period of time, the patient's body may get used to it. The sedation will need to be decreased slowly in these patients to avoid withdrawal symptoms. Patients may have subsequent hallucinations, delusion, depression, post traumatic disorders and cognitive problems.

The Joint Commission on Accreditation of Health Care Organization (Chicago, Jan 1, 2001)[2], has defined four levels of sedation: minimal, moderate, deep and general anaesthesia (Table 33.1). Sedated patients should be drowsy but arousable and able to follow commands. In certain patients, especially those who are asynchronous with controlled modes of mechanical ventilation or in whom decreased oxygen consumption is desired, a deeper level of sedation is required. In general, sedation should be accompanied by analgesia because analgesics potentiate the effects of sedatives, resulting in lower sedative dose requirements. Sedation needs vary over the course of a patient's stay in an ICU. In the acute phase, a profound stress response may require deeper sedation and higher doses of analgesics. When a plateau is reached, sedative and analgesic requirements may decrease, but delirium may emerge. In the recovery phase, sedation and analgesia are tapered and discontinued.

Table 33.1 : Levels of Sedation

Minimal sedation :	Patient responds normally to verbal commands. Cognitive functions may be impaired, but ventilatory and cardiovascular functions are unaffected.
Moderate sedation :	Patient responds purposefully to verbal commands with or without light tactile stimulation. Spontaneous ventilation is adequate and cardiovascular function is maintained.
Deep sedation :	Patient is not easily aroused but responds purposefully to painful stimulation. Patient may not be able to maintain a patent airway, and spontaneous ventilation may be adequate. Cardiovascular function usually is maintained.
Anaesthesia :	Consists of general anaesthesia and spinal or major regional anaesthesia. It does not include local anaesthesia. Patients are not arousable, even by painful stimulation. The patient often requires assistance in maintaining a patent airway and positive pressure ventilation. Cardiovascular function may be impaired.

In 1995, Society of Critical Care Medicine (SCCM) task force[3] recommended midazolam hydrochloride and propofol for short-term sedation, lorazepam for longer-term sedation, and haloperidol for delirium. Most ICUs do not follow these recommendations, and sedative and analgesic regimens vary widely. Lack of a standardized approach to sedation and analgesia can lead to polypharmacy over medication or under medication and increased cost.[4]

Several scales have been used to assess the adequacy of sedation in ICUs. The simple-to-use Ramsay scale (Table 33.2) is the most common graded scale; the desired score depends on the indication for sedation. With additive scales, the level of sedation is ranked by the sum of scores in several categories. The increased numbers of categories with additive scales improve validity but make this type of scale too cumbersome for routine use. Observational sedation scales are useless in patients receiving neuromuscular blocking agents. Blood pressure and heart rate are objective indicators, but may be affected by underlying illness and drugs. Crippen[5] pioneered the use of continuous neurologic monitoring with processed electroencephalography, particularly during neuromuscular blockade. Bispectral processed electroencephalographic monitoring has been correlated with observational sedation scales and is especially useful in deeply sedated or paralyzed patients.[6]

Table 33.2 : Modified Ramsay scale for rating sedation

Indication	Score
Anxious, agitated, restless	1
Awake, cooperative, oriented, tranquil	2
Semi asleep, but responds to commands	3
Asleep but responds briskly to glabellar tap or loud auditory stimulus	4
Asleep with sluggish or decreased response to glabellar tap or loud auditory stimulus	5
No response can be elicited	6

Benzodiazepines

The benzodiazepines, which have anxiolytic and amnesic properties and anticonvulsant effects, are commonly used for sedation in ICUs. They undergo hepatic metabolism, some to active metabolites that may accumulate in the presence of renal and hepatic insufficiency. The most reliable and effective route of administration is intravenous, because the absorption of oral and intramuscular doses may vary. Benzodiazepines may be given intravenously by either intermittent bolus dosing or continuous infusion. Disadvantages of intermittent boluses include the need of high nursing input and the risk of under dosage or over dosage.

With continuous infusions, bolus doses are given to obtain the desired level of sedation and infusion is used to maintain that level. The continuing need for infusion as well as the dose should be reassessed daily; the infusion rate is decreased when sedative requirements are stable over a 24 hour period.[7] Daily interruption of infusions, when feasible, may decrease the duration of mechanical ventilation and the length of ICU stay.[8] Tolerance occurs with prolonged administration and withdrawal syndrome may accompany rapid discontinuation of the drug.

Lorazepam

It is a more potent amnestic than diazepam. Lorazepam is metabolized by the liver to inactive metabolites. The half-life of lorazepam is prolonged in setting of renal failure. It is the benzodiazepine of choice in liver failure. It is water insoluble and is dissolved in a propylene glycol carrier.

Table 33.3 : Comparison of parenteral benzodiazepines

Drug	half-life hours	onset(min) dose	equivalent dose IV	bolus	comment
Diazepam	20–66	3–5	0.3–0.5	2–20	not recommended for continuous infusion
Lorazepam	10–20	10–20	0.05	1–4	drug of choice in hepatic failure; may accumulate in renal failure
Midazolam	1–4<3	0.15–0.3	3–5		peripheral distribution prolongs effects; hepatic and renal

Three benzodiazepines diazepam, lorazepam, and midazolam are available for parenteral use (Table 33.3). Onset and duration of action are determined by lipid solubility. Respiratory depression and hypotension are dose-dependent. Hypotension occurs primarily in hypovolemic patients and is potentiated by the concomitant use of opioids.

Diazepam

This water soluble drug is metabolized by the liver to an active metabolite, desmethyldiazepam, which has a half-life of 48–96 hours. Diazepam is not recommended for continuous infusion.

Midazolam

It is water soluble and can be administered intravenously without irritation. It is metabolized by the liver to the less potent 1-hydroxy-midazolam. Accumulation can occur in the setting of renal and hepatic failure. Midazolam is the most potent amnestic and produces greater decrease in blood pressure in hypovolemia than diazepam does. Despite the relatively short half-life of midazolam, extensive distribution can cause prolonged sedation. Recovery time is proportional to the infusion's duration; therefore, midazolam infusion generally should not exceed 48 hours.

Benzodiazepine Reversal

Flumazenil is a competitive antagonist of benzodiazepine effects. It is administered intravenously at a dose of 0.2 mg and increased to a maximum of 1 mg, which may be repeated at 20 minute intervals to maximum dose of 3 mg/hour. Caution is needed with long-term benzodiazepine use, because withdrawal seizures may occur.

Other Sedatives

Barbiturates and ketamine hydrochloride are no longer commonly used for sedation in ICUs. Etomidate, short acting sedative used for rapid sequence intubation, can produce adrenocortical suppression after a single dose, making it inappropriate for use in critically ill patients.[9]

Propofol

It has a rapid onset of action and short half-life. It has amnestic effects, but not to the degree of benzodiazepines. It is metabolized at least partially by the liver to inactive metabolite and excreted by the kidneys; however, the presence of renal or hepatic dysfunction does not significantly affect clearance. It can accumulate in peripheral tissues, prolonging sedative effects. Tolerance to the drug has been reported after more than 7 days of use but may occur sooner.

Adverse effects include hemodynamic and respiratory depression, pain with peripheral administration and green discolouration of the urine. Hypotension is dose and rate dependent. Propofol is dissolved in a lipid emulsion, and prolonged infusion requires frequent monitoring of triglyceride levels to avoid pancreatitis. This risk may be reduced by using the 2% rather than the 1% formulation.[10]

With Propofol the time to extubation is shorter once the drug is discontinued, but the degree of hypotension and cost are higher than with midazolam.

Haloperidol

It is a butyrophenone derivative with a half-life of 14 hours. It is used for the treatment of delirium in ICUs. Although not approved by the US FDA for intravenous administration, it has been shown in many studies to be safe when administered by this route.

Hypotension may occur in hypovolemic patients. QT-interval prolongation, torsades de pointes, and neuroleptic malignant syndrome are infrequent, but life threatening adverse effects. The recommended dose for intermittent intravenous administration is 1 to 10 mg every 4 to 12 hours.

Analgesia

Patients in ICUs may experience pain related to underlying illness or injury, medical procedures and therapies, causing anxiety and discomfort, interference with sleep, prevention of early mobilization, and augmentation of the stress response. In patients with multiple organ system derangements, treatment of pain may compromise other system functions (causing respiratory depression or hypotension), and agents must be chosen with this in mind.

Opioid analgesics are the drug of choice for pain relief in the critically ill. Opioid analgesics are metabolized primarily by the liver and excreted in the urine. Tolerance may develop with prolonged administration.

Route of administration vary, but narcotic analgesics are most commonly given intravenously, by either intermittent bolus or continuous infusion. The I.V. route is preferred in ICU patients because absorption may vary with other routes. In alert patients, continuous patient-controlled analgesia can be accomplished by I.V. or epidural administration. Patient-controlled analgesia allows adjustment of narcotic medication within present limits, decreases nursing burden and reduces patient anxiety over inadequate or untimely delivery of analgesics.

The intrathecal or epidural route can be used for administration of narcotics or local anesthetics. This mode is most effective in postoperative patients; it should be avoided in critically ill patients who are immunocompromised or who have coagulopathy, because epidural haematoma or abscess may result. Anaesthetics can cause early respiratory depression and narcotics can cause late respiratory depression.

The use of intermittent I.V. boluses requires constant vigilance and a constant level of analgesia is difficult to achieve. It is important that continuous infusion be preceded by bolus dosing to achieve the desired level of analgesia; a constant level can then be maintained with continuous infusion.

Monitoring of analgesia in the critically ill is difficult. Reliable, objective measures of pain are unavailable and underlying disease or medication may alter BP and heart rate, which are commonly used indicators in non communicative patients. The visual analogue scale is useful tool for assessing pain patients who are awake and communicative, which is often not the case in ICUs.

Side effects : The major dose limiting side effect of opioid analgesics is respiratory depression. Some narcotics, especially morphine and mepridine hydrochloride, may cause histamine release, resulting in pruritus, hypotension, and smooth muscle contraction. Opioids blunt the cough reflex and the sensation of dyspnoea. All narcotics, particularly the phenyl piperidine can cause muscle rigidity, which may interfere with respiration. Hypotension generally occurs only in hypovolemic patients or in patients receiving very large I.V. doses. Narcotics reduce gastrointestinal motility and may cause nausea, vomiting, or ileus. Smooth muscle contraction may result in contraction of bladder sphincter and urinary retention.

Morphine and Meperidine (Pethidine)

Morphine is the narcotic analgesic of choice in ICUs. It has a rather slow onset owing to its lipid solubility. The active metabolite of meperidine, normeperidine, can accumulate and cause tremor, pupillary dilatation, and seizures. Doses should be reduced in patients with renal insufficiency.

Phenyl Piperidine

These are mu-receptor agonists; include fentanyl, alfentanil HCl, remifentanil, and sufentanil citrate. They are more potent than morphine and have a faster onset of action. Fentanyl is the opioid analgesic of choice in patients with haemodynamic instability[3]. Despite the drug's short half-life, redistribution into peripheral tissues occur and can cause prolonged effects. Fentanyl has an active metabolite, that may accumulate in renal failure. Alfentanil has no active metabolite, making it the drug of choice in renal failure. All phenyl piperidine are considerably more expensive than morphine.

Butorphanol can provide an effective sedation as well as a pain relief when used as intravenous infusion in patients with prolonged stay.[11] It allows tolerance of endotracheal tube, patient does not fight with the ventilator and takes care of awareness during prolonged IPPV.

Narcotic Reversal

Naloxone hydrochloride, an opioid-receptor antagonist, reverse most of the effects of narcotics. Intravenous doses of 0.4 to 2.0 mg are used. Smaller doses can reverse respiratory depression without affecting analgesia.

Non Narcotic Agents

NSAIDs are mild analgesics that inhibit prostaglandin synthesis. Prostaglandins appear to be involved in the smooth muscle contraction seen in renal and biliary colic, conditions in which these agents are particularly effective. In addition to having anti- inflammatory activity, NSAIDs are antipyretic and inhibit platelet aggregation; they do not cause the sedation, respiratory depression and hypotension that are common with opioid analgesics. Major side effects are platelet dysfunction, renal dysfunction and gastrointestinal ulceration or irritation. NSAIDs are limited by the lack of I.V. formulation; however, ketorolac tromethamine may be administered intramuscularly or intravenously. In some patients, regionally injected local anaesthetic blocks can reduce or eliminate the need for narcotic analgesics, control postoperative pain, attenuate the neurohumoral response to stress and provide analgesia and anaesthesia for invasive procedures.

Neuromuscular Blockade

Appropriate sedation and analgesia methods are usually adequate to control agitation in patients in an ICU. However, neuromuscular blockade is necessary in certain situations[12].

- ★ Severe acute respiratory distress syndrome requiring inverse ratio ventilation or permissive hypercapnia
- ★ Severe respiratory failure requiring improved chest wall compliance
- ★ Facilitation of independent lung ventilation
- ★ Excessive shivering
- ★ Need for immobility (for MRI, CT, tracheostomy)
- ★ Tetanus or neuroleptic malignant syndrome.

Neuromuscular blocking agents should never be used without concurrent sedation and analgesia.

Neuromuscular blocking agents may be used to reduce oxygen consumption,[13] control intracranial pressures or facilitate endotracheal intubation, unconventional modes of mechanical ventilation or procedures that require complete immobility.

Vecuronium bromide, atracurium besylate and cisatracurium besylate are commonly used intermediate acting neuromuscular blocking agents. Vecuronium is effective in 3–5 minutes and has a duration of action of about 35 minutes. Vecuronium may accumulate in the setting of renal or hepatic failure. Atracurium and cisatracurium are degraded by Hoffman elimination and ester hydrolysis and, therefore, do not exhibit half-life prolongation in patients with renal or hepatic failure. Laudanosine, a metabolite may accumulate in renal failure and cause seizures; however, case reports suggest that clinical doses are unlikely to result in important central effects in humans.[14] Cisatracurium is more potent than atracurium and does not cause the hypotension seen with high doses of that drug. Onset and duration of action are similar to those of Vecuronium.

Pancuronium bromide, a long acting medication, is by far the least expensive neuromuscular blocking agent used for continuous infusion in ICUs. It has a vagolytic effect on the sinus node and blocks the reuptake of norepinephrine. Tachycardia and hypertensions are the major side effects. Resistance to paralytic effect may occur with prolonged use. Piperacuronium bromide and doxacurium chloride are more potent and long acting than pancuronium but are considerably more expensive.

Monitoring of Neuromuscular blocking agents: When neuromuscular blocking agents are used, the degree of paralysis should be monitored with a peripheral nerve stimulator. The two most common sites for twitch monitoring are the ulnar nerve and facial nerve. Four electrical impulses are delivered over 2 seconds, a sequence known as train of four. In the absence of neuromuscular blockade, muscle contraction occurs with each stimulus. The usual goal is to obtain one of four twitches, which corresponds to about 90% blockade.

If no twitches occur, the "tetanus mode" may be used. 5-second stimulation generates a sustained twitch, after which the train of four sequences is repeated. If no twitches occur, the patient is over paralyzed and the neuromuscular blocking agent is discontinued until two of four twitches return. If one or two twitches occur on post-tetanic train of four, the agent is held or decreased until one or two twitches return on simple train of four.

REFERENCES

1. Bion JE and Oh TE. Sedation in intensive care manual, 4 ed. Oh T editor. Oxford; Butterworth, Heinemann. 1998;673–678.

2. Adopted from joint committee on accreditation of health care org. standards and intents of sedation and analgesia. Comprehensive accreditation manual for hospitals: The Official Handbook. Chicago: The Joint Commission, Jan1'2001 Update.
3. Shapiro BA, Warren J, Egol AB, et al. Practice parameters for intravenous analgesia and sedation for adult patients in the intensive care unit; an executive summary. Society of critical care medicine. Crit Care Med 1995;23(9) 596–600.
4. Dasta JF, Fuhrman TM, McCandles C. Patterns of prescribing and administering drugs for agitation and pain inpatients in a surgical intensive care unit. Crit Care Med 1994;22(6): 974–80.
5. Crippen DW. Using bedside EEGs to monitor sedation during neuromuscular blockade: a new way to gauge therapeutic effectiveness. J Crit Illness 1997;12(8) : 519–524.
6. Riker RR, Simmons LE, Prato BS, et al. Assessing sedation levels in mechanically ventilated ICU patients with the bispectral index and sedation agitation scale. Crit Care Med 1998;26(1) A94.
7. Blanchard AR, Love AA, Southwood RL, et al. Standardized cost effective sedation guidelines in a tertiary medical intensive care unit. Crit Care Med 1999;27(12 suppl):A131.
8. Kress JP, Pohlman AS, O'Connor MF, et al. Daily interruption of sedative infusions in critically ill patients undergoing mechanical ventilation. N Engl J Med 2000;342(20):1471–7.
9. Moore RA, Allen MC, Wood PJ, et al. Perioperative endocrine effects of etomidate. Anaesthesia 1985;40(2):124–30.
10. McLeod G, Dick J, Wallis C, et al. Propofol 2% in critically ill patients; effects on lipids. Crit Care Med 1997;25(12): 1976–81.
11. Kumar P, Sharath R. Butarphanol continuous infusion in ICU(abstract) proceedings ISSPCON Kolkata,2004.
12. Blanchard AR. Sedation and analgesia in intensive care. Medications attenuate stress response in critical illness. Post Graduate Med. 2002;111(2):59–74.
13. Crone RK, Farnitol J. The effects of Pancuronium bromide on infants with hyaline membrane disease. J Pediatr 1980;97:991.
14. Gwinnutt CL, Eddleston JM, Edwards D, et al. Concentrations of atracurium and ludanosine in CSF and plasma in three intensive care patients. Br. J. Anaesth 1990;65(6): 829–32.

•••

TRAUMA AND PAIN

34

Introduction

Trauma knows no anatomical barriers. Depending on the site and severity of trauma, physiological changes occurring can affect recovery in such patients. Goal of pain management is not only to decrease patient's pain but also to return the patient to a more normal physiologic status. Pain relief following polytrauma is the most neglected and underestimated requirement of emergency trauma management. Most of the clinicians fail to recognize the significant detrimental impact that pain has upon the recovery of trauma patients. Many series, which followed polytrauma patients, noted a very high incidence of residual damage, up to 30–40% in the form of pain syndromes. Rationale behind active pain relief is two folds; firstly pain relief promotes ambulation and movements which in turn help in restoring pulmonary functions, decrease venous stasis, DVT and pulmonary embolism. Secondly LA and opioids used in peridural block, the nociceptive reflexes are thus preventing much of the physiological derangements seen after trauma.[1]

Pathophysiology of Pain in Polytrauma

Adverse physiologic effects of pain after trauma include:

1. decreased diaphragmatic contractility;
2. chest wall splinting;
3. tachycardia;
4. hypertension;
5. increased oxygen consumption;
6. hyperglycaemia;
7. ileus;
8. splanchnic hypoperfusion;
9. fluid retention;
10. immobility;
11. irritation, insomnia and other psychiatric problems.

Therefore, understanding of pain pathways and modalities of pain transmission from periphery towards CNS are very important. It helps in assessing the pain as well as formulating modalities of pain relief.[2] Sports injuries can result into chronic pain in shoulder and knee joint (Tables 34.1 and 34.2).

Methods of Assessment of Pain

Various objective and subjective methods like adjective rating scale (ARS), numerical rating scale (NRS) and visual analogue scale (VAS) can be applied for assessment of severity of pain.

Table 34.1 : Trauma score in critical care patients

Category	Value	Points	
Respiratory rate	10–24	4	A
	25–35	3	
	> 35	2	
	< 10	1	
	0	0	
Respiratory effort	Normal	1	B
	Retractive	0	
Systolic blood pressure	> 90	4	C
	70–89	3	
	50–69	2	
	< 50	1	
	0	0	
Capillary refill	Normal	2	D
Delayed >2 sec	Delayed	1	
	None	0	

Glasgow Coma Score (GCS)					
Eye opening					
Spontaneous	- 4	1	GCS Points		
To voice	- 3		14–15	5	E
To pain	- 2		11–13	4	
None	- 1		8–10	3	
Verbal response			5–7	2	
Oriented	- 5	2	3–4	1	
Confused	- 4				
Inappropriate words	- 3				
Incomprehensible	- 2				
None	- 1				
Motor response					
Obeys commands	- 6	3			
Localizes pain	- 5				
Withdraw (pain)	- 4				
Flexion (pain)	- 3				
Extension (pain)	- 2				
None	- 1				
Total GCS Points = (1) + (2) + (3)			Total trauma score points = A + B + C + D + E		

Adapted from Champion HR, Sacco WJ. Carnazzo AJ, et at. : The Trauma Score, Crit Care Med 1981; 9:672–676,

Principles of Management in Trauma and Sports Injuries

Basic principles of active pain relief service include:

1. Decrease in the production of chemicals, which sensitize peripheral nerves.
2. Blocking nociceptive neurotransmission within peripheral nerves[3].
3. Modulating pain perception at spinal cord and CNS[4].

Table 34.2 : Principles of disaster (trauma) resuscitation (Ist hour)

Stage		Possible Interventions
Life-supporting first aid	Airway breathing	Jaw thrust, head tilt, removal of basic life support, debris from pharynx, mouth-to-mouth ventilation or equivalent
	Circulation	Pulse check, closed cardiac compressions, control of external haemorrhage, leg elevation, immobilization of cervical spine
Advanced trauma	Airway	Intubation, surgical airway life support
	Circulation	Restoration of spontaneous circulation, fluid resuscitation, vasoactive agents, defibrillation, open chest compressions, treatment of pneumo/ hemothorax (military antishock trousers suit)
	Other systems	Cerebral preservation, degree of exposure, spinal cord injury precautions, thoracic/abdominal trauma evaluation, burn assessment, pain management, definitive studies (*e.g.*, angiography)

Factors deciding the methodology are:

1. Type of environment;
2. Automatic location;
3. Presence of complications like infection and coagulopathy;
4. History of drug abuse;
5. Psychological aspect – Phantom limb;
6. Regional techniques.

(A) Epidural/ spinal placement of analgesic drugs has opened up a new chapter in management of polytrauma. Epidural and spinal anaesthesia are not recommended as a sole anaesthetic technique in acute trauma management. Low quantity of drug is used as compared to systemic route and thus avoids very many deleterious side effects. Low dose local anaesthetic singly or in combination with opioids can be used in continuous infusion to provide long duration and better quality of analgesia. These methods have additional benefits in that they help in reducing incidence of DVT as well as improve tissue perfusion by sympathetic blockade especially in vascular surgery. Most trauma textbooks have strongly recommended their use in thoracic trauma management.

(B) **Regional Blocks:** Either continuous infusion nerve blocks or infiltration anaesthesia has definite role in patients with minor injuries, but not in the management of acute pain in polytrauma where more than one area is involved. Patients who can be managed with these techniques are not subjected to unnecessary general anaesthesia thus avoiding side effects.[3]

(C) **Acupuncture/TENS:** Its role in acute manage-ment is debatable, but do have an appreciable role in chronic cases.

(D) Hypnosis and psychotherapy.

(E) Cryo neurolysis.

(F) Intrapleural medication for rib fractures and lung contusion.

(G) Peripheral nerve blocks – ankle/wrist.

(H) Intercostal nerve block.

(I) Subcutaneous morphine.

(J) Cognitive, behavioural and physical therapy.

Drugs

1. **Opioids :** Morphine still remains the backbone as it can be given safely in many formulations. Most commonly used routes are PCA , I/V continuous infusions and epidural. Newer synthetic opioids like fentanyl, Su and alfentanyl are short acting and with few side effects. Respiratory depression occurs rarely but cannot be ignored and thus demands careful monitoring. Epidural administration can provide prolonged and excellent quantity analgesia with a low dose. PCA requires sophisticated equipments and is not practiced in India.[5]
2. **Local anaesthetics:** Lignocaine and bupivacaine are most commonly used LA drugs. Lignocaine has short duration of action and comparatively safer than bupivacaine. Continuous infusion of low dose solution through epidural catheter provides safe and excellent analgesia. Continuous axillary/femoral block gives sympathetic blockade necessary in vascular grafts.[2]
3. **NSAIDs:** In acute trauma NSAIDs have little role. Ketorolac and diclofenac are the only I.M. preparation available at present and useful in minor injuries. In cases with circulatory compromise these I.M. preparation gives erratic results and are not recommended.[2]
4. **Topical application:** Refrigerant anaesthetic sprays, vapocoolents, alternative delivery techniques for topical LA drugs.[2] Iontopheresis single dose injectors and tree oils have some role in such patients.
5. **Other drugs:** Varieties of oral adjuvants are available but useful in chronic pain. Anti-depressant and other psychotic drugs are useful in chronic pain syndrome following trauma. Adrenaline, clonidine, steroids, midazolam and neostigmine are few examples of adjuvants, which prolong duration of/or improve quality of analgesia.[6,7]
6. Physical therapy, in mobilization and exercise, heat and cold care are very useful in trauma and sports injuries.

A. Sports Injuries Resulting in Chronic Knee Pain

Anterior Pain

Patellar

Chrondromalacia patellae, recurrent dislocation, subluxation or tracking problems, myofascial dysfunction quadriceps

Infrapatellar

Bursitis

Tibial tubercle

Osgood-Schlatter's disease

Anteromedial/Anterolateral Pain

- Parapatellar

  Fat pad impingement, degenerative arthritis.
- Intermediate-internal derangement

  Meniscal tear, cruciate ligament tear, synovial pinching or tear, meniscal cyst, post-traumatic arthritis, osteochrondritis dissecans.
- Extreme lateral/medial

  Collateral ligament injury, pes anserinus bursitis or myofascial dysfunction adductor muscles, entrapment saphenous nerve in adbductor canal.

Posterior

- Baker's cyst, myofascial dysfunction hamstring or calf musculature.
- Reflex sympathetic dystrophy

B. Sports Injuries Resulting in Chronic Shoulder Pain

Subdeltoid/Subacromial Pain

Tendinitis, rotator cuff, subacromial bursitis, subdeltoid bursitis, brachial plexus injury, thoracic outlet (neurovascular compression) syndromes, cervical radiculopathy.

Anterior Pain

Bicipital tendinitis, dislocating biceps tendon, subscapular tendinitis, impingement coracoacromial ligment on biceps tendon, rotator cuff tear, shoulder subluxation, myofascial dysfunction (infraspinatus, deltoid, scaleni, supraspinatus, pectoralis major, pectoralis minor, biceps, coracobrachialis).

Posterior/Lateral Pain

Haematoma of deltoid muscle, myofascial dysfunction (deltoid, levator scapulae, supraspinatus, teres major, teres minor, subscapularis, serratus posterior, triceps, trapezius).

Pain at the start of throw or tennis serve

Rotator cuff tendinitis, subdeltoid bursitis, subacromial bursitis.

Pain at the end of throw or tennis serve

Insertional tear long head triceps, tear posterior capsule, posterior osteopytes.

Pain with movement/restricted movement

Post-traumatic arthritis, recurrent dislocation.

Reflex sympathetic dystrophy

Shoulder-hand syndrome

Burns

The management of burns include management of blood loss and pain in the initial phases. Later on infection and nutrition are managed.

Table 34.3 : Phases of burn management

Phase	Management issues
Resuscitation (First 24 hours)	Airway assessment, carboxyhaemoglobin level, 100% oxygen, pulmonary toilet, blood gases, chext X-ray management of adult respiratory distress syndrome. Haemodynamic assessment, Blood pressure above 90 systolic Urine output above 0.5 cc/kg/hr Pulse under 130, IV crystaloids and colloid for shock. Wound care
Postresuscitation (2 to 6 days)	Airway maintenance, pulmonary toilet, adequate gas exchange, infection control. Haemodynamic maintenance, fluid for hypovolemia, intropes for ↓ cardiac output, acid-base and electrolyte regulation. Nutritional support, wound care.
Inflammation (7 days to wound closure)	Prevention of nosocomial pneumonia, pulmonary toilet, infection control measures, appropriate antibiotics, prevention of adult respiratory distress syndrome. Adequate nutrition, parental if needed. Maintenance of adequate oxygen delivery, blood transfusions as needed.

Rehabilitation/wound remodeling	Prevention of pain, stress, sepsis. Restoration of function to affected area. Control of scarring/contractures. Restoration of whole patient to functional activity. Pain control. Psychological support.

Conclusion

No single drug or method can provide complete and satisfactory pain relief. Tailor made combinations of drug and the delivery systems provide maximum benefits and have few side effects. Continuous infusions of local anaesthetics and one of the opioid administrations through thoracic/lumbar epidural appears to be most effective method to provide pain relief in first few hours following trauma. For isolated limb injuries, involving vessels, continuous axillary/femoral sheath block with LA and opioid solution provide not only excellent analgesia, but also help in salvaging limb. Once patient recovers after surgical intervention, one can switch over to oral NSAIDs or any other method mentioned above. Prevention of post traumatic complication is prevented by early mobilization in trauma and sports injury.

REFERENCES

1. Rybrol, Schurizer BA, Peters et al. Post operative analgesia and lung functions: a comparison of intramuscular with epidural Ketamine. Acta. Anaesthesio Scand 198,26;514–518
2. Raj PP. Practical management of pain 3rd edi., St Louis, Mosby Year Book; 1998.
3. Kehleth. The endocrine metabolic response to post operative pain. Acta. Anaesthesio Scand (suppl) 1982;74:173–175.
4. Lund C, Selmar P, Hensen OB, et al. Effect of epidural bupivacaine on somatosensory evoke potential after dermatomal stimulation.Anesth. Analg. 1987; 66:34–38.
5. Mathor LE. Parentral opioids for post operative analgesia. Res. Anaesthe. 1982;7:144.
6. Islas JA, Astorgc J, Laredo M. Epidural Ketamine for control of post operative pain, Anesth. Analg. 1985;64: 1161–1162.
7. Kinahata LM. Spinal analgesia with Morphine and Clonidine. (editorial). Anesth. Analg. 1989; 65:194.
8. Maron RR. Orthopedic aspects of sports medicine. In Appenseller O (ed): Sports medicine, ed, Baltimore, Urban and Schwarzenberg 1988.
9. Callilet R. Soft tissue pain and disability. Philadelphia, F A Davis, 1983.

•••

LABOUR PAIN

35

Labour pain represents most common form of acute severe pain and lack of its treatment results in severe psychological effects lasting in late stage of life. The figure 35.1 shows the MPQ scores in various chronic pain syndromes, acute painful conditions and labour pain. The intensity of labour pain is at the top of the pole just before the pain due to causalgia and amputation of digits[1] (Fig. 35.1). Also the treatment of labour pain managing two patients instead of one, the mother and the newborn. In India there is still a lack of awareness for the need for relief of labour pain in patients and obstetricians. This is still taken as a normal part of joyous occasion of a new birth by the family. Obstetricians also are still devoting their attention to a safe birth, instead of treating mother's pain which is still taken as a necessary evil or a curse of God to the eve. This is depriving the mother of their basic right to have pain relief. However, the scenario is changing fast in the last decade. There are many labour pain relief epidural services in some of the teaching institutions, corporate hospitals and general practitioners of obstetrics. The initial hostility of obstetricians is fast receding because of the availability of safe pain relief modalities and demand from the mother for her pain relief. The author's initial effort to start epidural pain relief for labour pain failed after a few months of its start in 1980 due to resistance from obstetricians and anaesthesiologists. The reluctance to take the load of additional burden and internal political issues were the reasons. However, in the last decade there is gradual acceptance specially amongst the younger generation.

Pregnant patients are at a greater risk than non-pregnant patients of (1) Pulmonary aspiration of gastric contents following loss of protective laryngeal reflexes. (2) Symptomatic blockade accompanying epidural or intrathecal injection of local analgesics produce profound hypotension because of aorto caval compression by the gravid uterus affecting placental and foetal well being. So aorto caval compression is avoided by the left uterine displacement and ephidrine if blood pressure is reduced.[2] (3) Cardio toxicity of bupivacaine and other local anaesthetic toxicity is more profound. (4) Opioid therapy produces more profound nausea and vomiting. (5) Activation of herpes simplex labialis raises[3] concern regarding newborn infection.

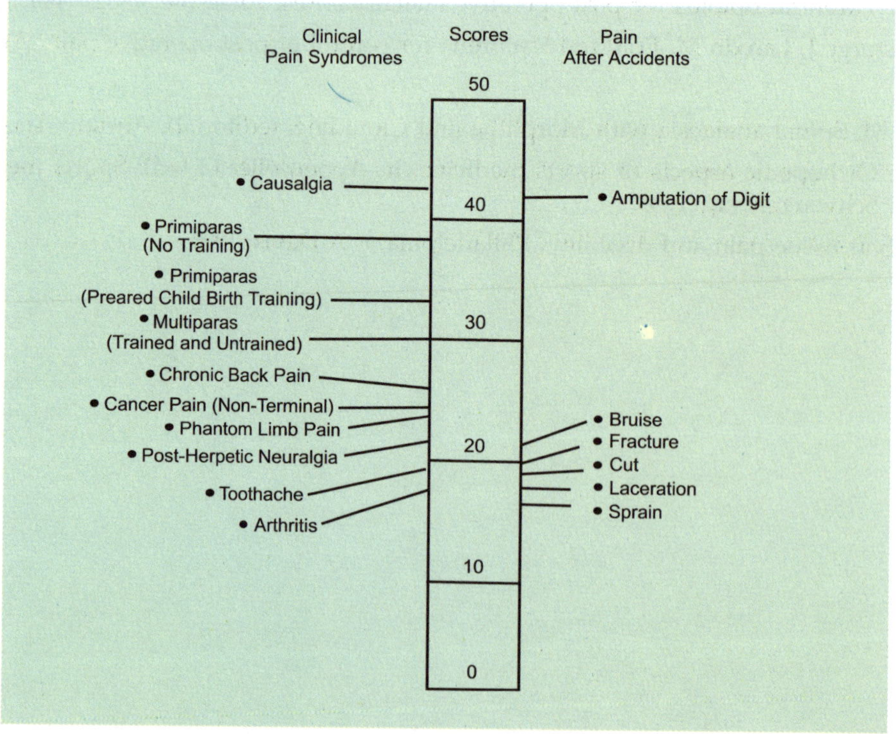

Fig. 35.1 : Comparison of labour pain with other conditions using MPQ

The neuro physiological mechanisms of labour pain are still unknown. The labour pain shares other characteristics of visceral pain *e.g.*, stretching, cutting and tearing of somatic structures providing increasing somatic input. The cutting of uterus itself is not painful[4]. The stimuli produce pain but not direct injury. This pain wears off an impending physical danger and beneficially alters behaviour allowing the women to seek shelter and aid from others. While a short painless labour is detrimental to perinatal course, the stress produced by labour may be detrimental to the foetus. The afferent fibres supplying the uterus and cervix are primarily unmyelinated A delta and C fibres travelling with sympathetic nerves, through uterine and cervical plexuses, the inferior, middle, superior hypogastric plexuses and the lumbar and thoracic sympathetic chain entering the cord via the 10th, 11th and 12th thoracic and 1st lumbar nerve routes.[2] The pain relief during the first stage of labour can be achieved by various blocks (Fig. 35.2). However, the role of labour pain of afferent fibres running with parasympathetic nerves is less certain. While there is no role of sensory fibres accompanying the parasympathetic pelvic nerves in women, vagal afferents excited by cardiac ischaemia activate a spinal pain suppression causing a painless silent myocardial ischaemia.[5]

Physiology of Labour Pain

Pain in First Stage of Labour

Uterine contractions cause stretching, tearing, distortion and possible ischaemia of uterine tissues, while simultaneous dilatation of cervix and stretching of lower uterine segment is occurring. The intensity of the pain increases progressively with the rising strength of contractions. These painful stimuli are transmitted by Aδ and C afferent fibres, which accompany sympathetic pathways through the pelvic, inferior, middle and superior hypogastric plexuses, the lumbar sympathetic chain, the white rami of spinal nerves T_{10}, T_{11}, T_{12} and L_1 and posterior root of these nerve roots of T_{11} and T_{12} are involved but as the intensity of contraction increases. T_{10} and L_1 are readmitted.

Backache may occur due to referred pain of uterus or cervix. It occurs at cutaneous innervation at T_{10}- L_1 or L_5S_1.

Pain in Second Stage of Labour

The pain caused by distension of the pelvic structure and perineum following descent of the presenting part is added to the uterine contraction, although, once cervical dilatation is complete, pain induced by contraction becomes less intense. The uterine pain continue to refer to T_{10}-L_1, while pain produced by stretching or pressure exerted on intra-pelvic structures, including peritoneum, bladder, urethra, rectum is referred to sacral segments. Pressure on roots of lumbosacral plexus is felt as low back pain or pain in thighs. Pain produced by stretching of perineum is trasmitted by pudendal nerve ($S_{2,\ 3,\ 4}$), posterior cutaneous nerve of thigh ($S_{2,\ 3}$), genitofemoral nerve ($L_{1,2}$) and the ilioinguinal nerve (L_2).

During 1st stage of labour, an epidural block limited to T_{11} and T_{12} initially and later extending to involve T_{10} to L_1 will usually be sufficient to provide excellent pain relief, while avoiding neural blockade of sacral segments. Premature sacral blockade can result in loss of stimulating effect upon contraction of Fergusons's reflex and loss of pelvic muscle tone, which aids the rotation of the presenting part.

Later in 1st stage and during the early part of 2nd stage pain often occurs in lower lumbar and sacral segments, so block can be extended. At this stage thoraco-lumbar block will be decaying, so that abdominal muscle strength will be adequate to permit voluntary expulsive efforts by mother.

Advantages of Pain Relief in Labour

Pain is a noxious and unpleasant stimulus, which produces fear and anxiety. Fear and anxiety exacerbate the pain of labour, but converse may also be true. Unrelieved stress in pregnant patients cause reduction in uterine blood flow, foetal heart rate and foetal oxygenation, which all return to normal when stress is removed.

Effective pain relief reduced plasma, noradrenaline prevents rise in 11-hydroxy corticosteroid, prevent metabolic acidosis developed by reducing the rate of rise of lactate, pyruvate and excess lactate levels and reduce maternal oxygen consumption by upto 15 per cent.

Effective epidural analgesia prevents the pain induced by hyperventilation and hypocapnia which can severe enough to produce tetany and also reduce the uteroplacental blood flow by upto 25%. Respiratory alkolosis further impairs foetomaternal gas exchange by shifting the oxyhaemoglobin dissociation curve to left and foetal PaO_2 may fall by upto 23%.

Basic Requirements of Obstetric Labour Analgesia

1. Safety.
2. Effective analgesia through painful periods of labour.
3. No depressant effects on maternal respiratory or cardiovascular system.
4. No depressant effects on the progress of labour.
5. No depressant effects on the baby before or after delivery.

6. No unpleasant maternal side effects.
7. High technical success rate.

Methods of Labour Analgesia

1. Non-pharmacological techniques.
2. Pharmacological techniques.

1. ***Non-pharmacological techniques include:***
   (*a*) Minimal training / equipments:
   - Emotional support
   - Touch and massage
   - Theurapeutic use of heat and cold
   - Hydrotherapy
   - Vertical position (Upright posture)

   (*b*) Specialized training/equipments:
   - Bio feedback
   - Transcutaneous electrical nerve stimulation (TENS)
   - Acupuncture
   - Hypnosis.

2. *Pharmacological Techniques*
   (*a*) **Systemic Analgesia Drugs:**

   Systemic drugs have been used to decrease the pain of child birth since 1847, when James Young Simpson used diethyl ether to anaesthetize a parturient with a deformed pelvis.

   Systemic analgesia (Table 35.1) remain common practice for several reasons:

1. Some conditions like haemorrhage, coagulopathy contraindicate the administration of epidural or spinal analgesia.
2. Epidural analgesia is not available in all hospitals.
3. Some patient deny invasive techniques.

Table 35.1 : Drugs used in labour pain

1. Opioids : Commonly used	– Pethidine 2.5–50 mg IV, 1–4 hourly	
	– Morphine 2–5 mg IV	
	– Pentazocine 10–20 mg IV	
	– Fentanyl 25–50 IV	
	– Butorphanol 0.51 mg IV	
2. Tranquilliser, Promethazine		
3. NSIADs		
4. Dissociative Drugs – Ketamine		
5. Other as a adjuvants.	– Barbiturates	– Pentobarbital
		– Secobarbital
	– Anthihistamines	– Hydroxyzine
	– Benzodiazepines	– Diazepam
		– Lorazepam
		– Midazolam
6. Entonox ($N_2O + O_2$) inhalation		

Epidural Labour Analgesia

Epidural analgesia is the most effective form of intrapartum analgesia currently available. In most cases, maternal request for pain relief represents a sufficient indication for administration of epidural analgesia.

The safe administration of epidural analgesia requires a complete preanaesthetic evaluation and the immediate availability of appropriate resuscitation equipments.

Indication

1. To treat pain experienced by a woman in labour.
2. It may facilitate a traumatic vaginal breech delivery or vaginal delivery of breech/twins/ preterm infant.
3. It facilitates control of blood pressure in pre-eclamptic women.
4. It also blunts the haemodynamic effects of uterine contractions, sudden increase in pre-load and the associated pain response (tachycardia, increased systemic vascular resistance, hypertension, hyperventilation) in patient with other medical complications (mitral stenosis, spinal cord injury, intracervical neurovascular disease, asthma).

Contraindications of Epidural Analgesia

1. Patient refusal or inability to co-operate.
2. Increased intracranial pressure secondary to a mass lesion.
3. Skin or soft tissue infection at the site of needle placement.
4. Frank coagulopathy.
5. Uncorrected maternal hypovolemia (*e.g.,* haemorrhage)
6. Inadequate training or experience in techniques.

Epidural Space in Pregnancy

- Intermittent obstruction of inferior vena cava by enlarging uterus encourages venous drainage through alternative pathways and so vertebral and azygous venous system dilate. The epidural veins are part of internal vertebral venous plexus and these veins become particularly engorged when mother is supine or during uterine contractions. The engorged veins act to reduce the volume of epidural space, so volume requirement of local anaesthetic agent is reduced. Segmental dose requirement is generally reduced in pregnancy and labour.
- In non-pregnant subject, pressure in labour epidural space is normally – 1 cm H_2O, whereas in early labour, between contractions, pressure in lateral position averages 1.63 cm H_2O and rises to between 4–10 cm H_2O by the end of first stage. Assuming the supine position will increase epidural space pressure by upto 50%, and this increase is proportional to the degree of inferior vena cava obstruction, uterine displacement will moderate the rise produced in this position. As pressure in epidural space is positive during labour, methods of identifying the space, which depends on negative pressure, should not be used.
- During contractions, the reflex increase in abdominal muscle tone and sudden efflux of blood from the contracting myometrium into the venous system contribute further rise in epidural space pressure from 2–8 cm H_2O, even in lateral position. Adequate pain relief epidurally minimise the pressure rise produced during contractions.
- The spread of local anaesthetic solution in the epidural space will be exaggerated during a contraction, so injection should not be made at this time. Also epidural veins will be greatly engorged and risk of puncture by needle or catheter will be increased, if either is inserted in epidural space during a contraction.

Methods of Identification of Epidural Space

Principally methods of identification of epidural space falls into two groups, those depending on loss of resistance as the needle pierces the ligamentum flavum and enters the epidural space and those relying upon negative pressure in the epidural space.

- In loss of resistance technique pressure should be exerted manually on the plunger of a glass syringe containing saline or air, as needle is advanced millimeter by millimeter. Mechanical aids of loss of resistance technique like Macintosh's (1953) needle with spring loaded stylet is not recommended as it is only reliable when it is kept in perfect working condition. Deflation of inflated tiny balloon attached to the epidural needle, on entering the epidural space can be useful aid as described by Macintosh (1950).[2]
- Negative pressure methods like hanging drop sign, Odom's indicator or Brook's modification of Odom's indicator are not recommended in late pregnancy or the patient in labour as the epidural space pressure will not be negative in these patients.

Ambulatory Epidural Analgesia or for Obstetric Analgesia (Walking Epidural)

Obstetric analgesia or "painless" delivery can be achieved by various techniques. The best results are obtained by epidural block and it still remains the "Gold Standard" of obstetric pain management.

The ideal procedure should:

1. Produce efficient "pain relief" with good co-operation from the patient.
2. Not depress the foetal respiration.
3. Not depress the uterus, thereby preventing prolonged labour.
4. B.P. fall to be avoided to safe guard foetal hypoxia.
5. Safer mother and child.

Success of the procedure is dependent on :

(a) Experienced anaesthesiologist.

(b) Willing patient.

(c) Patient's mental make up and positive attitude.

Walking epidural or Ambulatory Epidural Analgesia (AEA) as the title suggests, where expectant mother after receiving epidural block can sit up or walk around during the actual process of labour pain without feeling any discomfort or pain.[1]

Reportedly the aim and advantages achieved by "Ambulatory epidural analgesia" are to shorten labour.

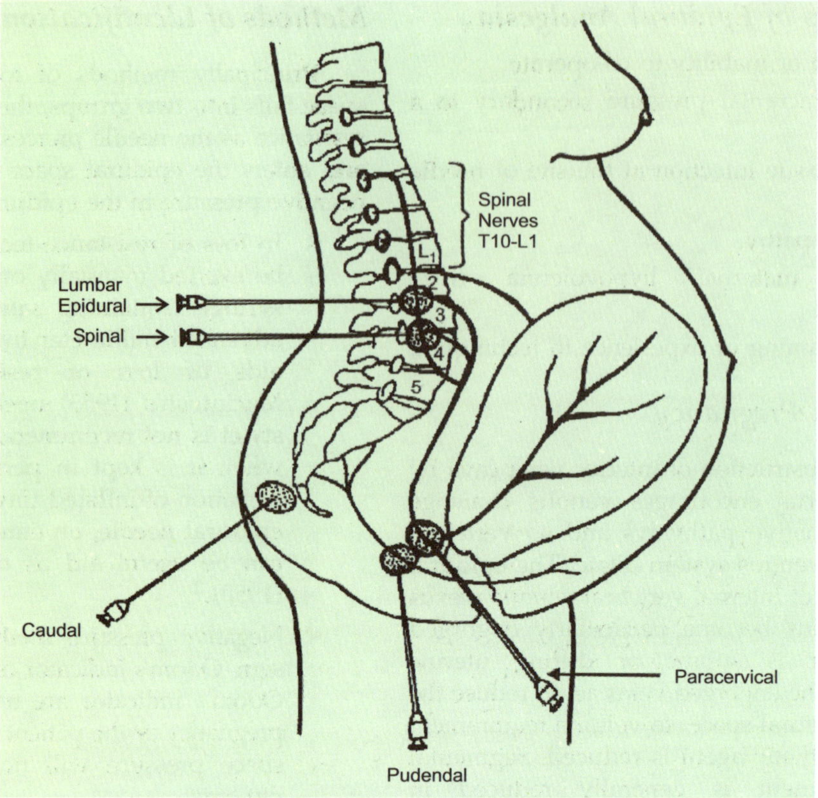

Fig. 35.2 : Regional obstetric analgesia

The patient can go to toilet, move limited, sit on a chair, read or write allowing ambulation.

The factors which are responsible to achieve shortening of labour after epidural block are:

(*a*) Confidence generated due to painless uterine contraction.

(*b*) Total maternal comfort.

(*c*) Increase in intensity of uterine contraction.

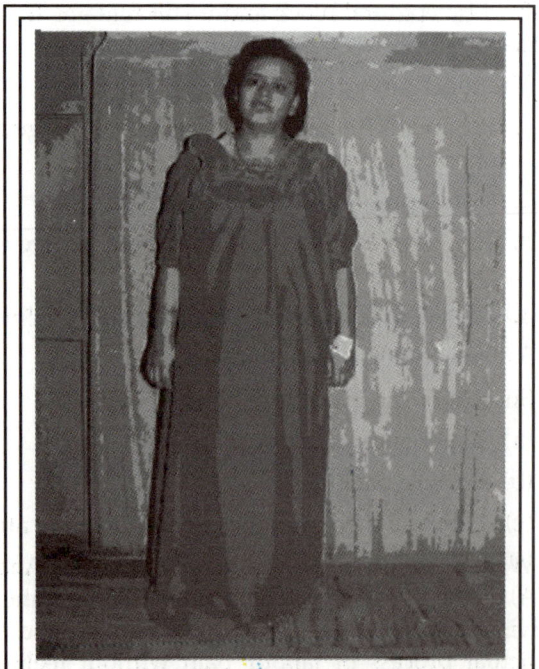

Fig 35.3 : Primigravidae after labour ambulatory epidural analgesia

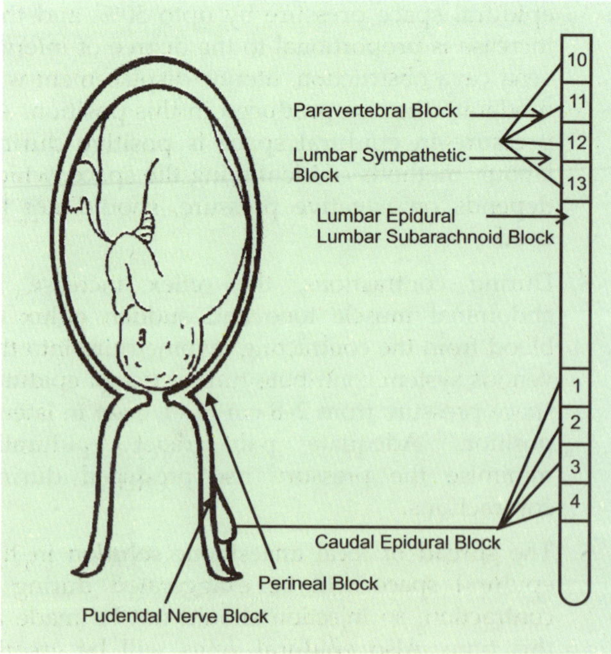

Fig 35.4 : Regional analgesia sites for labour pain

(*d*) Facilitates foetal head descent.

(*e*) Relaxes pelvic musculature.

(*f*) Inferior vena cava compression is avoided.

Technique

After taking all the aseptic precautions, lumbar epidural block is given in L2–L3 or L3–L4 space placing epidural catheter either in cephalic or caudal direction, depending on stage of labour the patient is in.

During the first stage of labour, the catheter is placed towards cephalic direction and as the labour advances and descent of foetal head is complete *i.e.*, head is fully engaged, the epidural catheter is placed towards caudal direction to achieve best results.

The twin catheter technique has been effectively used to obtain the advantages of selective block at different stages of labour. For walking epidural, this procedure is very effective.

The local anaesthetic drugs and their doses, duration of action and repeat doses are described as follows:

Drugs /strength/ initial dose/ duration /repeat dose through infusion pump.

(*a*) Bupivacaine/ 0.125%–0.25% / 10–18 mL/ 2 ½–3 hrs / 10 mL/hr

(*b*) Lignocaine hydrochloride (plain) / 0.75%–1% / 10–15 mL / 1–2 hrs / 7–10 mL/hr

(*c*) Combination– Bupivacaine 0.125% 5–7 mL 2 hrs 5–7 mL/hr + Fentanyl 2 mcg/mL and above[2].

Combination of bupivacaine and lignocaine is effective as lignocaine has rapid onset as compared to bupivacaine and bupivacaine has longer duration of action.

Addition of adrenaline with above drug is not recommended as it slows the uterine contractions, and may lead to uterine inertia, thereby prolonging labour.

Carbonated lignocaine solution has been better than normal lignocaine.

To achieve more effective response of the local drugs addition of fentanyl 100 mcg or fortwine 30 mg as a single dose or through continuous infusion of the mixture at a rate 10–15 mL per hour.[bupivacaine (0.125%) + 2 mcg/ mL fentanyl at 15–20 mL/hr].[2]

Results

(*a*) Shortening of labour, (1) in multipara–significant shortening (2) in nullipara no shortening of labour.

(*b*) Forceps application (1) in multipara– percentage is less in patient with walking epidural (2) in nullipara – no significant difference.[2]

(c) Efficacy of drugs available in the country is not up to international standard. As the strength of the drug (concentration) is reduced by diluting it, the anaesthesia becomes patchy and not very effective.

Local anaesthetic drug: Ropivacaine is more effective in ambulatory labour analgesia.

Effective dose is (0.07%) 15–20 mL. It is an amide type local anaesthetic agent possibly less motor block than other agents, duration similar to bupivacaine but lower toxicity. Available in 0.2–1% solution. Maximum dose: 3–4 mg/kg/4 hrs.

Neurexial analgesia is now very safe.

A low dose spinal / epidural regimen provides:

★ effective analgesia,
★ stable maternal haemodynamic,
★ few side effects which are tolerable.

Its complications due to:

★ invasive nature of technique,
★ patient characteristic,
★ medical malpractices.

Side Effects of Walking Epidural

As an epidural often slows a woman's labour, patient is three times more likely to be given an oxytocin drip to speed things up[3, 4]. The second stage of labour is particularly slowed, leading to a three times increased chance of forceps. Women having their first baby are particularly affected: choosing an epidural can reduce their chance of a normal delivery to less than 50%.

Walking is possible and safe for most and in a well equipped and staffed unit, parturients can be given a choice, if it is clear that walking will do no harm. However, safe ambulation with low dose CSE or epidural analgesia requires:

★ no postural hypotension or symptoms,
★ minimal or no motor block,
★ minimal or no proprioceptive block,
★ monitoring facilities including foetus,
★ co-operative, understanding parturients,
★ presenting part of foetus engaged and well applied to cervix.

Less common side effects for a woman having an epidural are:

Accidental puncture of the dura, or spinal cord coverings, which can cause a prolonged and sometimes severe headache (1 in 100).

Ongoing numb patches, which usually clear after 3 months (1 in 550): Weakness and loss of sensation in the areas affected by the epidural, (4–18 in 10,000) also usually resolved in 3 months.

Epidural abscess which needs urgent surgical intervention.

More serious but rare side effects include:

★ permanent nerve damage,
★ convulsions,
★ heart and breathing difficulties (1 in 20,000),
★ death attributable to epidural (1 in 200,000). When opiates are used, a woman may experience difficulty in breathing which comes on 6–12 hour later.

Effects of epidurals on babies

Although findings are not consistent, possible problems, such as rapid breathing in the first few hours[5] and vulnerability to low blood sugar suggests that these drugs have measurable effects on the newborn baby.

REFERENCES

1. Webb RJ , Cantor GS. Obstetrical epidural anesthesia in a rural Canadian hospital.Can J Anaesth 1991;39:390–393.
2. Kumar P, Pandya U. Role of Bupivacaine and Fentanyl in Painless labour. A thesis for M.D.Anaesthesia, Saurashtra University, Rajkot, 1999.
3. Ramin SM, Gambling DR, Lucas MJ et al. Randomized trial of epidural versus intravenous analgesia during labour. Obstet Gynecol 1995;86(5):783–789.
4. Howell CJ. Epidural versus non-epidural analgesia in labour. (Revised 6th May,1994) in : Keirse MJNG, Renfrew MJ, Neilson JP, Crowther C. (eds) Pregnancy and childbirth module. In: The Cochrane Pregnancy and childbirth Database. (Database on Disc and CD ROM) the Cochrane Colaboration : Issue 2, Oxford: Update software 1995 (available from BMJ publishing group, London).
5. Morikawa S, Ishikawa I, Kamatsuki H, et al. Neuro behaviour and mental development of newborn infants delivered under epidural analgesia with bupivacaine. Nippon Sanka 1990;42:1495–1502.

•••

OROFACIAL PAIN: DENTAL, VASCULAR AND NEUROPATHIC PAIN

36

Acute and Chronic Orofacial Pain

Acute orofacial pain is primarily associated with an inflammatory process within the teeth and their periodontal structures.[1] Acute and chronic manifestations of pain in the orofacial region, as in other body parts, differ from one another in their time course, aetiological mechanisms, response to therapy and behavioural reactions. The most prevalent chronic orofacial pain is musculoskeletal and originates from muscles, tendons and the temporomandibular joint. Primary vascular type orofacial pain (VOP) is another prevalent diagnostic entity typified by severe episodic, pulsatile pain accompanying autonomic signs and symptoms. Variable temporal patterns necessitate abortive or prophylactic modalities of treatment for VOP. Neuropathic orofacial pain (NOP) can be of the neuralgic paroxysmal type, as in trigeminal neuralgia, or of a continuous chronic nature, often associated with nerve injury, as in deafferentation pain.

Primary Vascular Type Craniofacial Pain

Primary vascular type craniofacial pain includes migraine, cluster headache (CH), and paroxysmal crania (Headache Classification Committee of the International Headache Society 1988)[1]. The aetiology of these headaches and facial pains is considered to be neurovascular, and they share signs and symptoms.[2] Common diagnostic features are: episodic pain that is unilateral, pulsatile, severe and may wake the patient from sleep. Accompanying phenomena include local autonomic signs (*e.g.*, tearing rhinorrhea) in paroxysmal hemicrania (PH) and cluster headache (CH), and systemic signs (*e.g.*, nausea, photophobia) in migraine. Atypical odontalgia has been described as a possible example of primary vascular-type pain in the mouth,[3] but recently vascular orofacial pain has been defined[4] which may represent an orofacial equivalent of primary vascular-type headaches. Although presenting similar signs and features, different entities of vascular-type craniofacial pain respond distinctively to therapy, stressing the importance of correct diagnosis.[5]

Table 36.1 : Signs and symptoms common to vascular-type craniofacial pain

Pain is:
- (*a*) periodic
- (*b*) severe
- (*c*) unilateral
- (*d*) pulsatile
- (*e*) wakes the patient from sleep

accompanied by:
- (*a*) local autonomic signs
  - (*i*) ocular: tearing, redness
  - (*ii*) nasal: rhinorrhea, congestion
  - (*iii*) local swelling or redness
- (*b*) systemic signs
  - (*i*) nausea, vomiting
  - (*ii*) photo/phonophobia

Table 36.2 : Differential diagnosis of primary vascular type craniofacial pain

	Migraine headache	Cluster headache	Paroxysmal hemicrania	Vascular orofacial pain
Age and sex				
Age of onset (years)	20–40	30–40	30–40	40–50
Male : female ratio	1:2	5:1	1:2	1:2.5
Location				
Laterality	unilateral, may change sides	unilateral, rarely changes sides	unilateral, rarely changes sides	mostly unilateral
Site	forehead, temple	orbital and periorbital	temporal and periauricular	intraoral and lower face
Time course				
Attack duration	hours to days	15–20 min	minutes	minutes to hour
periodicity	periodic chronic	periodic/ periodic	chronic/ chronic	periodic
Frequency of pain attacks	1-6/month	in clusters, 1–2/day	daily, 6–15/day	daily, varies in frequency
Character				
Type of pain	throbbing, deep	paroxysmal, boring	paroxysmal, lancinating	throbbing, may be paroxysmal
Pain intensity	moderate to severe	severe	severe	moderate to severe
Precipitating factors	stress, hunger, menstruation	alcohol	movement of head	sometimes cold foods
Associated signs	nausea, photophobia visual aura	lacrimation, rhinorrhea, ptosis, miosis	lacrimation, rhinorrhea, eye redness	Cheek swelling and redness, tearing

Migraine

Migraine with or without aura is a periodic, unilateral headache occurring mostly in the forehead and temple areas. Pain intensity is moderate to severe, usually throbbing, sometimes accompanied by photo- and phonophobia, and associated with nausea and occasional vomiting. The two forms of migraine — migraine with and without aura, are interrelated; one form may transform into the other, and both respond equally well to 5-hydroxytryptamine (5-HT) receptor agonists. Dilatation of large intra- and extracranial arteries occurs in both forms during an attack, but regional cerebral blood flow changes occur only in migraine with aura.

Migraine without Aura

An idiopathic, recurring headache disorder lasting 4–72 hours, migraine without aura is typically unilateral, pulsating in quality, of moderate to severe intensity aggravated by physical activity, and associated with nausea and sometimes vomiting and with photo- and phonophobia. Certain diagnostic criteria must be met to fulfill the definition of migraine without aura. (Headache Classification Committee of the International Headache Society 1988).[1] These include at least five attacks that have at least two of the following characteristics: (*a*) unilateral location, (*b*) pulsating quality, (*c*) moderate to severe intensity and (*d*) aggravation by physical activity.

Migraine with Aura

An idiopathic, recurring headache disorder, migraine with aura typically is associated with neurological symptoms (migraine with typical aura) and consists of one or more of the following: visual disturbances, unilateral paresthesia and/or numbness, unilateral weakness, and aphasia or unclassifiable speech difficulty. The aura lasts less than one hour and will be usually followed by the migraine without aura.

Epidemiology

Based on many studies a 1 - year prevalence in adults of about 10–15% has been suggested for migraine, including migraine both with and without aura.[6] The male to female ratio is about 1 to 3, with a prevalence of 5–8% in males and 15–25% in females. The female preponderance in migraine is more consistent across studies than the overall prevalence figure of migraine. The age of onset is early, and about half of cases start before the age of 20 years. Interestingly, no sex differences are apparent until age 11, after that age a female preponderance appears which may be linked to female hormones.[7] The 1-year prevalence of migraine with aura is approximately 2–4% which is lower than that of migraine without aura.

Precipitating factors: There are many precipitating factors, including emotional or psychological stress, menstruation, contraceptive medication, sleep (usually too long), fasting and fatigue. Other precipitating factors are associated with various foods and beverages such as chocolate, dairy products, alcohol, fruit, fried foods, tea, coffee, and seafood. Food additives such as nitrites, nitrates, and sodium glutamates are among well-known trigger factors.

Treatment: Migraine headaches can be treated either prophylactically or abortively. Frequency of attacks is the most important consideration for treatment approach. Abortive treatment, aimed at stopping the pain attack once it has started, is used when there are no more than three attacks per month. When four or more attacks occur per month, prophylactic treatment should be considered. Analgesics and anti-inflammatory drugs are to be considered first and if these are not effective the recently introduced 5-HT agonists such as sumatriptan should be utilized. On rare occasions opioids, preferably as an intranasal spray, may be considered. Combination drugs are also available, some of which contain ergotamine combined with other medications such as caffeine, codeine, and an antiemetic. Drug efficacy is greater when abortive therapy is initiated as early in the course of the attack as possible, and when a full dose is used.

In contrast to abortive treatment, which is used during the attack, prophylactic medication is taken on a daily basis in order to reduce the severity and frequency of potential migraine attacks. Three main groups are presently considered as most effective, with relatively few and minor side effects. These include β-adrenoceptor blocking drugs, tricyclic antidepressants, and anticonvulsants.

Table 36.3 : Treatment of primary vascular-type craniofacial pain

	Migraine headache	Cluster headache	Paroxysmal hemicrania pain	Vascular orofacial
Abortive	Triptans (sumatriptan, rizatriptan, zolmitriptan); NSAIDs (COX-1 or COX-2 inhibitors)	Oxygen (100%, 6 litres/ min for 15 min); sumatriptan; ergot	Indomethacin	NSAIDs (COX-1 or COX-2 inhibitors); other non-narcotic analgesics
Prophylactic	Amitriptyline; β blockers; valproates	Ergot, methysergide, lithium carbonate	Indomethacin	Amitriptyline; β blockers

Table 36.4 : Comparison of effect, adverse events and contraindication for different classes of drugs used in the preventive treatment of migraine

Class/substances	Attack frequency	Adverse events	Contraindications
Beta-Adrenoceptor Antagonists			
Propranolol : 80–160 mg per day Metoprolol : 100–200 mg per day Alcohols : 50–100 mg per day	50% reduction 50% reduction 50% reduction	Bradycardia Hyprotension Fatigue Sleep disturbances Dyspepsia Depression	Asthma Bradycardia Cardiac failure Hypoglycaemia
Calcium Channel Antagonists			
Florarizine : 5–10 mg × 1 per day	50% reduction	Sedation Weight gain Depression Sleep disturbance	Depression Parkinson disease
(Verapamil) : 120–240 mg × 2 per day	50% reduction	Constipation Bradycardia	Bradycardia Conduction defect
5-HT_2 Antagonists Pizocifon : 0.5–1 mg × 1–3 per day	50% reduction	Increased appetite Weight gain Drowsiness	Narrow-angle glaucoma? Prostatic hypertrophy?
Cyproheptsdine : 4 mg tablet × 2–4 per day	50% reduction		
5-HT Agonies			
Mythysergide : 1–2 mg × 1–3 per day (should be given for 4–6 months, stopped for 4–6 weeks and then restarted)	50–75% reduction	Nausea Sleep disturbance Peripheral vasoconstriction Retroperito-neal / pleuro-pulmonary fibrosis	Pregnancy Cardiac and peri-phereal vascular disorders.Impaired kidney or liver functions Collagen diseases
Anti-Epilleptics Sodium valproote : 300–500–600 mg × 1–3 per day	50–75% reduction	Nausea, Vomiting Tremour Weight gain/ loss	Pregnancy Thrombocytopenia Liver disease
Tricyclics (Amitriptyline : 10–100 mg per day	50% reduction	Sedation Weight gain Dry mouth Blurred vision	Narrow angle glaucoma Prostatic hypertro-phy. Recovery phase after myo-cardial infarction

Cluster Headache

Cluster headache (CH) is characterized by attacks of severe unilateral pain in the orbital and periorbital area. Pain lasts from 15 to 180 minutes and occurs from once every other day to as often as 8 times a day. Episodic CH refers to a temporal pattern consisting of a series of pain attacks, or "active" episodes, occurring in succession (hence clustering) over period of 4–12 weeks with "inactive" periods that lasts from 6–18 months. In the active period pain occurs daily or almost daily. About 10% of patients have a continuous on constantly active pattern known as chronic cluster headache.[8]

Pain pattern. Pain is unilateral, excruciatingly severe, and paroxysmal, occurs in the ocular, frontal, and temporal areas. In most cases, the pain starts in the orbital area, but as it continues and becomes more severe it radiates to the forehead, temporal region, upper and lower jaws, and, in some cases, to the neck and shoulder. Five pain attacks of this type are necessary to fulfill the diagnostic criteria for cluster headache. (Headache Classification Committee of the International Headache Society 1988).[1] Nocturnal attacks are typical and account for about 50% of attacks, with the highest frequency occurring toward early morning. Attacks tend to be shorter and less severe in intensity at the beginning and towards the end of each cluster period. However, the duration of each attack tends to lengthen during the course of the disease.[8]

Accompanying phenomena: Pain attacks are accompanied by ipsilateral conjunctival injection, lacrimation, stuffiness of the nose, and rhinorrhea. Forehead and facial sweating and eyelid oedema also occur. Ipsilateral ptosis and miosis may be associated with some attacks; occasionally, they persist after attacks and may remain permanently.

Precipitating factors: Alcohol precipitates attacks in the active period but not during the remission period. Histamine, administered intravenously or subcutaneously, and sublingual nitroglycerine also may precipitate an attack, and can be used as diagnostic tools.

Treatment: Treatment consists of abortive and prophylactic approaches. The most effective abortive treatment is the administration of 100% oxygen, through a loosely applied face mask, at a rate of 7–8 L/minute for 15 minutes.[9] Ergot preparations and subcutaneously administered sumatriptan have a beneficial effect.

Prophylactic treatment is administered during the active period. Ergot preparations should not exceed 10 mg per week, as higher doses may produce peripheral arterial spasm and necrosis. Methysergide

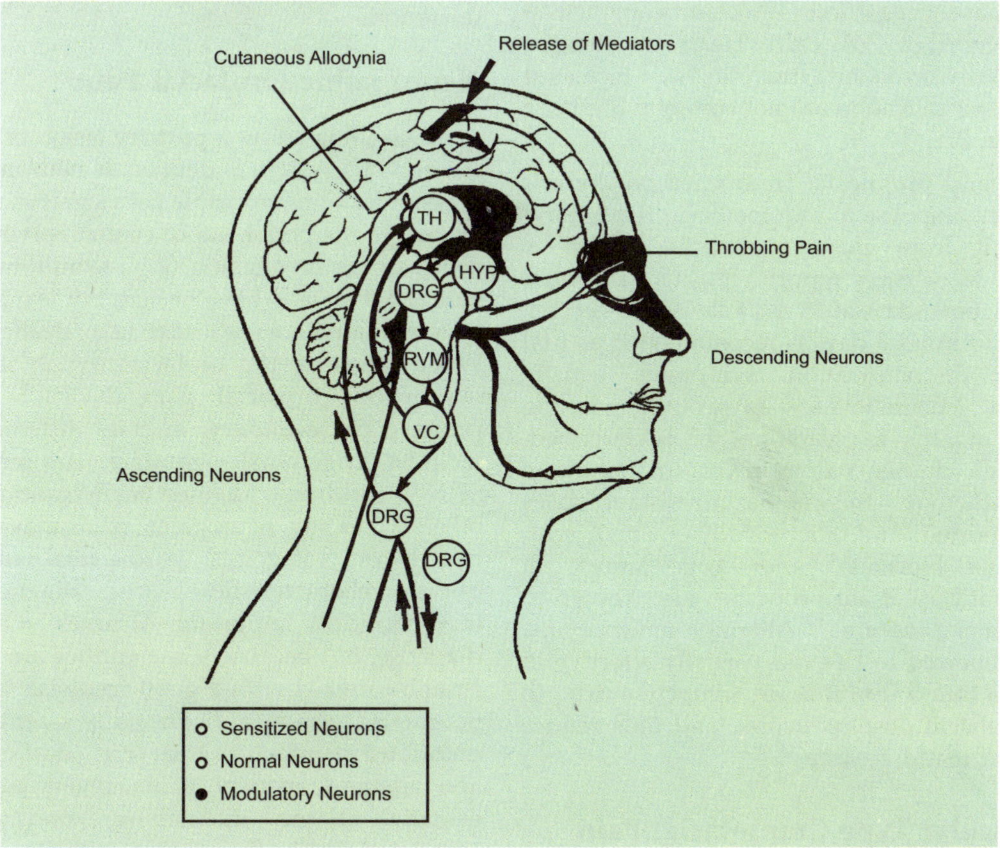

Fig. 36.1 : Showing ascending and descending pathways of migraine

can be administered only for short periods (weeks) to avoid retroperitoneal fibrosis. Lithium carbonate is utilized for the chronic type of cluster headache, but blood levels should be carefully monitored.[10]

Paroxysmal Hemicrania

Paroxysmal hemicrania (PH) is a vascular-type headache characterized by very frequent, short bouts of severe unilateral pain around the orbit and temple. Chronic and episodic forms, similar to cluster headache (CH) have been described. Associated signs include ipsilateral conjunctival injection and tearing with nasal congestion and rhinorrhea. The absolute response of PH to indomethacin therapy differentiates from CH.

Location: Pain occurs typically in the temporal, periauricular, and periorbital areas,[11] hence the term hemicrania. Referral to the shoulder, neck, and arm has been reported. Unlike CH, which may change sides, the vast majority of cases of PH do not. Most cases in PH are unilateral and do not become bilateral, but strong pain may cross the midline.[12]

Accompanying phenomena – As in other primary vascular-type headaches, PH is accompanied by a number of usually ipsilateral autonomic phenomena. These may occur bilaterally, but are more pronounced on the symptomatic side. The most commonly seen are lacrimation (62%), nasal congestion (42%), and conjunctival changes and rhinorrhea (36% each). Heart rate changes (bradycardia, tachycardia, or extrasystoles),[11] increased local sweating and salivation are not common but have been reported in PH.

Treatment and prognosis: Treatment is prophylactic with a consistent response to indomethacin that clearly distinguished it from cluster headache, which is nonresponsive. Most cases report a positive response within 24 hours, but 3 days at 75 mg followed, if needed, by 150 mg for a further 3 days is recommended as trial therapy.[13] On discontinuation, symptoms usually reappear within 12 hours to a few days, but long-lasting remission for months to years has been described. Persistently high dosage requirements may indicate underlying pathology. Indomethacin-resistant cases have been reported and successfully treated with calcium channel blockers[14] and acetazolamide (a diuretic with anticonvulsant properties also known to reduce intraocular pressure).[15] Although amitriptyline has not been reported to be even partially effective in PH, it has been found useful as an adjunctive drug to enable indomethacin dose reduction (and thus reduce side effects) and to aid in sleep.[16]

Primary Vascular Type Craniofacial Pain

There is unequivocal evidence for the evidence of sensory axons innervating cephalic blood vessels. Together they have been termed as trigeminovascular system.[17] These trigeminal axons relay nociceptive information to the central nervous system (CNS); when stimulated antidromically, they promote neurogenic inflammation, because this inflammation takes place within the restricted space of the cranium, the pain of migraine may be more severe than if it occurred in a more flexible space. Such pain mechanisms are possible in other craniofacial structures with confined spaces. Thus, the pain in cluster headache may be associated with a perivascular inflammatory process of the carotid artery in its bony canal or with increased intraocular pressure.[2] It is not surprising that such a neurogenic inflammatory process, when confined to another limited space, *i.e.*, the tooth-pulp chamber or inferior alveolar canal, may cause strong intraoral pain that mimics pulpitis. Evidence for a neurogenic inflammatory process within the tooth pulp may support possible mechanisms for a vascular-type dental orofacial pain. Nerve fibres exhibiting positive immunoreactivity to substance P and calcitonin gene related peptide have been demonstrated in the dental pulp and oral mucosa in several species, including humans.[18] Neurogenic inflammation in the trigeminovascular system seems to play a central role in the genesis of vascular type headaches, and the same mechanism could function in the oral mucosa and teeth. It is possible that pressure build-up plays a role in intrapulpal pain sensation.

Neuropathic Orofacial Pain

Pain initiated by a primary lesion or dysfunction of the nervous system is defined as neuropathic pain. The appearance of neuropathic pain signifies some abnormal process in the peripheral or central nervous system. This process may be ongoing (*e.g.*, symptomatic trigeminal neuralgia) or may have healed, but leaving the nervous system in a pathological state (*e.g.*, deafferentation pain). When affecting the orofacial region it is termed as neuropathic orofacial pain (NOP).[19] NOP may be primary or secondary, and its differential diagnosis includes trigeminal neuralgia, deafferentation pain, SUNCT syndrome (defined below), and neuritis, among others. Clinically, neuropathic pains may be divided into two broad categories: paroxysmal and continuous. These characteristics are diagnostically and therapeutically important. At times NOP is difficult to diagnose, but because some entities are therapeutically straightforward with a good response (*e.g.*, trigeminal neuralgia), accurate diagnosis is essential. Others are notoriously difficult to treat (*e.g.*, deafferentation pain), and adequate patient management and support are essential. Some threatening conditions may be associated with these pain entities, such as CNS tumours, systemic disease, or pressure on a peripheral nerve by space-occupying lesions.

SUNCT syndrome

Shortlasting, unilateral, neuralgiform headache attacks with conjunctival injection and tearing (the SUNCT syndrome) are considered to belong to the neuropathic pain entities. SUNCT is a unilateral craniofacial pain characterized by brief paroxysmal pain accompanied by ipsilateral local autonomic signs, usually conjunctival injection and lacrimation, nasal stuffiness.

Combination Syndromes

Cluster-tic syndrome and hemicrania-tic syndrome can occur in combination with trigeminal neuralgia.

Neuropathic craniofacial pain secondary to trauma

A total of 2% of all neuralgias in the orofacial region are thought to be secondary to pathological lesions. For example, TN occurring in young patients (especially 20–24 years) or presenting bilaterally may signify underlying disease, *i.e.*, multiple sclerosis or tumour. Accompanying phenomena such as sensory changes, muscle weakness, and autonomic signs should alert the clinician. Secondary neuropathic pain may also develop after trauma or viral infection.

Deafferentation

Mechanical injuries to peripheral nerves may ultimately lead to a variety of painful condition. Various factors will determine the quality of the pain and accompanying sensory changes. These factors include the severity and type of injury, the time elapsed since injury and the group of nerve fibres damaged. Involvement of the sympathetic nervous system may cause interaction and pain that is sympathetically "maintained."

Phantom Tooth Pain (Atypical Odontalgia)

International Association for Study of Pain (IASP) has defined atypical odontalgia as a severe throbbing pain in the tooth without major pathology. The high incidence of pain that is pulsatile and episodic, with pain that migrates and even changes sides, makes it likely that this may be a vascular phenomenon. Indeed, the term vascular toothache has been interchangeably used to describe this pain entity. However, this condition has also been referred to as phantom toothache, implying mechanism. The question whether atypical odontalgia is a vascular or neuropathic syndrome is a source of controversy. Indeed, many cases present with continuous pain that is contrary to a classical vascular-type pain. When the pain displays a constant, burning quality a neuropathic-type mechanism is likely to exist, and the term neuropathic orofacial pain is used, instead of atypical odontalgia. It is possible that cases of atypical odontalgia metamorphose into, or coexist with, neuropathic-type pains in response to repeated dental interventions aimed at pain relief.

Craniofacial Macrotrauma

Peripheral nerve injury has been implicated in post traumatic headache and facial pain. This may take the form of paroxysmal neuralgic pain or chronic deafferentation pain seen in more severe injuries. Even in relatively minor head trauma, widespread shearing may cause extensive axonal injury that is commonly known as diffuse axonal injury and may contribute to central mechanisms of post traumatic pain.

Nerve entrapment in scar tissue or direct nerve injury with aberrant regeneration and abnormal nerve activity due to neuroma formation, as seen in other traumatic neuropathic conditions, may be the peripheral pathological basis. Trigeminal nerve axons are less prone to developing ectopic hyperexcitability, suggesting that post-traumatic pain in the trigeminal region may be more infrequent than in other regions of the body.

Sympathetically Maintained Pain

Sympathetically mediated pain (SMP) refers to a group of disorders in which, as the name suggests, the sympathetic component of the autonomic nervous system is involved. IASP considers SMP to be a feature of complex regional pain syndromes, which include syndrome previously named reflex sympathetic dystrophy and causalgia. Local interaction at the injury site between sensory and sympathetic fibres initiates a positive feedback system that serves to maintain pain. Continued peripheral input probably results in central sensitization and peripheral sensory changes such as hyperesthesia, allodynia, and hyperpathia. Essentially, SMP is a descriptive term that is used for any pain condition that is sympathetically dependent and, therefore, relieved by sympatholytic procedures. It has not been widely studied in the head or face and mostly appears in case reports.

Other Clinical Syndromes Associated with Neuropathic Orofacial Pain

Multiple sclerosis, tumour of the brain and branches of trigeminal nerve, diabetes, herpes and geniculate neuralgia respond to treatment of cause.

Table 36.5 : Primary and secondary neuropathic orofacial pain

Primary	Secondary
Idiopathic neuralgias: Trigeminal Glossopharyngeal Geniculate	Post traumatic: Sympathetically independent Sympathetically mediated
Pretrigeminal neuralgia	Viral: Postherpetic Geniculate
SUNCT syndrome	Neural tumours Central Peripheral
Combinations: Cluster-tic Chronic paroxysmal Hemicrania-tic	Systemic disease: Multiple sclerosis Mixed connective tissue disease Diabetes

REFERENCES

1. Headache Classification Committee of the International Headache Society. Classification and diagnostic criteria for headache disorders, cranial neuralgias and facial pain. Cephalgia 1988;7:1–96.
2. Pareja JA, Pareja J, Palomo T, Cabarello V, Pamo M. SUNCT syndrome: repetitive and overlapping attacks. Headache 1994;34:114–116.
3. Rees RT, Harris M. Atypical odontalgia. Br. J. Oral Surg 1978;16:212–218.
4. Benoliel R, Elishoov H, Sharav Y. The diagnosis and treatment of persistent pain following trauma to the head and neck. J Oral Maxillofacial surg 1994;85:158–161.
5. Sharav Y, Benoliel R. Primary vascular-type craniofacial pain. Compendium Cont Educ Dent 2001; 22: 119–132.
6. Rasmussen BK, Breslau N. Migraine, epidemiology. In: Olesen J, Tfelt-Hansen P, Welch KMA (Eds). The headaches, New York: Raven press, 1993; pp 169–173.
7. Bille B. Migraine in school children. Acta Paediatr 1962; 51 (suppl 136).
8. Nappi G, Russell D. Cluster headache clinical features. In: Olesen J, Tfelt-Hansen P, Welch KMA (Eds). The headaches, New York: Raven press, 1993; pp 97–104.
9. Ekbom K, Sakai F. Cluster headache, management. In: Olesen J, Tfelt-Hansen P, Welch KMA (Eds). The headaches, New York: Raven press, 1993; pp 591–599.
10. Kudrow L. Lithium prophylaxis for chronic cluster headache. Headache 1977; 17:15–18.
11. Haggag KJ. Russell D. Chronic paroxysmal hemicrania. In: Olesen J, Tfelt-Hansen P, Welch KMA (Eds). The headaches; New York, Raven press, 1993, pp 601–6-8.
12. Kudrow DB, Kudrow L. Successful aspirin prophylaxis in a child with chronic paroxysmal hemicrania. Headache 1989;29; 280–281.

13. Pareja J, Sjaastad O. Chronic paroxysmal hemicrania and hemicrania continua. Interval between indomethacin administration and response. Headache; 1996, 36:20–23.
14. Shabbir N, McAbee G. Adolescent chronic paroxysmal hemicrania responsive to verapamil monotherapy. Headache, 1994; 34: 209–210.
15. Warner JS, Wamil AW, McLean MJ. Acetazolamide for the treatment of chronic paroxysmal hemicrania. Headache, 1994; 34:597–599.
16. Benoliel R, SharavY. Trigeminal neuralgia with lacrimation or SUNCT syndrome. Cephalgia 1998a; 18:85–90.
17. Moskowitz MA. The trigeminovascular system. In: Olesen J, Tfelt-Hansen P, Welch KMA (Eds). The headaches, New York: Raven press, 1993; pp 97–104.
18. Wakisaka S. Neuropeptides in the dental pulp: distribution, origins, and correlation. J Endodontics 1990; 16:67–69.
19. Benoliel R, Sharav Y. Neuropathic orofacial pain. Compendium Cont Educ Dent 1998c; 19:1099–1116.

•••

MANAGEMENT OF PAIN OF PELVIC ORIGIN

37

Pelvic pain is one of the most common problems affecting women of reproductive age. For clinical purposes, pelvic pain can be divided into acute and chronic presentations. Acute pelvic pain refers to pain symptoms below the umbilicus that have been present for less than six months. Chronic pelvic pain refers to menstrual or non-menstrual pain of at least six months duration occurring below the umbilicus. The most common causes of acute pelvic pain include the early stages of diseases that cause chronic pelvic and problems caused by ectopic pregnancy, spontaneous abortion, ovarian cyst, endometritis, appendicitis and urinary tract calculus. The most common causes of chronic pelvic pain are endometriosis, chronic PID, adenomyosis, uterine leiomyomata, irritable bowel syndrome, interstitial cystitis, diverticulitis and fibromyalgia. Some women with chronic pelvic pain also have concomitant psychosocial problems such as depression, somatisation, narcotic dependency and history of physical and sexual abuse.

Epidemiology

Several population surveys have reported on the prevalence of chronic pelvic pain (CPP) among women of reproductive age. In one study of 2016 women responding to a written questionnaire, 24% reported that they had a history of constant or intermittent pelvic pain of greater than six month duration that was not exclusively associated with menstrual periods. Of the women with chronic pelvic pain, 25% reported that they also had IBS, and 9% reported that they also had genitourinary tract symptoms. In a telephone survey of 5263 women of reproductive age, 15% reported chronic pelvic pain that was active during the past three months. In this study, 61% of the women reported that a cause of their chronic pelvic pain had not been clearly identified. In a survey of the medical records of 284, 162 female patients aged 12 to 70 in the UK, the incidence of chronic pelvic pain was 38.3 per 1000 women.[1]

Aetiology

Many disease processes can present as chronic pelvic pain. These conditions primarily consist of gynaecologic, gastrointestinal and urologic diseases. The relative frequency of the causes of pelvic pain is strongly influenced by the local patients, referral patterns and the speciality focus of the practice. For example, in population with a low incidence of STD, endometriosis is often the most common cause of chronic pelvic pain.[2,3] In contrast, in populations with a high prevalence of STD, chronic PID is most common cause of chronic pelvic pain.[4]

Classification of Chronic Pelvic Pain Syndrome

1. **Pelvic pain syndrome:**
   (*a*) Urological Bladder pain syndrome *e.g.*, interstitial cystitis
   Urethral pain syndrome
   Penile pain syndrome
   Prostate pain syndrome
   Scrotal pain syndrome *e.g.*, testicular pain syndrome, post vasectomy pain syndrome, epididymal pain syndrome
   (*b*) Gynaecological Endometriosis associated pain syndrome
   Vaginal pain syndrome
   Vulvar pain syndrome *e.g.*, general vulvar pain syndrome
   Localized vulvar pain syndrome (vestibular pain, clitoral pain syndrome)
   (*c*) Anorectal proctalgia fugax
   Anorectal pain syndrome
   Anismus
2. **Others:** (*a*) Neurological – pudendal pain syndrome
   (*b*) Muscular–perineal pain syndrome, pelvic floor muscle pain
   (*c*) Urological–Infective cystitis, prostatitis, urethritis epididymo orchitis
   (*d*) Gynaecological–endometriosis
   (*e*) Anorectal–proctitis, haemorrhoids, anal fissure

(*f*) Neurological–pudenal neuropathy, sacral spinal cord pathology

(*g*) Others–vascular, cutaneous and psychiatric.

The pelvic viscera receive their innervation via autonomic nervous system. The sympathetic portion originates from the thoracolumbar area of the spinal cord. The parasympathetic supply follows the distribution of the vagal nerve in combination with parasympathetic fibres from S1, S2 and S3. The autonomic nerve fibres enter the pelvis by following several routes. Most of them contribute to the formation of the superior hypogastric plexus.

Non Gynaecologic Causes of Pelvic Pain

Gastrointestinal

Irritable bowel syndrome (IBS) affects an estimated 15% of adults, affecting twice as many women as men. Patients present with chronic or recurring abdominal pain associated with altered bowel habits (diarrhoea, constipation or both) and bloating.[5] The pathophysiology of IBS is felt to be multifactorial, involving altered bowel motility, visceral hypersensitivity and psychosocial factors.[6]

The Manning diagnostic criteria are widely used and have been validated through factor analysis. A diagnosis of (IBS) is likely in patients with abdominal pain with two or more associated symptoms – pain relieved by defecation, pain associated with loose or more frequent stools, abdominal distension, feeling of incomplete evacuation or mucus in stools.

Urogenital

Pain management in urological patients is a subject afflicted by failure to identify its pathophysiological origins. The problem is most commonly experienced in "interstitial cystitis" or "chronic prostates". These terms reflect the clinical interpretation of the symptoms described by the patients.

Interstitial Cystitis (IC)

Interstitial cystitis is a poorly understood chronic inflammatory condition of the bladder. Altered bladder permeability from a defective gycosaminoglycan mucus layer has been proposed as the aetiology of this condition. However, it is not known if this is the cause or an effect of interstitial cystitis. Epidemiologic data showing an association between IC and autoimmune diseases have led to theories that IC may be immunologically mediated.

No micro-organism has been found to be the cause of IC. Although cultures of urine from a minority of IC patients may contain bacteria, antibiotic treatment is ineffective in this disease.

Inflammation seems to be an essential part of the picture in classic IC. Histological examination of bladder lesions has revealed pain cystitis and perineural inflammatory infiltrates of lymphocytes and plasma cells. Inflammation is scant in non-ulcer IC.[7]

Mast cells are multifunctional immune cells that contain highly potent inflammatory mediators such as histamine, leukotrienes, serotonin and cytokines. Many of the symptoms and findings in classic IC such as pain, frequency, oedema, fibrosis and neovascularisation in the lamina propria may be due to the release of mast cell derived factors.[8]

Toxic constituents in the urine may cause injury to the bladder in IC. One hypothesis is that heat labile, cationic urine components of low molecular weight may exert a cytotoxic effect, defective constitutive cytokine production may decrease mucosal defences to toxic agents.[13]

A decrease in the microvascular density in the suburothelium has been observed. In a 1999 study, it was found that bladder perfusion decreased with bladder filling in IC patients, but that the opposite occurred in controls.[14]

Clinical Features and Diagnosis

Patients report severe pelvic pain with bladder filled that is relieved by voiding. Pain may also be described as pelvic, vaginal or perineal, prompting evaluation for a gynaecologic aetiology and delaying diagnosis. Diagnostic criteria for interstitial cystitis are symptoms of frequency, pain and urgency–findings of low bladder capacity on voiding diary or urodynamic assessment, and the characteristic cystoscopic appearance with Hunner ulcers and granulations.

Initial Evaluation

Should include a urine analysis, urine culture and cytology. A voiding diary is helpful in the initial evaluation of these patients. In women with interstitial cystitis, voiding diaries usually demonstrate 20 or more voids in 24 hours with 3 or more voids at night and average volumes of 100 mL. Cystoscopy is important to exclude stone, foreign body or carcinoma and may show characteristic findings. Sensitivity to intracellular potassium has been proposed as a diagnostic test but does not add significantly to the sensitivity or specificity of diagnosis.

Treatment Approaches

These include systemic agent, instillation therapy and surgical management. Trials of systemic agents including antihistamines, azothioprine, corticosteroids, heparin, pentosanpolysulphate and tricyclic compounds have shown inconsistent benefits. Placebo effect and intermittent remission rates of upto 50% with an average duration of 8 months complicate the ability to assess effectiveness in small studies that are often not blinded or randomized. Dimethyl sulphoxide has been used for intravesical therapy with response rates of 50% to 90%, although the majority of studies are uncontrolled. DMSO is teratogenic in animals and should be avoided in pregnancy.

Cystodissection

Performed at the time of diagnostic cystoscopy, may provide short-term relief to 20 to 30% of patients. Surgical treatments include urinary diversion procedures, augmentation cystoplasty and denervation procedures. These are generally reserved for severe disease that is unresponsive to other therapies.[15]

A frequently cited report by Bumpus claims imprecisely that hydro distension achieved symptom improvement in 100 patients over several months. Dunn claimed to have achieved complete absence of symptoms in 16 of 25 patients during a mean follow-up of 14 months using the helmstein method, where an intravesical balloon is distended at the level of systolic blood pressure for three hours[16].

Acupuncture

In non-curable and agonizing diseases such as IC, desperate patients frequently seek access to complimentary medicine such as acupuncture. However, scientific evidence for such treatments is often poor.

Supra trigonal cystectomy with subsequent bladder augmentation represents the most favoured continence-preserving technique for the surgical management of IC. The therapeutic success of supra trigonal cystectomy has been reported in numerous studies.

Chronic Prostatitis

A syndrome in men, characterized by chronic perineal and penile pain with varying degrees of urinary and sexual dysfunction, is generally recognized without difficulty by clinicians and often labelled as chronic prostatitis. As the cause of the most prevalent, non bacterial, forms of the condition remains unknown, and, therefore, no definitive diagnostic tests exists, diagnosis has relied on a combination of clinical features, exclusion of other diagnoses (such as bladder outlet obstruction) and the results of investigations, especially the four glass test (Stamey). However, there is no generally agreed clinical definition that brings together the symptomatic features and investigative findings, so it is difficult to make reliable comparisons among the many descriptive and therapeutic studies in 30 years of medical literature or to draw many conclusions.

Treatment

For the few patients with bacterial prostatitis, antibiotic selection should be guided by the sensitivities of the organisms cultured from urine or prostatic secretions and an agent with good prostatic penetration, usually a quinolones such as ciprofloxacin would be the agent of choice.[21] One month of initial therapy is suggested by existing studies, but upto a third of patients may relapse and need more prolonged courses or suppressive antibiotic treatment.[22]

The treatment of the non infective syndrome is more problematic. Although the condition is so common, there are no published large scale randomized treatment trials. Small controlled trials and observation studies have suggested a place for selected antibiotics (which may act by non antimicrobial mechanisms such as anti-inflammatory effects) including doxycycline, erythromycin and ofloxacin, (blockers such as terazosin, transurethral microwave thermotherapy and allopurinol).[27] However, no highly effective therapy has been identified. A review of the literature suggest that alpha blockers, muscle relaxants and various physical therapies improve symptoms.

Scrotal Pain

Acute scrotal pain includes torsion of the testis or appendices and requires immediate diagnostic and therapeutic attention. Although it is not life threatening its manifestations affect the patients quality of life. It can be unilateral or bilateral and continuous or intermittent. It is not uncommon for examination to localize the site and distinguish between testicular and epididymal pain.

Mechanism

Afferent innervation of testis is via Genitofemoral nerve which has a femoral branch to the skin of the ventro medial region of the thigh and a genital branch to the scrotal region. The Ilioinguinal nerve conveys sensations from the groin region. The Ilioinguinal and Genitofemoral nerves are, however, subject to a great deal of anatomic variability.[28]

According to the traditional view the testis perceive sympathetic input from the para aortic ganglia. Studies using biochemical methods indicate that efferent fibres reaching the testis derive from major pelvic and accessory pelvic ganglia.[29]

Treatment

Patients with extra genital disease are treated according to the cause. Patients without identifiable lesions must primarily be treated conservatively (adjuvant antibiotics, analgesics, TENS, nerve blocks) of Genitofemoral or Ilioinguinal nerve. If these are unsuccessful sugery can be considered. However, the results of epididymectomy and orchidectomy are poor (20% and 60% success rates, respectively). Microsurgical testicular denervation represents another therapeutic option and favourable results have been reported. It has been suggested that patients with micro calcifications should be kept under surveilence because of a possible increased risk of testicular malignancy. Ganglion of Impar block with local anaesthetic has been used successfully in relieving chronic scrotal pain. If required the block is repeated and neurolysis of the ganglion of Impar is performed for chronic pain, if other methods fail to provide adequate pain relief.

Urethral Syndrome

Urethral syndrome represents a less well defined entity. Positive diagnostic signs are urethral tenderness or pain on palpation and slightly inflamed urethral mucosa found during endoscopy. In clinical practice, the diagnosis of urethral syndrome is commonly given to patients who present with the symptoms of dysuria (with or without frequency, nocturia, urgency and urge in continence) in the absence of evidence of urinary infection. It is the later phase that results in difficulties because the methods typically used to identify urinary infection are extremely insensitive.

Dysuria is pain or discomfort experienced in association with micturition. The classical symptom of a burning sensation in the urethra during voiding caused by infection is well known. Less appreciated is the external dysuria experienced by women with vaginitis when urine passes over the labia.

Urethral trauma arising from intercourse may cause pain and dysuria. This used to be called as "Honeymoon cystitis", and a friction and trauma to the urethra may be the cause in the absence of infection. Women with pelvic floor dysfunction sometimes describe the symptoms, as do post menopausal women in whom the trauma is associated with estrogen deficiency, loss of lubrication and vaginal dryness.

Gynaecological Causes of Pelvic Pain

Pelvic pain is a common complaint among women. Nearly 10% of all American women aged 18 to 50 suffer from chronic pelvic pain.

Endometriosis

It is a major cause of pelvic pain characterized by the presence of functional endometrial glands and stroma outside the uterine cavity. Although many lesions have a characteristic appearance, histologic examination improves the accuracy of the diagnosis. These lesions are typically found in the pelvis, but may be located on the bowel, bladder or remote locations such as lung. These lesions are hormonally responsive, typically resulting in pain that worsens just before and with menses. Approximately 40% of women with endometriosis have physical findings consistent with this disorder. Physical findings that are present in some women with endometriosis include 1. uterosacral ligament nodularity, tenderness or thickening 2. an adnexal mass 3. lateral displacement of the cervix and 4. cervical stenosis.

Adenomyosis

It is characterized by the presence of endometrial glands within the myometrium, resulting most frequently in severe dysmenorrhoea and menorrhagia. Women with adenomyosis typically have a slightly enlarged, globular, tender uterus on physical examination. Adenomyosis may also be suggested by ultrasound or MRI but the diagnosis remains clinical with pathological confirmation.

Chronic pain after PID may result from persistent or recurrent infection or be caused by scarring, tissue damage and adhesions. Chlamydial infection may be asymptomatic in women, thus no acute episode may precede the chronic sequelae. Additionally with improved antibiotic treatment and radiologic and laparoscopic abscess drainage, more woman with acute PID and tubo- ovarian abscess are managed conservatively.

Pelvic adhesions may result from previous infection, scarring from endometriosis and surgery. Pain is most likely to occur from adhesions when they are extensive or result in fixation of internal organs.

Evaluation of Gynaecologic Chronic Pelvic Pain

In the initial evaluation, the history helps to identify causes of pain that are hormonally responsive. For example, pelvic pain that is more intense just before or during the first few days of menses is likely caused by endometriosis or adenomyosis. Woman with endometriosis report premenstrual spotting, dyspareunia, dyschezia, poor relief of symptoms with non-steroidal anti-inflammatory drugs, progressively worsening symptoms, inability to attend work or school during menses, and the presence of pelvic pain unrelated to menses. Non-hormonally responsive disease should be considered for pain that is not related to menses. This category includes both gynaecologic causes of pelvic pain (*e.g.*, chronic PID and pelvic adhesions) and non-gynaecologic causes (*e.g.*, IBS, diverticulitis, fibromyalgia or interstitial cystitis).

Laboratory and Imaging Test

These are useful in the evaluation of woman with chronic pelvic pain, include WBC count, urinalysis, tests for chlamydia and gonorrhoea, pregnancy test and pelvic ultrasound. Pelvic ultrasound is highly sensitive for detecting pelvic masses, including ovarian cysts and uterine leiomyomas. Endometriosis cysts of the ovary (endometriomas) often have a characteristic ultrasound appearance that allows for an ultrasound diagnosis. Sonography is very useful for identifying small pelvic masses (<4 cm in diameter) that are often not palpable on bimanual pelvic examination. For many cases of chronic pelvic pain such as endometriosis and chronic PID, a surgical procedure such as laparoscopy is required to make a definitive diagnosis.

Treatment of Gynaecologic Chronic Pelvic Pain

Many authorities believe that resection/ablation of endometriosis lesions improves pelvic pain caused by endometriosis. A non-hysterectomy approach to the treatment of chronic pelvic pain is nerve transection procedures. **Laparoscopic ureterosacral nerve ablation (LUNA)** involves the destruction of the uterine nerve fibres that exit the uterus through the uterosacral ligament.

Presacral neurectomy refers to the interruption of the sympathetic innervation of the uterus at the level of superior hypogastric plexus. Prospective and retrospective cohort studies suggest that hysterectomy is effective in relieving chronic pelvic pain from many diverse aetiologies.

Danazol is a derivative of testosterone and has moderate affinity for the androgen receptor. At doses used in clinical practice (200–800 mg daily) danazol suppresses endometriosis lesions by suppressing LH, FSH and the estrogen secretion and by blocking estrogen action in the lesions.

Symphysis Pubis Dysfunction

One problem that many pregnant women about is pubic pain which is caused by pelvic girdle area not working in the way it should, probably because of hormones, mis- alignment of the pelvis, or on interaction of the two. Any activity that involves lifting one leg at a time or parting the legs tends to be particularly painful. Pregnancy hormones including progesterone tend to loosen the ligaments of the body in preparation for birth and especially woman whose joints are flexible before pregnancy are more susceptible to the effects of hormones.

Quite often it is a self limiting and pain disappears within few weeks of delivery. Avoid the use of vaccum extractor and forceps, as these may necessitate opening the legs wider than pubic symphysis can safely tolerate. Epidural is to be avoided if at all possible as this is often associated with more severe damage. It seems logical that an elective caesarean section might prevent damage to the pubic symphysis, but in reality the problem is caused during pregnancy and elective caesarean wont fix it.

Levator Ani Syndrome

This has been described in association with a variety of organic conditions but also occurs under circumstances in which organic disorders are absent and the pathophysiology is uncertain. The pain is often described as dull aching or pressure like discomfort in the rectum, lasting several hours. Prolonged sitting and the act of defecation have been described as precipitating factors. Several studies have suggested that increased anal canal pressures and increased EMG activities often are present.

As is often the case with poorly understood entities a wide variety of treatments alone or in combination, have been reported to be effective. The use of muscle relaxants such as diazepam and methocarbomol in addition to massage and sitz bath was reported to be effective, although not by all investigators. Electro galvanic stimulation through a rectal probe produced 80%–90% improvement of symptoms in unselected patients. Surgical division of puborectalis muscle showed initial optimistic results but subsequent studies reported a high incidence of incontinence for liquid or gas.

Proctalgia Fugax

It is an obscure disorder that was first described more than 100 years ago and is characterized by sudden severe pain in the rectal area lasting several seconds or minutes, then disappearing completely, leaving the patient asymptomatic until the next episode. In contrast to levator ani syndrome patients are often asymptomatic when examined, and there are no characteristic findings to improve diagnostic certainity. In two uncontrolled studies of patients with proctalgia fugax who sought medical attention, a high percentage were found to have high scores for anxiety, hypochondriasis, perfectionist tendencies and somatization. There have been reports of benefits with clonidine, nitrates, diltiazem and caudal epidural block. The presence of psychological dysfunction should lead to consideration of antidepressants anxiolysis or psychotherapy where appropriate.

Pudendal Nerve Entrapment

Pain caused by entrapment of pudendal nerve is confined mainly to the perineal region. It is positional in nature exacerbated by sitting and partially relieved by standing or recumbent. The diagnosis is confirmed by nerve conduction studies which shows distal motor latency for the offending nerve. There was a report of surgical decompression of the pudendal nerve which was found to be flattened in the pudendal canal of Alcock and in contact with the sharp inferior border of sacrospinous ligament. After surgical decompression and rehabilitation, the patient experienced significant relief of pain and returned to normal activity.

Musculoskeletal

Fibromyalgia is a chronic condition that presents with diffuse musculoskeletal pain. There are 9 defined anatomic tender points providing 18 possible sites of excessive tenderness. Excessive tenderness in 11 or more of 18 along with fatigue is considered diagnostic. Fibromyalgia symptomatology has been associated with patients who suffer from chronic pelvic pain.

In myofascial pain syndromes, the tenderness is confined to one anatomic region. Palpation of trigger points produces a characteristic and reproducible pain pattern. In patients with chronic pelvic pain, trigger points are commonly found in back and abdomen. Topical medications and trigger point injections have been used to treat this disorder alongwith NSAIDs.

Role of Neural Blockade

Neural blockade can be used for diagnostic as well therapeutic purposes in the management of pain which originates from the pelvis. This can be used to differentiate the origin of the pain, central from peripheral and visceral from somatic. The process of therapeutic blocks should only be undertaken after evaluating the underlying pathology. Peripheral nerve blocks have a very limited applications. Most of the structures are innervated by sympathetic nerves. However, **pudendal nerve block** for entrapment of pudendal nerve is a definite option and block of this nerve with local anaesthetic along with steroid provides effective pain relief. Similarly **Ilioinguinal nerve block** in a patient following its entrapment in inguinal hernia surgery does produce good pain relief.

Sympathetic nerve blocks have been used effectively in the management of pelvic pain not responding to other means. **Superior Hypogastric plexus** block is an important tool in the pelvic pain management of cancer origin. This plexus is located retroperitoneally at the lower half of the fifth lumbar and the upper part of the first sacral vertebra. This is connected above with another sympathetic plexus–celiac plexus. Superior hypogastric plexus provides sympathetic innervation to fundus of the uterus, fallopian tubes, broad ligament, part of the urinary bladder and the distal part of colon. The block of the plexuses performed either under X-ray control or this can be guided by CT. After a diagnostic block with local anaesthetic, neurolytic agent is then injected. A further confirmation of the position of the needle is achieved by using contrast media and visualizing it spread under fluoroscopy.

Ganglion of Wallther (ganglion Impar) is the termination of the sympathetic chain. It is located at the sacrococcygeal junction and a block of this ganglion is used to relieve the pain in the perineal regions and the genitals. Patients with malignancy of rectum, urinary bladder, colon and cervix have shown appreciable pain relief with blocking ganglion of Impar.

Epidural Block

The role of this block lies only in terminal patients, where other treatment options have failed or not possible. The other role of epidural block lies in distinguishing between central and peripheral origin of the chronic pelvic pain. Differential epidural block can be used to help clarify the segmental level of origin, after administering graded dosages through an indwelling epidural catheter. If it is decided to keep an indwelling catheter for more than a few days, infection through the catheter should be carefully guarded against.

Intrathecal / Epidural Opioids

This is an option when other palliative measures of pain control have failed to produce desired pain relief. This has an inherent danger of producing respiratory depression. For long-term pain relief, epidural catheter is tunnelled and there is an option of implantation of injection port.

Summary

Chronic pelvic pain is difficult to diagnose and to treat because of the multiple and often overlapping causes. A systemic approach aids in the thorough evaluation and appropriate therapy. At the initial visit, a thorough history should be taken and complete physical examination performed. Screening for coexisting conditions, such as depression, narcotic abuse is crucial, so these issues may be addressed immediately while additional causes for pelvic pain are evaluated.

REFERENCES

1. Zondervan KT, Yudkin PL, Vessey MP et al. Prevalence and incidence of chronic pelvic pain in primary care: Evidence from a national general practice data base. Br J Obs Gynecol 1999;106:1149–55.
2. Koninckx PR, Meuleman C, Demeyere S et al. Suggestive evidence that pelvic endometriosis is a progressive disease. Whereas deeply infiltrating endometriosis is associated with pelvic pain. Fertil Sterile 1991; 55: 759–65.

3. Ling FW. Randomized control trial of depot leprolide in patients with chronic pelvic pain and clinically suspected endometriosis. Obs Gynecol 1999;93:51–8.
4. Stacey CM, Munday PE. Abdominal pain in women attending a genitor urinary medicine clinic: who has PID? In J SID AIDS 1994;5:338–42.
5. Horwitz BJ, Fisher RS. Current concepts: the irritable bowel syndrome. New Engl J Med 2001;334:1846–50.
6. Manning AP, Thompson WG, Heaton KW et al. Towards a positive diagnosis of irritable bowel. BMJ 1978;2:653–4.
7. Fall M, Johansson SL, Aldenborg F. Chronic interstitial cystitis– a heterogenous syndrome. J Uro 1987;137:35–8.
8. Peeker R, Enerback L, Fall M, Alderborg F. Recruitment, distribution and phenotypes of mast cells in interstitial cystitis. J Uro 2000;163:1009–15.
9. Mattila J, Linder E. Immunoglobin deposit in bladder epithelium and vessels in interstitial cystitis; possible relationship to circulating anti intermediate filament auto antibodies. Clin Immunol Immuno Pathol 1984;32:81–9.
10. Hang L, Wullt B, Shen Z, Karpman D, Svanborg C. Cytokine repertoire of epithelial cells lining the human urinary tract. J Uro 1998;159:2185–92.
11. Pontari MA, Hanno PM, Reggieri MR. Comparison of bladder blood flow in patients with/ without interstitial cystitis. J Uro 1999;162:330–4.
12. Hanno PM. Diagnosis of interstitial cystitis. Uro Clin North Amerc. 1994;21:63–6.
13. Peters K, Diokno A, Steinert B, Yuchico M, Mitchell B, Krohta S, Gillette B, Gonzalez J. The efficacy of intravesical Tice strain bacillus Calmet Geurine in the treatment of interstitial cystitis. A double blind, prospective placebo control trial. J Uro 1997;157;2090–2094.
14. Nickel JC, Prostatitis. Evolving management strategies. Uro Clin North Amerc. 1999;26;737–51.
15. Schaeffer AJ, Darras FS. The efficacy of norfloxacin in the treatment of chronic bacterial prostatitis refractory to cotrimoxazole and /or carbenacillin. J Uro 1990;144:690–3.
16. Meares EJ. Prostatitis and related disorders in : Walsh PC, Retik AS, Stamey TA, Vaughan EDG, ad. Campbell's urology Philadelphia:WVSaunders.1992;p807.
17. Rouviere H, Delmas A .In:anatomy human volume –2 : Parris Masson. 1985;557.
18. Rab M, Ebmer And J, Dellon AL. Anatomic variability of illioinguinal and genito femoral nerve.Implications for the treatment of groin pain. Plast Reconstr Surg 2001;108:1618–23.
19. Gray CL, Powell CR, Amling CL. Outcomes for surgical management of orchalgia in patients with identifiable intrascrotal lesions. Eur Uro J 2001;39:455–9.
20. Padmore DE, Norman RW, Millard OH. Analysis of indications for and outcomes of epididymectomy. J Uro 1996;156:95–6.
21. Westrom L, Joeseof R, Reynolds G et al . Pelvic inflammatory disease and fertility. Sex Trans Dis 1992,19;185–92.
22. Peters AA, Trinbos-kemper GC, Admiral C et al. A randomized clinical trial and the benefits of adhesiolysis in patients with intraperitoneal adhesions and chronic pelvic pain. Br J Obs Gynecol. 1992;99:59–62.
23. Rao SSC, Hatfield RA. Paroxysmal anal hyperkinesis; a characteristic feature of proctalgia fugax. Gut 1996; 39:609–612.
24. Wallace WC, Madden WM. Experience with partial resection of the puborectalis muscles. Dis Colon Rectum 1969;12:196–200.
25. Barnes PRH et al. Experience of posterior division of puborectalis muscle in the management of chronic constipation. Br J Surg 1985; 72:475–477.
26. Thompson WG. Proctalgia Fugax. Dig Dis Sci; 1981; 26:1121–1124.
27. Pilling LF, Swenson WM, Hill JR. The psychological aspect of proctalgia Fugax. Dis Colon Rectum1972; 8:372–376.
28. Amarnath L, Welder SD. Caudal epidural block in the management of proctalgia fugax. Am J Pain Management. 1994; 4:153–155,
29. Ramsden CE. Pudendal nerve entrapment. Am J Phys Med Rehabl—01-JUN-2003;82(6): 479–84.
30. Applegate W V. Abdominal cutaneous nerve entrapment syndrome. Surgery. 1972;71:118–24.
31. Beard RW. Chronic pelvic pain. Br J Obs Gynecol 1998;105:8–10.

•••

38

MECHANISM OF VISCERAL PAIN

Visceral pain is the most common form of pain produced by disease and need immediate medical attention. Most of the knowledge about the visceral pain is based on the basic mechanisms of pain derived from the experimental studies of somatic nociception.

Superficial pain is well localized and evokes specific protective reflexes, but deep pains are characterized by poor localization, tonic increase in muscle tone and evoke strong autonomic responses *e.g.*, changes in respiration, heart rate, blood pressure. Deep pain also evokes stronger emotional responses.

Pain arising from internal organs differs in important ways from that arising from somatic structures. Visceral pain is difficult to localize and is diffuse in character. It is often associated with greater autonomic and motor responses than somatic pain. Unlike somatic structures, the principle conscious sensations that arise from the internal organs are discomfort and pain.

All viscera receive dual innervations involving both cranial and spinal nerves with secondary interneuron in the medullary and spinal dorsal horn. They have additional sensory neurons with cell bodies in and on the viscera themselves, in the ganglia near the viscera (celiac, inferior mesenteric ganglia) or may have cell bodies in the sympathetic chain (para vertebral ganglia).

Visceral pain is an important component of the normal sensory repertoire of all human beings and is treated by different specialists differently, but more effective relief of visceral pain requires deep knowledge of the causation of pain of internal origin.

Mechanism of somatic and visceral pain are different, so the information obtained on one cannot be inter-related and interpreted for the other. However, more is learnt about the mechanism of somatic and visceral sensations, more it is realized that apart from various similarities, many important differences exist.

Most human visceral pain models have been applied to GIT, and relied mainly on mechanical and electrical stimuli.

Visceral Sensory Neurons[2]

Axons of visceral sensory neurons are mostly either in myelinated A delta fibres or unmyelinated C fibres, the proportion of C fibres predominating generally. Further it is seen that high threshold fibres are neither uniformly C fibres nor the low threshold fibres contain predominantly A delta fibres. Similarly the conduction velocity and spontaneous activity of visceral C or A delta fibres is not same.[3]

Causes of True Visceral Pain

Any stimulus that excites pain nerve endings in diffuse area of the viscera causes visceral pain. Various causes are:

1. Ischaemia, because of the formation of acid metabolic end products or tissue degenerative products like bradykinin, proteolytic enzymes or others.
2. Chemical stimuli–proteolytic acidic gastric juice leaks through a ruptured gastric or duodenal ulcer causing wide spread visceral peritonitis, stimulating broad areas of pain fibres.
3. Spasm of the hollow viscus–spasm of the portion of the gut, gall bladder,[4] bile duct, ureter etc, can cause pain by mechanical stimulation of the painful nerve endings. Pain from a spastic viscus is in the form of cramps (increasing and then subsiding), occurs intermittently and is seen during gastro-enteritis, constipation, menstruation, parturition, gall bladder and ureteric colics.
4. Over distension of a hollow viscus–over filling over stretches the tissues or can cause collapse of blood vessels causing ischaemic pain.

Peripheral Mechanisms of Visceral Pain[5]

Visceral afferents possess many of the characteristics of nociceptors. The mechanosensitive afferent fibres, innervating most of the hollow viscera exists in two types. Some fibres have low thresholds for response (<5mm Hg of distending pressure) but encode distending stimulus intensity into the noxious range, others have thresholds for response that falls in noxious range (>30 mm Hg of distending pressure).

These observations suggest that both low and high threshold mechanosensitive visceral afferent fibres contribute to discomfort and pain and all the visceral afferent fibres function as nociceptors.

Endogenous algogen bradykinin excites both splanchnic and vagal afferent fibres. The effect of bradykinin on vagal afferent fibres was indirect (secondary to, longitudinal muscle contractions) and the direct action on splanchnic nerve afferents is mediated by beta-2 bradykinin receptors.

Similarly, a central modulation has been proposed to explain pain associated with the respiratory system. Lungs and bronchi are innervated by vagal and sympathetic afferent fibres. Vagal fibres identified as mechanosensitive afferents, respond to stretch (inflation or deflation of the lungs) and chemo-receptors called J-receptors respond to varied algogenic chemicals *e.g.*, bradykinin, prostaglandin, serotonin and capsaicin.

Visceral Hyperalgesia[6]

Ritchie was the first to document the presence of visceral hyperalgesia in patients with irritable bowel syndrome. Two mechanisms are responsible:

★ Peripheral mechanism sensitizes the afferent fibres innervating the insulted tissues.

★ Central mechanism involves changes in the[7] excitability of spinal and supraspinal neurons.

Tenderness of colon during abdominal distension can be reproduced by sigmoid distension at endoscopies in more than 50% of suffering patients and similarly during oesophageal distending pressure of 8 mL volume.

Sensory Versus Afferent[2]

Three different groups of internal organs can be distinguished depending on the kind of sensation evoked from them.

1. Organs from which pain is the only sensation that can be evoked. Largest group includes heart, blood vessels, respiratory airways, stomach, biliary system, small intestine, pancreas, ureter and internal reproductive organs.
2. Organs from which painful and non-painful sensations can be evoked: oesophagus, colon, rectum and urinary bladder.
3. Another new type of sensory receptor contributes to the signalling of chronic visceral pain, to long-term alteration of spinal reflexes and abnormal autonomic regulation of internal organs.

Non-painful sensations are related to digestive or excretory functions. The afferents are those that evoke regulatory reflexes and those mediate painful and non-painful sensations. These afferents could form single, two or exist in three separate groups.

Silent Receptors

These have no spontaneous activity, nor respond to acute high intensity mechanical stimulation in normal circumstances, but become active after inflammation of the peripheral organs. These afferents are functionally different from the rest of visceral afferents and are mainly concerned with stimuli such as tissue injury and inflammation. These are present in most viscera *e.g.*, colon and bladder and contribute to signalling of chronic visceral pain, to long-term alterations of spinal reflexes.

Sensitization of Visceral Sensory Receptors

Cutaneous nociceptors possess the capacity to increase their excitability following intense noxious stimulation or local injury by, (*a*) lowering of threshold, (*b*) an increase in supra threshold responsiveness, (*c*) development of nociceptors sensitization. The response closely matches the cutaneous hyperalgesia, that is characterized by decrease in pain threshold and increased pain sensation around the injured site. There is an increase in body of evidence to show that central mechanisms are responsible for secondary hyperalgesia by the arrival to the CNS of nociceptive afferent barrage from the injured site.[7] Thus inflammation of the gastric mucosa or bladder evokes painful sensation which can be depicted as cutaneous representation. Although central mechanism plays vital role in moderating this sensation, there is increased afferent activity due to the sensitization of visceral sensory receptors.

Table 38.1 : Thoracoabdominal pain

Visceral	Referred	Musculoskeletal	Neurogenic	Cutaneous	Miscellaneous
Thoracic					
Lung/trachea Carcinoma (Pancoast) Pneumonial/	Shoulder Shoulder- hand syndrome	Bony origin rib/ sternum Costochondritis (Tietze's	Herpes zoster Acute Postherpetic syndrome	Scars	Vascular Angina Pulmonary infarc Aortic

Pleurisy Heart Myocarditis; Mediastinitis; Angina Oesophagus Carcinoma; Oesophagitis	Patietal pleura irritation Diaphragmatic irritation Angina Midthoracic Angina Gastro-oesopha- geal reflux joint disease Bone metastases Soft tissue: muscle ligaments, breast Post-trauma Postsurgical	syndrome) Vertebrae Disk disease Facet syndrome Compression fracture Osteoporosis steroids Degenerative	Causalgia Post-trauma Postsurgical Myelopathies Demyelination Spinal cord Injury		Infectious disease Metastatic disease
Upper mid abdomen					
Pancrease Pancreatitis, acute Carcinoma	Midepigastric Gall bladder PUD	Rectus abdominis syndrome Hernias: Umbilical	Herpes zoster Acute Postherpetic syndrome	Scars	Porphyria Vascular occlusion Sickle cell anaemia
Stomach Carcinoma; Gastric and duodenal ulcerations; Gastritis Liver Hepatitis; Carcinoma Gall bladder Cholelithasis; Cholecystitis, Carcinoma Intestine Crohn's disease Acute; Obstruction; Herniation; Volvulus; Adhesions Chronic; Carcinoma Carcinoma Kidney/Ureters Nephrolithiasis; Carcinoma; Polycystic disease;	Periumbilical Renal Appendicitis Flank Pancreatic Renal (chro- nic renal insufficiency)	Ventral	Causalgia Diabetic neuropathy Myelopathies		SMA syndrome Irritable bowel Toxins: Pharmacologic Pharmacolo- gical Environment

Pyleonephritis Miscellaneous Postsurgical **Low abdomen** **Pelvic** Bladder Carcinoma; Cystitis Testicles/ Ovary Post-trauma; Torsion; Tubo-ovarian abscess Prostate Carcinoma Uterus/Cervix Carcinoma; Endometritis Miscellaneous Endometriosis; Ectopic pregnancy; Postsurgical phantom syndrome Inguinal hernia	Dysmenorrhoea Postsurgical phantom syndrome (S/P hyster-ectomy; S/P orchiectomy) Lower back pain	SI joint dysfunction Organ prolapse Pelvic metastases	Postherpetic syndrome Causalgia	Scars	Porphyria

Altered Visceral Sensation after Repetitive Stimulation or Inflammation

It is a common clinical observation that is persistent and intense stimulation of the viscera and inflammation results in increased pain sensitivity. Similarly the condition like irritable bowel syndrome and irritable stomach syndrome are characterized by painful sensation in the absence of any injury.

Excitability Changes of Visceral Sensory Receptors

Several electrophysiological studies have reported the responses of visceral afferent fibres to (*a*) repetitive stimulation of their receptive endings (*b*) local or systemic administration of algesic chemicals (*c*) ischaemia or hypoxia.[7] Effects of hypoxia on visceral afferents include initial sensitization producing increased afferent inflow from the hypoxic viscus which in turn evokes reflexes aimed at restoring normal blood flow and in addition ischaemic pain.

Biochemistry of Visceral Pain

When tissue is injured, a host of potential sensitizing chemicals are released or synthesized at the site of injury or released from circulating cells attracted to the site of injury. These include amines (histamines, serotonin), peptides (substance-p, CRGP), bradykinin, cytokines, prostaglandins and leucotrienes, excitatory amino acids (glutamate) and free radicals. Two distinct biochemical classes of fine unmyelinated primary afferents are present and differ from each other. These peptides and non peptide groups differ anatomically and contain different neuro transmitters. Biochemical identification of visceral afferents suggests that peptides are particularly important for the transmission of information from viscera. Bradykinin NK-2 receptors are also implicated in visceral nociception and to control intestinal motility or colon distension.

Spinal Mechanism of Visceral Pain

Hyperalgesia following a noxious stimulus consists of two components[7] (*a*) primary hyperalgesia (*b*) secondary hyperalgesia. The mechanisms that underlie primary and secondary hyperalgesia are sensitization of nociceptors and increase in the excitability of central (spinal) neurons respectively. After a tissue injury, there is an increase of afferent barrage arriving at the spinal cord in addition to the release of chemical mediators of nociception leading to increased excitability of neurons on which these afferents terminate.[6]

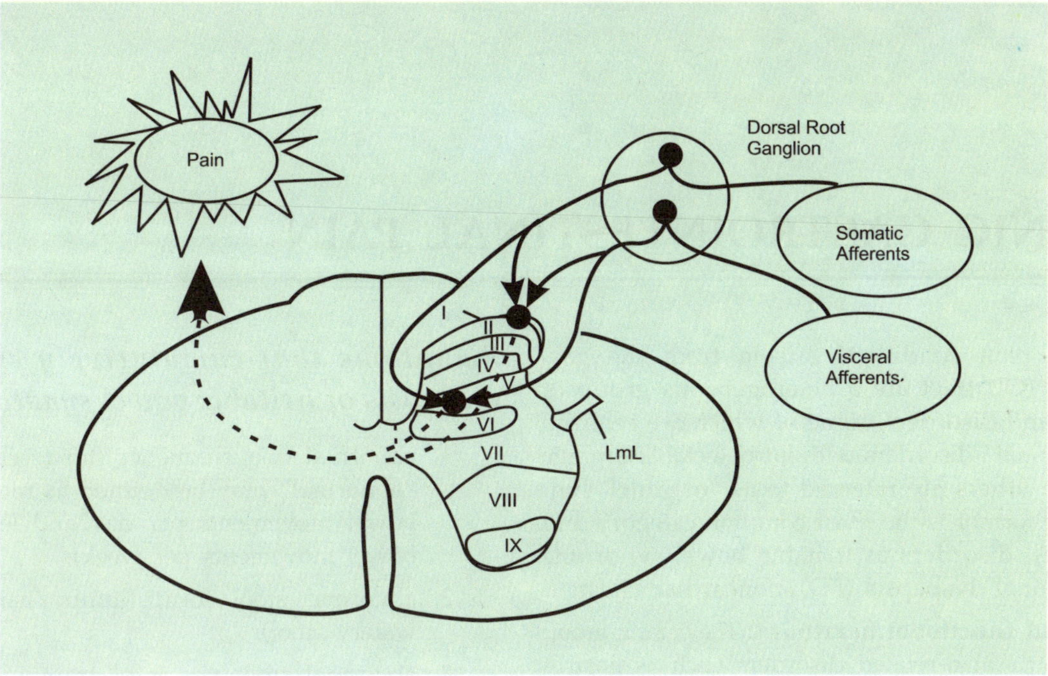

Fig. 38.1 : Viscerosomatic convergence of primary afferent fibres onto dorsal horn output of these neurons contribute to perception of visceral pain

Central Mechanism of Visceral Pain

Prolonged noxious stimulation of the viscera increases the excitability of viscerosomatic neurons in the spinal cord inflammation of the viscera leading to increased responsiveness of the spinal cord neurons. "Wind up" is regarded as a display of central sensitization but visceral nociceptive neurons which are quite capable of showing increased excitability on prolonged noxious stimulation, do not "wind up" as is seen with somatic neurons.

Repetitive noxious stimulation increases the excitability of spinal cord nociceptive neurons due to activated neuronal discharges or release of certain neuro-transmitter or both. Positive feedback loops increase excitability especially on visceral nociceptive neurons and is responsible for the enhanced motor and the autonomic reflexes. Post synaptic release of neurotransmitter enhances the excitability further following prolonged stimulation.[8]

Role of peripheral NMDA receptors is important in normal visceral pain transmission and might be responsible for the peripheral sensitization and visceral hyperalgesia. The existence of neuronal mechanisms capable of painful raising the question of pain memory has been seen. Pain could be induced by micro stimulation of the thalamus many years after actual event. These are mainly seen for visceral pain. Cortical specialization in the sensory discriminative, affective and cognitive areas of the cortex could account for the perceptual differences observed between somatic and visceral pain.

REFERENCES

1. Cervero F. Visceral hyperalgesia revised. Lancet 2000; 356:1127.
2. Cervero F. Mechanism of visceral pain–updated review. Refreshers course syllabus. Pain 2002;40:403–411.
3. Glamberardino MA. Recent and forgotten aspect of visceral pain. Eur J. Pain. 1999;3:77–92.
4. Gordon A, Irving. Acute pancreatitis. Pain.1997;45:319–333.
5. Guyton and Hall. Text book of medical physiology. Visceral pain. 10th ed. 2000:48:557–559.
6. Houghton AK, Wang C C et al. Do nociceptive signals from pancreas travel in dorsal column? Pain 2001;89:207– 220.
7. Laird JMA, Martinez- Caro L. A new model of visceral pain and reffered hyperalgesia. Pain 2001a:92:335–342.
8. Nessij and Gebhart GF. Visceral pain – A review of experimental studies. (review article). Pain. 1990;41:1 67– 234.

•••

CHRONIC GASTROINTESTINAL PAIN

39

Chronic pain conditions arising from the gastrointestinal (GI) tract are a heterogeneous group of syndromes and disorders, some of which are referred to as "functional" disorders without detectable organic cause, while others are referred to as "organic" syndromes. The former is the most common category and includes such disorders as irritable bowel syndrome (IBS), functional dyspepsia (FD), noncardiac chest.

Pain, and functional heartburn: The organic group includes gastric acid-related disorders such as gastro-oesophageal reflux disease, peptic ulcer disease, and chronic pancreatitis. IBS is likely to represent a heterogeneous group of disorders based on their pathophysiology and aetiology, all presenting with various combinations of abdominal pain, discomfort and altered GI function (such as altered bowel habits, difficulty in swallowing, and vomiting). Substantial evidence supports the concept that IBS overlaps with the other functional GI disorders (in particular FD and noncardiac chest pain), reflecting possible similar pathophysiology and suggesting similar treatments.

According to Rome II criteria IBS is now understood in terms of multiple pathophysiological determinants contributing to a common set of symptoms, rather than being considered a single disease entity. It is defined as a "group of functional bowel disorders in which abdominal discomfort or pain is associated with defecation or a change in bowel habit, and with features of disordered defecation."[1]

Rome II Diagnostic Criteria for Irritable Bowel Syndrome[2]

Atleast 12 weeks, which need not be consecutive, in the preceding 12 months of abdominal pain that has two out of three features:

1. relieved with defecation; and/or
2. onset associated with a change in frequency of stool; and/or
3. onset associated with a change in form (appearance) of stool.

Symptoms that cumulatively support the diagnosis of irritable bowel syndrome

1. abnormal stool frequency (for research purposes "abnormal" may be defined as more than three bowel movements per day and less than three bowel movements per week);
2. abnormal stool form (lumpy/hard or loose/watery stool);
3. abnormal stool passage (straining, urgency, or feeling of incomplete evacuation);
4. passage of mucus;
5. bloating or feeling of abdominal distension.

The diagnosis of a functional bowel disorder always presumes the absence of a structural or biochemical explanation for the symptoms.

Evolving Pathophysiological Models for Functional GI Disorders

Different conceptual models for IBS pathophysiology have been proposed to take into account the available body of pathophysiological and epidemiological data at a given time. While traditional reductionistic models had focused primarily on isolated peripheral aspects of IBS, such as epithelial function ("mucous colitis"), GI motility ("spastic colon"), or a combination of both ("spastic colitis"), more recent conceptual models of visceral hypersensitivity and postinfective IBS (PI-IBS) have taken into account both peripheral and central dimensions of the disorder.[3]

Post Infective IBS

Studies on function and tissue in PI-IBS patients have shown changes in intestinal motility and epithelial function, including increased intestinal permeability and bile acid malabsorption and increased numbers of colonic enteroendocrine cells. Histological evidence suggests alterations in mucosal function in PI-IBS, including an increased expression of interleukin 1â mRNA, increased cellularity of the lamina propria and an increase in CD3-reactive lymphocytes. The implication of stressful life events in the development of PI-IBS suggests a convergence of central and peripheral mechanisms in the expression of this syndrome.[3]

Interaction Between CNS-Directed and Gut-Directed Pathogenetic Mechanisms

A series of observations support bidirectional interactions between the central nervous system (CNS) and the immune system, as well as between CNS and the enterochromaffin cells of the gut. Mast cell degranulation in the gut occurs in response to psychological stress and can even result from Pavlovian conditioning. Mast cell products released in the gut (such as proteases or histamine) have the potential of activating and/or sensitizing visceral fibres. Altered stress responsiveness can be associated with increased permeability of the intestine, altering the access of luminal organisms and antigens to the gut immune system and thereby increasing susceptibility to inflammatory triggers in the gut lumen. Alternatively, immune cell products including different cytokines and chemokines released in the gut may have profound influences on the responsiveness of central stress circuits, including gene expression of corticotrophin-releasing factor (CRF) and vasopressin.[5] While acute peripheral inflammation may be associated with an upregulation of central stress responsiveness, chronic inflammatory processes such as rheumatoid arthritis or ulcerative colitis may be associated with a downregulation.[4]

Diagnosis of Most Common Syndromes

The diagnostic approach to patients presenting with abdominal pain differs widely depending on the acuteness or chronicity of symptom presentation. In the case of acute abdominal pain, the symptom is usually an indicator of underlying acute pathology such as inflammation, ulceration or perforation. A combination of physical examination and targeted endoscopic and radiological investigations are generally successful in identifying the underlying pathology and providing the basis for specific therapies. In the case of chronic pain, the approach is fundamentally different. A diagnosis is based on identifying positive symptoms consistent with the condition and excluding, in a cost effective manner, other conditions with similar clinical presentations. When "alarm features" such as weight loss, persistent diarrhoea, and family history of colon cancer are excluded, the specificity of the symptom based Rome I criteria for IBS exceeds 98%, and hence the risk of missing organic disease is low. Routine laboratory tests, including blood tests and stool analysis, are performed during the initial presentation of the patient. Depending on the primary symptom presentation and the patient's age and specific history, targeted standard endoscopic/radiologic examinations are performed with the goal of ruling out the most likely organic causes for the pain, such as peptic ulcer disease, erosive oesophagitis, malignancies and inflammatory bowel diseases.

Current and Future Therapies

Pharmacological Therapies

In the absence of published results from well designed clinical trials, it is a fair statement that less than a handful of drugs are better than placebo in the treatment of functional GI disorders. Little evidence supports superiority over placebo for any of the most commonly used drugs, such as antispasmodics and fibre in the treatment of chronic functional abdominal pain. Clinical evidence and meta analysis suggest that low doses of tricyclic antidepressants may be beneficial, even in patients without a diagnosis of depression or anxiety disorder. In contrast, there is no evidence for the effectiveness of selective serotonin reuptake inhibitors in patients without comorbid affective disorders.[6]

A series of drugs have recently been developed that are targeted at different serotonin receptors in the gut, in particular the 5-HT_3 and 5-HT_4 receptors. The first new effective drug for abdominal pain and diarrhoea was lotronex (alosetron HCl), a selective 5-HT_3 receptor antagonist.[7] However, potentially serious side effects observed in a small number of patients prompted the manufacturer to withdraw the drug. New targets for drug development for IBS include the neurokinin receptors, the cholecystokinin receptors and the corticotropin releasing factor (CRF) receptor.

Non Pharmacological Therapies

Evidence for the effectiveness of non-pharmacological interventions in the treatment of IBS is weak, even though clinically, many physicians see improvement with a variety of interventions. Several psychological treatments including cognitive behavioural therapy and hypnotherapy have been effective in controlled trials.

REFERENCES

1. Thompson W G, Longsterth GF, Drossman. Functional bowel disorders, GUT, 1999; 45:1143–1147.
2. Thompson W G, Longsterth GF, Drossman. Functional bowel disorders, Dorrsmann ga, Vora, Talley, N.J,(eds). Rome II. Functional GIT disorders diagnosis, pathophysiology and treatment, A multinational consensus, 2nd edition, McLeen; Degnon Associates,2000; pp 351–432.

3. Gwee KA. 1999. The role of psychological and biological factors in post infective gut dysfunctions. Gut 1999; 44;400–406.

4. MacQueen G, Marshall J,Perdue Segal S, et al. Pavlovian conditioning of RET mucosal mast cells to secerete mast cell protease II. Science 1989; 243:83–85.

5. Kresse et al. Millian M, Saperas et al.Colitis induces CRF expression in hypothalamic megalcellular neurons and blunts CRF gene response to stress in rats. Am.J. Physiol.Gastroinest Liver. Physiol.2001;281:G1203–G113.

6. Boyer WF. Potential indications for selective serotonin reuptake inhibitors, Int. Clin. Psycho Pharm, 1992;6: 5– 12.

7. Blanchard EB, Schwartz SP, Schultz M et al. Two controlled evaluation of multicomponent of psychological treatment of IBS. Behave Res. Ther. 1992; 30: 175–189.

•••

40

ACUTE DENTAL PAIN

Usually, dental pain is a result of dental caries. Initially, when the carious lesion is confined to the dentine, pain is evoked due to changes in temperature or exposure to sweet substances. As the lesion penetrates deeper into the tooth, the pain produced by these stimuli become stronger and lasts longer (hyperalgesia). Eventually, when the carious lesion affects the tooth pulp, an inflammatory process develops (pulpitis), which is associated with acute, intermittent spontaneous pain. Following pulp necrosis, micro-organisms and products of tissue disintegration invade the area around the root apex (periapical periodontitis) and the tooth becomes very sensitive to chewing, touch and percussion. At that stage the explosive, intermittent pain, typical of pulpitis, acquires a continuous boring nature and the tooth is no longer sensitive to changes in temperature. In clinical practice the demarcation between these various stages is sometimes indistinct; *e.g.*, the tooth may be sensitive simultaneously to temperature changes and to chewing.

Dentinal Pain

Pain originating in dentine is a sharp, deep, sensation. It is usually evoked by an external stimulus and subsides within a few seconds. Such stimuli are normally produced by food and drinks that are hot, cold, sweet or sour and the pain evoked by such stimuli indicate a hyperalgesic state of the tooth. The pain is poorly localized and the patient may not be able to distinguish whether it originates from the lower or upper jaw. Duplication of pain produced by control application of cold or hot stimuli to various teeth in the suspected area can aid in identifying the affected tooth.

Dentinal pain due to caries is best treated by removal of the carious lesion and restoration of the tooth. Sensitivity usually disappears within a day.

Table 40.1 : Differential diagnosis of dental and periodontal pain

Pain origin	Localization	Character	Intensity	Intensifiers	Associated Signs	Radiology
Dental						
Dentinal	poor	Evoked, does not outlast stimulus	Mild to moderate	Hot, cold, sweet or sour food	Caries, exposed dentine, defective restorations	Interproximal caries, defective restorations
Pulpal	Very poor	Spontaneous, explosive, intermittent	Moderate to severe	Heat, cold, sometimes chewing	Deep caries, extensive restorations	Deep caries or restoration with pulp exposure
Periodontal						
Periapical	Good	Continues for hours; deep and boring	Moderate to severe	Chewing	Periapical tenderness, redness and swelling	Usually no periapical changes at acute stage
Lateral	Good	Continues for hours; deep and boring	Moderate to severe	Chewing	Periodontal tenderness, redness, swelling, tooth mobility	Sometimes alveolar bone resorption

Pulpal Pain

Pain associated with pulp pathology (pulpitis) is spontaneous, strong and often throbbing and is exacerbated by temperature changes, sweet foods and pressure on the carious lesion. When pain is evoked it outlasts the stimulus and can be excruciating for many minutes. Similar to dentine pain, localization of pulpal pain is poor and seems to be even worse when pain becomes more intense. Pain may be described by patients in different ways. It may manifest as a continuous dull ache and can be periodically exacerbated for short or long periods of minutes to hours.[2] Pain may increase and throb when the patient lies down and in many instances it wakes the patient from sleep.[1] The pain of pulpitis is frequently not continuous and abates spontaneously; the precise explanation for such abatement is not clear. Localization of the affected tooth is achieved through hot and cold application and by percussion. Depending on the prognosis of the pulp (reversible or irreversible pulpitis) and that of the tooth, treatment may aim at conserving the pulp, extirpating it, or extracting the tooth. Pulpal pain usually disappears immediately after effective treatment.

Table 40.2 : Acute and chronic orofacial pain features

	Acute	Chronic
Time course	Short (hours to days)	Long (months to years)
Aetiology	Peripheral inflammatory	Central neuropathic
Response to:		
analgesics	Good	poor
psychrotopics	poor	moderate to good
Behavioural response "behaviour"	anxiety, "guarding"	depression, "illness"

Periodontal Pain

Periodontal pain usually results from an acute inflammatory process of the gingiva, periodontal ligament and alveolar bone due to bacterial infection. Pain is readily localized and the affected teeth are very tender to pressure. Two pathological pathways are common with pain resulting from either (1) pulp infection and pulp necrosis that results in periapical inflammation; or (2) periodontal infection with pocket formation that results in a lateral periodontal abscess. Although pain characteristics, ability to localize the pain, and pain producing situations are similar in both cases, treatment differs for aetiological reasons and these categories are therefore, discussed separately.

Acute Periapical Periodontitis

Pain is spontaneous and moderate to severe in intensity for extended periods of time (hours). Pain is exacerbated by biting on the tooth and, in more advanced cases even by closing the mouth and bringing the affected tooth in contact with the opposing teeth. In these cases, the tooth feels extruded and is sensitive to touch. Frequently the patient reports that pulpal pain preceded the pain originating from the periapical area. Localization of pain originating from the periapical area is usually precise; in this respect periodontal pain differs from the poorly localized dentinal and pulpal pain. However, although the patient is able to indicate affected tooth, in approximately half the cases that pain is diffuse and spreads into the jaw on the affected side of the face.[1]

During examination the affected tooth is readily located by means of tooth percussion. The periapical vestibular area may be tender to palpation. The pulp of the affected tooth is non-vital and therefore, does not respond to thermal changes or to electrical pulp stimulation. In more severe, purulent cases (acute periapical abscess) there is swelling of the face associated with cellulitis, sometimes accompanied by fever and malaise. The affected tooth may be extruded and mobile.

Treatment is aimed at the source of irritation in the pulp chamber and the root canal, which are open and debrided to allow drainage. Grinding the tooth to prevent contact with the opposing teeth helps to relieve pain. If cellulitis, fever and malaise are present, systemic administration of antibiotics is recommended. Soft tissue incision and drainage are very effective when a fluctuating abscess is present. Pain usually subsides within 24–48 hours.

Lateral Periodontal Abscess

Pain characteristics are similar to those of acute periapical periodontitis. Pain is continuous, well localized, and moderate to severe in intensity; it is exacerbated by biting on the affected tooth. Examination may show swelling and redness of the gingiva, usually located more coronally than in the case of acute periapical lesion. The affected tooth is sensitive to percussion and is often mobile and slightly extruded. In more severe cases, cellulitis, fever, and malaise may occur. A deep periodontal pocket (over 6 mm) is usually located around the tooth; probing of this pocket usually results in pus exudation. The tooth pulp, however, is usually vital, *i.e.*, it reacts to temperature changes and electrical stimulation. Gentle irrigation and curettage of the pocket should be performed. The tooth should be ground in order to prevent contact with the opposing tooth. When cellulitis, fever, and malaise are present, systemic antibiotic administration is recommended. Pain usually subsides within 24 hours of treatment.

Gingival Pain

Gingival pain may occur as a result of mechanical irritation, acute inflammation associated with a gingival pocket or acute bacterial or viral infection.[3]

Food Impaction

Gingival pain caused by food impaction is characterized by localized pain between two adjacent teeth especially after meals, and particularly when food is fibrous. The pain is annoying with a feeling of pressure and discomfort. Pain gradually disappears until evoked again at the next meal and may be relieved by removing the food impacted between the teeth. Upon examination, a faulty contact between two adjacent teeth is usually noticed, where food tends to get trapped. The gingival papilla is inflamed, tender to touch and bleeds easily. The cause of the faulty contact between the teeth is often a carious lesion, and restoring the tooth will eliminate the pain.

Pericoronitis

This severe pain is usually located at the distal end of the arch of teeth at the lower jaw. Pain is spontaneous, exacerbated by closing the mouth and aggravated by swallowing and may be associated with trismus. Upon examination, a flap of gingiva over a partially erupted tooth is acutely inflamed, red and oedematous. Occasionally, fever and malaise are associated with this infection. Treatment includes irrigation of debris between the flap and the affected tooth and eliminating contact with the opposing tooth (by grinding or extraction). Systemic antibiotic administration is commonly recommended especially when trismus occurs.

Acute Necrotizing Ulcerative Gingivitis

Soreness and pain are felt at the margin of the gums. Pain is intensified by eating and brushing the teeth and is accompanied by gingival bleeding. Metallic taste is sometimes experienced, and usually there is a fetid smell from the mouth. Necrosis and ulceration are noticed upon examination of the marginal gingival, with different degrees of gingival papillary destruction and adherent greyish slough represents the pseudomembrane that is present in the acute stage of the disease. Swabbing this slough is associated with pain and bleeding. Although basically this is bacterial disease that responds to antibiotics, it is not clear whether the bacteria initiate the disease or are merely secondary to underlying local or systemic factors. Treatment includes swabbing and gently irrigating the ulcerative lesions, preferably with an oxidizing agent (hydrogen peroxide, scaling and cleaning the teeth). Systemic antibiotics are recommended when fever and malaise are present.

REFERENCES

1. Sharav Y, Levine RE, Tekert A, et al. The spatial intensity and unpleasantness of acute dental pain.Pain 1984;20:363–366.
2. Cohen S. Endodontic diagnosis In: Cohen S Burns RC (Eds). Pathways of the pulp, 7th ed. St. Louis, CV Mosby 1996.
3. Sharav Y. Orofacial pain; dental, vascular and neuropathic pain. 2002 – An updated review. Refresher course syllabus. Giamberardino MA, (Eds) IASP Press, Seattle, 2002.

•••

ISCHAEMIC PAIN

41

Chronic critical limb ischaemia is manifested by pain at rest, non healing wounds and gangrene. Ischaemic rest pain is typically described as a burning pain in the arch or distal foot that occurs while the patient is recumbent but is relieved when the patient returns to a position in which the feet are dependent. Objective haemodynamic parameters that support the diagnosis of critical limb ischaemia include an ankle-brachial index of 0.4 or less, an ankle systolic pressure of 50 mm Hg or less, or a toe systolic pressure of 30 mm Hg or less. Intervention may include conservative therapy, revascularization or amputation. Progressive gangrene, rapidly enlarging wounds or continuous ischaemic rest pain can signify a threat to the limb and suggest the need for revascularization in patients without prohibitive operative risks.

Risk Factors

Chronic critical limb ischaemia is the end result of arterial occlusive disease, most commonly atherosclerosis. In addition to it in association with hypertension, hypercholesterolemia, cigarette smoking and diabetes, less frequent causes of chronic critical limb ischaemia include Burger's disease, or thromboangiitis obliterans and some forms of arteritis.[1]Diabetes is a particularly important risk factor because it is frequently associated with severe peripheral arterial disease. Atherosclerosis develops at a younger age in patients with diabetes and progresses rapidly. Moreover, atherosclerosis affects more distal vessels in patients with diabetes; the profunda femoris, popliteal and tibial arteries are frequently affected, while the aorta and iliac arteries are minimally narrowed. These distal lesions are less amenable to revascularization. Atherosclerosis in distal arteries in combination with diabetic neuropathy contributes to the higher rates of limb loss in diabetic patients compared with non-diabetic patients.

Clinical Presentation

The development of chronic critical limb ischaemia usually requires multiple sites of arterial obstruction that severely reduce blood flow to the tissues. Critical tissue ischaemia is manifested clinically as rest pain, non-healing wounds or tissue necrosis (gangrene).

Ischaemic rest pain is classically described as burning pain in the ball of the foot and toes that is worse at night when the patient is in bed. The pain is exacerbated by the recumbent position because of the loss of gravity assisted flow to the foot. Ischaemic rest pain is located in the foot where tissue is farthest from the heart and distal to the arterial occlusions.[2] Patients with ischaemic rest pain often need to dangle their legs over the side of the bed or sleep in a recliner to regain gravity augmented blood flow and relieve the pain. Patients who keep their legs in a dependent position for comfort often present with considerable oedema of the feet and ankles.

Non-healing wounds are usually found in areas of foot trauma caused by improperly fitting shoes or injury. A wound is generally considered to be non-healing, if it fails to respond to a 4–12 weeks trial of conservative therapy.

Gangrene is usually found on the toes. It develops when the blood supply is so low that spontaneous necrosis occurs in the most poorly perfused tissues.

Diagnosis

The presence of rest pain can sometimes be difficult to discern in patients with other chronic leg pain such as that caused by peripheral neuropathy. Labelling a wound as non-healing can also be a subjective assessment. However, a number of physical findings and objective haemodynamic parameters can be used to substantiate a diagnosis of chronic critical limb ischaemia. Typical physical findings include absent or diminished pedal pulses, shiny smooth skin of the feet and legs, and muscle wasting of calves.

Differential Diagnosis

Ischaemic rest pain may be confused with night cramps, arthritis or diabetic neuropathy. Night cramps occur in the calf muscles; they usually awaken the patient from sleep and are relieved by massaging the muscle, by walking or by using antispasmodic agents. Patients with arthritis of the metatarsal bones may have pain in the foot. The distinguishing characteristic of the arthritic pain is that it usually occurs intermittently and at sporadic intervals, whereas ischaemic rest pain consistently occurs after a specific interval of recumbency. Diabetic neuropathy may also present with pain in the foot and is occasionally associated with diminished pulses and trophic skin changes. This pain, however, is not steadfastly associated with recumbency.

Ischaemic rest pain: Patients with ischaemic rest pain should be given pain medication as necessary, and any underlying systemic cause of inadequate blood flow such as CCF, should be corrected. If pain persists after 4–8 weeks of conservative therapy with pain medication and interventions to optimize the patient's overall condition, the possibility of operative intervention should be explained to the patient including the risks and benefits of the procedure.

Surgical intervention includes revascularization and amputation. Arteriography is often performed for further evaluation and planning of revascularization. Some centres are utilizing magnetic resonance angiography as an alternative or supplement to ateriography to minimize the risk of dye exposure.

Non-healing wounds: Conservative therapies include teaching the patient ways to avoid trauma to the wound site, including the wearing of properly fitting shoes. Dressings should be changed frequently; the patient should be seen weekly until the wound heals. Progressive gangrene, rapidly enlarging wounds and continuous ischaemic rest pain unrelieved by dependency are each unstable condition that can rapidly lead to limb loss and require urgent intervention.

Revascularization: Surgical interventions include revascularization or amputation. If the patient wants to undergo revascularization and is an acceptable operative candidate arteriography is often performed for further evaluation and planning of revascularization. Limb preservation by means of revascularization is cost effective, leads to a better quality of life for most patients and is associated with lower perioperative morbidity and mortality than amputation.

REFERENCES

1. Rybrol, Schurizer BA, Peters et al. Post operative analgesia and lung functions: a comparison of intramuscular with epidural ketamine. Acta Anesthesio Scand 198;26:514–518.
2. Raj PP. Practical management of pain 3rd edi., St Louis, Mosby Year Books; 1998.
3. Kehlet H; The endocrine metabolic response to postoperative pain. Acta Anesthesio Scand (suppl) 1982;74:173–175.
4. Lund C, Selmar P, Hensen OB et al. Effect of epidural bupivacaine on somatosensory evoke potential after dermatomal stimulation.Anesth. Analg. 1987;66:34–38.
5. Mather LE, Parentral opioids for postoperative analgesia. Res Anaesthe. 1982;7:144.
6. Islas JA, Astorgc J, Laredo M. Epidural Ketamine for control of postoperative pain, Anaesth. Analg. 1985; 64:1161–1162.
7. Kinahata LM. Spinal analgesia with morphine and clonidine. (editorial). Anesth Analg 1989; 65:194.
8. Maron RR. Orthopedic aspects of sports medicine. In : Sports medicine. Appenzelbro (ed). Baltimore, Urban and Schwarzenberg 1988.
9. Callilet R. Soft tissue pain and disability. Philadelphia, F A Davis, 1983.

•••

TEMPOROMANDIBULAR DISORDERS

42

Pain in the musculoskeletal system is among the most common types of painful disorders in the body, including the orofacial region. The temporomandibular disorders (TMD) are currently viewed as a cluster of related pain conditions in the masticatory muscles, temporomandibular joint (TMJ) and associated structures, *i.e.*, they are considered as a form of musculoskeletal pain.

Mechanism of Orofacial Musculoskeletal Pain

A mechanism-based classification of orofacial musculoskeletal pain will at least require a detailed description and evaluation of both spontaneous pains (*e.g.*, intensity, quality, and localization) and stimulus-evoked pain (*e.g.*, responses to different stimulus modalities).

Intensity of Spontaneous TMD Pain

TMD pain can be persistent and constant, but there can also be substantial variation across time with exacerbations and spontaneous remission. Standard descriptions of persistent (TMD) pain usually state that the intensity ranges from mild to moderate to strong or even excruciating levels of pain and that the pain is often exacerbated by muscle function[1] of perceived pain intensity, requires the use of standardized scales, such as verbal descriptor scales of visual analogue scales (VAS) .[2] A survey of recent clinical studies on persistent TMD pain indicated that the average pain level measured on a 100-mm VAS with the jaws at rest ranges between 30 mm and 50 mm.[3] VAS scores greater than 30 mm, probably represents at least moderate pain levels. The perceived pain intensity of TMD generally fluctuates with significant differences between the lowest, highest and average pain, VAS scores during a week and between different facial sites. The use of diaries also can be helpful to estimate the pain because the perceived pain intensity of TMD patients can change over time simply due to regression of the mean. Furthermore, the memory of pretreatment jaw-muscle pain is significantly dependent on the past and present levels of pain[4] showed that the experimental chewing increased the levels of pain in a majority of patients with persistent jaw-muscle pain.

Quality of Spontaneous TMD Pain

The usual way to describe persistent TMD pain is, as deep, dull ache, sometimes with a boring, pressing or tightening type of pain. The McGill Pain Questionnaire (MPQ), originally introduced as an attempt to provide a detailed description of the quality of pain,[5] has become the most frequently used pain questionnaire.

In a sample of 200 patients with persistent facial pain including TMD pain, Turp et al. (1997) found that more than 30% of subjects used the words 'aching', 'tight', 'throbbing', 'tender', 'exhausting', 'nagging', 'sharp' and 'tiring'. The choice of 'radiating' (26%) and 'pressing' (22%) seems rather specific for TMD pain conditions compared to other pain conditions.[6] The quality of pain appears to be markedly different between patients with myofascial TMD pain and pain in the TMJ.[7] It is unclear whether this difference can be explained by activation of different nociceptive fibres in the muscle and joint tissue or by higher-order cognitive-emotional differences. Thus, certain words seem to be specifically related to the description of persistent TMD pain, but no word is specifically indicative of this pain condition in a similar way that 'pulsating' has been tied to migraine and 'pressing' and 'tightening' to tension-type headache.

Pain drawings made by patients are simple, but useful tools to illustrate the localization and extent of pain areas in general. Pain drawings completed on a systematic basis by patients with pain complaints in the craniofacial region have revealed that only about 19% have pain confined to this region, whereas 66% have widespread referred pain outside the craniofacial and cervical regions.[7]

The various theories on referred pain mechanisms have been reviewed recently.[3] There is a general agreement that the diffuse nature and poor localization of muscle pain is related to central convergence of afferent fibres onto common central neurons because this feature will in effect reduce the spatial resolution of somatosensory information. The nociceptive afferents from muscles, joints, skin and viscera converge onto common projection neurons. It is nevertheless unclear why muscle or joint pain can be referred to the skin, whereas the reverse is seldom encountered. Differences between cutaneous and muscular nociceptive afferents in terms of somatotopic organization, sizes of receptive fields, and laminar distribution of their terminals may explain the predominant referral of muscle pain[10]. Other mechanisms than central convergence are also likely to be involved in the expression of referred pain, because there is normally a time delay between the onset of local and referred pain. One possibility is that the nociceptive barrage from muscle tissue opens up latent connections, in a form of central divergence.[8] The synaptic connections between neurons that originally had no effective drive from the myositis-induced muscle may now become effective. The neurobiology subserving such mechanisms is probably related to central sensitization of second-order neurons and the development of hyperexcitability.

Table 42.1 : Possible strategies for non-surgical management of temporomandibular disorders

Physical	Pharmacological	Psychological
Stretch therapy	Topical NSAIDs	Information
Jaw exercises	Oral NSAIDs	Counselling
Massage	Acetaminophen	Education
Ultrasound	Glucocorticosteroids	Stress management biofeedback
Heat/cold	Muscle relaxants	Relaxation
TENS	Benzodiazepines	Cognitive-behavioural therapy
Soft laser	Tricyclic anti-depressants	Psychotherapy
Acupuncture		
Oral splints	Opioids	

Management of Orofacial Musculoskeletal Pain

Because the underlying mechanism of TMD pain is only partially understood, it is difficult to design therapy to cure the pain. Instead a more realistic goal will be to alleviate pain. Thus, the management strategies for TMD pain follow the same principles of management of other musculoskeletal pain conditions and may be physically, pharmacologically and psychologically oriented (Table 42.1).

Physical Management of TMD Pain

There may be a significant reduction in perceived pain intensity following the intervention (*e.g.*, acupuncture, biofeedback or splints), but that there may only be marginal or even no difference when the active treatment is compared to a placebo control. Thus, the specificity of many of the proposed treatments appears to be remarkably low. Oral splints have also been used extensively for management or even for 'curing' TMD pain.

Pharmacological Management of TMD Pain

Nonsteroidal anti-inflammatory drugs (NSAIDs) like ibuprofen in combination with diazepam provide significantly better pain relief compared to ibuprofen alone or placebo. A short-acting benzodiazepine, triazolam, improved sleep, but failed to provide significant pain relief in TMD patients. A combination of acetaminophen, codeine and doxylamine succinate (antihistaminic) provided significant pain relief than placebo in another study in mixed TMD patients.

Psychological Management of TMD Pain

Systematic studies on the efficacy of psychological management of TMD pain are rather scarce. A combination of biofeedback, stress management, and oral splints provides significant and long-lasting pain relief in TMD pain patients.[2] It appears to be important to tailor the treatment to each individual patient and not to consider psychological interventions on TMD pain as a treatment of last resort, but rather use it concurrently with biomedical and dental treatments.

Surgical Management of Pain

In some selected cases with persistent pain in the TMJ and restrictions in movement, which have not responded adequately to conservative treatment, surgical approaches may be recommended to alleviate the symptoms. The procedures range from irrigation of the upper joint space of the TMJ (arthrocentesis), direct inspection, lysis and lavage (arthroscopy), to positional changes in the condyle (modified condylotomy) or removal of the disk (diskectomy). It is clear treat that irrespective of the specific procedure, the success rate is close to 80% or more.

REFERENCES

1. Okeson JP. Bell's orofacial pains. Chicago.Quintessence, 1995.
2. Grace Ly RH. Studies of pain in normal man. In:Wall PD, Melzack.R.(Ed). Textbook of pain Edinburgh; Churchill Livingstone 1994; 315–336.
3. Svennsson and Graven-Nielsien T. Craniofacial muscle pain. Review of Mechanisms. J. Orofacial pain, 2001;17:2–10.
4. Feine JS, Laigne GJ, Dao TTT et al. Memories of chronic pain and perceptions of relief. Pain 1998;77: 137–141.
5. Melzack R. The MacGill pain Questionnaire; Measured properties and scoring methods. Pain 1975; 1:277–300.
6. Turp JC, Kowalzki CJ, Stohler CS. Pain descriptors characteristics of persistent facial pain. J. Orofac Pain. 1997;11: 285–290.
7. Mogini F, Italiano M. TMJ disorders in myogenic facial pain;A Discriminative analysis using MPQ. Pain 2001; 91: 323–330.
8. Mens S, Hoheisel U, Kaske et al. Muscle pain: Basic mechanisms and clinical correlate in Jenson TS, Turner JA et al. Eds,Proceedings of 8th World Congress of Pain, Progress in pain research and management, Vol 8 Seattle : IASP: Press, 1997; 479–4996.

•••

PAIN MANAGEMENT IN AIDS

43

Acquired immunodeficiency syndrome is caused by HIV-1 and HIV-2 viruses. HIV type 1 is a retrovirus containing RNA, core protein and a reverse transcriptase enzyme allowing virus to assemble DNA from its RNA. The new viral DNA incorporates into the host DNA, encoding for viral replication. The RNA also contains genes that regulate HIV synthesis, determine virus infectivity and down regulate HIV replication.[1] HIV surface glycoproteins bind to lymphocytes, monocyte macrophage cells and control nervous cells leading to immune system defects and incompetence.[2] The HIV infection progress slow or fast depending on the antigenic infections, genetic predisposition, environmental factors etc.[3]

HIV infection presents clinically in several different forms:

1. Asymptomatic
2. Acute HIV disease
3. Lymphadenopathy
4. Severe infections (Pneumocystis carinii) or mild infections (Candida)
5. Tumours – Kaposi sarcoma
6. Autoimmune–Idiopathic thrombocytopenic purpura
7. Systemic symptoms only – fever, chills, fatigue
8. Neurological – HIV encephalopathy
9. Psychiatric disorders (depression)
10. Renal – HIV nephropathy.

Diagnosis

1. HIV antibody test – Enzyme linked immunosorbent assay (ELISA).
2. The Western Blot – more specific test.[5]

HIV Encephalopathy[6]

Aetiopathogenesis

1. Neural death from HIV infection.
2. Neuronal dysfunction.
3. Alteration of CNS trophic factors, nerve growth factor, resulting in neuronal death or dysfunction.
4. An alteration of neurotransmitter production and release.
5. Blockade of neuroreceptor for neurotransmitter or trophic factors resulting in cellular dysfunction or death.
6. Altered neuronal function following elaboration of alpha interferon and inter-leukin 2a.

Table 43.1 : Chronologic list of HIV Associations

Preoperative visit	
Anaemia	Azidothymidine (AZT) effect
Ataxia, paresis	Vascular myelopathy
Azotemia	Nephropathy
Behaviour (high-risk)	HIV infection
Cough	Bronchitis or pneumonitis from opportunistic infection
Dysaesthesias paresthesias (distal)	Predominantly sensory neuropathy; herpes zoster
Fatigue	Anaemia; electrolyte imbalance from vomiting or diarrhoea
Fever, headache	Aseptic meningitis
Mentation (altered)	HIV encephalopathy; increased intracranial pressure from a mass
Plaques (white, tongue)	Oral hairy leukoplakia
Papules (red, palate)	Kaposi sarcoma
Radiculopathy	Herpes zoster

Syncope, orthostatic hypotension	Autonomic neuropathy; dehydration
Weakness (motor)	Guillain-Barre syndrome
Resuscitation	
Intubation, catheters	Fluid exposure; induction of infection
Traumatic wounds	Fluid exposure
Preinduction	
Catheters	Fluid exposure; induction of infection
Peridural access	Thrombocytopenia, coagulation abnormalities; progressive neurological disease; immune compromise; induction of bacterial infection, assessment of peripheral nervous system
Induction	
Analgesics	Possible suppression of immune function; tolerance from IV drug abuse
Hypnosedatives or inhalation agents	Exacerbation of encephalopathy; oversensitivity from CNS disease
Oxygen	Compensation for V/Q mismatch (opportunistic infection)
Succinylcholine	Hyperkalemia from neuromuscular disease or vacuolar myelopathy
Enflurane	Seizure
Nitrous oxide	Leukopenia
Nondepolarizing muscle relaxants	Aberrant neuromuscular function (neuromuscular junction spared)
Cardiac arrest	Autonomic neuropathy
Intraoperative	
Oxygen	Oxygen desaturation from pulmonary disease; compromised CNS, function; anaemia
Analgesics	Opioids versus local anaesthetics
Arrhythmias	Antiviral drug interaction or side effects, cocanine abuse; cardiomyopathy
Ventricular failure	Wall motion or valve abnormalities; pericardial effusion
Aerosolized blood	Orthopaedic or cardiothoracic surgery
Liver metabolism	Alcohol abuse; antifungal agents
Emergence	
Extubation	Fluid exposure
Ventilation	Prolonged
Postoperative	
Analgesics	Opioids versus local anaesthetic; consider best opiate route
Assessment	Neurological alterations (central or peripheral nervous system)

Clinical Features

Symptoms vary from headache, behavioural changes, encephalopathy, grand mal seizures (encephalitis), syncope, limb weakness, trunkal rash, weight loss, cough, chest pain, azotemia, accidental fracture, myalgia (myopathy), sleep disorders, hallucinations (psychological disorders), spastic paresis, ataxia and dementia (myelopathy).

Diagnosis of HIV Encephalopathy[7]

There is evidence of peripheral neuropathy in 50–90% which is either

(*a*) Immune mediated – Guillain-Barre syndrome, Demyelinating polyneuropathy.

(*b*) Vasculitis - Multiple mononeuropathy.

(*c*) Dying back neuropathy – Sensory neuropathy.

(*d*) Ischaemic neuropathy – Herpes zoster.

Symptoms

Cognitive – confusion, slowed thinking.

Behavioural – depression, personality change.

Signs

Motor – clumsiness, limb weakness.

EEG shows background slowing.

Coagulation abnormalities – thrombocytopenia, prolonged prothrombin time, increased bleeding time.

CSF – increased protein, mononuclear cells and IgG levels.

CT scan – subcortical brain atrophy (SBA).

MRI – SBA and periventricular demyelination.

Autonomic Nervous System Changes in HIV Infection (65% incidence in AIDS)

1. Bradycardia and hypotension followed by syncope, general anaesthesia, intrathecal or epidural analgesia results in cardiac arrest.
2. Autonomic dysfunction – diarrhoea, sweating and impotence.

Neuromuscular Junction

Polymyositis, muscle weakness, increased CPK, inflammatory myopathy with perivascular and interstitial infiltrates.

Pain Management

Parasthesias, dysaethesias and burning, all produce discomfort even if patient doesn't complain of pain. These symptoms don't respond to analgesics. Local anaesthetic blocks can treat pain due to reflex sympathetic dystrophy, herpes,[8] peripheral neuropathy and Guillain-Barre syndrome. The treatment includes local infiltration, somatic nerve blocks, sympathetic nerve blocks and epidural blocks. However, somatic nerve blocks *e.g.*, intercostal block only produce a numbness.

Local Infiltration

Subcutaneous infiltration of bupivacaine 0.25% 20 mL with 80 mg methyl-prednisolone[9] repeated 2–4 days in herpes.

Sympathetic Nerve Blocks

For example, Stellate ganglion for face, neck, upper thorax and lumbar sympathetic block for abdomen or lower limbs can relieve dysaesthesias[10] after herpes and sensory neuropathy.

Epidural Blocks

Used for herpes or abdominal pain, Guillain-Barre (GB), syndrome and neuropathy. Bupivacaine 0.25% 10 mL, every week till pain and lesions disappear.

Potential Peridural Neurological Concerns with HIV Infection

An infection, neurological disease, coagulation disturbance contraindicate epidural injection.

CNS – HIV infection, increased intracranial pressure from a tumour, local anaesthetic systemic toxicity.

PNS – (Guillain-Barre) syndrome
Local anaesthetic neural toxicity
Epidural catheter neural injury or exacerbation of neural disease
Vascular neuropathy
Intraneural injection injury.

Epidural Complications

1. Anterior spinal artery occlusion
2. Epidural haematoma
3. Epidural abscess
4. Spinal cord or nerve root injury
5. Intravascular injection
6. Infectious contamination of spinal fluid
7. Dural puncture headache or unexplained subarachnoid drug effect.

Psychological Disturbances in AIDS Patients

1. Adjustment disorders – anxiety
2. Major depression, delirium, dementia, treatment related (chemotherapy), previous psychiatric illness, stress. There may be malignancy associated psychosocial factors *e.g.*, type C or lack of emotional expression – apathy, hopelessness, passive are also found in cancer. Thus a multi disciplinary approach to patient management in AIDS as adviced is a better option[7].
   (*a*) Physician evaluation – pain, history
   (*b*) Refer to a mental health provider, psychosocial evaluation for emotional, psychological problems is done and treated by counselling, stress management, biofeedback, imagery, hypnosis, meditation.
   (*c*) Medication therapy – for sleep, depression, anxiety, muscle relaxation techniques, anti–inflammatory analgesics *e.g.*, paracetamol and PCA, local topical applications.
   (*d*) Physiotherapy for tension, muscle strain compensation, dysfunction, stretching exercises, strengthening exercises, heat, TENS.
   (*e*) Sympathetic nerve blocks, local anaesthetic injections to relieve muscle spasm.
   (*f*) Management of primary disease – antiviral drugs, immunology, coagulation management, infection treatment, ventilatory sup-

port in G-B syndrome, interferon, radiotherapy in cancer. This includes management of symptomatic relief of symptoms[2] other than pain.

The obstetric anaesthesia can be managed for labour and delivery by regional anaesthesia techniques taking adequate precautions.

REFERENCES

1. Ho DD, Pomerantz RJ, Kaplan JC. Pathogenesis of infection with human immunodeficiency virus. N. Engl J Med. 1987; 317: 278–286.
2. Boisun DL, Lane HC, Fauci AS. Immuno pathogenesis of the AIDS. Ann Int. Med. 1985; 103: 704–709.
3. Haverkos HW. Factors assosciated with the pathogenesis of AIDS. J. Infectious Dis. 1987; 156: 251–257.
4. Saxon A, Campon V. AIDS. State of the art. J. Allergy Clin Immunol. 1988; 81: 796–802.
5. Burger J R. The neurological complication of HIV infection. Acta Neurscand. 1988; 116: 40–76.
6. Dalakas M, Wichman A, Sever J. AIDS and the nervous system. JAMA, 1989; 261: 2396–9.
7. Janisse T. Pain management of AIDS pt. In practical management of pain. Raj PP (ed.), St. Louis, Mosby Year Books, 1992; 546–573.
8. Ebstein E. Triamcinolone- procaine in the treatment of zoster and post herpetic neuralgia. Calfornia medicine. 1971; 115(2): 6–10.
9. Parkins HM, Hanlon PR. Epidural injection of local anaesthetics and steroid for relief of pain secondary to herpes zoster. Arch surg. 1978; 113: 253–254.
10. Higa K, Dan K, Manabe H et al. Factors influencing the duration of treatment of acute herpetic pain. Antibody titres. Pain. 1988; 32: 147–157.

•••

AGEING AND PAIN

44

There is a prevalence of muscloskeletal and joint pain of the neck, back, hip and knee and stiff joints on awakening in older (above 75 years) as compared to patients with mean age of 40 years, according to National Health Nutritional Survey[1] [epidemiologic follow-up study in 1982-1984.] even in cases where prevalence of pain was not higher in the older group, the intensity of pain was reported as more severe as were symptoms associated with depression and limitations of activities of daily living. Musculoskeletal pain has more impact in the old age.[2]

Laboratory studies showed effect of age on psycho-physical of pain sensitivity as below:

1. Thermal
   (*a*) Radiant heat: Response slightly higher pain, sensory and reactionary thresholds in elderly patients.
   (*b*) Contact heat: In sensory threshold, no age effects.
   (*c*) Cold pressor: Tolerance is lower in males while minimal increase in females with increasing age.
2. Electrical shock
   (*a*) Cutaneous: sensory threshold and tolerance is lower in elderly.
   (*b*) Tooth: In sensory thresholds, no age effects, lower discrimination accuracy in elderly, and response bias not affected.
3. Pressure on tendoachilles: Tolerance lower in elderly, sensory threshold higher.

Osteoarthritis is most common joint disorders in the elderly and has considerable effect on illness behaviour and suffering.[3] This is more prevalent in knee joint in the female population due to physiologic, psychological and social factors.

There are no age differences in pain sensitivity.

Presbyalgos – Age in later years of life systematically influencing pain sensitivity and perception is termed presbyalgos. The presbyopia above 55 years of age is loss of visual accommodation, compounded buy lens opaqueness is a frequent problem.

Presbyaccusis – is the progressive loss of higher frequency sounds, decreased speech recognition is due to peripheral changes in the labyrinth.[4]

Causes of presbyalgos:

1. Age dependent loss of receptors for pain (nociceptors).
2. Changes in primary nociceptors afferents.
3. Changes in more central mechanisms subserving pain sensation and perception.
4. Changes in descending pain control mechanisms.
5. Birth cohort differences in socio-cultural history that influence the meaning of pain.

Dementia

Effect of dementia on pain sensibilities and expression is unclear. Wide distribution of cerebral degenerative, loss of communicative and cognitive skills, as well as failure of basic reflexes (gag reflex) critical to survival in later stages of dementia leads to altered pain sensation. Pain assessment can be improved following newer pharmacological agents for symptomatic treatment of dementia. The pain perception, characterized by indifference leads to misdiagnosis of fracture of major bones simply because of pain is not reported.[5] The cure providers should be more educated, more efficient methods to assess and treat the pain in the older patients is needed.

Psychosocial problems of pain in elderly from family interviews showed the following results:

Loneliness and social isolation.

Learned helplessness.

Acute stress and anxiety.

Maladaptive environment.

Autonomous depression.

Personality disorder.

Organic syndrome.

Hypochondriasis.

Management was done by:

Increased family interactions.

Time-limited psychotherapy.

Behaviour modification through family.

Good communication from physician.

Benzodiazepines.

Antidepressant therapy.

Special Considerations in Geriatric Pain Assessment[6]

1. General considerations:
   (*a*) recognize that age itself does not reduce pain sensitivity;
   (*b*) recognize that there is no evidence that age per se influences qualitative properties of pain;
   (*c*) recognize the importance of encouraging the patient to discussing the pain.
2. Co-morbidity: illness and symptoms presentations in elderly who is often characterized by multiplicity, duplicity and chronicity.
3. Mental status : cognitive impairment assessment *e.g.*, dementia.
4. Depression : pain as a source of depression.
5. Activities of daily living : differentiate between limitations caused by painful or non-pain related dysfunction. The former leads to depression.
6. Medications : assess all current and recent medications (check the brown pill bag).
7. Family and social support systems should be maintained.

REFERENCES

1. National Health nutritional survey (NHA WES) I Epidemiologic follow up study (1982 – 1984); Plan and operation of the National Health and Nutritional Survey I (epidemiologic follow up study (1982-10/984) Vital Health Statistics Series I, No. 22, DHSS Pub No. (DHS) 87-1324.
2. Harkins SW, Price DD, Bush FM, et al. Geriatric pain In: Wall PD, Melzack R, (Eds). Textbook of Pain Edinburgh, Churchill-Livingstone, 1994: 769–784.
3. Hockbergh MC, Lawrence RC, Everett DF et al. Epidemiological associations of pain in osteoarthritis of knee: Data from the National Health and Nutritional Examination Survey and National Health and Nutritional Examination I. Epidemiologic follow up survey semin. Arthritis Rheum. 1989; (suppl 2):4–9.
4. Gordon – Salant S. Hearing. In : Encyclopedia of gerontology. Borren J(Ed) San Diego. Academic press, 1996; 643–654.
5. Fisher – Morris M, Gallantly A. The experience and expression of pain in Alzheimer patients. Age aging. 1997;26:497–500.
6. Harkin SW, Scott RB. Pain and presbyalgos In. Barren J(ed). Encyclopedia of gerontology. Borren J(Ed) San Diego. Academic press, 1996; 247–260.

●●●

SECTION–VII

Acute Pain

PHYSIOLOGICAL RESPONSE TO ACUTE PAIN

45

The physiological sensory and emotional experience of pain are associated with actual or potential tissue damage with histamine, serotonin, bradykinin, 5-HT, substance P and generation of noxious stimuli. The later may be manifested as increased muscle and sympathetic tone leading to increased metabolism and oxygen consumption.

Primary Afferent Mechanisms

Thinly myelinated Aδ fibres and unmyelinated C fibres, innervating skin and viscera give rise to pain and autonomic motor responses *e.g.*, changes in BP, heart rate and respiration. These afferents also release peptide transmitters *e.g.*, tachykinins, substance P, neurokinin and calcitonin, gene related peptides (CGRP). These substances cause hyperemia, plasma extravasation and leukocyte adhesion. The final contribution to the triple response includes the axon reflex "flare", contraction of smooth muscle in the airways, urinary bladder, iris and other tissues. These effects serve to increase the blood flow to an area and stimulate immune cell response. This may be beneficial local response to defend the tissue against the injury but in chronic inflammatory disease this persistent neurogenic component (bradykinin, 5-HT) exacerbate the inflammation leading to tissue damage. The inflamed tissue accumulates these inflammatory mediators leading to reduced pH in stomach, bladder and muscles, causing inflammation in these organs. Neuropeptides like CGRP release from sensory nerve endings by action potential invading the collateral fibres antidromically or by local reflex mechanisms trigger by raising concentration of free intracellular Ca^{++} ions (Fig. 45.1).

Respiratory Effects

Pulmonary changes during acute pain involving upper abdomen and thorax include reduced vital capacity, TV, RV, FRC and FEV_1. The cause of this is a reflex mediated increase in tone in abdominal muscles during expiration and a decrease in diaphragmatic function.[2] These result in reduced pulmonary compliance, muscle splinting, inability to breath, cough deeply and in some cases hypoxemia, hypercarbia, retention of secretions, atelectasis and pneumonia. Increase in muscle tone contributes to increased oxygen consumption and lactic acid production.

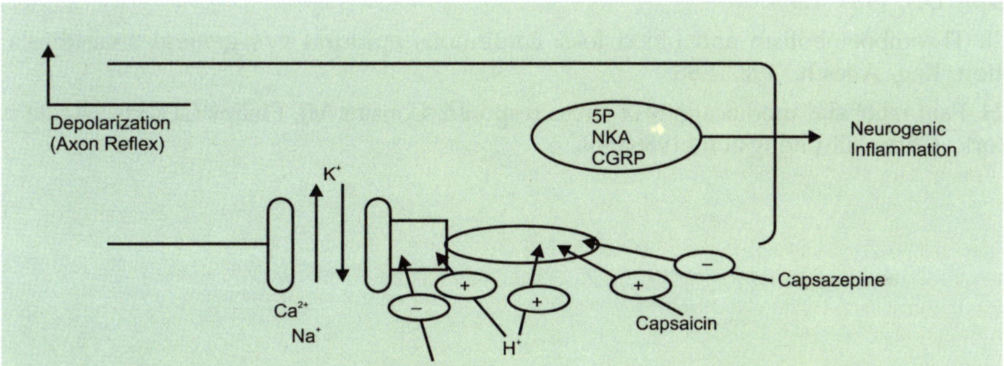

Fig. 45.1 : Physiology of nociceptive receptors

Cardio Vascular Effects

Pain stimulates sympathetic neurones and leading to tachycardia, increase in SV, cardiac work and myocardial O_2 consumption. The reduced fear of aggravating pain reduces physical activity, venous stasis and platelet aggregation and thus increasing the risk of myocardial ischaemia, infarction or deep vein thrombosis.[4]

Gastrointestinal Effects

Ileus, nausea and vomiting following pain is due to nociceptive impulses from viscera and somatic structures (*e.g.*, surgical pain). Post operative epidural analgesia have shown to be of improving the bowel functions.

Urinary Retention

Pain reduces the motility of the urethra and the bladder leading to urinary retention.

Stress Responses

The tissue injury associated with acute pain leads to adaptive neuroendocrine, immunologic and intracellular biochemical signals. The neuroendocrine response to pain involves hypothalamic pituitary endocrinal sympathoadrenal interactions. This subsequently results in increased sympathetic tone, hypothalamic stimulation, increased catecholamines and catabolic hormones secretion (cortisol, ACTH, ADH, GH,cAMP, glucagon, Aldosterone, renin Angiotensin II). Further there is a decreased secretion of anabolic hormones (insulin, testosterone). The effect of these changes include sodium and water retention and increased blood glucose, free fatty acids, ketone bodies and lactate. Metabolism and oxygen consumption are increased and metabolic substrates are mobilized from storage depots.[5]

Paediatric Patients

Acute pain causes suffering and physiologic abnormalities in children and neonates similar to those that occur in adults. Because of developmental, cognitive and emotional differences the assessment of pain in paediatric patients becomes more difficult.

Elderly Patients

The elderly patients may have more systemic diseases (*e.g.*, cardiac, pulmonary and endocrine). The different attitude and expectations about their treatment can also have a bearing on physiological status of these patients. There is no information available on their different pain threshold than young patients, though pain is less reported in elderly.

REFERENCES

1. Charlton JE. Treatment of Postoperative Pain, In: Pain 2002 an updated review. Giamamberardino MA {ed} SAN Diego. IASP Press. 2002.
2. Duggan J, Drummond BF. Activity of lower intercostal and abdominal muscle after surgery in humans. Anesth Analg 1987; 66, 852.
3. Ford GT, Whitelaw WH, Rosenal TW. Diaphragm function after upper abdominal surgery in humans. Am Rev Respir Dis, 1983: 127,431.
4. Modig J. Thromboembolism and blood loss: continuous epidural v/s general anaesthesia with controlled ventilation. Reg, Anesth.; 1982;1:88.
5. Kehlet H. Pain relief and modifications of stress response. Cousins MJ, Philips GD(eds): Acute pain management New York, Churchill-Livingstone:1986;p49.

•••

ACUTE PAIN SERVICES

46

It has been two decades approximately since the introduction of acute pain services. Originally considered to be the panacea for acute pain, management of acute pain patients continues to be problematic.[1] It is timely to re-examine the role and lacunae of acute pain services.

Inadequacies: National Health and Medical Research Council (1999)[2] documented these inadequacies.

Table 46.1 : Reasons for ineffective analgesia[2]

- Misconception. Pain intensity can be assessed by observation alone.
- The common idea that pain is merely a symptom and not harmful in itself.
- The mistaken impression that analgesia makes accurate diagnosis difficult or impossible.
- Fear of potential addiction to opioids.
- Concerns about respiratory depression and other opioid related side effects such as nausea and vomiting.
- Lack of understanding of the pharmacokinetics of various agents.
- Lack of appreciation of variability in analgesic response to opioids.
- Prescription for opioids that include the use of inappropriate doses and/or dose intervals.
- Misinterpretation of doctor's orders by nursing staff., including use of lower ranges of opioid doses and delaying opioid administration.
- The mistaken belief that patient weight is the best predictor of opioid requirements.
- Patients' difficulty in communicating their need for analgesia.

Substantial evidence has mounted to show that clinician's insufficient knowledge about pain mechanisms and management, in combination with erroneous beliefs and attitude towards pain and its management, in particular opioids, leads to suboptimal pain management.[3]

The increased understanding due to enhanced research, multimodal strategies, pre-emptive analgesia, appreciation of neuropathic pain as a result of nerve injury and the adoption of multidisciplinary approach have become the working fundamentals of present day acute pain services.[4] However, in spite of all standardized clinical, investigative and education programmes, the patients are still experiencing inadequate pain relief.[1]

Although an improved pain relief based on protocols and directing consistent standards of safe and effective care has resulted in improved patient outcome,[5] many lessons have been learnt as the nature and role of these services evolved along with the controversies generated (Table 46.2) over the past two decades.

Table 46.2 : Controversies surrounding an expanded role for acute pain management services[4]

- Abandonment of the "classical" concept of an acute pain service.
- "Individualized" treatment approaches.
- Education implications.
- Case managers.
- Multidisciplinary approach.

A. Barriers

1. Poor knowledge of pain control by physicians and nurses is still the major barrier to improving pain management.
2. The sociopolitical factors, myths and misconceptions are the newly identified institutional barrier to change.
3. Issues such as restrictions on drug administration, complicated paper work, inadequate funding, lack of institutional commitment and accountability, importance of pain management along with other various clinical activities.
4. Rising patient acuity and number of patients, shortage of qualified nurses and difficulty in getting nurses to attend training courses dictate the need for more radical steps, if there is to be a lasting and meaningful change.[7]

In an attempt to address institutional barriers and increased clinical accountability American Pain Society recommended the introduction of Pain intensity rating as a routine part of assessment.

1. Pain as a 'fifth vital sign' will make it 'visible', thereby raising its awareness.
2. Focus on revising the prescribed guidelines and on encouraging evidence based practice. By questioning the use of weak opioids for moderate to severe pain; oral morphine was successfully used in acute pain in children simply by providing prescribing guidelines to all prescribers.

B. Nurse Based Services

Rawal (1999)[8] – considers the most economically justified and efficacious model of delivering pain relief service provided by a nurse based anaesthesiologist supervised team. This overcomes the institutional barriers about additional costs of a new pain service in an already constrained budget. However, the **Nurse Based Services** suffers from:

1. Nursing practices, hospital protocols, delayed administration of analgesics due to hospital rules classifying opioids by statute as "controlled drugs" under narcotics act. The procurement of opioids from a locked cupboard, checking it against the prescription signed by an authorized person, prepare the medication and give it to the correct patient, complete the documents and lock the medications away. In a busy ward, this leads to a delay time of approximately 30 (minutes) to 1 hour, so the drug is not selected for administration.
2. This is compounded by double checking procedures (by 2 nurses) as in Australia. Mann and Redwood (2000)[6] did away with double checking procedures after 100% nursing staff reported a significant improvement in services. This case illustrates how professionals might negotiate their own institutional barriers despite major professional and legal implications.
3. Davies et al. 1999[9] described how in 506 patients in a teaching hospital, epidural catheters used for pain relief, were removed because of nursing resource constraints, hence depriving the patients of good pain relief. Attaining excellent analgesia depends on **more than simply selecting the right modality**. Issues like staff training, placement and organization of service delivery still remains.
4. Patients are still unwilling to communicate with the nursing staff about their pain because of perceived busyness of staff.[10]
5. Nurses are less concerned with patients' pain once continuous form of therapy *e.g.*, epidural infusions, PCA are commenced despite the need for continuous assessment.[11] Some nurses and doctors abrogate their responsibility by relying solely on machines and drugs to solve the pain problem.
6. Pain management needs to be formalized as an integral part of the organizational structure, with a commitment from hospital administrators to account for the patient nurse ratio for a better assessment, evaluation and management. This can be helped by achieving good outcomes.[11]

C. Local Factors

Worldwide proliferation of clinical guidelines for acute pain management, the continued prevalence of acute pain, highlight their inadequacy as these ignore the impact of contextual influences *e.g.*, local influences and barriers on clinicians decision making. Taking stock of contemporary pain management literature will lead to enhancing the current modus operandi of the Acute Pain Services, by evolving beyond their foundational state, tackle some very difficult issues causing obstacles.[7]

D. On Demand (PRN) Analgesic Delivery

Although on demand I.M. analgesic administration is a simple, inexpensive and widely employed method, the delays in analgesic dosing due to patients waiting as long as possible, expecting that pain medications will be delivered immediately on request, which is highly unlikely in a busy ward.

Secondly, PRN dosing 3–4 hours is unable to maintain therapeutic plasma concentration only 30% of this time interval. The individual differences between peak plasma concentrations vary 3 to 5 fold and time to peak activity, 7 to 10 folds. This along with nurse's response leads to 30 minutes to an hour delay in analgesic administration.[13]

E. Under Medication

Under medication of post-operative, burn and trauma patients occurs due to caregiver's fear that pain medication may mask changes in status and risk, patient addiction in spite of no reported cases of iatrogenic addiction ever reported. Pain due to cough, deep breathing, rib fractures were not treated adequately, manipulative procedures require more analgesic than normal analgesic drug doses.[14]

F. Variables Influencing Pain Relief[15]

Certain variables requiring different doses of attention are often overlooked. These are as follows:

1. **Old age** alters opioid dose response reducing the requirement.
2. **Weight:** Although analgesic drugs are administered on an mg/kg basis there is no evidence to link body weight to individual dose requirements and plasma concentrations.
3. **Culture:** A fact that patients react to pain according to what it means to them emotionally and how they are taught to respond, should be better recognized and assessed.
4. **Gender:** There are conflicting reports about influence of gender on self administered dose of analgesics. Male patients may self administer more analgesics to achieve desired results.
5. **Psychological factors:** Earlier evaluations showed that anxious patients reported higher pain scores and analgesic consumption. However, highly aggressive and angry patients tend to consume more medication than patients with passive coping styles. The aggressive patients demonstrated a tendency to be highly motivated and enjoy self administration of drugs.
6. **Pharmacokinetic alterations associated with major organ failures:** The fact that analgesic's hepatic uptake and clearance is delayed with increasing side effects in major organ failure *e.g.*, hepatic, renal or cardiac. Dose adjustment is of critical importance in the already compromised organ function.
7. **History of substance abuse opioid tolerance** leads to withholding IV- PCA. A well supervised setting allows PCA use successfully. A fact that these patients require increased amounts of drugs to compensate for baseline requirements and for controlling the pain following surgery or trauma is often over looked.
8. **Pharmacodynamics and other variables:** Alterations in blood brain barrier, cross tolerance and level of endogenous opioids may be responsible for inter-patient variability in pain perception and analgesic response. A correlation between CSF and plasma level concentrations of endogenous opioids in adult and children has been reported and not often found out.

Recognition of the Problem

Department of Health and Human Services, USA, in 1992 introduced the clinic practice guidelines for acute pain, focusing attention on under medication and benefits associated with optical control.[15]

The guidelines goal was to:

1. reduce severity of pain,
2. introduce more effective methods,
3. educate patients that marked increase in pain intensity should not be tolerated and educate caregivers about importance of prompt evaluation and treatment,
4. contribute to fewer complications, improved outcome and shortened hospital stay.

The guidelines emphasized that:

Pain management should be considered to be essential part of physician's commitment to patient care, and recommended an organized, individual approach to pain control, with clear lines of responsibility, frequent assessment and treatment. Governmental recognition of the problem was followed quickly by reviewers in medical and lay press, which reshaped attitudes about, and expectations of acute pain control.

Possible Role Expansion of Acute Pain Management Services[11]

- Recognition of pain as a continuum. Not readily classified as acute or chronic.
- Major surgery–post operative care by anaesthesiologists and nurses.
- Opioid tolerance/abuse must be properly understood.
- Palliative care in cancer patients by managing pain along with GIT, renal, psychological problems contributing towards improving quality of life at the end stages.
- Acute and chronic pain – backache, cancer, myalgia, trauma.
- Neuropathic pain- diabetes, nerve injury, iatrogenic, alcohol neurolysis.

Hopeful signs[17]

1. Commission on Accreditation of Health Care Organizations implemented new statutes "to assess and control pain".
2. The American Academy of Pediatrics made a statement calling on physicians to do more to control children's pain.
3. Veterans Health Administration published VHA National Pain Management strategy advocating proper treatment of pain as "there were some incredible inconsistencies in the way our patients were treated for pain".
4. Dr. Robert D Kerns, PhD, Chief of Psychology Service at Connecticut Health care system proposed a strategy for transforming pain into a vital sign, just as important as temperature, pulse and blood pressure. In early 2000, says Kerns, only 50% of medical care givers were aware of

the pain problem. Now the figure has jumped to about 5%. His subsequent goals include education of all clinical staff and expanded research on pain management.

5. International Association for Study of Pain decided in 2003 about a proposal to celebrate Global Pain Awareness Week (6-13 September, every year) by all IASP chapters.
6. Pain clinic OPD and pain curriculum for post graduate students in the field of Anaesthesiology has been included in MCI requirements for recognition for medical institutions.
7. Indian Society for Study of Pain ISSP was started in 1984 with only 3 centres giving pain relief in whole of India. Now through its growth there are pain clinics in almost all medical colleges and major cities. The morphine availability laws were gradually simplified through the efforts of ISSP and WHO, thus easy for a practitioner to procure morphine after obtaining a narcotics license from the District Drug Inspector.[18]

REFERENCES

1. Mann E and Redwood S. Improving pain management. Breaking down the Invisible barrier. Brit. J. Nurs 200; 9(19):2067–2071.
2. National Health and Medical Research Council. Acute Pain Management. Scientific Evidence: Commonwealth of Australia, 1999.
3. Mark R and Sachar E. Under treatment of medical in patients with narcotic analgesics. Ann. Intern Med. 1973; 78173–181.
4. Hyang N, Cunningham F, Laurite C. Can we do better with post-operative pain management? Am J Surg 2001; 182: 440–8.
5. Harmer M and Davies K. The effect of education, assessment and standardized prescription on post-operative pain management. Anesthesiology, 1998; 53:424–30.
6. Taylor J and Wilson S. Focus on nursing clinical challenges. In: LumbyJ, Picore; D (Eds). Managing pain. Allen and Unwin, 2002; pp 3–17.
7. Bucknall T, Manias E, Bott M. Acute pain management: implications of scientific evidence for nursing practice in the post operative context. Int J Nurs Pract, 2001; 7: 266–73.
8. Rawal N. Ten years of acute pain service- achievements and challenges. Ref Anaesth Pain Med. 1999; 24(1): 68–73.
9. Davies H, McLeod G, Bannister J, McCrae W. Obstacles in organization of service delivery reduce the potential of epidural analgesia. BMJ, 1999; 319:1499–1500.
10. Carr E, Thomas V. Anticipating and experiencing post-operative pain: the patients' perspective. J Clin Nurs 1897; 6:191–201.
11. Lantry GL. Post-operative pain: Toward contemporary Acute Pain Services. In: Pain 2002– An Updated Review: Refresher Course Syllabus. Ca lamborardino MA(Ed) IASP Press, Seattle, 2002; 357–62.
12. Owen H, McMillan V, and Rogowsky D. Post-operative pain Therapy: A survey of patients' expectations and their experiences. Pain. 1990; 41:303.
13. Graves DA, Arrigo JM, Foster TS et al. Relationship between plasma morphine concentrations and pharmacological side effects. Clin Pharmac. 1985; 4:41.
14. Gwirz KH, Young JV, Walker SG et al. Intrathecal opioid analgesia for acute post-operative pain: Experience with $, 1334 surgical patients. Anesthesiology 1995; 83: A780.
15. Sinatra RS. Acute pain management and Acute Pain Services. In: Neural Blockade in clinical Anaesthesia and Management of Pain. 3rd Ed., Cousins MJ and Bridenbough, PO (Eds), Lippincott-Raven, Philadelphia, 198, 793–835.
16. Cart DB, Jacox A, Chapman RC et al. Acute Pain Management in infants, children and adolescents: Operative and medical procedures, Department of Health and Human Service. Pub. No. 92-0032, Agency for Health and Human Services. Rockville, MD; 1992.
17. Rebecca AC. Overcoming barriers to pain relief. Psychologists are among those knocking down the obstacles to successful pain treatment. Monitor on Psychology 2002; 33(4), 410.
18. Kumar P. A Handbook of Management of cancer pain and related symptoms: Morphine Availability in India. Samvedna, New Delhi; 2003.

•••

47

POST-OPERATIVE PAIN

The pathophysiology of pain and its malefic consequences upon recovery after surgery are the same anywhere in the world, but the resources available to relieve pain may be markedly different.

Henrik Kehlet[1] has demonstrated repeatedly that major surgical operations are still followed by unpleasant sequelae such as pain, reduced organ function, and a prolonged hospital stay. This is still the case despite the introduction of patient-controlled analgesia and multidisciplinary acute pain teams. It has been assumed that simply by ensuring that sufficient pain relief is not only available, but also given, then the optimal clinical outcome will occur. Yet this is manifestly not so, and it is now obvious that other factors must not only be considered, but also incorporated in our post-operative care plans if we are to improve outcome and shorten hospital stay.

Pathophysiology of Acute Post-operative Pain

The response to surgical trauma has been characterized as having two phases. An initial "shock" phase occurs where metabolic rate is reduced and with it most other physiological processes. In practical terms, this phase is brief and it is the second phase. The so-called "flow" phase, that dominates for days, or even weeks, depending upon the magnitude of the procedure and the presence or absence of complications. Characteristically, both metabolic rate and cardiac output rise. Plasma levels of catabolic hormones such as adrenocorticotrophic hormone (ACTH), cortisol, catecholamines, antidiuretic hormone (ADH), renin, angiotensin, aldosterone, and growth hormone rise, whereas anabolic active hormones such as insulin and testosterone start to fall.

The consequences are seen in alterations in glucose homeostasis, with increases in total body utilization of glucose. Lipid turnover and oxidation are enhanced, and there is usually a small increase in protein turnover and breakdown. In major trauma, however, the increase in protein breakdown can be much larger and of far greater significance. Post-surgical changes normally include a shift in the fluid and electrolyte balance toward sodium and water retention, with potassium retention and an increase in vascular permeability to albumin. These changes are coupled with a general "defence mode" of the body's immune mechanisms as shown by inhibition of fibrinolysis, increased coagulability, and other changes in immune function.

The responses to the surgical stimulus are endocrine, metabolic and inflammatory, and to a greater or lesser extent, post-operative pain relief will be directed at reducing these responses. Any injury, whether elective or traumatic, will follow basic pathways, and the greater the injury, the greater the intensity of the stress response. Thus any superficial surgery, including procedures with a short duration or those that do not involve a body cavity, will only show a relatively transient response. Conversely, operations involving the thorax or abdomen may lead to a profound response in which the flow phase can last for days, or even weeks if complications ensue.[2]

Reduction in the Stress Response

For many years researchers have suggested that reduction in the stress response will reduce post-operative organ dysfunction and that this, in turn, will lead to an improved outcome. Painstaking work, chiefly by Kehlet and his co-workers, have shown that only regional anaesthetic techniques will reduce the surgical stress response.[1] To be effective fully, the regional technique should be continuous. Several studies show that continuous epidural analgesia over a period of up to 48 hours is effective in modulating the stress response to lower limb and abdominal surgery.

Epidural opioid techniques have less effect upon the stress response and are comparable with the use of other, more conventional techniques.

Pre-emptive Analgesia

There have been many studies of identical amounts of different analgesic agents delivered before and after the painful stimulus. None have shown any benefit, with the exception of some studies where local anaesthetic techniques have been started before the procedure and then continued into the post-operative period. Various analgesics prevent the excitability of neurons due to release of amino acids and peptides (which in turn excite cells and trigger a cascade of changes in the cell. *e.g.*, entry of Ca^{++} ions, unmasking of NMDA receptors, release of nitric oxide and novel proteins, lasting for a few hours.

Types of Analgesia

Acetaminophen and NSAIDs

Acetaminophen (paracetamol) is devoid of anti-inflammatory activity, but is a most effective analgesic that has minimal side effects in clinical doses. This drug is the foundation of any analgesic regime and should be used routinely as part of the basic treatment of acute pain.

Non steroidal anti-inflammatory drugs (NSAIDs) are also a standard treatment for post-operative pain. Drugs in this group are also extremely effective but suffer from the drawback of having a substantial side effect profile. These agents may have significant central actions in addition to their recognized peripheral activity.[3] Acetaminophen and NSAIDs do not appear to have any effect upon the surgical stress response or upon organ dysfunction. Their main benefit appears to lie in providing moderate pain relief that will reduce opioid requirements by 20-30%.

As is the case for acetaminophen, having NSAIDs available to treat acute pain may offer benefits that greatly outweigh their risks, provided that these are borne in mind. Choice of drug will remain dependent upon availability, desired route of delivery, length of action and cost (Table 47.1) .

Table 47.1 : Monitoring and documentation of post-operative analgesia

Analgesic Medication:
Name, Concentration and dose of drug
Settings of PCA device (if used), demand dose lockout internal, continuous infusion
Amount of drug administered
Intervals of drug dose set in hours
Supplemental analgesics
Routine Monitoring:
Vital signs: Temperature, heart rate, blood pressure, respiratory rate
Analgesia
Pain at rest, with activity
Pain relief– Percentage, score
Supplement analgesics
Side Effects:
Cardiovascular: hypotension, bradycardia, ↑PR.
Respiratory status: Respiratory rate, level of sedation
Nausea and vomitting, pruritus, urinary retention
Neurological–Motor and sensory function and level.
Epidural haematoma
Treatment advise/Protocol
Treating side effects
CNS depressants concurrent use
Contact the physician incharge
Emergency analgesic, if other methods fail.

Table 47.2 : Equianalgesic doses of opioids

Drug	Parenteral	Route Oral (m.g.)	PCA bolus
Morphine	10	30	0.01–0.03 mg/kg
Codeine	130	200	–
Fentanyl	0.1	–	0.5–1 mcg/kg
Pethidine	75	300	0.2–0.5 mg/kg
Methadone	10	20	0.01–0.03 mg/kg
Oxy morphone	1	–	0.01 mg/kg
Levorphanol	2	4	–
Alfentanyl	0.1–0.2	–	0.1–0.2 mg
Buprenorphine	0.1–0.3	–	0.3–0.1 mg
Pentazocine	5–30 mg	–	0.1–0.4 mg/kg.

Opioids

Opioids are the main method of controlling acute post-operative pain. Morphine and its derivatives and synthetic compounds such as meperidine (Pethidine) and fentanyl are capable of excellent pain relief by a variety of routes. Despite this, there remain significant numbers of patients who do not receive adequate pain relief. Reasons for this include poor understanding of the drugs by both patients and staff. The length of action may be overestimated and the dosage prescribed inadequate. Clinicians may fail to assess and compensate for interpatient variability. Too many prescribing regimens are of the "one size fits all" type and may reflect knowledge deficits or prescribing prejudices. There may be inappropriate concerns about the dangers associated with opioids and reluctance on the part of the patient to ask for effective doses because of real or perceived problems such as nausea and vomiting or addiction.

1. The most common way of achieving effective pain relief is for small amounts of opioid to be given intravenously. Thereafter, intermittent intramuscular injections of opioid can be used to maintain pain relief. This approach is usually unsatisfactory when given on a p.r.n. basis, because the patient's reluctance to ask for medication, the time taken for the staff to respond, prepare, and administer the drug, and the onset time of the drug build an inertia into the system that guarantees a poor result. Fixed-interval prescribing would be better, but interpatient variability makes it difficult to achieve optimal pain relief, making it a risky prescribing strategy. In addition, any method of pain relief that requires frequent intramuscular injections will be unpopular with both patients and staff.

Continuous subcutaneous infusions have been suggested as an alternative, but problems associated with achieving an adequate loading dose and variability in individual kinetics mean that close monitoring is required throughout the time the infusion is in use. The same concerns apply to continuous intravenous infusions. The situation has led to the use of patient-controlled intravenous injection of opioids, where patients are allowed to self-administer analgesics in accordance with their own needs. In theory this should mean the elimination of individual variations in kinetics and allow each patient to titrate the analgesia to the level of control they desire.

Patient-controlled analgesia (PCA) has been compared with conventional methods of analgesia in several studies (reviewed by McIntyre[4]) with only minor differences between techniques. Most studies favour PCA, and the general belief seems to be that this method of analgesic delivery can match patient need in a more flexible manner. PCA is essentially maintenance therapy and is most effective if pain is controlled initially with intravenous boluses given by medical or nursing staff. (Table 47.2)

Table: 47.3 : Relative efficacy of analgesics in terms of number of patients who must be treated to obtain more than 50% pain relief (NNT). In the post-operative period

Drug	Mean NNT
Codeine (60 mg)	9.1
Codeine + rectaminophen (60 mg) (100 mg)	2.2
Dictofenac (50 mg)	2.3
Rofecoxib (50 mg)	2.3
Ibuprofen (600 mg)	2.4
Ketorolac (10 mg)	2.6
Pethidine (100 mg)	2.9
Morphine (10 mg I M)	2.9
Paracetamol (1000 mg)	3.8
Aspirin (1000 mg)	4.0
Tramadol (100 mg)	4.8
Dextropropoxyphene (65 mg)	7.7
A lower NNT means higher analgesic efficacy.	

Regional Anaesthesia

The use of regional anaesthesia in its many different forms has become widespread in the last two decades. Its popularity is mainly due to its suitability for use in short-stay surgery, but in addition there is increasing recognition of the increased post-operative morbidity caused by the routine use of large doses of opioids. Local anaesthesia can be delivered peripherally as an infiltration, a discrete nerve block, or a plexus blockade, or centrally in the form of spinal or epidural blockade.

The safety and efficacy of epidural analgesia has been reviewed by Wheatly and his colleagues (2001).[5] The use of local anaesthetic (LA) agents alone is not widely practiced because of a significant failure rate associated with regression of the sensory blockade. In addition, other problems may be associated with motor block and there may be falls in blood pressure related to accompanying sympathetic blockade. Similarly, the sole use of opioids has no clear benefits, and it is more usual for an opioid and LA combination to be given epidurally.[6]

A combination of opioid and LA provides better pain relief than PCA with intravenous morphine.[5] There seems no doubt that the administration of the two types of drugs together reduces the requirement for opioids. This reduction is found no matter which opioid is used. Optimal LA concentration is usually not more than 0.1% of bupivacaine.

Continuous Infusion

Post-operative epidural analgesia may be given as a continuous infusion, by bolus injections, or as a combination of both techniques in the form of patient-controlled epidural analgesia (PCEA). A continuous infusion is an effective way of maintaining an adequate level of analgesia, but bolus doses are required to re-establish that level if the block regresses and analgesia becomes inadequate. Thus PCEA is becoming used more frequently, which is in keeping with the principle of allowing patients to control their own pain relief.

Central blockade is in the form of spinal or epidural anaesthesia is less suitable for day-case or short-stay surgery than is local infiltration or peripheral or plexus nerve block. Regional anaesthesia is particularly suited for this type of surgery as it offers excellent operating conditions and the possibility of prolonged and highly effective post-operative analgesia.[6] The technique chosen should be appropriate to the proposed surgery (including the use of a tourniquet) and the intra operative block may be different from that needed for post-operative pain management. For example, surgery of the hand or foot may be carried out under plexus blockade with a short of medium acting LA acting agent, and post-operative pain can be controlled by use of a long acting LA drug administered as a peripheral nerve block or infiltrated locally at the site of the surgery.[7] This method will last far longer than the "definitive" block for the surgery and will avoid the complications associated with residual motor blockade as well as the need to protect the limb during this period.

Advantages

The use of regional anaesthetic techniques for any surgery may offer many advantages:

1. Patients remain oriented and alert and be discharged early with effective pain control.
2. The requirement for opioids will be reduced.
3. The side effects associated with the use of these agents such as nausea and vomiting, will be reduced. Poor pain control and nausea and vomiting are the most common reasons for unplanned admission after short-stay surgery.
4. The increased use of day stay surgery will have economic benefits for the health care system.

Wider acceptance of this form of surgery requires surgeon and patient education, better planning of patient throughout, and adequate post-operative monitoring to ensure that analgesia remains optimal after the patient is discharged from hospital. There is even evidence that long-term outcome can be influenced positively by the use of a regional anaesthetic technique for a short time post-operatively.

In summary, despite the ready availability of practice guidelines to treat acute post surgical pain (American Society of Anesthesiologists 1995), disappointingly few studies confirm the clinical prejudice that effective pain control will benefit patient and improve outcome. Nonetheless, the necessary evidence is appearing slowly. In practical terms, the judicious use of peripheral and centrally acting analgesics in combination with LA techniques will offer the patient the best pain relief, permit early mobilization and rehabilitation, and lead to the best outcome. Improved outcome, in turn, will have long-term health and economic benefits.

REFERENCES

1. Kehlet H. Multimodal approach to control post-operative pathophysiology and rehabilitation.Br J Anaesth 1997; 78: 606-617.
2. Beal AL, Cerra FB. Multiple organ failure syndromes in the 1990's. Systemic inflammatory response and organ dysfunction. JAMA 1994; 271: 226–230.
3. McCormack K. Non steroidal anti-inflammatory drugs and spinal nociceptive processing. Pain 1994; 59:9–43.
4. McIntyre PE. Safety and efficacy of patient- controlled analgesia. Br J Anaesth 2001; 87:36–46.
5. Wheatley RG, Schug SA, Watson D. Safety and efficacy of post-operative epidural analgesia. Br J Anaesth 2001;87:47–61.
6. Miniche S, Mikkelsen S, Wetterslev J, Dahl JB. A qualitative systematic review of incisional local anaesthesia for postoperative pain relief after abdominal operations. Br J Anaesth 1998;81:377-383.
7. American Society of Anesthesiologists. Practice guidelines for acute pain management in the perioperative setting. Anesthesiology 1995; 82:1071-1081.

•••

PAIN IN CHILDREN

48

Magnitude and Nature of the Problem

Surprisingly little is known about the prevalence of acute, recurrent, and chronic pain in children, despite the inevitability and frequency of painful injuries and diseases, a potential for long-term impairment and disability, and the striking immediate and potentially substantial long-term behavioural and social consequences.[1] The challenges of collecting epidemiological data are compounded by the highly variable impact of the injuries and diseases associated with pain on subjective experiences of pain and suffering, physical and psychological impairment, and restriction in lifestyle and social roles.

Clinically Significant Acute Pain

The incidence and prevalence of clinically significant bouts of acute pain have been difficult to establish. Case identification largely depends upon the child experiencing sufficient discomfort to require medical consultation. This domain largely concerns pain associated with the onset of disease, with injury from trauma, and arising from medical procedures. Pain resulting from procedures (*e.g.*, surgery, radiation therapy, chemotherapy or amputation) can include diagnostic, prophylactic, and treatment interventions.[2]

Chronic Pain

An understanding of the epidemiology of chronic pain in children is slowly emerging. P.A. McGrath (1999)[3] reviewed the prevalence of different types of children's chronic pain related to disease and trauma, nonspecific factors and emotional distress. Chronic pain was defined "as any prolonged pain that lasts a minimum of 3 months or any pain that recurs through a minimum period of 3 months".

Table 48.1 : Prevalence of data on diseases related to paediatric pain[3]

Sources of pain	Prevalence per 100,000
Chronic disease	
Arthritis	3-460
Sickle cell disease	28-120
Fibromyalgia	57
Cancer (pain from disease and therapy)	unknown
Numerous others (*e.g.*, haemophilia)	unknown
Trauma-related (nociceptive/neuropathic)	
Reflex sympathetic dystrophy	unknown
Phantom limb pain (high among amputees)	unknown
Chronic non specific pain	
Knee pain	3,900-18,500
Back pain	2,800-7,800
Dysmenorrheal	7,200-7,900
Recurrent pain	
Migraine headache	1,400-37,000
Recurrent abdominal pain	6,000-15,000
Recurrent limb pain	4,200-33,600
Mental health-related	
Somatization complaints	estimates vary

While the data are not wholly satisfactory, they indicate that pain is a common experience for children. Pain remains a cardinal symptom of disease and the principle motivation for consultation with primary care practitioners. Health care practitioners caring for a broad range of conditions will encounter pain and must have competence in its assessment and management. The personal and social consequences of pain have the potential to be substantial, but will vary with the type of pain. The emotional, behavioural, social and familial consequences of chronic pain are more likely to be severe for children who become obliged to abandon their usual roles in schools and with friends. The impact of school absence is progressive and cumulative. Chronic pain can have a profound effect on adolescence as they are challenged at this time of life to establish independent social roles and lives. There is substantial risk of depression and other forms of comorbidity emerging to further compound these difficulties.

A Socio Communications Model of Children's Pain

The model of pain proposed here not only attends to the experience of pain and its determinants but also examines how the subjective experience is behaviourally expressed, how others attend to and interpret these expressions when attributing pain to the child and how these understandings affect the nature and quality of care provided for that child. (Fig. 48.1).

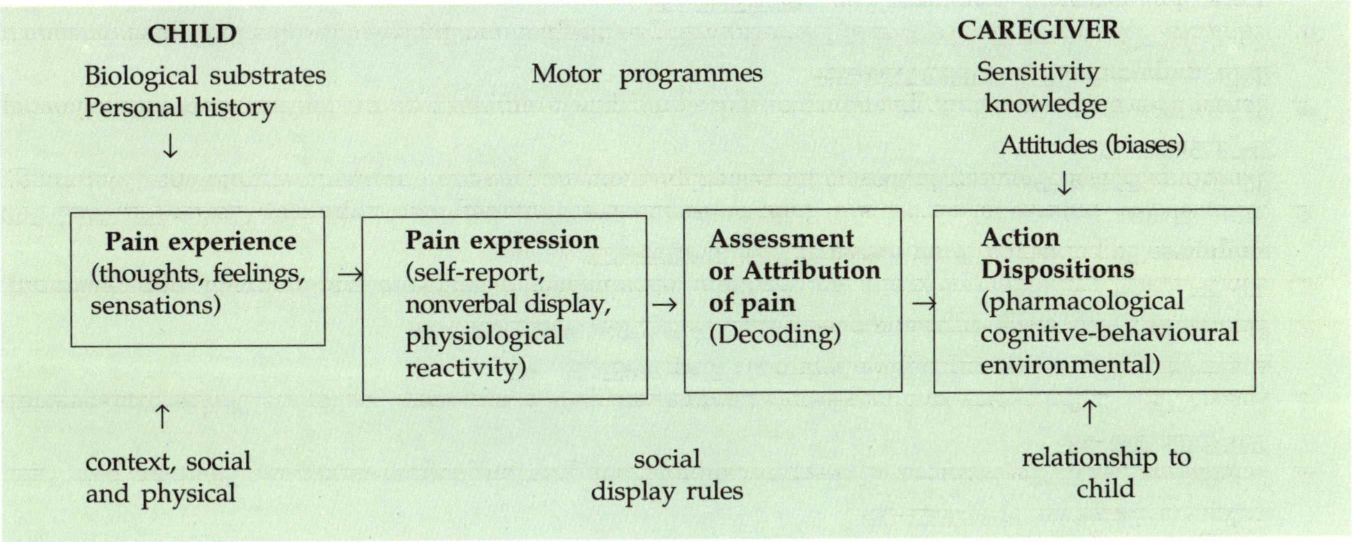

Fig. 48.1 : The world of a child in pain : a socio communications model

REFERENCES

1. Anand KS, Craig KD. New perspectives on the definition of pain. Pain 1996;67:3–6.
2. Goodman JE, McGrath PJ. The epidemiology of pain in children and adolescents: a review. Pain 1991;46: 247–264.
3. Goodman JE, McGrath PJ. The impact of mothers' behavior on childrens' pain during a cold pressor task. Presented at the annual convention of the Canadian psychological association, Halifax, Nova Scotia, 1999.
4. Craig KD, Lelley CM, Gilbert CA. Social barriers to optimal pain management in infants and children. Clin J Pain 1996; 12:232–242.

•••

SECTION–VIII

Neuropathic Pain

49

PHANTOM LIMB PAIN

Phantom limb sensation is the occurrence of a specific sensation in an amputated limb. Phantom limb pain refers to painful sensations in the missing limb and needs to be differentiated from stump pain which refers to pain in the actual stump.

The literature shows a major discrepancy about the incidence and the treatment of phantom limb pain, with earlier reports in the region of 0.5%–10%.[1,2] Later studies report a more realistic incidence of 60%–80%.[3,4] It is proposed that the variants may be due to the different ways of estimating pain intensity.[5,6,7]

Moreover there are other important factors that determine the incidence.

1. Age, gender, level or side of amputation, have no influence on the incidence of phantom limb pain,[8] though it was earlier reported to be much less seen in younger children.
2. Cause of amputation. Elective surgical amputation versus traumatic amputation also seems to have no difference in incidence,[5] but amputations for a painful pathology result in more vivid, intense and long lasting phantom.
3. Temporal profile: Incidence of the condition decreases with time. While 33% of patients experience the phantom immediately after cessation of anaesthesia, another 32% developed pain within the first 24 hours. Onset is delayed by a few days to weeks in 34% of patients.
4. In congenital amputees, the presence of phantom limb pain seems to be much less than the above mentioned types.[9]

Time course of phantom limb pain: The appearance of significant phantom limb pain usually occurs within the first week post amputation,[6] though an earlier prospective study found that 48% of amputees developed it within the first 24 hours, 83% with 96 hours and less than 10% after 1 week.

Phantom limb pain may follow a regressional pathway after many years and may burn itself out, though there is some controversy regarding this. Houghton in his retrospective study asked amputees to assess their phantom limb pain at different times after the amputation and the VAS decreased from 4 immediately after the surgery to a value of 1 five years later (scale 0–10).[3] Nikolajsen found that there was no decline in time, but the duration of each attack decreased significantly.[4]

Clinical Features

Pain

Many expressions have been used to describe phantom limb pain. These include a shooting pain, tingling, pricking, pins and needles, burning, cramping, squeezing or itching. It is also described as an electric shock down the limb and is "extremely painful". Very seldom does a patient experience a continuous pain. It is usually intermittent and individual attacks last seconds, minutes or hours, rarely extending for days or weeks.[2,4] The location of the pain is mainly distal in the amputated limb.[6] In a study of 64 above knee amputations where 66% had pain in the foot or toes, 39% had additional pain in the calves and only 6% had additional pain as high as the thigh.[1]

Non Painful Sensations

After studying phantom limb pain after upper limb amputations demonstrated that increased intensity of phantom limb pain is associated with more intense non painful limb sensations.[2,4] Changes in the length, size, temperature, volume or position of the phantom limb are commonly described. The phantom may also show movement both voluntary and involuntary and may assume the same painful posture as that of the real limb prior to amputation, especially if the limb had been immobilized for a prolonged period. Even when a deformed limb is amputated, the deformity is carried onto the phantom. Superadded phantom sensations can also occur like the experience of a ring, wrist watch, strap, shoe, plaster cast, etc.[10,11,12]

Telescoping

About one third of patients with phantom limb show a bizarre phenomena called telescoping, which involves gradual shrinkage of the distal parts of the phantom onto the stump, and in some cases may feel the hand or foot protruding from the stump. Telescoping was thought to be inversely related to phantom limb pain.[13,14,15]

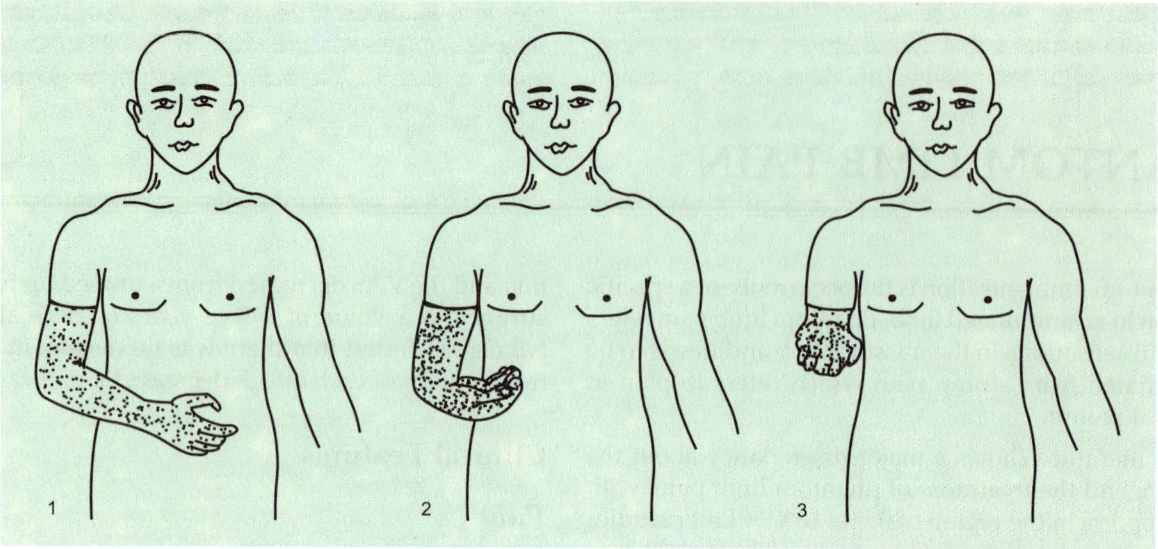

Fig. 49.1 : During telescoping of the phantom limb, the original phantom (l) begins to shorten (2). The most highly innervated areas (thands) remain, while the mid-portion of the phantom limb shortens in length. The phantom limb may continue to shorten until the phantom hand is perceived to be directly attached to the stump (3)

Pre-amputation Pain and Phantom Limb Pain

The correlation between existing pain before amputation and phantom limb pain has been studied extensively.[15,16] Parkes reported that pre amputation pain increased the phantom limb pain.[17] In a later study Wall failed to find such a relation in a study on 25 amputees who had an amputation due to cancer. In a study of 176 vascular amputees, it was found that there was significant relation between existing pre-amputation and the phantom limb pain immediately after and upto 2 years.[15] Several cases have been reported of continuation of pre-amputation pain into the phantom limb pain situation like that experienced of a painful dressing done earlier[15]. Other descriptions include the reactivation of pain experienced years before the amputation.

Stump Pain and Phantom Limb Pain[16,17,18]

Phantom limb pain differs from stump pain in intensity and quality, the former being consistently expressed with more sensory adjectives and the latter in more effective terms. Though phantom limb constitutes a percept generated by a complex perceptual neural network, its incidence is positively correlated with the occurrence and the intensity of stump pain. Phantom limb pain occurs in conjunction with stump pain in about one-third of amputee and is exaggerated by episodes of stump pain[19,20], such as blood flow and muscle tension changes, could be involved in phantom limb pain. Phantom fades more rapidly with a healthy stump requiring analgesics *e.g.*, fentanyl.[21]

Pathophysiology

Considerable progress has been made in elucidating the pathophysiology of phantom limb pain since the times when it was thought to be a primarily psychological disorder–a manifestation of either some mental-emotional problem or a basic personality structure.[22,23]

Phantom limb pain is now established to be a real problem resulting from complex interaction between peripheral and central mechanisms.[22] It is based on the hypothesis that phantom limb pain cannot be explained by a single mechanism and is due to simultaneous neuronal inputs from peripheral nerves and sensitized spinal cells activating neural networks in widespread nerve regions of the brain that subserve the somato-sensory pain memories.

Increased cortical excitability has been demonstrated in phantom limb patients compared to pain free amputees. Injury induced, long lasting central neuroplasticity accounts for sustained persistence of phantom limb pain in the absence of peripheral inputs. Clinically this results in hyperalgesia and allodynia. Anatomical substrates of central hyper excitability might be the activation of widespread network of neurons producing a spreading facilitation of adjacent neurons thus inducing a process of cortical reorganization.

Somatosensory Memories

Somatosensory memories have been reported in patients with a loss of afferent input such as amputation, brachial plexus avulsion, spinal cord injury and spinal anaesthesia. This, however, is not restricted to phantom limb patients. Somatosensory memories in patients who have undergone deafferentiation but still have the real limb, are similar to those in amputees.

Factors Influencing Development of Somatosensory Memories

- ★ Pre-amputation pain: Pain is the most crucial factor necessary for the development of somatosensory memories.
- ★ Temporal relation between pain and amputation: When pain is experienced in a limb at or near the time of amputation there is high probability that it will persist into the phantom limb. If there is a discontinuity between the experience of pain and amputation the likelihood of that pain becoming incorporated into the phantom limb is reduced.
- ★ Duration of pre-amputation pain: The length of time reported to be painful before amputation is not related to the persistence of pain after amputation.
- ★ Type and location of pre-amputation experience: Many types of pain or body regions have the potential to become represented as a phantom pain following amputation.
- ★ Intensity of pre-amputation pain: Severe pains are represented more frequently. Development of somatosensory memories may depend on a mechanism whose threshold is sensitive to a combination of intensity and duration so that intense pains of short duration and long lasting mild pains produce sufficient excitation to produce long-term central changes.
- ★ Psychopathology and emotional disturbance: Subjects cannot be differentiated on the basis of personality.
- ★ Input from modalities other than somesthesia: Activation of pain memory after amputation may be facilitated by integration of multi model inputs established prior to amputation.

Mechanism

When pain is experienced before amputation, the sensory qualities of pain are neurally represented. Pain information is encoded in terms of spatial and temporal pattern of the nerve impulses, which in turn depend upon the quality, intensity and body location of the lesion. The strength of encoding depends on both the intensity and the temporal qualities of pain. This somatosensory memory once formed can be activated even when only some of its elements are present in the sensory output. The loss of normal afferent inputs following amputation releases the tonic inhibition of previously established somatosensory representation, allowing it to persist unchecked. The affective or emotional tone that accompanies the experience is generated on a moment to moment basis by the joint function of intensity, quality, location of the somtosensory component, personal meaning of pain and other cognitive evaluative factors that determine pain experience.[23]

Implications for Treatment

The concept of somatosensory memories has significant implications for potential therapeutic strategies. Since pre-operative pain significantly contributes to the development of the phantom, patients should be free of pain as long as possible prior to amputation in order to prevent the formation of somatosensory memory. Pain experienced just before the amputation is more likely to result in a phantom. Therefore, injury barrage produced during amputation may also produce long lasting changes which are experienced as phantom limb phenomenon. Use of combined G/A or subarachnoid block during amputation should be more effective than G/A alone. G/A does not block formation of somatosensory memory components since its formation is independent of conscious awareness of pain.

Management

Advancements in the understanding of the pathophysiology of phantom limb pain is tempered with by the fact that only 7% of patients are helped with therapy. Sherman and Sherman found that of the 61% amputees with phantom limb pain who underwent consultation, only 17% were actually treated.[20]

Acute Management

Primary anaesthetic intervention is the cornerstone of phantom pain management. Rapid and effective pain reduction in the pre-amputation period, will effectively reduce phantom limb pain by preventing the formation of somatosensory memories. Epidural and intrathecal infusions of local anaesthetics and opioids remain the modalities of choice. One advantage of this approach is that the catheter can be used for the operative phase. The epidural of intrathecal infusions should be continued for 2-3 days after the surgery. Reduction in incidence of post-operative phantom limb pain was observed when regional anaesthesia was used. Where pain relief was provided by regional analgesia for 3 days before surgery and extended to provide anaesthesia for the procedure, no post-operative phantom or stump pain occurred for upto one year. Pre-operative epidural infusion of bupivacaine, clonidine and diamorphine remains a promising choice.

Further management of pain in the post-operative period is by use of opiods, local anaesthetics and beta blockers. Intravenous infusions of calcitonin and oral opiods can be of value in the acute phase.

REFERENCES

1. Ewalt JR et al. The Phantom limb. Psychosomatic medicine,1947;9:118–123.
2. Bach S, Noreng MF, Tjellden NU. Phantom limb pain in amputees during the first twelve months following limb amputation, after peri operative lumbar blockade. Pain, 1988;33:297–301.
3. Houghton AD et al. Phantom pain: Natural history and association with rehabilitation. Annals of the Royal college of Surgeons. 1994;76:22–25.
4. Nikolajsen L et al. The influence of preamputation pain on post amputation stump and Phantom pain. Pain, 1997a;72: 393–405.
5. Jensen T S et al. Immediate and long-term phantom limb pain in amputees : incidence, clinical characteristics and relationship to pre amputation limb pain. Pain, 1985; 21: 267.
6. Simmel ML. The reality of phantom sensation. Social Res, 1962;29:337–56.
7. Flor H et al. Cortical reorganization and phantom phenomenon in congenital and traumatic upper extremity amputees. Experimental Brain Research.1998;119:205–212.
8. Mithcell SW. Injuries of nerves and their consequences. Philadelphia: Lippincott, Carlen PL, Wall PD, Nadrovna H et al. Phantom limbs and the related phenomenon in recent traumatic amputations. Neurology, 1978:28:211–7.
9. Jensen TS et al. Phantom limb, phantom pain and stump pain in amputees during the first six months following limb amputation. Pain 1983;17:243-256.
10. Montoya P, Larbig W, Grulke N et al. The relationship of the phantom limb pain to other limb phenomenon in upper limb extremity amputees. Pain, 1997;72:87–93.
11. Jensen PS, Nikolajsen L. Phantom pain and other phenomenon. Textbook of Pain.Eds. Wall PD, Melzack R. 4th ed. 1999.Churchill Livingstone, New York.
12. Katz J. Psycho physiological contributions to phantom limbs. Can J Psychiatry,1992:37.
13. Weiss SA, Fishman S. Extended and telescoped phantom limbs in unilateral amputees. J Abn Soc Psychol, 1963:66.
14. Ramachandran VS, Hirstein W.The perception of phantom limbs: the D.O.Hebb lecture. Brain,1998:121.
15. Wall R et al. Does pre-amputation pain influence phantom limb pain in cancer patients? Southern Medical Journal.1985;78:34–36.
16. Hill A, Niven C A, Knussen C. Pain memories in Phantom limbs: A case history. Pain, 1996;66:381–384.
17. Parkes C. Factors determining the persistence of phantom limb pain in the amputee. J Psychosom Res, 1973;17:97–108.
18. Wall PD. The prevention of post-operative pain. Pain, 1988;33:289–90.
19. Katz J, Melzack R. Pain memories in phantom limbs:Review and the clinical observations. Can J Psychiatry, 1990:43.
20. Sherman R, Sherman C. Prevalence and characteristics of chronic phantom limb pain among American veterans; results of a trial survey. Am J Phys Med 1983; 62:227–238.
21. Jahangiri M, et al. Prevention of phantom pain after major lower limb amputation by epidural infusion of diamorphine, Clonidine and bupivacaine.Ann R Coll Surg Engl. 1994;76:32-48.
22. Baron R, Wasner G, Lindner V. Optimal treatment of phantom limb pain in the elderly. Drugs Aging. 1998;12(5):361–76.
23. Sherman RA. Phantom limb pain. Mechanism based management. Clin Pediatr Med Surg. 1994:11(1):85–106.

REFLEX SYMPATHATIC DYSTROPHIES

50

Two major syndromes are recognized; causalgia and reflex sympathetic dystrophies (RSD). There are major similarities between the two syndromes and there are reasonable grounds to believe that similar pathophysiological mechanisms are involved in the genesis of both conditions, which involve abnormal neural activity of both the peripheral and central nervous systems. The most important fact is that though the causative factors may be different, effective pain relief can be achieved in both syndromes by early sympathetic interruption. However, there remain some significant differences between the two conditions in clinical presentation, pathophysiology and managements.

The International Association for the Study of Pain has prepared a classification of chronic pain and descriptions of chronic pain syndromes.[1] The definitions for causalgia and reflex sympathetic dystrophy are as follows: **Causalgia**, sustained burning pain, allodynia, and hyperpathia after a traumatic nerve lesion, often combined with vasomotor and sudomotor dysfunction and later trophic changes. **Reflex sympathetic dystrophy**, continuous pain in a portion of an extremity after trauma, which may include a fracture but does not include a major nerve, associated with sympathetic hyperactivity.

Aetiology

It is obvious that the sympathetic nervous system plays an important role in the genesis of causalgia and RDS. However, the exact mechanism and the various contributions of the sympathetic, peripheral and central nervous systems have yet to be delineated. For example, it is not clear whether the beneficial effects of sympathetic blockade are mediated by blockade of sympathetic efferents or by interruption of afferent fibres travelling in the sympathetic chain.

There is some evidence that suggests that certain types of pain may be mediated by afferent fibres in the sympathetic chain. For their part the sympathetic efferents may be responsible for segmental and suprasegmental discharges which produce vasoconstriction and ischaemia, thus causing further activation of nociceptors, and leading to a "vicious circle" of response that leads to the severe changes of advanced disease.

Various other models have been proposed involving modulation of nociceptors sensitivity by sympathetic fibres. One such model suggests that discharges in sympathetic efferents activate adjacent "pain afferents" by electrical (ephaptic) "cross-talk". There are substantial flaws in this hypothesis, but recent studies by Devor have suggested that "cross-talk" does occur, but that this is chemical rather than electrical.[2]

The role of the central nervous system is the subject of debate as well.[3] There is no doubt that prolonged pain from sympathetic overactivity such as is seen in these two conditions appears capable of causing profound change in the central nervous system. The most recent attempt to draw together the many factors involved in the genesis of causalgia and RDS is that of Roberts.[4] This hypothesis suggests that the initial trauma activates unmyelinated C nociceptors. These activate and sensitizes wide dynamic range (WDR) neurons in the dorsal horn whose axons ascent to the higher centres. This sensitization of the WDR neurons becomes persistent so that they become responsive to activity in large diameter A mechanoreceptor afferents. These are activated by light touch and thus produce allodynia. In addition, the sensitized WDR neurons also respond to mechanoreceptor in the absence of cutaneous stimulation, thus causing spontaneous sympathetically generated pain, what Roberts has termed "sympathetically maintained pain".

Causalgia

In the vast majority of cases, causalgia presents after nerve injury. This is usually partial and is classically seen after high velocity missile injury or after a blast injury close to a nerve trunk. The nerves involved are usually of brachial plexus; particularly those components that form the median nerve, median nerve itself, or sciatic nerve and its two major branches. The injury is frequently high, well above elbow or knee.

Invariably the pain develops almost immediately after the injury. It is characterized as **burning**, and its nature is described as constant, severe and diffuse. The site is usually distal to the injury, and there is frequently an associated allodynia and hyperpathia. Although a few patients experience a spontaneous remission of their symptoms, if the pathological process is permitted to continue unchecked, there will be vasomotor and sudomotor disturbances, and consequently trophic changes will appear. The unremitting and severe nature of the pain make marked physical and emotional changes likely. Bonica has argued that the diagnosis of causalgia cannot be made unless it can be shown that blockade of all sympathetic pathways to the limb produce a dramatic and total relief of pain and most of associated symptomatology.[5]

Incidence

Most of the information about the incidence of causalgia is from studies carried out in wartime. From several studies carried out during World War II, it appears that the incidence of causalgia varies between 2% to 5%. A more recent study from the Vietnam war suggests an incidence of 1.5%. It has been suggested that this apparent reduction from earlier series may be due to two factors: more rapid hospitalization and more rapid diagnosis and treatment. Some authors have suggested that the disease is self-limiting, but practical experience suggests that this is not true, and that many cases will progress to almost total incapacity, which may last many years, if left untreated.

Area Involved

Data from published work supports the contention of Sunderland[6] that the nerves most commonly involved are median, sciatic and its two main branches, and brachial plexus. He believes that these nerves are most at risk as they carry the bulk of the sensory fibers and postganglionic supply to the hand and foot respectively. However, causalgia can involve other nerves and cases have been reported involving trigeminal, greater occipital and intercostals nerves and the cauda equina.

Nature of the Pain

The characteristic pain appears immediately or within a few days in 80% of cases. The description is one of **burning** pain felt **superficially** in the distal part of the limb. It is often reported as being most intense in those areas used frequently, such as the tips of the fingers, the palm of the hand and the toes and sole of the foot. The severity of the pain had been shown to be extremely severe in a study using the McGill Pain Questionnaire, being well in excess of that encountered with other conditions, such as back pain, post-herpetic neuralgia and cancer pain. In addition, patients with causalgia complain of other **deep** components to their pain, which may be episodic and described as stabbing, tearing, crushing, bursting or throbbing.

Initially, the pain is limited to the distribution of the involved nerve, but if the disease is left untreated the symptoms will spread to the entire limb and the pain will become far more diffused in nature with radiation to more distant areas.

The burning nature of the pain may lead patients to seek relief by wrapping with towel round the limb. However, the response to changes in temperature is not predictable, and the sensation of heat probably reflects sensory damage rather than vascular disturbance. Even the slightest sensory stimulus may provoke an increase in pain. This does not necessarily have to be sensory, even auditory or visual stimuli by any form of movement and the lightest touch may be agonizing. This in turn, lead to rapid involvement of distant structures as, for example, where a frozen shoulder is secondary to causalgia primarily involving the hand.

Neurological and Tropic Changes

Disuse is probably a major contributing factor in the sensory and motor changes seen as causalgia progresses into chronicity. The sensory changes are almost impossible to catalogue as the allodynia and hyperpathia make examination so distressing to the patient. Disturbance of vasomotor and sudomotor function are common. Generally it has been felt that the usual course of events was for an initial period of sympathetic activity, as manifest by vasodilatation, warmth and increased sweating, to be followed by progressive vasoconstriction and cold. However, there are plenty of data that suggest that this is not always the case. However, it should be emphasized that their absence does not make the diagnosis less likely.

Trophic changes are only seen in later stages of the disease and are probably almost entirely due to the disuse. Classically the skin is shiny and atrophic, and often there is a hair loss and coarse development of the nails, which may remain uncut to avoid provocation of the pain. There is fixation and fibrosis of the joint capsule and associated muscular atrophy. This process may even go so far as to produce contractions and subluxations in severe and prolonged cases. There may be osteoporotic changes in bone of the involved limb. Frequently these changes are irreversible, and their presence indicates that prior therapy was ineffective. In general, those patients treated early will not develop trophic changes, thus early and aggressive treatment is required if disabling consequences are to be avoided. In addition, those patients who develop chronic and emotional problems. However, it should be emphasized that behavioural abnormalities which appear to be present in cases of causalgia, for example, protecting the limb at all costs, avoiding company and wrapping wet towels around the limb, will immediately disappear when pain relief is obtained.

Treatment

The relief of pain by sympathetic blockade is a diagnostic feature of the disease. If the pain is not relieved by sympathetic blockade, it is not causalgia. Thus, sympathetic blockade by one method or another should be regarded as being the primary treatment for causalgia.

In the first instance diagnostic blockade is most easily carried out by blockade of the appropriate sympathetic supply by the injection of local anaesthetic. For diagnostic purposes it is of paramount importance to ensure that the sympathetic denervation is complete, by the measurement of galvanic skin resistance or a similar test of sympathetic function. Practical experience suggests that even in the most experienced hands, complete sympathetic blockade is not achieved every time, and this may lead to misdiagnosis, which in turn may lead to mistreatment, the worst possible outcome for the patient.

Having confirmed that the pain is relieved by sympathetic blockade, the next step is to decide which form of interruption of the sympathetic pathways is the most appropriate. This can be achieved by serial sympathetic blocks using local anaesthetic, by intravenous regional sympathetic blockade, by surgical or chemical sympathectomy or by use of systemic drugs. In all cases the aim is to produce pain relief, thus enabling an aggressive programme of physical therapy to be instituted, which is of paramount importance in the re-establishment of normal function in the involved limb.

Local Anaesthetic Blockade

It is possible to obtain total cure of the symptomatology of causalgia by performing serial local anaesthetic blockade. The blocks should be carried out daily, or on alternate days, and use a long–acting local anaesthetic such as bupivacaine. Alternatively, a catheter technique of infusion of local anaesthetic could be employed. This method of treatment is most effective in milder cases and those where it is possible to initiate treatment early. The number of patients who benefit from this approach is of the order of 20%.

Intravenous Regional Sympathetic Blockade (IRSB)

This technique was first described by Hamington-Kiff over ten years ago.[7] Essentially, this technique necessitates the injection of guanethidine into a vein in the involved limb whilst the circulation is occluded by tourniquet, in a manner similar to that used when performing Bier's block. It is alleged that the guanethidine will produce a long lasting sympathetic blockade by displacing noradrenaline from the sympathetic nerve ending, and the drug will become bound at the receptor preventing reuptake, and resulting in a prolonged blockade of adrenergic sympathetic nerve function. The blockade and pain relief may last many hours or even days. It has the considerable advantage of being simple to perform, and uses a minimum of equipment, but cannot be used for the treatment of causalgia in areas that cannot have the circulation occluded by tourniquet.

Sympathectomy

Surgical sympathectomy has been regarded for many years as the treatment of choice for causalgia. The results have been reviewed by Bonica.[5] The majority of series report a high success rate, on the order of 90%. However, there are reports that show less success. This may be because of incomplete sympathectomy, or be due to other factors such as the involvement of central nervous system. Sympathectomy could also be achieved by the use of neurolytic agents such as alcohol or phenol, but there are almost no reports of this method being used to treat causalgia.

Systemic Drugs

There are reports of the successful management of causalgia with oral propanolol and phenoxybenzamine. There are theoretical reasons for believing that other drugs may have some part to play in the management of causalgia, based on experiences in the treatment of reflex sympathetic dystrophy.

Other Methods

Physical therapy must accompany any attempt at therapy by other means, and must be started as soon as possible. The importance of the role of physical therapy is shown by the reports of cures of milder cases of causalgia by physical therapy alone. It is the restoration of function and return to normal activity that lead to prolonged pain relief in both causalgia and RSD. Sympathetic blockade and relief of pain make it possible to carry out the physical therapy. However, if this is not carried out, little overall benefit will be obtained from the block alone.

Other methods that have been used to treat causalgia are trans-cutaneous electric nerve stimulation (TENS) and dorsal column stimulation. As with any disease process there is no specific treatment that will abolish all pain, and adjuvant therapy may well be needed to help other problems. These may range from treatment of psychiatric or psychological handicap to use of strong opioids to treat accompanying pains.

Reflex Sympathetic Dystrophy (RSD)

The majority of cases of RSD follow trauma. The precipitating event is usually a strain/sprain injury, or one that involves a crush injury.[8] However, the initial trauma does not have to be severe, and RSD can follow the most minor events such as cuts or bruises. RSD can also occur as a result of surgery, or some other medical intervention such as manipulation, or the application of a plaster cast. Thus there is the potential for medico legal action.[9] RSD can be a consequence of certain medical conditions and has been reported after myocardial infarction, cerebrovascular accidents, cancer and other illnesses.

RSD can present in many different forms, ranging from a clinical picture indistinguishable from causalgia, to a mild form with only slight abnormalities in sensation and function. Severe RSD, like causalgia, presents as a severe burning pain, which is exacerbated by the slightest stimulus. There is associated allodynia and hyperpathia, there may be marked vasomotor and sudomotor disturbances and little to distinguish it from causalgia other than the lack of neural injury. It has been argued that RSD develops later than causalgia, after a few weeks or months, and that the severity is much less initially than that seen with causalgia. This distinction seems to be entirely academic and of no practical significance.

Moderate RSD is characterized by a diffuse burning pain, which is also described as being dull, throbbing and aching. There are varying degrees of vasomotor and sudomotor disturbances. **Mild** RSD is the most common, and without doubt the most commonly missed form, and represents the borderline between the normal response to the injury and the more severe presentations mentioned earlier. If there is the slightest suspicion of RSD it is prudent to institute therapy. With less severe forms of RSD one part of the symptomatology may be out of proportion to the other. For example, one patient may present with pain as the predominant feature, another with a limb that is cold, cyanosed and with excessive sweating, showing increased vasomotor activity.

Perhaps the most important thing to note about both the pain and the other physical findings in RSD is that they do not follow any segmental or dermatomal pattern, and have a tendency to spread proximally. This may represent a disease process that initially involves the sympathetic nervous system, but in which central nervous system effects play an increasing role as the disease becomes chronic.

Time Course of Physical Findings

Changes will be dependent upon the severity of the disease and whether or not treatment is instituted. The first changes may appear days to months after the injury and may be so distant from the precipitating event that the connection may not be made. The patient may experience the characteristic pain, associated with allodynia and hyperpathia. There is localized swelling and oedema with loss of the nail angle and skin increases, and there may be muscle spasm. The pain is diffuse but localized, and the skin is usually warm, dry and pink. As the problem becomes more chronic, the pain involves a larger area and the skin involvement changes to become cold, sweaty and cyanosed. The first early trophic changes to skin and nails can be observed.

With further disease progression true dystrophic changes begin. If the disease has been untreated this takes about 3 to 6 months. There is a constant burning, throbbing pain with marked sensitivity of the skin, which is cold and cyanosed. The limb may be oedematous but this is no longer pitting and is of brawny type. There is loss of hair, and the nails are brittle and cracked. An X-ray shows early osteoporotic change.

In the final stages the pain and cutaneous sensitivity may be less of a feature. There are irreversible changes present in skin and underlying tissues. The skin is a now smooth and glossy, and covers digit that are thin and pointed due to loss of the subcutaneous fat pads. There is muscle atrophy; particularly of the small muscles and there may be joint contractures and subluxations. X-rays show marked osteoporosis and demineralization of bone. When the disease has been present for a prolonged period of time there is the risk of associated psychiatric or psychological problems. These may require treatment but it should be remembered that they are usually secondary to the original problem and not the cause of it.

A high index of suspicion should accompany the complaint of persistent pain after minor trauma, surgery or disease, especially where this is accompanied by vasomotor or sudomotor changes, prolonged loss of function and early trophic changes. If available, X-rays, scintigraphy[10] and thermography may be useful in establishing the diagnosis.

Treatment

The same principles apply to the treatment of RSD as apply to causalgia. Early and aggressive treatment must be the primary aim.

The actual treatment selected will depend upon the severity of the disease and the time since the development of the symptoms. For mild cases physiotherapy alone may prove sufficient, but the usual method of treatment is sympathetic blockade in combination with physiotherapy during the time when the block is working. As with causalgia, the blocks should be carried out daily or on alternate days, and should be continued until such time as pain relief is obtained or there is no further improvement with each block. Duration of pain relief may vary from the length of action of the drug used to several days. Local anaesthetic infusions or IRSB may yield longer acting pain relief.

In cases where sympathetic blockade produces good pain relief of limited duration, sympathectomy should be considered.

RSD has been successfully treated with other noninvasive methods. There have been reports of the successful use of TENS in patients as young as 9 years of age. Most reports of the use of TENS claim high success rates, but follow-up is limited and it appears that there may be a fall off in response, similar to that seen when other conditions are treated by TENS.

Many drugs have been tried in the treatment of RSD. Among those claimed to be effective are propanolol, phenoxybenzamine, prazosin, high dose corticosteroids, calcium channel blockers, guanithedine[11] and tricyclic antidepressants. Data are limited and many of claimed results await confirmation.

REFERENCES

1. Merskey H., ed. Classification of chronic pain: descriptions of chronic pain syndromes and definitions of pain terms. Pain, suppl 3 (1986); S28–S29.
2. Devor M. Nerve pathophysiology and mechanisms of pain in causalgia. J. Auton. Nerv. Sys., 7(1983); 371–384.
3. Schott GD. Mechanisms of causalgia and related clinical conditions: the role of central and of sympathetic nervous systems, Brain. 109(1986); 717–738.
4. Roberts WJ. A hypothesis on the physiological basis for causalgia and related pains. Pain, 24 (1986); 297–311.
5. Bonica JJ. Causalgia and other reflex sympathetic dystrophies. In: Bonica JJ, Liebeskind JC, Albe-Fesssard D. eds. Advances in Pain Research and Therapy, vol. 3, Raven Press, New York, 1979; pp. 141–166.
6. Sunderland S. Nerves and Nerve Injuries, Livingstone, Edinburgh, 1968.
7. Hamington-Kiff JG. Pharmacological target blocks in hand surgery and rehabilitation, J. Hand Surg., 9 (1984); 29–36.
8. Rowlington JC. The sympathetic dystrophies, Int. Anesthesiol. Clin., 21 (1983); 117–129.
9. Horowitz SH. Iatrogenic causalgia: classification, clinical findings, and legal ramifications, Arch. Neurol., 41(1904); 821–824.
10. Holder LE, Mackinnon SE. Reflex sympathetic dystrophy in the hands: clinical and scintigraphic criteria. Radiology, 152 (1984) 517–522.
11. Bonelli S, Conoscente G, Movilia PG, Restelli L, Francussi B, Grossi E. Regional intravenous guanethidine vs. stellate ganglion block in reflex sympathetic dystrophies: a randomized trial, Pain, 16 (1983); 297–307.

•••

MANAGEMENT OF NEUROPATHIC PAIN

51

Introduction

Trauma or disease affecting peripheral nerves frequently results in the development of chronic, often intractable pain *i.e.,* neuropathic pain syndromes. While nociceptive pain is the result of stimulation of nervous system, the neuropathic pain is caused by the dysfunction of nervous system itself – thus chronic pain following nerve injury is a paradox. General consensus is that both central and peripheral nervous systems play roles in neuropathic pain syndromes. The various aetiological factors are direct trauma, ischaemia, infection, metabolic diseases and tumour invasion.[1] It is associated with (*a*) spontaneuos paraesthesia -dysaesthesia and pain (*b*) pain evoked by movement (*c*) tenderness over partly denervated body part. Chronic neuropathic pain is a negative pain as it does not signal to any potentially harmful environmental stimuli or disease process rather renders the patient debilitated and disabled. Except for certain conditions such as trigeminal neuralgia treatment of neuropathic pain is largely empirical and often unsatisfactory. Recent clinical trials with newer drugs have made definite improvements in medical management of neuropathic pain.[2]

Mechanisms of Neuropathic Pain

Both peripheral and central mechanisms play equally important roles.

Peripheral Mechanisms

1. *Abnormal Sodium Channels and Ectopicneural activity*

Early theory of neuropathic pain mechanism that has been accepted till date is ectopic neural activity due to neuroma formation, with spontaneous impulse originating at the site of injury or in the dorsal root ganglia. Abnormal or dysfunctional sodium channels have been implicated as the cause of ectopic activity and explain the benefit of sodium-channel blocking agents such as lidocaine, mexiletine, phenytoin and carbamazepime.[2] Recent evidence of tricyclic antidepressants acting as sodium-channel blockers explains the immediate analgesic effect with these drugs in neuropathic pain.[3]

2. *Sympathetic Dysfunction*

Animal studies have confirmed that damaged primary afferent fibres acquire adrenergic sensitivity and surviving afferents develop noradrenergic sensitivity. Causalgia is the classical example of sympathetically maintained pain (SMP) associated with nerve injury. Newer terminology include – complex regional pain syndrome (CRPS-type 1 and 2). Most patients obtain virtually complete pain relief with sympathetic blocks.[2]

3. *Neurogenic Inflammation*

(*a*) Following neural injury, inflammatory neuropeptides (*e.g.,* substance P) and prostaglandins (*e.g.,* PGE_2) may be released from primary afferent nociceptors and sympathetic post-ganglionic neurons. This explains the clinical response to NSAIDs, lidocaine and capsaicin. (*b*) The connective tissue sheath surrounding a peripheral nerve is innervated by primary nociceptive afferents called nervi nervorum which may enter the nerve trunk with the endovascular bundle. Compression and inflammation of the sheath may render the whole nerve tender and painful.

Central Mechanisms

1. **Central Sensitization :** Occurs in any situation with prolonged or intense C fibre input. In Postherpetic neuralgia (PHN), where there is ongoing C fibre activity, central sensitization play a significant role in maintaining pain. Secondly, with central sensitization large diameter and low threshold Aβ mechanoceptors become capable of generating pain. Both substance P and glutamate acting at the NMDA receptor contribute to central sensitization and are potential therapeutic targets in neuropathic pain.

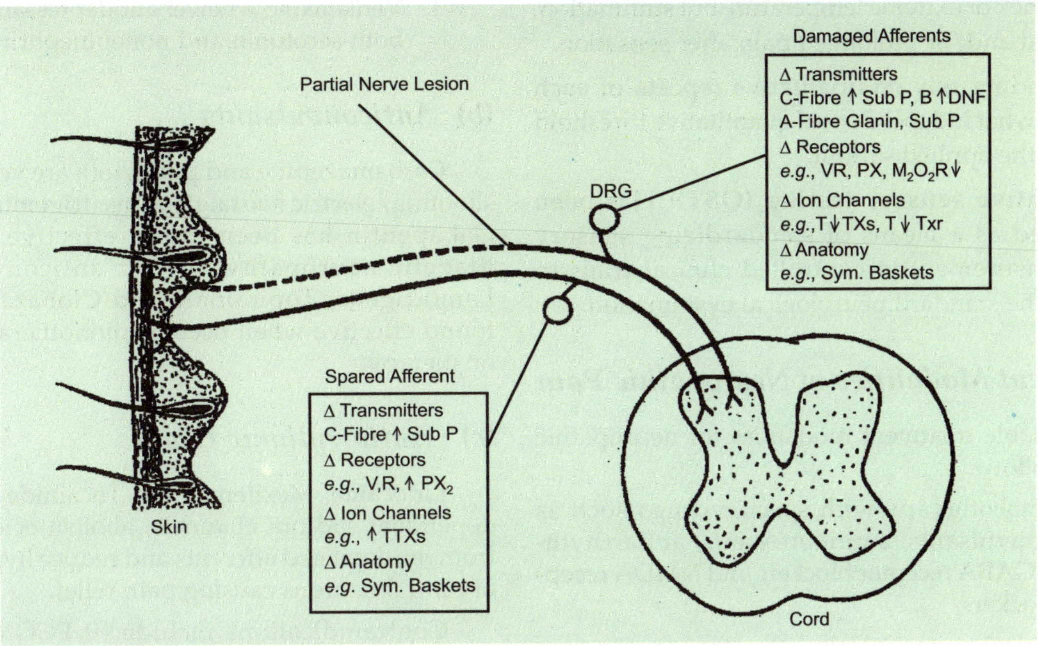

Fig. 51.1 : Changes in gene expression in sensory neurons in neuropathic pain showing damaged and spared neurons in the same peripheral nerve. BDNF = Brain derived neurotrophic factor MOR = mu opioid receptor. TTXr = Tetradotoxin resistant, TTXs = tetrodotoxin sensitive

2. **Deafferentation hyperactivity :** Deafferentation produces hyperactivity in dorsal horn cells. Following dorsal rhizotomy or peripheral nerve damage, many dorsal horn cells begin to fire spontaneously at high frequencies. Pain is a characteristic sequela of the deafferentation in branchial plexus avulsion.
3. **Reorganization of central connections :** After peripheral nerve damage, there is loss of central terminals of unmyelinated primary afferents but large diameter Aβ afferents start to respond maximally to gentle mechanical stimulation and sprout to directly innervate the deafferented nociceptive dorsal horn neurons.
4. **Loss of inhibitory large fibre afferents :** According to Gate Contol hypothesis, it is proposed that pain in nerve injury is due to selective damage of pain-inhibiting large diameter myelinated sensory axons. In fact, transcutaneous electrical nerve stimulation (TENS) is seen to produce traumatic pain relief in pain traumatic mononeuropathis and dorsal column stimulation selectively activating the central branches of large diameter afferents has been found effective in patients with neuropathic pain. It has been established that presence of large-fibre peripheral mononeuropathy is a definite risk factor for developing PHN.

Management of Neuropathic Pain

Successful management depends upon (A) proper clinical assessment and (B) application of proper treatment modality.

A. Clinical Assessment

History: Detailed history taking is very important. Neuropathic pain has certain clinical characteristics such as:

1. Delay in onset of pain following injury or disease process.
2. Localisation of pain in an area of sensory deficit.
3. Unprovoked spontaneous paroxysm of pain at rest with a tendency to disturb sleep.
4. Change in the character of pain from the time of onset.
5. Pain may be constant and steady or intermittent and stabbing often described as burning, sharp, shooting, unusual tingling, crawling or electrical in nature; may be relieved by applying pressure.

Clinical examination: With attention to somatosensory system is important.

Common clinical features are:

1. Positive sensory features in absence of any clinically evident swelling or inflammation.
2. Allodynia with pain in response to normally innocuous stimuli such as light touch and temperature.
3. Hyperalgesia with a lower threshold of pain.
4. Dynamic rather static allodynia with evoked pain worse with light brushing than with pressure; pain relieved by pressure.
5. Hyperpathia with an increase in threshold of pain in response to normally painful stimuli such as

pin prick or extreme temperature but summation, spread and/or prolonged pain after sensation.

These finding rely on qualitative reports of each patient, somewhat independent of quantitative threshold of pain from the applied stimuli.

Quantitative sensory testing (QST): Has been recommended as a means of standardizing sensory function measurement in controlled clinical trials to supplement the standard neurological examination.

B. Treatment Modalities of Neuropathic Pain

The available treatment modalities for neuropathic pain are as follows:

1. Pharmacotherapy with specific drugs such as anticonvulsants, antidepressants, antiarrhythmics, GABA receptor blockers and NMDA receptor blockers.
2. Stimulation techniques *e.g.*, transcutaneous electrical nerve stimulation (TENS), dorsal column stimulation and thalamic stimulation.
3. Chemical neurolysis (anhydrous glycerol, aqueous phenol, alcohol, steroid and aminoglycosides etc.)
4. Neurosurgical destructive procedures.

1. Pharmacotherapy

(a) *Antidepressants*

1. **Tricyclic antidepressants** (TCA) are currently the best documented therapy for neuropathic pain. Commonly used drugs are Amitriptyline, Desipramine and Nortriptyline. These are inhibitors of the re-uptake of monoaminergic transmitters and they potentiate the effects of biogenic amines in CNS-pain modulating pathways. Amitriptyline (75-150 mg/day) is used effectively in diabetic neuropathy and post-herpetic neuralgia. Improvement of sleep, mood and anxiety are the added benefits.

Mechanism of action : (*i*) block serotonin and norepinephrine re-uptake (*ii*) block voltage dependent Na^+ channels, (*iii*) act as α-adrenergic receptor blocker.

Side effects are (*i*) orthostatic hypotension (*ii*) sedation (*iii*) urinary retention and (*iv*) cardiac conduction abnormality.

2. Serotonin selective re-uptake inhibitors (SSRI) : *e.g.*, Fluoxetine and Paroxetin SSRIs have virtually none of the serious side effects common with TCAs. These are non-sedating and devoid of adrenergic, histaminergic and muscarinic side effects.
3. Venlafaxine, a newer antidepressant which blocks both serotonin and nonepinephrine re-uptake.

(b) *Anticonvulsants*

Carbamazepine and phenytoin are very effective in shooting/electric neuralgic pains (trigeminal neuralgia). Gabapentin has been found effective in PHN and diabetic neuropathy. Newer anticonvulsants like Lamotrigene, Topiramate and Clobazam have been found effective when used as monotherapy or as add-on therapy.

(c) *Antiarrythmic Drugs*

Lidocaine, Mexiletine and Tocainide block voltage dependent sodium channels, abolish ectopic impulses from the damaged afferents and reduce hyperexcitability of central neurons causing pain relief.

Contraindications include (*i*) ECG abnormalities (*ii*) decreased LV function and (*iii*) coronary heart disease.

(d) *Drugs acting on GABA Receptors*

Drugs affecting GABAergic transmission have been found to alleviate neuropathic pain. Presently available agents are:

(*a*) Baclofen – a GABA-B receptor agonist (*b*) Valproic acid decrease GABA metabolism and increases post-synaptic GABA activity (*c*) Vigabatrine inhibits GABA transferase (*d*) Benzodiazepines (clonazepam) bind to specific GABA-A receptor and facilitate the effects of GABA.

(e) *Opioids*

Use of opioids in neuropathic pain is controversial. Recent studies have demonstrated beneficial effects of morphine/fentanyl infusion, oral oxycodone/tramadol, intrathecal morphine in painful diabetic neuropathy, PHN and various other neuropathic syndromes.

(f) *NMDA receptor antagonists*

These drugs block the excitatory Glutamate receptors in the CNS. Clinically available drugs include – ketamine, dextromethorphan, memantin and amantidine.

(g) *Levodopa*

It has been found to be very effective in suppressing dysaesthesias in restless leg syndrome, acute herpes zoster pain and diabetic neuropathy. The mechanism is not known.

(*h*) *Topical Agents*

Allodynia is a common feature in neuropathic pain. Capsaicin is an agonist of vallinoid receptor present on sensitive terminal of primary nociceptive afferents. Repeated or prolonged application of capsaicin inactivates the receptor terminals and produce analgesia. Local anaesthics and cyclo-oxygenase inhibitors are also found to be effective when applied topically.

2. *Stimulation Techniques*

TENS has been found to be effective in focal nerve injuries. Dorsal column stimulation and deep brain stimulations are invasive procedures which may be used in special cases of intractable neuropathic pain but the limitations include – dislocation of electrodes, infection, bleeding and prohibitive cost.

3. *Chemical Neurolysis*

Entrapment neuropathy can be successfully treated by neurolysis. Gasserian gangliolysis with anhydrous glycerol produces satisfactory pain relief in trigeminal neuralgia. Patients with SMP syndromes may obtain significant relief by sympathetic blocks with alcohol or local anaesthetics.

4. *Neurosurgical Procedures*

Neurectomy, rhizotomy, dorsal root entry zone lesions, cordotomy and thalamotomy may produce short-term pain relief. These destructive techniques might increase the amount of deaffentation, giving rise to more severe pain and, therefore, not advocated in neuropathic pain. But only in case of trigeminal neuralgia where aetiology is transposition and vascular compression, microvascular decompression is an effective treatment option.

Conclusion

The perception and management of neuropathic pain still remains a challenge because of the reasons that (*a*) the pathophysiology is complex and not clear; (*b*) Both central and peripheral neural mechanisms are involved; (*c*) pain is refractory to commonly used analgesics and (*d*) proposed medications/therapies have limitations. Therefore, proper clinical assessment, optimum planning of therapeutic approach and careful monitoring are the keys to successful management.

REFERENCES

1. Bennett GF. Neuropathic pain.In: A textbook of pain. Wall PD, Melzack R. 3rd ed. Churchill Livingstone, 1994; pg 202.
2. Dellemijn PLI, Fields HL, Allen RR, Mckay WR, Rowbotham MC. The interpretation of pain relief and sensory changes following sympathetic blocade. Brain, 1994;117:1475–1487.
3. Devor M, Keller CH, Deerinck TJ, Ellisman MH. Sodium channel accumulation on axolemma of afferent endings in nerve ending neuromas in Apteronotus, NeurosciLett 1989; 102:149–154.
4. England JD, Gamboni F, Levingson SR. Immunocytochemical localization of sodium channels form along demyelinated axons. Brain Res. 1991; 549:334–337.
5. Kingery WS. A critical review of controlled clinical trials for peripheral neuropathic pain and complex regional pain syndromes. Pain 73:123.

•••

CRANIAL NEURALGIAS

52

Neuralgia is defined as pain, more precisely paroxysmal pain, in the distribution of peripheral nerves. If pain occurs in the distribution of cranial nerves this is Cranial Neuralgia. The various forms of cranial neuralgias and also some of the other types of facial pain have been outlined under the following headings:

1. Tic-like Pain of Cranial Nerve Origin or the Classical Cranial Neuralgia

Included in this rubric are the followings:

A. Trigeminal neuralgia
B. Glossopharyngeal neuralgia
C. Nervus intermedius neuralgia
D. Occipital neuralgia
E. Superior laryngeal neuralgia
F. Other neuralgias.

A *Trigeminal Neuralgia*

John Fothergill first described trigeminal neuralgia, or tic douloureux, the most common facial neuralgia in 1773. With an annual incidence of approximately 4.5 per 1 lac,[1,2] the disorder usually occurs in middle and late age but even young adults and children can be affected.[3,4] The male to female ratio of occurrence is 1:1.6.

The symptoms include paroxysm of pain in the distribution of the second and third divisions of the trigeminal nerve. The first division can be involved in about 5 % of cases. The pain is described as lancinating, shooting or electric shock like. It typically lasts for several seconds to two minutes but can occur repetitively many times an hour through out the day and night and might last for weeks at a time. After attacks that occur over several hours the facial pain might linger continuously. The severe paroxysm causes the patient to wince, giving rise to term Tic. The pain can be initiated or triggered by stimulation within any area of the affected nerve(s) in the form of light touch, eating, talking, shaving, yawning, or brushing of teeth. The disorder is episodic with relapses and remissions over many years. The periods of remissions might last for months to years. The reason for the relapses and remissions is unknown. The large majority of trigeminal neuralgia is unilateral but bilateral neuralgia is present in 3-5% cases.

Trigeminal neuralgia is classified as being primary (idiopathic) or secondary to structural intracranial lesions. Lesions responsible for secondary trigeminal neuralgia include a meningioma, schwanoma, malignant infiltration of the nerve or skull base, basilar artery aneurysm or pontine lesions. The pontine lesions may be infarcts, demyelinating disease or other infiltrating lesions. Demyelinating diseases can cause bilateral trigeminal neuralgia. In primary trigeminal neuralgia, physical examination is usually negative with normal sensory and motor functions. With secondary trigeminal neuralgia, however, there might be associated sensory or motor deficit in the trigeminal distribution or beyond. The aetiology of primary trigeminal neuralgia is still under debate, although many cases are thought to be related to vascular compression of the trigeminal routes at the root entry zone as originally described by Dandy[5] and popularized by Jannetta.[6] Brisman and colleagues[7] reported that high resolution MRI with gadolinium demonstrated vascular compre-ssion of the trigeminal nerve in 59% of their patients.

B. *Glossopharyngeal Neuralgia*

This pain syndrome has similar pain characteristic to trigeminal neuralgia, but the distribution of pain is localized to the glossopharyngeal nerve. The pain is paroxysmal, has a lancinating / sharp quality, and is localized to the throat, posterior third of tongue, tonsillar region, nasopharynx, larynx and ear. The pain can be triggered by swallowing, chewing, laughing, yawning, and talking. Rarely the pain may be bilateral. Bradycardia and syncope can be associated with a paroxysm of pain.

For most cases, the neuralgia is primary with no specific aetiology, although there is some evidence to suggest the presence of micro vascular compression of the auriculo pharyngeal branch of 9th and 10th cranial nerves to be the underlying lesion. There are no demonstrable abnormalities on clinical examination in patients with glossopharyngeal neuralgia. Secondary glossopharyngeal neuralgia occurs in structural lesion like neoplasm of the oropharynx and skull base. The clinical examination in that case demonstrates sensory or motor neurological deficit in the 9th and 10th cranial distribution.

Treatment: Includes carbamazepine, phenytoin, gabapentin, clonazepam or baclofen individually or in combination. If these treatments do not adequately control the patient's symptoms, consideration should be given to intracranial section of glossopharyngeal nerve and the upper rootlets of the vagus nerve, which relieves the pain in the majority of patients. Micro vascular decompression of the root entry zone of the glossopharyngeal nerve has also been reported to alleviate the pain.[8]

C. *Nervus Intermedius Neuralgia of Hunt (Geniculate Neuralgia)*

This exceedingly rare pain syndrome, which tends to affect patients of middle age, involves the pinna of the ear and the auditory canal and has been related to neuralgia of the geniculate ganglion and nervus intermedius. Yentur and Yegul[9] reported a case of nervus intermedius neuralgia following herpes zoster infection, although in most cases no clear aetiology is known. The clinical features of this disorder are paroxysms of pain lasting for seconds to minutes. Longer, more persistent burning / sharp pain has also been described and occassionally abnormalities of lacrimation, salivation and taste can be associated. The pain is triggered by light touch within the posterior aspect of the auditory canal. Though some patients with this disorder respond to treatment with carbamazepine, Lovely and Jannetta reported favourable pain relief with excision of nervus intermedius and geniculate ganglion.[10]

D. *Occipital Neuralgia*

A paroxysmal pain disorder in the distribution of the greater, lesser or third occipital nerves can occur unilaterally or sometimes bilaterally, and is associated occassionally with sensory loss in the distribution of the affected nerve(s). The pain in occipital neuralgia is sharp shooting / lancinating in quality, although a more constant dull ache may be present in the appropriate distribution. The affected nerve(s) will be tender to palpation with reproduction of pain, with percussion of involved nerve. Trauma to the occipital region can occassionally be the initiating event, but the condition most frequently starts spontaneously.[11]

Treatment: Carbamazepine can eliminate or reduce the pain in some patients. Effective but often only temporary treatment may be accomplished with local anaesthetic injections alone or in combination with a corticosteroid injection. Sectioning of the nerve is futile and this can promote the development of a neuroma or anaesthesia dolorosa.

E. *Superior Laryngeal Neuralgia*

Here the neuralgic pain occurs in the throat, submandibular region and below ear. The precipitating factors are swallowing, shouting, turning of the head, upper respiratory tract infection, tonsillectomy, and carotid end arterectomy. Structural lesions must be excluded through appropriate investigations. Treatment typically consists of local nerve block or ablation of the superior laryngeal nerve.

F. *Other Neuralgias*

Neuralgias involving the nasocilliary and supraorbital nerves have been described and are rare. They differ only in location in that the symptoms occur in the distribution of each respective nerve. The pain is again paroxysmal and lancinating in nature. Structural lesions must be eliminated through thorough investigations before making a diagnosis. Treatment typically consists of local nerve block or ablation of the appropriate nerve as the last resort.

2. Persistent Pain of Cranial Nerve Origin

Various pathological lesions of cranial nerves such as demyelination, inflammation, infarction or compression may lead to persistent pain.

(*a*) **Demyelination** of optic nerve or optic neuritis is manifested with blurred vision and associated pain during eye movement.

(*b*) **Infarction:** Oculomotor nerve commonly suffers from ischaemic damage in hypertensive or in diabetic patients. This is manifested by oculomotor palsy and periocular pain.

(*c*) **Inflammation:** This is exemplified by herpes zoster infection of the posterior root ganglia and is characterized by pain and skin eruption in the distribution of the affected ganglia.[12] Sometime the motor roots are also involved. Herpes zoster primarily affects the spinal ganglia, but in 20% the cranial ganglia are affected. The common cranial nerves affected are the trigeminal (ophthalmic zoster) and the facial (otic zoster or Ramsay Hunt syndrome) nerves. In ophthalmic zoster, the most commonly affected is the ophthalmic division. Along with pain in the nerve distribution there may be pan ophthalmitis and corneal scarring in the eye and at times oculomotor nerve paresis. In Ramsay Hunt Syndrome, there is pain and rash in the tympanic membrane, external auditory canal and at times the outer surface of ear lobe. Sometimes C_1 and C_2 cervical routes are also involved besides there is lower motor type of facial palsy and in 50% cases loss of taste in the anterior two third of the tongue.

(*d*) **Compression/ distortion of cranial nerves and C_2, C_3 nerve roots :** Some of the examples are cited below,

★ Tolosa-Hunt Syndrome[13] due to granulomatous inflammation in the cavernous sinus and superior orbital fissure. The ipsilateral 2nd, 3rd, 4th, 5th and 6th cranial nerves may be involved individually or in various combinations. The pain is retro or periorbital and may radiate to frontotemporal region of the affected side. The condition responds well to corticosteroids.

★ Neck-Tongue syndrome[14] is an uncommon disorder manifested by acute unilateral occipital pain and numbness of the ipsilateral tongue precipitated by sudden rotational movement of the head. The symptoms are due to transient sublaxation of the atlanto – axial joint that stretches the joint capsule and the C_2 ventral ramus (which contains proprioceptive fibres from the tongue originating from the lingual nerve to the hypoglossal nerve to the C_2 root).

★ Gradenigo syndrome: Lesions of the apex of the petrous temporal bone, such as middle ear infection or tumour can cause pain referred to frontotemporal region and ear, associated with 6th cranial nerve palsy.

★ Raeder Para trigeminal syndrome: Due to tumour or granulomatous lesion in the parasellar region, there is unilateral frontotemporal and maxillary pain with affection of sympathetic plexus around internal carotid artery, evidenced by ptosis and miosis.

3. Headache and Facial Pain of Central Origin

(A) **Anaesthesia dolorosa:** This is pain in the region of 5th cranial nerve distribution on the face. This type of pain, allodynia and sensory deficit some times occurs after radio frequency thermocoagulation or after gamma-knife stereo tactic radio surgery of trigeminal neuralgia, if the posterior nerve roots are damaged. This is deafferentation pain secondary to posterior rhizotomy.

(B) **Thalamic pain:** In central nervous system lesion, such pain may occur due to damage of the second order trigeminal neurons, spinothalamic tract or ventrobasal nucleus of thalamus.

4. Atypical Facial Pain

Atypical facial pain is a term given to patients who do not fall into the diagnostic categories of the other possible aetiologies of facial pain and where exhaustive radiological and other investigations have failed to yield a root cause for the patient's symptoms. The patients tend to be female and middle aged. The pain in this disorder is typically described as intense, deep and constant pain that is burning or aching in nature and is poorly localized.[15] The pain is typically unilateral but may occur bilaterally. The pain can be associated with parasthesia, numbness and tenderness, but these symptoms as well as the pain do not follow anatomic patterns.[16] There are no triggers for the pain of atypical facial pain as in the neuralgic disorders. The aetiology of atypical facial pain remains unknown. There is a high incidence of depression and anxiety in patients with the diagnosis of atypical facial pain.[17] Treatment typically consists of tricyclic antidepressants, monoamine oxidase inhibitors (MAOIs), or benzodiazepines.

Conclusion

Unlike arthropathic and many other common painful disorders, the neuralgic pain responds effectively to tricyclic antedepressants or to anticonvulsants like carbamazepine, gabapentin, topiramate and lamotrigene. In case of those not responding satisfactorily to pharmacotherapy, elegant surgical procedure like micro vascular decompression or gamma-knife radio surgery may prove invaluable. Although cranial neuralgias are commonly primary disorders, structural intracranial lesions may at times lead to neuralgia[18]. Therefore, appropriate neuro imaging and other investigations are necessary to ascertain the underlying diagnosis for proper treatment.

REFERENCES

1. Yoshimasu F, Kurland L, Elveback L. Tic Douloureux in Rochester, Minnesota, 1945-1969. Neurology 1972; 22: 952–6.
2. Katusic S, Williams D, Beard C, Bergstralh E, Kurland L. Epidemiology and clinical features of idiopathic trigeminal neuralgia. Similarities and differences, Rochester, Minnesota, 1945-1984. Neuro Epidemiology 1991;10:276–81.
3. Mason W, Kollros P, Janetta P. Trigeminal neuralgia and its treatment in a 13-month-old: a review and case report. J Cranio Mandib Disord 1991;5:213–6.

4. Childs A, Meaney J, Ferrie C, Holland P. Neurovascular compression of the trigeminal and Glossopharyngeal nerve. 3 case reports. Arch Dis Child 2000 ; 82: 311–5.
5. Dandy W. Concerning the cause of trigeminal neuralgia. Am J Surg 1934;24:477.
6. Janetta P. Structural mechanisms of trigeminal neuralgia: arterial compression of the trigeminal nerve at the pons in a patient with trigeminal neuralgia. J Neuro surg 1967;26 (suppl): 159–62.
7. Brisman R , Khandji A G, Mooij RBM. Trigeminal nerve-blood vessel relationship, as revealed by high resolution magnetic resonance imaging and its effect on pain relief after Gamma knife radio surgery for trigeminal neuralgia. Neuro surgery 2002;50:1261–7.
8. Fraioli B, Esposito V, Ferrante L, Trubiani L, Lunardi P. Micro surgical treatment of Glossopharyngeal neuralgia: case reports. Neuro surgery 1989;25:630–2.
9. Yentur E, Yegul L. Nervus intermedius neuralgia: uncommon pain syndrome with uncommon etiology. J Pain Symp Manage 2000;19:407–8.
10. Lovely T, Janetta P. Surgical Management of geniculate neuralgia. Am J Otol 1997;18:512–7.
11. Victor M, Ropper A. Headache and other cranial facial pains. Adams and Victor's principles of neurology. New York: McGraw Hill.pp 175-203.
12. Gilldon DH. Varicella Zoster. Virus infection. In Vinken PJ, Bruyn GW, Klawans HL, McKendall RR. Eds. Viral disease. Handbook of clinical neurology. Vol.56. New York: Elsevier Science, 1989;229–247.
13. Averbuch-Heller L, Daroff RB. Painful ophthalmoplegias, Tolosa Hunt syndrome, an ophthalmoplegic migraine. In :Goadsby PJ, Silberstein SD, Eds. Headache, Boston: Butterworth-Heinemann, 1997;285–297.
14. Lance JW, Antony W. Neck tongue syndrome on sudden turning of head. J Neurol Neuro surg Psychiatry 1980;43:97–101.
15. Paulson GW. Atypical facial pain. Oral Surg Oral Med Oral Pathol.1977; 43:338–41.
16. Loeser J. Tic Douloureux and atypical facial pain. In: Wall PD, Melzack R, editors. Textbook of pain Edinburgh: Churchill Livingstone : 1994;pp.699–710.
17. Lacelles R. Atypical facial pain and depression. Br J Psychiatry 1966;112:651–9.
18. Turp J, Gobtti J. Trigeminal neuralgia versus atypical facial pain. A review of the literature and case report. Oral Surg Oral Med Oral Pathol 1996;81:424–32.

•••

TRIGEMINAL NEURALGIA : CURRENT PERSPECTIVES

53

Trigeminal Neuralgia (Tic Douloureux) is one of the most painful conditions which can be treated by medications and surgical skills. Lack of knowledge of the natural history of this neuralgia has laid erroneous claims for therapeutic efficacies. Inadequate long-term follow-up of the patients has led to inflated claims for the efficacy of the procedure.

Signs and Symptoms

★ Electric shock like brief stabbing pain.
★ Pain free interval between attacks.
★ Unilateral pain during any one attack (bilateral 3%).
★ Abrupt onset and equally abrupt termination.
★ Pain restricted to trigeminal nerve distribution.
★ Minimal or no sensory loss in trigeminal nerve distribution.
★ Triggered by non-painful stimuli from remote area.

Differential Diagnosis

1. Vascular headache and face pain may be intermittent but lasts for hours with burning, dysaesthesia, rhinitis, lacrimation and sweating. This is in cluster or random without sensory loss.
2. Myofascial pain originates in TM joint or muscles of mastication. Pain may be bilateral, aching, cramping, local tender area and without sensory loss.
3. Local pathology in paranasal sinuses, jaws, teeth and pharynx causes severe pain without trigger. Pain is throbbing, aching or burning in nature with a local tenderness at the area of involvement.

Laboratory Tests

Usually clinical examinations sufficient for diagnosis except in cases of neurological involvement, where MRI, CT Scan may reveal arterial loop impinging upon the trigeminal nerve as it exits pons.[1] MRI can reveal other causes like multiple sclerosis, angiomas or tumour. Further tests like angiography and myelography may also be indicated.[2, 3]

Prognosis

Usually occurs in old age. Intermittent pain with spontaneous remission which may last for years. Patients may responds to medical and surgical treatment.

Therapy

Since trigeminal neuralgia is a central pain, tranquillizers and antedepressants may help, while antinociceptives like NSAIDs which act on tissue injury site are not helpful to these patients.[4, 5]

Table 53.1 : Medication used in trigeminal neuralgia

Generic name	Dose in mg / day	Side effects
Carbamazepine (10%)	600–1200	Nausea, vomiting, dizziness, hepatic, haemato suppression
Phenytoin (25%)	300–500	Nausea, dizziness, ataxia
Mephenesin	5–15	Dizziness, somnolence
Gabapentin	300–400	Dizziness, somnolence
Baclofen	40–80	Dizziness, somnolence, nausea

Nerve Blocks

Blocking of the cervical or trigeminal nerves may provide pain relief. Alcohol block by skilled operators provide good initial success and low complication rate. The relief lasts for a few months to a year. There is anaesthesia in the division of the nerve blocked. The other neurolytics like phenol, chlorocresol have also been used with a varying success rate. Blocking of individual branches of the trigeminal nerve is technically a simple and safe method, especially when used with the aid of nerve locator. Further infraorbital, supraorbital branches can also be blocked with neurolytic drugs (a few drops) safely with the help of a nerve locator when pain is present after the block of main division.

craniectomy with decompression of the trigeminal nerve is the surgical treatment of choice.

Sectioning of the preganglionic fibres of the corresponding division of trigeminal nerve through Frazier's transtemporal extradural approach seemed to give lasting relief from pain, but was associated with loss of sensation in the distribution of the sectioned division and dysaethesia in some of the patients.[8]

Trigeminal neuralgia is said to be a result of demyelination that sets in from compression of the trigeminal nerve at its root entry zone into the brainstem. This compression is believed to be done to a vascular loop from anterior inferior cerebellar artery (AICA) that presses on the trigeminal nerve at its root entry zone. The com-

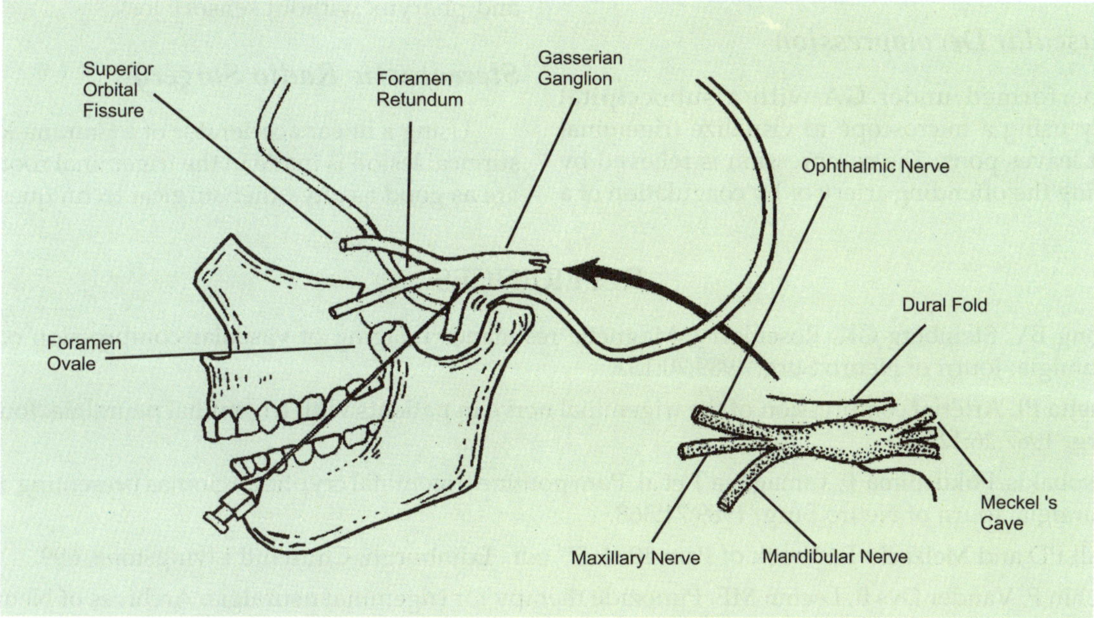

Fig. 53.1 : Gasserian ganglion – Origin and branches of trigeminal nerve

pression and pulsation of the arterial loop. The arterial loop may be demonstrated in a good MRI.

This belief in vascular compression has led to the surgery of micro vascular decompression (MVD) of the trigeminal nerve using Dandy's posterior fossa approach. When a definite vascular compression by a vessel grooving the nerve at its root entry zone is seen, the vessel to maintain permanent separation.

Micro vascular decompression of the trigeminal nerve has now become a procedure of choice. It seems to give relief without any sensory loss or disturbing dysaesthesia. Only 25% – 27% of patients are said to have a recurrence when followed over years. The recurrence occurs possibly in those in whom the vessel has not caused grooving of the nerve and is simply lying on the nerve. In such cases where definite vascular compression is not seen, it is better to section the fibres of the affected divisions and have permanent relief from pain. Though associated with sensory loss in the distribution of the corresponding divisions.

Sphenopalatine Ganglion Block

Has been modified by the author in leftover pain after maxillary nerve block in neuralgia when a pain in the region of an area above the centre of upper lip, just below the tip of nose is present. This block can also be indicated in hyperhydrosis. A small cotton wick 4–5 cm long is winded down as in a oil lamp wick and inserted into the naris involved. This is a non-invasive method for the tough left-over pain in maxillary neuralgia. Alternatively anaesthetist can put a small cotton pledget on the middle turbinate under vision through a nasal speculum. The local analgesic instillation break the cycle of pain which disappears after 3–4 days. The wick method used by the author has been the simplicity of removal of the wick and again putting another wick by the patient him/herself at home.

Surgical Therapy

A surgical procedure is warranted when pharmacological therapy has failed. Gangliolysis and suboccipital

Cryotherapy

By using a cooling probe, the peripheral branches of the trigeminal nerve are damaged. The effect may last upto one year along with a transient sensory loss.

Gangliolysis

Since nerve avulsions, rhizotomy, alcohol injections produce anaesthesia dolorosa, painful parasthesia and keratitis, Gangliolysis has been performed with 80% success rate. Needle is introduced under fluoroscopic control into foramen ovale. Paraesthesia on stimulation of area with 60 Hz current indicates needle is in proper place and radio-frequency lesion is made.[8]

Micro Vascular Decompression

It is performed under GA with a suboccipital craniotomy using a microscope to visualize trigeminal nerve as it leaves pons. The compression is relieved by repositioning the offending artery or by coagulation of a vein. 5-year success rate is about 85% and usually without sensory loss.

Retrogasserian Neurotomy

Sectioning the trigeminal root between the ganglion and the pons, if micro vascular decompression fails. It is approached through posterior fossae. Partial rhizotomy is also performed to reduce anaesthesia dolorosa. Peripheral neurectomy of the branches of trigeminal nerve provides short term relief.

Trigeminal Tractotomy

A section of trigeminal tract in the medulla, produces loss of pain and temperature sensation in ipsilateral face and pharynx without sensory loss.

Stereotactic Radio Surgery

Using a linear accelerator of a Gamma-knife, a radio surgical lesion is made in the trigeminal root. The results are as good as any other surgical techniques.

REFERENCES

1. Wong BY, Steinberg GK, Rosenlarry. Magnetic resonance imaging of vascular compression on trigeminal neuralgia. Journ of Neuro Surg. 1989;70:132.
2. Janetta PJ. Arterial compression of the trigeminal nerve in patients with trigeminal neuralgia. Journ of Neuro Surg. 1967;26:129.
3. Tusubakis, Fukushima T, Tamagava T et al. Para pontine trigeminal cryptic angiomas presenting as trigeminal neuralgia. Journ of Neuro Surg. 1989;71:368.
4. Wall PD and Melzack. Textbook of Pain 1964. 3rd edi.. Edinburgh, Churchill Livingstone, 699.
5. Lashin F, Vander Dys B, Lechin ME. Pimozide therapy for trigeminal neuralgia. Archives of Neurology 1989; 46:960.
6. Mullen S, Lichtor T. Percutaneous micro compression of the trigeminal nerve. Journ of Neuro surg. 1983;59:1007.
7. Kumar P, Lyngdoh N. Role of PNS as an aid in trigeminal neuralgia. Ind pain, 2005; 19 (1); 20–24.
8. Bhagwati SN. Management of trigeminal neuralgia. Proceedings of CME – PAIN, XVII ISSPCON, Jamnagar, 2002.

•••

TREATMENT OF POST-HERPETIC NEURALGIA

54

The incidence of herpes zoster in the community is about one case per thousand population, and most of these are concentrated on the over sixty age group, where the incidence is about one per hundred.[1]

The pattern of incidence of the pain syndrome is similar to that of the disease, with the main incidence being in the older age groups, where over 50% may go on to suffer persistent pain.

To manage the pain syndrome, it is necessary to understand the pathology and how this in turn leads to the various pain mechanisms.

Herpes zoster presents as a pain, which is succeeded by a vesicular rash along the cutaneous distribution of a nerve. It is almost invariably one nerve root that is involved, apart from the trigeminal nerve where often only the ophthalmic division is affected.

The infection is caused by the **Varicella** virus which has lain dormant in a posterior root ganglion since a previous chickenpox infection, and has been reactivated by some immune-suppressing life event.

Precise descriptions of the pathology are rare because most patients die at home and are not subject to post-mortem examination, but some studies do exist and it has been shown that the infection starts in the dorsal root ganglion cell, spreads to the adjacent dorsal horn cells and along the ascending columns for one or two spinal segments[2].

The main spread of the infection is along the peripheral nerve, with demyelination and wallerian degeneration right out to the cutaneous nerve endings, and the skin eruption appearing at that site.

This is a total neuritis from the posterior horn cell to the skin with varying degrees of destruction, and possibly some spread of the inflammation into the spinal cord. The balance of the neuronal destruction is of the large diameter sensory fibres causing deafferentation of the control systems in the posterior horn cells.

All this is accompanied by severe pain which requires management with strong analgesics in full doses.

Common sense and published work suggest that active treatment of the acute infection should reduce the incidence of long-term pain, and application of idoxuridine solution to the vesicles and systemic anti-viral medications such as amantadine appear to reduce the incidence of the post-herpetic pain syndrome.[3]

History

The patient will always give a history of an acute attack of zoster, though it may have been many years previously. The description of the pain may vary due to the variable nature of the disease and he may need some leading questions to bring out all the information required. As most people are not accustomed to describing what they all admit is a most peculiar pain, it is helpful to present a choice of words such as are available in the McGill Questionnaire. This should in turn give details of the nature of the pain; typically this will be of the following:

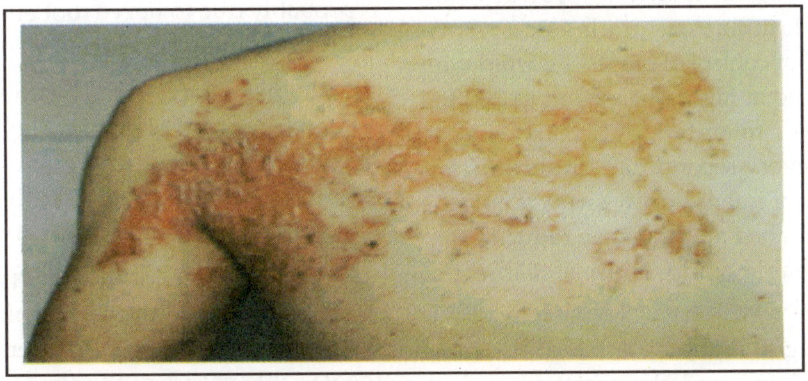

Fig. 54.1 : The figure shows aberrant vesicles in other areas of the body, usually associated with haematogenous dissemination

1. Spontaneous posterior horn cell activity leading to bursts of pain and to a vibrating jaggy pain referred to the stigmatized area.
2. Reflex sympathetic dystrophy with burning pain in the segment due to overactivity of the sympathetic control systems.
3. Hypersensitivity in the scarred area due to continuing inflammatory changes in the nerve endings and continued release of histamine and bradykinin. With complete nerve destruction, these symptoms may become quiescent and the area may become numb.
4. That the whole syndrome goes dormant during sleep is another common feature and an important management ploy.

Management

It is most important that the patient should understand from the beginning that there is no cure for this condition and that normal healing has been completed and further spontaneous improvement is unlikely. The only treatment justified at this stage is that aimed at symptom control and each symptom may need to be managed separately.

The first step is to explain this complex pathology as simply as possible to the patient and to highlight the points in the history that will facilitate non drug management. If sleeping normal, with or without mild hypnotics, this is a great aid to their accepting relaxation and avoidance of stress, instructions.

The incurable nature of the condition at this stage must be accepted. But with this, the availability of control can be explained, with the need to accept that the treatment will be ongoing into the foreseeable future. Like diabetes, it is a life sentence.

Drug management starts with withdrawal of all opiates and anti-inflammatory analgesics. Anti-convulsant medication for control of bursts is started with sodium valproate 200 mg at night, increasing to 200 mg morning and evening if tolerated, and increasing in increments of 200 mg every second day until control is achieved. If side effects of intense drowsiness occur, the patient should be kept in bed and the dose reduced step by step until a reasonable compromise is achieved. Adjusting may take a few weeks.

Amitriptyline 25 mg at night is started at the same time. This helps to achieve good sleep pattern and an improvement in the autonomic control. If necessary increase to 50 mg after one week. External electrical stimulation is most effective, if started after establishment of anti-convulsant medication. In the majority of patients where the deafferentiation is incomplete, the stimulus is best applied along the injured nerve. This may be either slow rhythm electrical needle acupuncture or TENS. Intermittent treatment is adequate either at the clinic or the patient's home.

If burning is very troublesome and the disease is relatively recent, sympathetic ganglion blockade combined with a desensitizing programme is indicated, and repeat block after three days, if necessary.

If the scarred area is very sensitive despite the above procedures subcutaneous infiltration with local anaesthetic and dilute triamcinolone solution with further desensitizing is indicated.

As with any patient who has had a long-standing chronic pain, psychological changes may have taken place. Attention to the language used to describe the pain and observation of any odd behaviour are essential. No amount of medication or stimulation will get a severely depressed or neurotic patient back to normal but a combination of the programme described above with behaviour modification and mental stimulation can achieve a lot. The most common presentations are either a complete withdrawal from family, or the assumption of bizarre forms of dress due to the hypersensitivity, or the use of the pain to manipulate others. Here education of family as well as patients is necessary to achieve control.

Reasons for Failure

In such a complex syndrome as post-herpetic pain, it is very easy to oversimplify in order to establish a programme for management. If patients don't fit, first check the diagnosis. Elderly people have many causes of aches and pains and in particular for girdle pain. If the pain is made worse by weight-bearing and movement, it is probably due to nerve root entrapment at the vertebral column and may be relieved by epidural steroid injection.

Herpes zoster may be the first manifestation of secondary spread of breast cancer—another potent cause of pain. These and others need not mean that pain control cannot be achieved, but that the symptom pattern may have to be reassessed and treatment modified.

A wide variety of treatments have been described by various authors for the control of post-herpetic pain. Most of these fail to stand-up to scientific scrutiny because of the variable nature of the syndrome and the difficulty in doing controlled studies in elderly patients.[4] The presenting symptoms when they are analysed are capable of being controlled by accepted techniques of pain management, but each patient's precise treatment will probably differ from any others. Some patients manage very well on relaxation and no drugs, others who only need stimulation, and others who do very well on anti-convulsants and amitriptyline in quite small doses. The security of having a place to go where their condition is understood is important to all and it is an essential part of their management.

REFERENCES

1. Rogozzino MW, et al. Medicine Baltimore, 61 (1982); 310–316.
2. Head H. Brain, 3 (1900); 353–523.
3. Juel Jenson et al. Br. Med. J., 4 (1970); 776–780.
4. Loeser JD.Treatment of herpes-zoster in elderly patients. Pain, 25 (1986); 149–164.

•••

SECTION–IX

Low Back Pain

55

LOW BACK PAIN (NEUROLOGICAL ASPECTS)

Low back pain is a common health problem. About 65% to 80% of the world's population develops back pain at some point during their lives. The surgical subspecialties of orthopeadics and neurosurgery are most frequently associated with low back pain evaluation and treatment though majority of patients don't require surgical intervention[1].

As many as 90% of patients with back pain have a mechanical reason for their pain.[2] Mechanical low back pain may be defined as pain secondary to overuse of a normal anatomic structure or pain secondary to trauma or deformity of an anatomic structure.[3,4] Careful clinical evaluation helps separate patients with mechanical back pain from those with nonmechanical back pain.[2]

The **clinical history** is an essential step in evaluating patients with low back pain. The age of a patient is helpful in determining the potential cause of back pain. The sex of the patient may also help select potential cause of low back pain.[3] However, no difference in sex, age and occupation wise difference in low backache patients, was observed by Kumar et al.[4]

The **duration and location of pain** help decide the subsequent kinds of questions that the evaluating physician will ask. Mechanical low back pain tends to have an onset associated with a physical task and is usually of short duration (days or weeks). Medical causes of low back pain tend to have a more gradual onset with no identifiable precipitating factor.

Most back pain is limited to the lumbosacral area of the low back. Radiation of pain in the thighs or the knees may be related to referred pain from elements of the spine (muscle, ligaments or apophysical joints). Pain that radiates from the low back to below the knees is usually neurogenic in origin and support a pathologic process effecting spinal nerve roots.

The **history** is directed towards understanding the chronologic developments of low back pain, its character and response to therapy. The anatomic structures of the lumbosacral spine receive specific types of sensory innervations that are associated with distinct qualities of pain. The major categories of pain include superficial somatic, deep somatic (spondylogenic) radicular, neurogenic, visceral referred and psychogenic[4].

In patients with a history suggestive of mechanical low back pain, the physical examination should concentrate or the evaluation of musculoskeletal and neural tissues of the lumbosacral spine.[3]

There are many **causes of backache**. The common causes are PID, facet joint degeneration, arachnoidits, pelvis lesions and tuberculosis. Whereas uncommon causes are cauda equine tumours, AVM, primary and secondary spinal tumours, ankylosing spondylitis and osteomyelitis. The cause of backache is detected by ruling out the causes one by one. This is done by proper history, clinical examination and investigations (Fig. 55.1).

Among **neurological examinations**, SLR-test, motor-sensory deficit, examination of deep tendon reflexes and Babinski reflex are the main cardinal points to be seen carefully.

As far as investigation is concerned plain X-ray particulary latral view is the basic requirement, whereas myelogram, CT scan, CT myelogram are further necessity according to the need. But recently MRI has revolutionized the radiographic evaluation of the lumboscaral spine. MRI has a number of advantages compared to other radiological techniques. MRI is able to define bony and soft tissue structures without intrathecal contrast. The entire length of the spinal cord and canal may be evaluated in multiple planes.

MRI has become the primary imaging modality for the study of spine. MRI is an excellent technique to view the spinal cord. MRI identifies syrinx, cord infarctions, cord injury, multiple sclerosis, demyelination and intramedullary tumours. The development of contrast media (gadolinium) has improved the characterization of spinal cord tumours. MRI can detect infection of the spine very well. It's a very useful technique for mechanical disorders of the spine like disc prolapse, spondylolisthesis, various spondylitic changes and fractures. Thus a consensus is growing that MRI is the most useful technique for lumbar spine imaging.

But MRI findings are only significant in patients with correlating clinical symptoms and signs. We may find substantial abnormalities of herniated disc and spinal stenosis, whereas actual clinical findings are minimal. Therefore, the finding of an abnormal disc is more reliable in symptomatic individual.

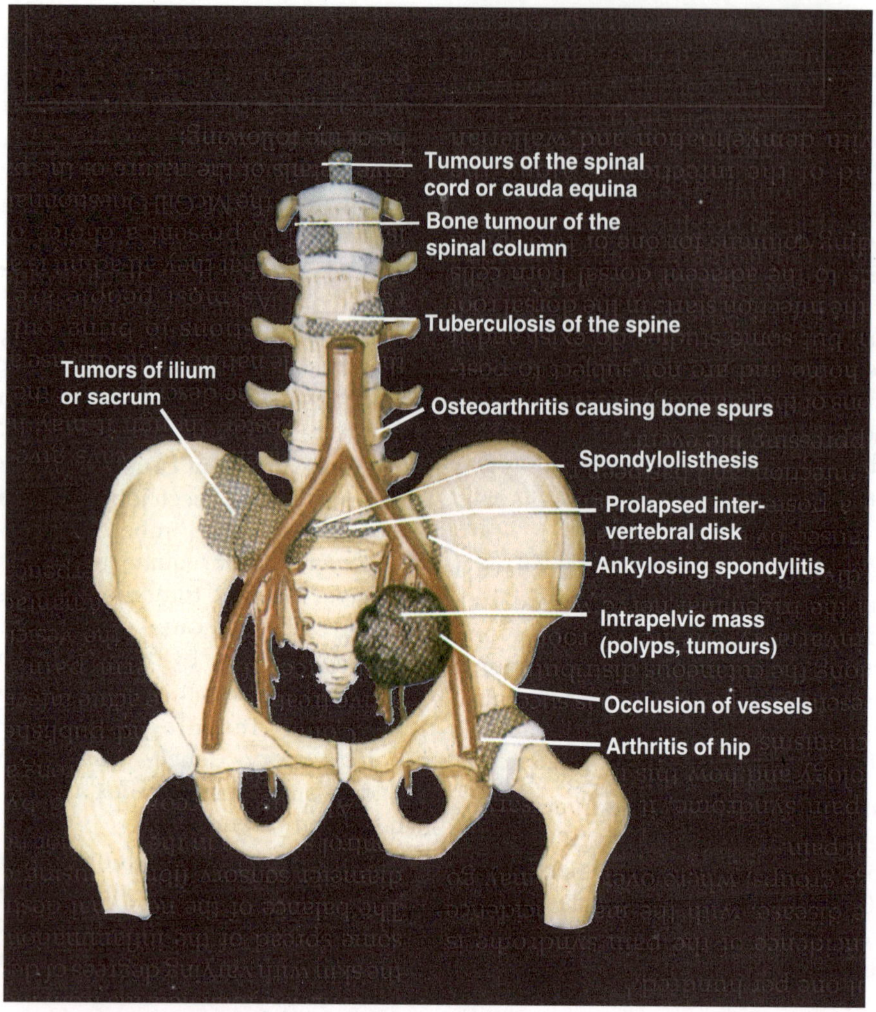

Fig. 55.1 : Causes of pain in the lower back and leg

A number of other radiographic techniques are available for the evaluation of lumbosacral spine. These are spinal angiography, discography, thermography, etc. These are used infrequently compared to the X-ray, CT or MRI. Similarly majority of patients don't require laboratory studies with their initial evaluation.

Electrodiagnostic studies are extensions of the neurologic examination and provide a means to identify nerve and muscle damage. These tests can confirm the clinical suspicion of nerve root compression, define the distribution and severity of involvement and document or exclude other illness of nerves or muscles that contribute to the patient's symptoms and signs. These tests include evaluation of electrical activity generated by muscle fibres at rest and during contraction (electromyography) and speed of conduction of impulses electrically generated in peripheral nerves (nerve conduction studies).

Electrodiagnostic tests are most helpful in documenting, objectively, neurophysiologic abnormalities in a patient where clinical examination (pain radiation, sensory changes, muscular weakness) does not necessarily indicate nerve root dysfunction.

Electromyography (EMG) is the test most commonly ordered to document the presence of a radiculopathy. EMG findings are based upon the interpretation of the observer. The experience of the examiner is very important in obtaining the most accurate information from the EMG evaluation. As opposed to EMG, nerve conduction tests become abnormal as soon as nerve damage occurs.

The limitations of electrodiagnostic studies must be considered when evaluating patients with low back pain. These studies do not determine a specific diagnosis. Localization of the lesion is not easy since most muscles in the lower extremity are innervated by two or more nerve roots.

Despite these limitations, electodiagnostic tests remain an important part of the investigation of low back pain patients. An abnormal EMG is corroborative evidence of organic diseases and helps the physician determine who is a potential candidate for surgical intervention. Electromyography changes may recede with resolution of the nerve impingement. However, patients with a good operative decompression with relief of symptoms may have EMG abnormalities persist 1 year after surgery. In patients without neurologic dysfunction, EMG and nerve conduction tests are normal.

Management : After investigating such patient of LBP utmost care should be taken in deciding treatment. First of all decision should be made between conservative and operative line of treatment. It depends on the aetiology of LBP, age of the patient, clinical findings, radiological investigations, associated medical condition and obesity.

Conservative therapy includes rest, physiotherapy, simple analgesics and vitamin B_1, B_6 and B_{12}. Candidates with acute pain without neurological deficit can be very well treated with bed rest and analgesics, whereas those with chronic history needs supervised physiotherapy. The need of analgesics should be restricted as far as possible. Simple, tolerable and non-toxic analgesics would be worthwhile to use rather than sophisticated research product having inadequate trials. Opioides are useful in a patient with psychosocial factor.

Patient with obesity requires dietary restriction and weight reduction. The use of steroid should be reserved only for emergency situation or while deciding conservative treatment in cases with neurological deficit. The combination of epidural steroids, oral analgesics helps in breaking the cycle of pain, allowing early ambulation and recovery.[4,6]

The role of physiotherapy is significant while treating patient conservatively.

The aim of physiotherapy is to restore function and to educate patients in their biomechanical capabilities. The modalities used include moist heat, traction, diathermy, electrical nerve stimulation[4] and massage. Maintaining the lumbar spine in a reduced lordotic curve (physiologically supine with slight knee flexion) is usually comfortable and the pelvic tilt position increases nutrition and circulation to the spine. Patients should be cautioned not to lift heavy and bulky objects without assistance. Acute conditions responded better to physiotherapy (Interferential current), while chronic conditions responded better to epidural steroids.[4, 6]

Decision for operative line of treatment is a challenging task to a neurosurgeon or orthopaedic surgeon particularly in a borderline case. Patient of LBP without neurological deficit should be treated conservatively as far as possible.

Principles of operation depends on the aetiology. Those with mechanical compression having benign etiology (disc prolapse, listhesis, etc.) needs to be decompressed adequately, whereas mechanical compression with aggressive disease can be operated conservatively.

Several different factors may lead to persistent pain following lumbar spine surgery. This is classically known as failed back surgery syndrome (FBSS). There are several different causes of FBSS, includes misdiagnosis, in appropriate operation, surgical complication and psychosocial problems. The best treatment of FBSS is prevention. Proper selection of patients for surgery is the primary determinant of successful outcome.

REFERENCES

1. Raj PP. Practical management of pain, 3rd ed, St Louis, Mosby Year Book. 1998.
2. Loeser JA, Bonica's management of pain, 3rd ed, Philadelphia, Lippincott-William and Wilkins, 2001.
3. Wall PD and Melzack R. Textbook of pain (3rd) ed Edinburg Churchill, Livingstone, 1994.
4. Kumar P. Socioindividual predictors in low back pain in relation to epidural steroids vs IFT. Indpain 2004; 18(2): 21–26.
5. Kumar Pramod. Atlas on peripheral nerve blocks, Jamnagar ISSP Con 2002.
6. Kumar P et al. Comparison of epidural triamcinalone versus physiotherapy in low backache. Proceedings of XIX ISSPCON 2005, Pune.

•••

EPIDURAL MEDICATION FOR BACK PAIN

56

Lowback pain and sciatica continues to challenge the physicians in the areas of aetiopathogenesis, diagnosis and therapy.[1] Epidural steroids has been used with varying success rate for the treatment of low backache (Table 56.1). Lack of controlled trials, protocols and identification of various factors, which influence ultimate outcome raises doubt regarding the efficacy of the use of steroids[2,3,4]. Study of various factors like aetiopathogenesis, chronicity of pain, route of medication, the volume and dose of methyl prednisolone depot (Table 56.2) and lastly evolving an appropriate index for evaluation of pain relief (Pain Relief Score)[5,6] has tremendously improved the management of low backache. Furthermore, the use of image intensifier or CT guidance resulted in accurate localisation and deposition of depo-medrol close to the site of pathology.

Table 56.1 : Results of various studies

Author	Route	Drug	Result
Winnie et al.[3] (1972)	Lumbar Epidural	Depomedrol	63%
Brevik et al.[2] (1976)	Caudal	Depomedrol	63%
Rastogi et al.[6] (1994)	Lumbar (n = 103)	Depomedrol	71.2%
	Caudal (n = 31)	Depomedrol	87%
Swerdlow et al. (1978)[4]	Epidural	Depomedrol	67%
Kumar P. et al.[11](2001)	Epidural Lumbar	Wycort, depomederol	60%
Kumar P.et al.[12](2005)	Epidural Lumbar	Triamcenalone	63%

Indications

Patients with compressive myelopathy with or without radiculopathy responds well to the epidural steroids.[7] Best results seen in patients having LBA of acute onset followed by subacute origin.[8] Patients with chronic LBA show poor response with epidural steroids. Indication are as follows:

Best Response

Acute PID

Spondylolisthesis

Spinal fracture

Coccidynia

Intermediate Response

Idiopathic

Lumbar spondylosis

Ankylosing spondylitis

Poor or No Response

Lumbar canal stenosis (LCS)

Facet join involvement

Table 56.2 : Factors effecting epidural steroid treatment

Factors:

1. Chronicity of pain
   Acute/subacute/chronic
2. Vol/conc. of drug:

   80–120/10 mL (Localised)
   80–120/20 mL (Generalised)
3. Use of Image – intensifier/CT
4. Site/nature of pathology
   Localised/General
5. Route of Medication,
   site of epidural injection
   Lumbar/Caudal

Table 56.3 : Diagnosis of low backache

* Clinical history and examination–Accidental fall or jerk, tender area, SLR, radiation, paresthesia.
* X-ray spine (L_1-S_2) AP, Lateral for disc compression, bone defects.
* Myelogram–for blockade of flow of radio-opaque dye.
* CT–for extent and localisation of the lesion.
* MRI–for accurate localisation of the lesion.
* Epiduroscopy/Epidurography– for accurate localisation and treatment.
* NCV/H-reflex by electrophysiological studies.

Epidural injections have been recommended to deliver drug to the area of the affected nerve roots, thereby decreasing the systemic effect of the administered steroid. White and collegues[8] showed that epidural steroid was most effective in the presence of nerve root irritation as evidenced clinically by signs of root irritation (positive SLR), radicular pain, dermatomal hyper aesthesia, weakness of muscle group innervated by the involved nerve roots, decreased deep tendon reflexes or electrophysiologically by changes in H-reflex or NCV. Kepes and Duncalf [9] reviewed literature on epidural steroid and concluded that its use was not scientifically proven. On other hand several studies demonstrated success rate ranging from 67% to as good as 87%.[2-6] There are several prospective, randomized controlled studies on the use of epidural steroid injections with disc pathology.[2,10,11]

Rastogi et al. (1994)[6] studied the influence of various factors like chronicity or duration of symptom, site and nature of pathology, route of medication, drug (triamcinaone or methyl prednisolone), dosage and volume, and the use of image intensifier. Chronicity or duration of symptom directly influence the outcome as best result seen in acute or when symptoms are <3 months old (Table 56.4) and worst result in chronic or > 12 months old symptoms.

Principles of Management

The essential principles of management of LBA with epidural steroids are more or less similar to the principles used elsewhere. These include an accurate diagnosis based on clinical, radiological or electrophysiological investigations (Table 56.3).The basic aim of clinical examination and investigations is to arrive at the nature of the disease as well as the site of lesion.[8] Epidural steroids are contraindicated in patients with tubercular pathology. After the diagnosis is confirmed and after explaining the procedure and prognosis to the patients the epidural depomedrol is deposited close to the site of pathology preferably under image intensifier or CT with or without radio-opaque dye (urographin). In the absence of image intensifier or CT the cathether tip may be placed close to the site of pathology by approximately measuring distance from the skin.

Table 56.5 : Indications for epidural steroid therapy

* **Selection of patients :**
  - Compressive myelopathy
  - L_5-S_1, Radioculopathy
  - PID/Post herpectic/spondylolisthesis
  - Coccyodynia/Secondaries spine
  - Post laminectomy
* Ischaemic Myelopathy - LCS
* Facet joint involvement
* Idiopathic

Methyl prednisolone when injected epidurally stays for more than 2 weeks and thereby exerting slow sustained effect. Dictum is that the epidural depomedrol or kenacort should be repeated at least for three times at an interval of one month provided there is some improvement following first injection. The use of oral analgesic combination along with steroid helps in breaking the cycle of pain, and increased mobility of the patient.[11] If there is no response following first few injections revise your diagnosis and consider for other modalities of treatment (Facet Rhizotomy or Laminectomy).

Table 56.4 : Relation of duration of symptoms to the success rate

Duration of symptom months	Success rate
<3	83-100%
3-6	67-81%
6-12	44-69%
7-12	46-58%

The nature of pathology broadly speaking compressive myelopathy or ischaemic myelopathy as seen in cases of lumbar canal stenosis (LCS) influences the ultimate outcome. Patients presenting with compressive myelopathy respond well to epidural steroids while patients with ischaemic pathology (LCS) associated with poor outcome. Patients with facet joint involvement or root canal stenosis are unlikely to respond to epidural steroids. Methyl prednisolone or triamcinolone can be used and seems to be equally effective.[11, 12] The epidural injection of triamcinolone or methyl prednisolone does not cause significant inflammatory changes in the spinal nerve root or meninges. Most of the patients take several days to respond to epidural steroid injection. Green PWD et al[10] noted that 37% of their patients responded to steroid within 2 days, 59% noted relief between 4-6 days and 4% after 6 days. Epidural methyl prednisolone depot exert continuous effect for nearly 3 weeks as evidenced by suppression of plasma cortisol levels as an indirect evidence.[9] This is the reason why epidural methyl prednisolone should be repeated at an interval of one month. Other factors like dose and volume or route of medication (lumbar or caudal) should be taken in account while planning the management. The accuracy in placement of drug close to pathology using an image-intensifier or CT definitely makes difference. Using a radio-opaque dye (Radio-opaque 300/350) through a needle or epidural cathether not only improve the accuracy in placement of drug but also gives a diagnostic clue on epidurogram, large central disc may call for surgery in near future. Lack of uniform criteria for the assessment of response or pain relief has led to confusion among the workers. For the sake of uniformity Rastogi et al. (1994)[6] proposed Pain Relief Score (PRS) based on pain relief, duration of pain relief and improvement in neurological status.

Maximum score : 10

0–5 : Poor/unsatisfactory pain relief

6–8 : Good

8–10 : Excellent

Recently, cervical and lumbar epidural steroids injections have been used successfully in the treatment of Bechterew's syndrome[7] (Ankylosing spondylitis). Use of thoracic or lumbar epidural in secondaries spine is limited. Rastogi et al.[6] showed good relief of pain in 4/7 patients and complete reversal of neurological deficit (paresis, bladder and bowel involvement) in 1/7 cases. Patients with post laminectomy syndrome are also benefited with epidural depomedrol as 7/8 patients showed good relief of pain.

Table 56.6 : Pain relief score (PRS)[6]

Pain Relief Percentage	Improvement in neurological deficit	Duration of pain relief months	Score
0	No change	0	0
1-25	Improvement	0-3	1
26-50	Normal	4-6	2
51-75	-	7-11	3
76-100	-	>12	4

Epidural methyl prednisolone depot has definite value in the management of chronic low back pain. Long-term relief of pain and improvement in mobility can be achieved using epidural steroid provided emphasis is laid on proper selection of patients[11] understanding often underlying pathology and last but not the least the placement of drug in the proximity of the lesion using image intensifier or CT guidance.

However, depot preperations of steroids may lead to irritation of nerves, so use of water soluble triamcenalone is preferred specially in chronic pain syndromes. The acute conditions respond better to the use of oral analgesics and physiotherapy with low amplitude current.[12]

REFERENCES

1. Goeberg HW, Jillo SJ, Gordener WJ, et al. Pain radiculopathy treated with epidural injection of procaine and hydrocortisone acetate. Results 113 patients. Anaesth, Analg. 1961;40: 130–4.
2. Brevik. H, Helsa PE, Molnar l et al. Treatment of Chronic low back pain and sciatic: Comparison of Caudal epidural injection of bupivacaine and methyl prednisolone with bupivacaine followed by saline. Adv, Pain Res, Ther, 1976;1:927–31.

3. Winnie AP, Hartman JI, Meyers Hl, et al. Pain Clinic II, intradural and extradural corticosteroid for sciatica. Anaesth Analg, 1972;51:990–9.
4. Swerdlow M, Sayle-Creer WA. Study of extradural medication in the relief of the lumbosciatic syndrome. Anaesthesia. 1970;5: 341–5.
5. Rastogi V. Epidural medication for back pain. Proceedings of XVI ISSPCON 2002, Jamnagar.
6. Rastogi V, Krishna M, Sarar SK, et al. Factors influencing the pain relief obtained with methyl prednisolone in low back pain and sciatica. The Pain Clinic.1994; 7:291–95.
7. Stav A, Ovadia L, Stemberg A, et al. Cervical and lumbar epidural steroid injections for pain relief in patients with Bechterew's syndrome. Preliminary study.The Pain Clinic.1994;7;283–89.
8. White AH, Derby R, Wynne GS . Epidural injections for diagnosis and treatment of low back pain. Spine 1980;5: 78–86.
9. Kepes ER, Duncalf D. Treatment of backache with spinal injections of local anaesthetics, spinal and systemic. Pain, 1985;22:33–47.
10. Green PWD, et al. The role of epidural cortisone injection in the treatment of discogenic low back pain. Clin Orlhop 1980;153:121–125.
11. Kumar P, Seema Parekh. Epidural steroids in low backache, Dissertation for M.D Anaesthesiology, Saurashtra University, Rajkot. 2001.
12. Kumar P, Adarsh CS. Comparison of epidural triamcenalone versus physiotherapy in low backache. Proceedings XIX ISSPCON 2005, Pune.
13. Kumar Pramod. Socio individual predictors in low back pain in relation to epidural steroids versus interferental therapy. Ind pain 2004;18(2):21-26.

•••

SURGICAL MANAGEMENT OF LOW BACK PAIN

57

Back pain is now considered as a modern international epidemic because more than 80% of the population have the experience of backache sometimes in their life. The early Greeks recognized this as a disease. They prescribed rest and massage for remedy. Since then, many authors tried to find out the real cause behind it *e.g.*, traumatic ruptures of disc tumours or tuberculosis. Openheim and Krause in 1909 for the first time successfully removed herniated disc for back pain. Mixer and Barr in 1934 established the relationship between sciatica and disc herniation and recommended surgical excision of disc. As medicine advances number of diagnostic devices have been available to find out the pathological factors causing backache.[1]

Low back pain has been understood better now and after numerous prospective clinical studies, it has been observed that surgical treatment is necessary in less than 10% cases. It is also a fact that surgery for backache is performed mainly for lumbar disc diseases and tuberculosis of spine. Other indications for operations are spondylolisthesis and spondylolysis, lumbar spinal stenosis, spinal tumours and failed spine surgery.[2] It is really important to know when should a patient be considered for surgical treatment. Usually the clinicians think of operations for backache on the following conditions:

1. Pain not responding to repeated conservative care.
2. Progressive weakness of the lower limbs.
3. Bladder or bowel dysfunction.
4. Instability of the spine.

Lumbar Disc Disease

Lumbar disc disease is most common in third and fourth decade of life. The pain in disc herniation is intermittent in nature and aggravated by straining, sneezing or coughing. It is relieved by rest and especially in the semi-Fowler position. Other symptoms may be weakness of lower limbs and paraesthesia. In high or midline lumbar disc herniation there may be numbness and weakness in the involved leg and occasionally pain in the groin or testicle. In massive intervertebral disc extrusion, symptoms of cauda equina syndrome like saddle anaesthesia, bilateral ankle are flexia and bladder disturbances may be present. Usually 95% of the lumbar disc herniation occurs at L4 - L5 level and straight leg raising test is positive.[2]

Disc removal is mandatory and urgent in cauda equina syndrome with neurological deficit. But in otherwise healthy people, an ideal patient for disc surgery should have the follwing criteria.[2]

1. Back pain with predominant unilateral leg pains extending below knee for at least 6 weeks.
2. Pain recurs after a minimum of 6 to 8 weeks of conservative treatment and it is relieved with anti-inflammatory drugs or epidural steroids.
3. Should have signs of sciatic irritation and neurological impairment.
4. CT, Lumbar MRI or Myelography should confirm the level of lesion and consistent with clinical findings.
5. Psychologic testing should show a hysteria or hypochondriasis T score of 75 or less.

In doubtful cases discography can be performed before surgery. But this technique should be applied for the patients who did not respond to repeated conservative treatment. To identify accurately the source of pain injections of local anaesthetic or contrast media in various specific anatomic areas may be useful.

However, before surgery both the patient and the surgeon must realize that disc surgery is not a cure but may provide symptomatic relief.[3]

Different Types of Operations for Disc

1. **Open disc surgery :** Through a midline incision 5–10 cm long on the back over the involved segment disc is removed.
2. **Micro lumbar disc excision :** Here incision is very small about 2.5 cm, but it requires an operative microscope for better visualization of the structures.
3. **Percutanous lumbar discectomy :** Many surgeons also practice it, but the results are variable.

4. **Chemonucleolysis** : A proteolytic enzyme chymopapain is injected into the disc and materials are aspirated out. It is not so popular in USA for the complication of transverse myelitis, but still it is practiced in Europe. In India it is not at all popular.

Post-operative Management

On the first post-operative day the patient is allowed to stand. Isometric abdominal and lower extremity exercises are re-instituted. Lifting, bending and stooping are gradually restored after sixth week.

Complications of disc surgeries are:

1. Cauda equina syndrome
2. Thrombophlebitis
3. Pulmonary embolism
4. Wound infection
5. Pyogenic spondylitis
6. Post-operative discitis
7. Dural tears
8. Nerve root injury
9. C.S.F. fistula
10. Lacerations of abdominal vessels
11. Injury to abdominal viscera.

Tuberculosis of Spine

The spine is the most common site of skeletal tuberculosis. More than 2 million people with active spinal tuberculosis are living in the world today. Dorsolumbar spine is affected mostly with low back pain. Striking features of this condition is a long history of ill-health and backache. Deformity is dominant feature in some cases. Occasionally the patient presents with cold abscess pointing in the groin or with paraesthesia and weakness of the legs. Vertebral collapse with diminution of disc space is the typical radiological finding. Late diagnosis and missed diagnosis are quite common because other clinical conditions like pyogenic and fungal infections, secondary metastatic disease, primary tumours of bone such as osteosarcoma, chondrosarcoma, myeloma, eosinophillic granuloma, aneurysmal bone cyst, sarcoidosis, giant cell tumour and Scheurmann's disease may show the features of spinal tuberculosis. In doubtful cases, CT, MRI and CT guided needle biopsy are helpful for proper diagnosis and treatment.

Surgery offers good result in advanced disease, but it requires skill and good O.T. facilities. The principles of surgeries are:

1. Abscess drainage
2. Radical debridement and arthrodesis

Paravertebral abscesses are drained easily from back through a small incision but repeated aspiration is very often practiced to avoid chronic discharging sinus. Psoas abscesses are entirely extraperitoneal and it is drained through Pethl's triangle by a lateral incision along the crest of the ilium.

Thoracolumbar area of the spine (D_{12}-L_2) is exposed through an incision along the eleventh rib and the lower lumbar vertebrae are exposed through renal approach. All debris, pus and sequestrated bone and disc are removed by suction. After radical debridement bone grafts are placed for fusion of the vertebrae.

After operation patient is placed in anterior or posterior plaster shell bed. The time of immobilization after surgery is about 3 1/2 months. Mobilization is then started gradually and antitubercular drugs are continued.

Spondylolisthesis and Spondyloysis

Spondylolisthesis is defined as an anterior or posterior slip of one vertebra on another and spondylolysis is unilateral or bilateral defect of pars interarticularis without displacement of vertebra[4]. Symptoms begin insidiously during the second or third decade as an intermittent dull ache in the lower back. Pain aggravates during walking and standing and may radiate to the buttocks and thighs. Later, unilateral sciatica may develop. Plain radiographs are the best way to diagnose spondylolithesis or spondylolysis. Myelography and three dimensional C.T. help to identify the intraspinal and extraspinal effects of spondylolisthesis which may be of surgical significance.

Surgery is not always necessary in spondyloloisthesis. When persistent pain in low back, buttocks and thighs incapacitiate a person for heavy work, surgery may be considered. In general, the younger the patient with painful spondylolisthesis the more definite is the indication for surgery, and the more likely is surgery to be successful. For sedentary workers surgery is indicated when spondylolisthesis is associated with sciatica. For adolescents, severe hamstring tightness is often an indication for spinal fusion. In fact, about 20% of patients with symptomatic spondylolisthesis require surgery and the rest can be treated well by conservative method.

Posterolateral fusion of the unstable spine is the treatment of choice by many surgeons. When symptoms of pressure on nerve roots are present, the fifth lumbar and first sacral roots should be inspected and the herniated intervertebral disc and fibrocartilaginous tissues around them should be excised before posterior fusion is performed. Various internal fixation devices are used currently to enhance the fusion.

Lumbar Spinal Stenosis

Narrowing of the spinal canal occurs in different pathological conditions especially due to hypertrophy at the posterior disc margin and the facet joints.[5]

Most of patients are male aged over 50 and they complain of aching, heaviness, numbness and paraesthesia in the thighs and legs, the pain is relieved by sitting, squatting or leaning against a wall to flex the spine. About one third of the patients complain of leg pain on walking (Neurogenic claudication) and relieved by standing. Claudication is more frequent in central or advanced stenosis. Moderate lateral canal stenosis and foraminal stenosis may present features of osteoarthritis of hip.

Radiographs will show the evidence of degeneration changes of the spine. For more reliable information and diagnosis myelography with metrizamide, CT and MRI are helpful.

Primary indications for surgery in spinal stenosis.

1. Increasing backache and leg pain.
2. Back Pain Resistant to conservative treatment.

But before surgery patient should be convinced about the possible results of surgery, because rate of improvement is not more than 70 to 86% in any of the series.[3]

Principles of Spinal Stenosis Surgery

1. It is better to identify the source of pain preoperatively using root blocks.
2. Specific attention should be directed to that area.
3. Spinal stabilization is required if two or more facet joints are removed.
4. Surgeon should be prepared for spinal fusion where findings at surgery requires more radical approach.

Operative Procedures

1. Midline decompression (neural arch resection)
2. Selective decompression as decided preoperatively
3. Spinal fusion with decompression.

Tumours of the Spine

Both benign and malignant tumours are found in different anatomical areas of the spine. Surgery depends on the nature of the tumour and its anatomical locations.

Some of the tumours like aneurysmal bone cyst, G.C.T. and other were once considered inaccessible surgically when found in the vertebrae.

Significant advances in anterior spinal surgery have made possible the resection of vertebral bodies with minimal morbidity. Metastatic lesions are forty times more common than primary malignant tumours of the spine. Removal of the tumour (when possible), decompression of the spinal cord and reconstruction of the structural defect are the basic goals of a surgical resection for metastatic lesions of the spine.[6] Mostly it affect the vertebral body and 70% of patients having neurological compromise.

Failed Spine Surgery

It is a very difficult situation when a surgeon faces such a problem. Under that circumstances, one has to look for:

1. Any new problem.
2. Previously undiagnosed or untreated problem.

In repeat surgery usually scarring, previous infection, pseudarthrosis and adverse psychologic factors of the patients are encountered. All investigations are repeated along with complete re-evaluation of the present clinical condition. Efforts should be made towards identification of the source of pain with the use of differential spinal, root blocks, facet blocks and discograms.[7] Nonoperative treatment should be attempted before the surgery is contemplated. Patients should know the prognosis of the repeat surgery because satisfactory results are obtaiend in 31% to 80%.[8]

REFERENCES

1. Goldthwait E. Low-Back lesions. J.Bone Joint Surg 1937; 19:810.
2. Nachemson A. The lumbar spine and orthopaedic challenge. Spine 1976;1:59.
3. Spengler DM, Freeman C, Westbrook R, and Miller JW. Low-back pain following multiple lumbar spine procedures. Failure of initial selection. Spine 1980; 5:356.
4. Eisenstein SM., Parry C.R. The lumbar facet arthorsis syndrome. Journal of Bone and Joint Surgery: 1987; 69B, 3–7.
5. Appley AG. Apley's System of Orthopaedics and Fractures: 7th edition; Louis, Solomon, 1993.
6. Grenshaw AH. Cambell's Operative Orthopaedics. Vol. 58th Edition 1992; pp3715–3775.
7. Wilkinson HA. Failed Back Syndrome, Etiology and Therapy. Harperand Row, 1983.
8. Ray et al. Surgical management of low back pain. Proceedings of XVI ISSPCON 2002, Jamnagar.

PHYSICAL THERAPY AND I.F.T

58

Applied Role of Interferential Current

There are very **commonest risk factors** which may be responsible for back pain *e.g.*:

- ★ Heavy manual work
- ★ Mismatched body strength and sudden movements
- ★ Long sitting and sedentary habits
- ★ Faulty postural habits
- ★ Obesity
- ★ Muscular insufficiency and multiple pregnancies
- ★ Emotional disturbances.

But, physiotherapy provides non drug, non invasive remedial approach to pain relief.

Foundation of physiotherapy can be traced to Romans and Greeks who in 250AD used electric fish for relief of pain due to gout, headache. By 19th Century, physiotherapist centred on the ability of electrical energy to relieve pain by using different modalities and by 21st century, recent advances are laser therapy, long wave therapy, interferential therapy which are used for immediate and long lasting pain relief.[1]

In 1849 – W.F.Chanang – Medical application of electricity.

In 1867 – G.M. Beard – First time made medical use of electricity.

In 1945 – Haiship – Dynawave neuromuscular stimulator.

In 1949 – Hans Nemec had first time successfully discovered interferential current therapy and its applications.[1]

'Interferential current therapy is a form of electrical treatment in which two medium frequency currents are used to produce a low frequency effect."

Skin impedance is much greater with low frequency currents and much smaller with higher frequency currents -

$$Z = \frac{1}{2\ JJFC}$$

where, Z = skin interference (in ohms)

F = frequency in Hz

C = skin capacitance in microfarads

This gives skin resistance at 50 Hz - 3200 ohms and at 4000 Hz = 40 ohms/100 cm^2.

Low frequency currents, due to high skin resistance, require a high current intensity to achieve the desired effect, and this causes marked stimulation to the patient.

Medium frequency currents, due to low skin resistance, requires a low current intensity to achieve the desired effects, which results in less sensory discomfort.

High frequency currents such as short wave diathermy and microwave, have frequencies too high to stimulate skin or muscle and produce only thermal effect.

If two medium frequency currents at constant intensity, but different frequencies are applied to body at same time, the intensity of the combined current will increase and decrease rhythmically. The combined current has a frequency equal to the difference between the two medium frequencies known as **Beat Frequency** and this is the **Interference Effect**.

Vector Effect

The interference field is rotated to an angle of 45° in each direction; the field thus covers a wide area. This is useful in diffuse pathology or if the site of the lesion cannot be accurately localized.

Parameters : Endomed 582 (Multiple stimulator)

Intensity	0–100 mA
Frequency	4000–5000 Hz
Pulse duration	125 μ sec
Beat frequency	0–299 Hz
Treatment time	15–30 minutes
Mode	Bipolar, Quadripolar
Poles	Four (2 positive; 2 negative)

It should be kept 10 feet away from short wave diathermy and ultrasound because of their magnetic effects.

Technique of Treatment

- ★ The patient is positioned comfortably in prone position and the skin is prepared as for any low frequency stimulation; it is washed with spirit and any skin lesions insulated with petroleum jelly.
- ★ The site for treatment is accurately located and the two pairs of electrodes positioned by the side of "trigger point" so that crossing point of the two currents is over or within the lesion.
- ★ The patient is warned that he will feel a tingling sensation which should not be too uncomfortable or burning.
- ★ In interferential equipment one frequency is fixed at 4000 Hz (generated by one pair of electrodes) and the other is variable between 4000 Hz and 4200 Hz (second pair of electrodes). By selecting the variable frequency, a beat frequency between 0 and 200 Hz may be generated, then patient experiences a mild tingling sensation.
- ★ The current should be sufficient to produce motor stimulation; if this is required.
- ★ After three to five minutes of treatment, it is common for the machine to be turned down, patient is asked to lie supine for 10 minute.
- ★ By increasing secretion of enkephalins and associated vasodilatation, circulation improves and pain is relieved.

Physiological Effect (Clayton)[1]

The physiological effects vary with such factors such as the magnitude of current, whether rhythmic or constant modes are used, the frequency range used and the accuracy of electrode positioning.

A. Relief of Pain : If constant beat of around 100 Hz is used, this causes a tingling sensation which after 15 minutes treatment can produce relief of pain for upto one hour.

B. Motor stimulation : If a rhythmic frequency between 1 and 10 Hz is used. The contraction is produced with minimal sensory stimulation and can be of deeply placed muscles, *e.g.*, those of pelvic floor.

C. Absorption of exudate : This is accelerated by a frequency of 1–10 Hz (rhythmic) as a rhythmical pumping action is produced which assists the normal absorption of exudate.

D. Increased blood flow, thus improved circulation.

E. Flush out oedema and decrease swelling.

F. Adhesion break-up.

G. Muscle re-education and relaxation of muscle spasms.

H. Prevention of joint contracture.

I. Maintaining or increasing range of motion.

Indications

1. Pain relief : Pain of sympathetic origin such as causalgia, neuralgia, pain from herpes zoster, amputation stump complications and recent injuries.
2. Myofasical pain syndrome : This is an extremely common painful condition of muscle, skin, fascia, tendons, periosteum or ligaments. The painful area is called "Trigger point". Patient suffers from deep dull aching pain worsened by activity or movement. IFT relieves pain spasm cycle, thereby providing permanent relief for the syndrome.
3. Back pain or disc lesions : It is useful for relief of acute back pain where the pain is localized to the back or referred down to a lower limb.
4. Swelling : It aids absorption of exudate particularly for haematomas.
5. Stress incontinence : The muscle stimulating frequencies aid weak pelvic floor muscles.
6. Sudeck's atrophy : This responds to interferential when other modalities have failed, but treatment may need to be prolonged.
7. Ligamentous and muscle injuries : It can be given in acute or chronic condition to relieve pain, promote healing and restore function. Treatment can be given with strapping in place.
8. Rheumatic conditions : Relief of pain arising from osteoarthritis, rheumatoid arthritis and ankylosing spondylitis may be obtained, with a resulting increase in function.
9. It can also be used for adjunctive treatment of post traumatic pain syndromes.

Contraindications

1. Pacemakers : Patients with pacemakers should avoid high and medium frequency currents.
2. Malignancy : Spread of the diseases may occur.
3. Pregnancy : Treatment should not be given to the pelvic organs during pregnancy.
4. Bacterial or viral infections : Treatment may cause spread of infection.
5. Thrombosis : Interferential tends to spread the blood clot and is contraindicated in deep venous thrombosis or thrombophlebitis. The heart and stellate ganglion should also be avoided.
6. Stroke.
7. Seizures.
8. Cardiac arrhythmias : Patient may have chance of developing dysrhythmias because disturbances in cardiac rhythm.

9 September 2005 12:30:11

9. Eyes or internal use.
10. Open wounds.
11. Tetany : Caution should be exercised in dosing.

Complications (Clayton)[1]

Only real danger with inferential currents is electrical burns, if bare electrode touches the skin or if the electrodes on the skin are too close, allowing a skin current to pass between them rather than through the deeper tissues.

Advantages

★ Medium frequency current is found effective for pain modulating and even has nerve block effect.

★ It gives long lasting pain relief as well as good relief in post-operative pain.

★ When combined therapy with ultrasound is used, it has been found to be very useful in tennis elbow and trigger points in muscles.

Other Physiotherapy exercises

Spine is an integrated organ and the vertebrae are chained together to work in a synchronized manner. Therefore, excluding neck or back from the management of either is often futile.[1,2]

A. *General Rules for Exercises*

1. Always exercise in fresh air with the room properly ventilated.
2. Don't exercise with full stomach, keep atleast 2 hours gap after meals.
3. Be in a free and relaxed mood during exercise.
4. Wear loose garments.
5. Exercise on a hard surface or thin matress.
6. Don't over do exercises, especially in the beginning.
7. Each exercise should last 10 seconds (7 seconds hold, 3 seconds relax) and be repeated 5–10 times each.
8. For self check and safety follow the exercise pulse rate guidelines.

B. *Exercises for Back*

1. Lie on back, arms above the head, knees bent, move one knees as far as you can towards chest and at the same time stretch out the other leg. Return and repeat alternately. (Fig. 58.1)

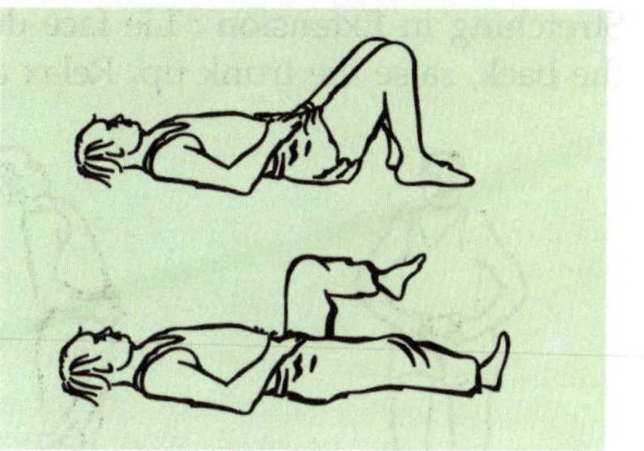

Fig. 58.1 : Back exercise

2. Lie on back with knees bent, bring both knees upto chest and with the hands clasped, pull the knees further towards the chest, keep shoulders flat on the mat. Relax and repeat. (Fig. 58.2).

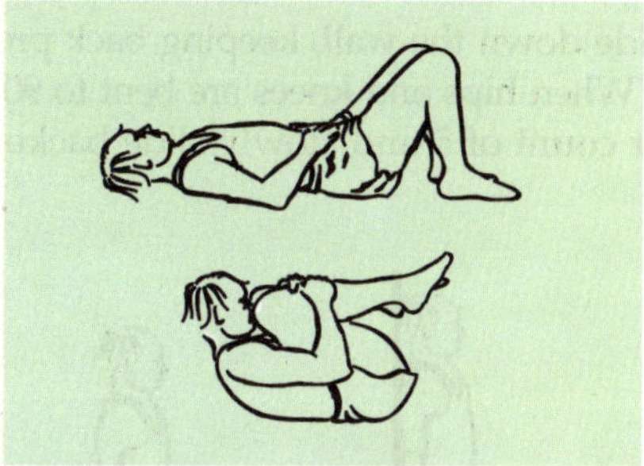

Fig. 58.2 : Back exercise

3. Abdominal muscle contraction : Lie on the back with arms on chest and knees bent.

   Contract abdominal muscles towards the spine by raising the head, hold for the count of ten and relax.

   Contract buttock muscles strongly and hold for the count of ten. Relax. (Fig. 58.3).

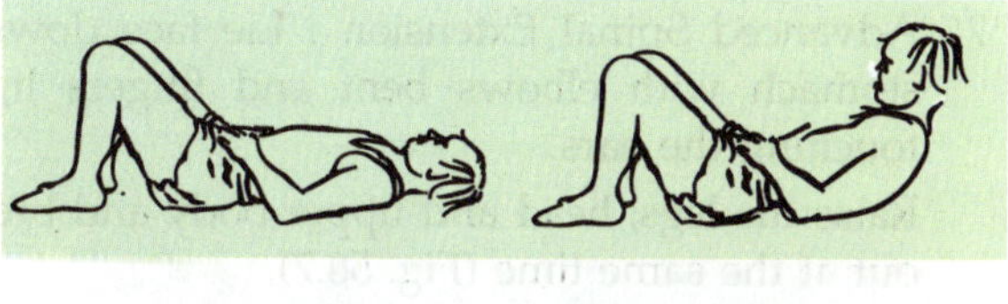

Fig. 58.3 : Abdominal muscle contraction

4. Lie on back with knees bent, hold the body flat as in No. 3, then slowly rise upto reach your knees with finger tips. Relax and repeat.

   Raise the legs without bending at the knee joints, kept for 5-10 seconds (Fig. 58.4).

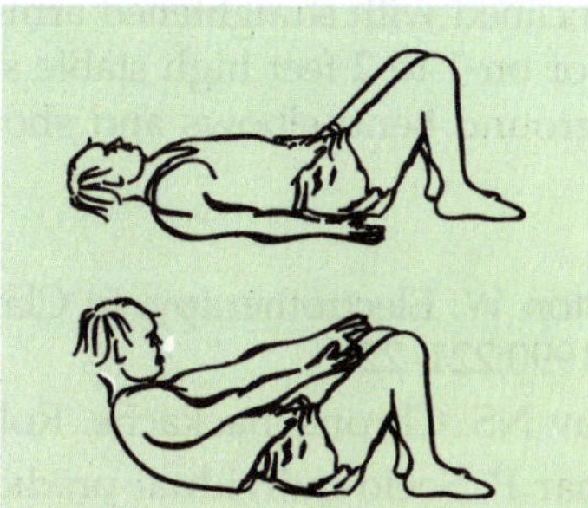

Fig. 58.4 : Abdominal muscle contraction

5. Stretching in Extension : Lie face down, hand at the back, raise the trunk up. Relax and repeat.

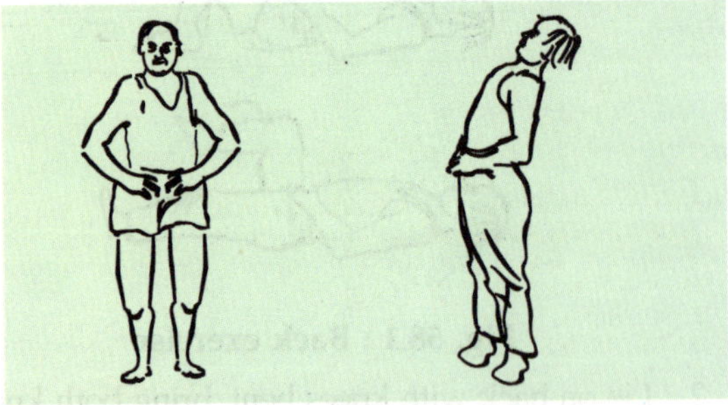

Fig. 58.5 : Wall side exercise

6. Wall Side : Stand with back pressed against wall and feet spaced one foot apart (Fig. 58.5).

   Slide down the wall, keeping back pressed against it. When hips and knees are bent to 90° angle, hold for count of 5 and slowly slide backup (Fig. 58.6).

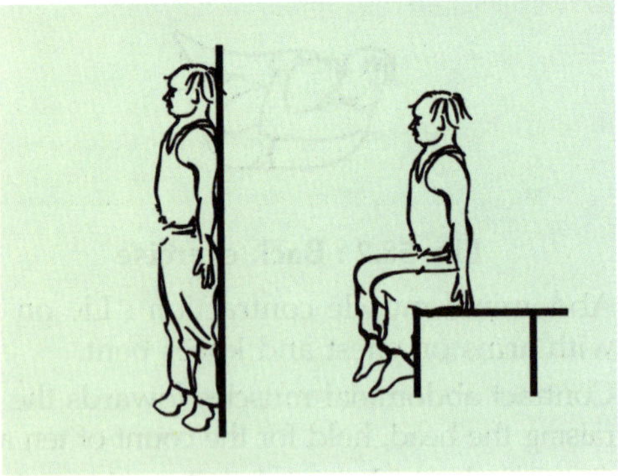

Fig. 58.6 : Wall side and sitting up side

7. Advanced Spinal Extension : Lie face down on stomach with elbows bent and fingers lightly touching the ears.

   Raise the legs, head and upper body and breathe out at the same time (Fig. 58.7).

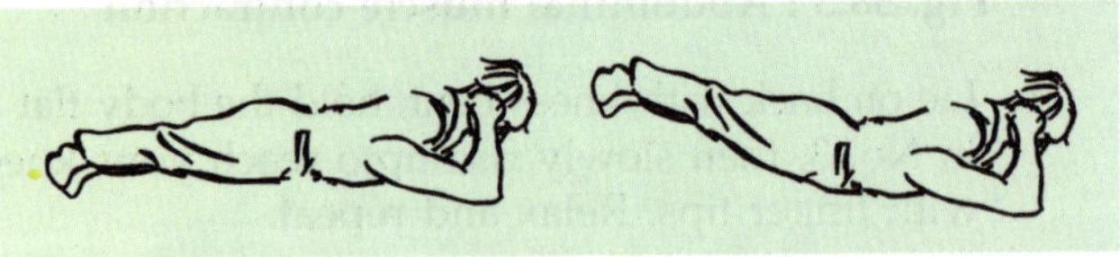

Fig. 58.7 : Advanced spinal extension

8. Lie inclined with straightened arms resting on bed end or on 1 to 2 feet high stable support, toes on the ground bend elbows and shoulders to lower whole body slowly. Relax and repeat with abdomen held straight (Fig. 58.8.)

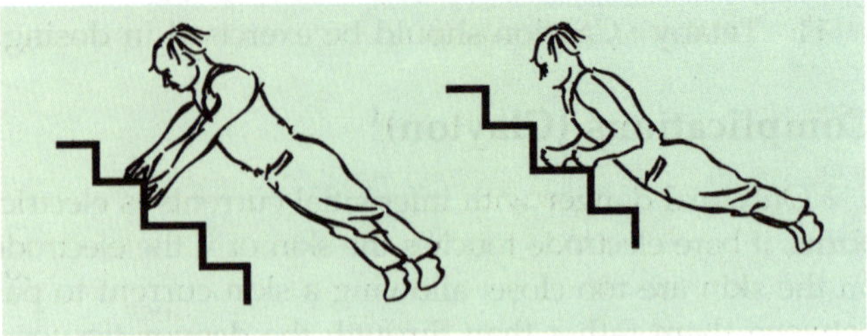

Fig. 58.8 : Upper spinal exercise

9. Sit-ups : Stand with arms stretched.

   Squat and straighten the hollow in the back. Return to sitting position (Fig. 58.9).

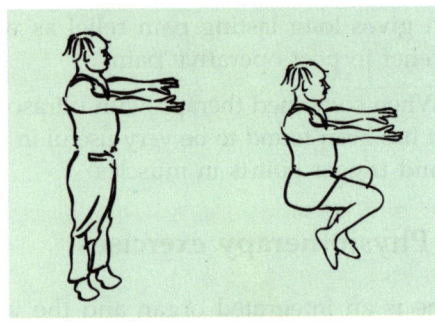

Fig. 58.9 : Sit ups

10. Intermediate spinal extension : Lie on stomach. Use arms to slowly raise shoulders and then slowly raise the legs stretched without bending at the knees. Count ten. Relax and repeat (Fig. 58.10).
11. Chest physiotherapy : Lying supine with knees bend.

    Deep breathing exercises with hands over upper abdomen – air fill under the hands and then sigh out feeling the hands sink down to encourage full, chest expansion.
12. Physiotherapy of the leg muscles – lying supine with feet spread 6" apart. Move the toes at the ankle to forward and backward and than rotate the feet at ankle joints.

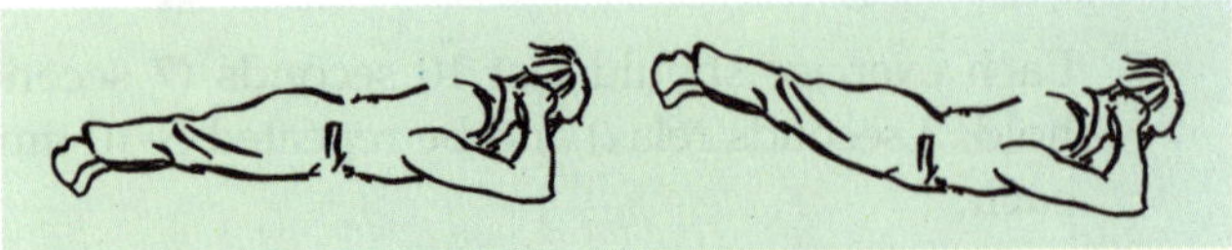

Fig. 58.10 : Intermediate spine exercise

REFERENCES

1. Clayton W. Electrotherapy. In Clayton's Physiotherapy. Wood KM, Norenberg AJ. (Editors), Atlanta, Raven 4 ed, 1990;221–228.
2. Yadav NS. Chronic backache. Role of physiotherapy. Ind. J. Pain 1994;8(2):15–21.
3. Kumar P. Socio-individual predictors in low back pain in relation to epidural steroids versus interferential therapy. Ind pain. 2005, 18(2); 21–26

•••

59

FACET BLOCK

A large percentage of low back pain is idiopathic and in many cases the sources of pain may be in and around the facet joint, joint capsule, musculotendinous junctions or ligaments. Pain may have an inflammatory component making joints more sensitive to movements than normal joints. Increasing the background neutral discharge in joints. The facet joint capsule contains low and high threshold mechanoreceptors, the former being proprio receptors while later being nociceptors. The surrounding musculotendinous units also have the same type of receptors with a higher proportion of proprio receptors. The neurons of the spinal tissues are chemosensitive to kaolin, substance P, activating both types of neurons, while the injection of bradykinin and serotonin, chemical mediators of inflammation activate units of facet joint and spinal cord.

Spinal loading or mechanical stimulation does maintain the discharge of the putative nociceptors which incidentally is maintained in case of chemical mediators. In an inflammed tissue there was a generally high spontaneous discharge rates which increased with stimulation. The inflammed tissue showed vigorous multi unit response to stress by moving the facet joint. Local analgesics and hydrocortisone can reduce the discharge rates from the inflamed tissue. The degenerative changes and associated muscle spasm developing when a facet joint is involved in a sprain from a free fall or violent twisting motion are formed as facet syndrome.[1]

Anatomy

Apophyseal (facet) articulators are formed by the superior articular facet of one vertebrae and the inferior articular facet of adjacent vertebrae above. The articular surfaces are covered by hyaline cartilage, the joints lined by synovium, innervated by dorsal ramus branches to its own level and to the level below figure 59.2. The lumbar facet joints are best visualized with 30° to 45° obliquity.

Facet Syndrome: Pathogenesis

Sudden jerk due to vehicle, athletic or occupational resulting in over riding of superior on the inferior articular facet in cervical, thoracic and lumbar regions. Degenerative changes *e.g.*, joint capsular hypertrophy, osteophyte formation and increased fibrous layer formation leading to muscle spasm on ipsilateral side.[2]

Clinical Features

1. Muscle spasm on ipsilateral side.
2. Local tenderness on palpation of transverse process.
3. Decreased range of motion involved level
4. Pain due to rotating motion and hyperextension. The pain is dull, aching, radiating to the occipital region, shoulder in cervical facet, to chest in thoracic and to back, hip and thigh in case of lumbar facet arthropathy. There is depressed straight leg raising test and depressed deep tendon reflexes.

Diagnosis is based on history, physical examination and X-ray and CT scan evaluation. Myelography is done to investigate this protrusion or any other changes in the joint. CT and MRI can demonstrate the changes in the facet joint at any level of the spine. Discography has also been used in differentiating facet joint from the disc protrusion patients. Electromyographic techniques are useful in identifying sites of nerve root damage.

The recording of selective somatosensory evoked potentials have been useful in demonstrating sites of nerve lesions.

Treatment

Conservative measures such as local heat, fraction, non-steroidal inflammatory drugs, local myofascial trigger points, infection and local infection in paravertebral muscles.

Arthrography with local anaesthetic and steroid injections under fluoroscopy may be of benefit upto 1 year pain relief.[3] Because of possibility of subarachnoid and epidural injection, it is done under fluoroscopy.

Manual manipulation may be required to reduce subluxation.

The facet arthrography: Conventional X-ray have poor correlation with clinical symptoms. CT scan may better correlate with symptoms.

Facet arthropathy with injection of local anaesthetic and anti-inflammatory agent is a diagnostic procedure which is diagnostic as well as therapeutic procedure overlying infection of overlying tissues is a contraindication.

Radiographic Facet Injection

Facet joints can be approached from posterior approach. Patient is placed in prone position on the X-ray

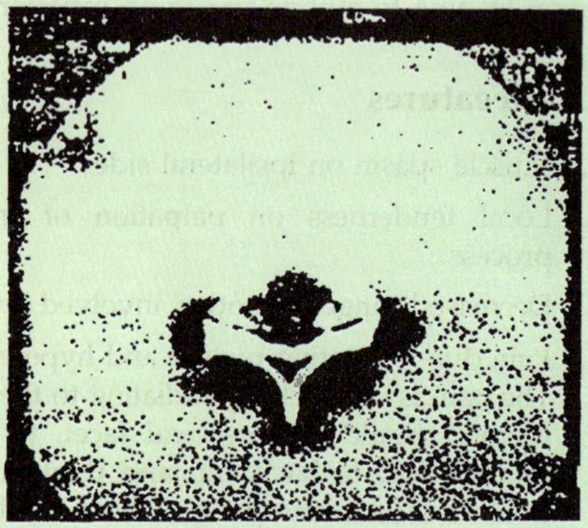

Fig. 59.1. (*a*) : Computed tomogram through the midcervical region showing the facet joints oriented in the coronal plane.

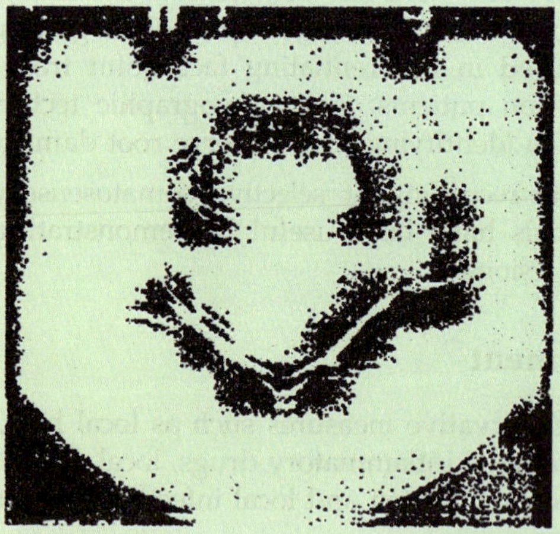

Fig. 59.1. (*b*) : Midthoracic CT

table. The symptomatic site is rotated while visualizing the facet joint under fluoroscopy to determine the obliquity. The best obliquity is 45° demonstrating anterior position of the joint. At L_5-S_1 posterior ilium should not be positioned above facet joint, observed under too obliquity.

After positioning the patient a wedge is placed beneath the abdomen, the hip and knee on the affected side are flexed, decreasing the lordosis. Skin is marked where the needles are to be inserted. A 22 SG spinal needle is directed vertically towards the facet joint and local anaesthetic 1.5 cc of 0.5% bupivacaine with 20 mg methyl prednisolone acetate or triamcinolone

The latter is now preferred to oil depot solutions of hydrocortisone and methyl prednisolone acetate for

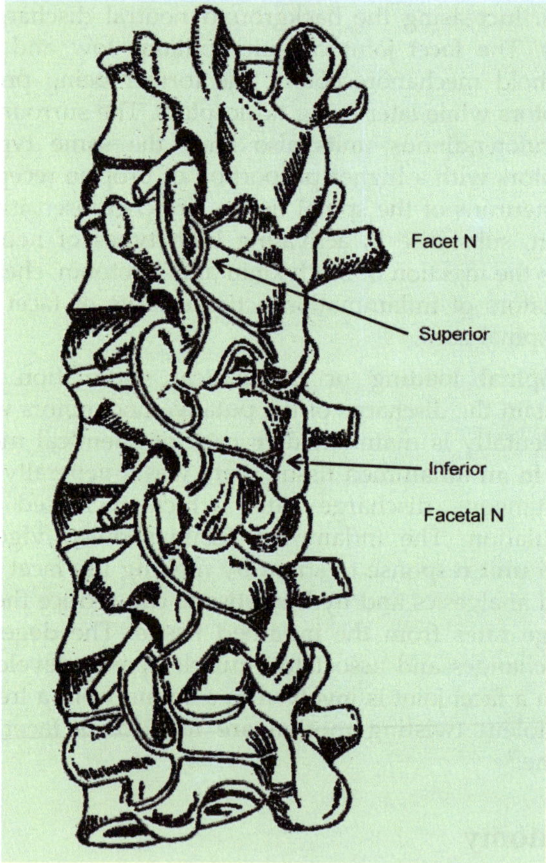

Fig. 59.2 : Each articular facet is innervated by inches from the posterior camus at the same level and the level above, resulting in a dual nerve supply.

the fear of irritation of nerve roots by oily solution. A puncture of joint capsule can be felt as it enters the capsule and then advanced into the facet joint and carefully aspirated and 1 cc of contrast media is injected. There is an immediate pain response relief following facet injection of local anaesthetic steroids. With a 30% relief upto 6 months, with 50–60% of immediate relief.

REFERENCES

1. Gharmley RK. Low back pain with special reference to the articular facets with presentation of an operative procedure. JAMA 1993;101:1773–1777.
2. Raj PP. Practical management of pain 2nd ed, St. Louis, Mosby year book 1992.
3. Carrera GF. Lumbar facet joint injection in low back pain and sciatica. Radiology 1980;137:665–667.

•••

FAILED BACK SURGERY SYNDROME

60

Failed back surgery syndrome (FBSS) refers specifically to persistent or recurrent chronic debilitating low back pain after one or more surgical procedures on lumbosacral spine, such as diskectomy, laminectomy and lumbosacral fusion.[1]

Failed back syndrome : Commonly refers to the same condition, although it more properly describes persistent back pain after unspecified treatment. Failed back, this term is commonly used to refer to both circumstances, but actually it implies functional **failure** of the back, as opposed to failure of treatment or surgery.

Incidence of FBSS : With Indian data on FBSS, being not available, it is to highlight that in US, where spine surgery exceed 300,000 operations per year, 10-40% of lumbar spine operations result in FBSS. In the context of more than 25% point prevalence and more than 80% lifetime incidence of low back pain in general population, the impact of this figures is of great concern.[2]

New invasive procedures such as percutaneous diskectomy and chemonucleolysis, while reducing some morbidity, have broaden the indications for treatment and thus added new categories of treatment failures.

Aetiology of FBSS

★ Inappropriate or premature selection of patients for surgery is a most common cause of FBSS.[3]

★ The second most common cause of FBSS is persistence of pain due to irreversible neural injury which can occur despite appropriate patient selection and successful performance of the surgery. It is always nice to tell the patient preoperatively, that main goal of surgery is to prevent further worsening rather than reverse existing damage.

★ Loss of primary afferent neurons (due to spinal cord compression by herniated disc) has been shown to be a risk factor for causing neuropathic pain after neuronal injuries. Several post injuries responses may be operative and this includes central sensitization, complex pharmacological changes and anatomic changes like sprouting of non-nociceptive mechanoreceptor neurons into nociceptive pathways within the substantia gelatinosa.[4]

★ Relative less common causes of FBSS is inadequate surgery like the persistence of unrecognized lateral recess stenosis or lateral disc herniation or a sequestered free disc fragment can be missed.

★ FBSS can also results from new pathologic process initiated by the primary surgeon. During spinal surgery, damage to nerves, dura, joints and muscles can produce pain. There have been reports of creation of segmental instability after generous laminectomy, pars fractures or pseudo-arthrosis after an inadequate fusion.[5]

★ FBSS can be result of extensive fusion or extensive instrumentation which tends to produce a loss of normal lumbar lordosis (Flat Back Syndrome), accelerates degenerative changes and leads to new pain problems.

★ Invasive diagnostic studies or fluoroscopic procedures can also occasionally causes chronic painful complications. This includes infection or arachnoiditis from procedures such as provocative discography, administration of epidural steroids and, myelography, which have been indicated in parts by the transition from oil based to water soluble contrast media.

Pseudo Failed Back Surgery Syndrome

Here the pain that accompanies axonal regeneration can be mistaken for FBSS pain. Axonal regeneration is usually associated with persistence or worsening of pain. This is due to accumulation of sensory.transductive molecules at the distal ends (growth cones) of the regenerating axons. The pain physician can identify how far regeneration has proceeded by tapping over the peripheral nerve until paresthesias are produced (Tinel's sign). The maximum rate of regeneration corresponds to the rate of fast anterograde axonal transport (approximately 1 mm per day) and thus this phase of recovery can last for months or more than a year. Hence this pain and paresthesia must be distinguished from FBSS pain, as in fact they are signs of recovery. They should not be considered an indication of worsening nor provoke reoperation.

Evaluation of Patient with FBSS

Because poor diagnostic evaluation, leading to inappropriate primary surgery is one of the common causes of FBSS, it is imperative that further diagnostic evaluation be correctly performed and interpreted despite the added complexity of diagnosis of FBSS patients. Hence FBSS patients should be referred to tertiary pain clinic centre specialized in dealing with difficult pain patients and equipped for specialized diagnostic testing. The progression of pain syndrome including pain free interval and effects of various treatments should be noted. Disease related to psychiatric problem should be clarified.

Physical Examination

This should include pertinent musculoskeletal neurologic, and tension signs, and also functional signs. It is essential to detect physical finding predictive of poor outcome, of a repeat surgical procedure. Abnormalities such as weakness or sensory loss that appears and disappears at various times, change location are suggestive of secondary gain or psychological problem and argue against repeat surgery.

Patchy "non-anatomic" sensory loss is common with lumbar arachnoiditis. Hyperalgesia after nerve injury can be present as superficial lumbosacral spine tenderness.

In patients with prior surgery, it can be difficult to distinguish among residual effects after successful treatment (for *e.g.*, persistent foot drop after nerve root compression), abnormalities remain untreated (*e.g.*, lateral recess stenosis) and iatrogenic problems. Deep tendon reflex, in particular, often remain abnormal despite adequate surgical decompression, with or without persistent pain, and so, although objective they have limited specificity.

Radiological Investigations

Myelography combines with CT in assessing cases for re operation.[3] In current practice CT has been largely supplemented by gadolinium-enhanced MRI. The association between pathological findings on MRI and clinical symptoms, however, is not always clear even when the identification of pathology is accurate, as confirmed by repeated surgery.

MRI avoids the possibility of subarachnoid contrast induced arachnoid fibrosis. MRI has limitation, however, in defining bony anatomy which often can be better visualized by plain X-ray and CT.

Ancillary Aids to Diagnosis

In FBSS patients, EMG is useful in differentiating acute and chronic muscle denervation. Nerve conduction studies can be helpful in assessing the location and severity of damage to nerve roots.

The small diameter axons conducting nociceptive impulses are better assessed in small punch skin biopsies which, when immuno labelled to permit visualization and counting of small nociceptive endings in the skin. Also in chronic back pain patients (and in FBSS), relief of pain and improvement of cognitive functions go hand in hand.

Psychological Testing

The standardized psychological testing has been helpful in identifying comorbidities requiring treatment, but in patients who were identified as candidates for a specific procedure, (*e.g.*, spinal cord stimulation) it explained a very small fraction of the variance in treatment outcome. Hence its prognostic value is limited, at least in patients carefully selected by other means.

Diagnostic Blocks

A series of nerve root blocks can be useful in the evaluation of FBSS patients with multi level anatomic abnormalities. By knowing which abnormalities are contributing to a patient's pain syndrome, surgery can be limited to those levels rather than undertaking a higher risk, multi level procedure.

Provocative Discography (PD)

The basic idea of performing PD is to determine whether mechanical loading of individual discs reproduces an individual patient's characteristic pain. Negative results of discography are helpful in avoiding further unnecessary surgery in FBSS patients. Overall, discography remains, in spite of 30 years use, a diagnostic study of uncertain reliability.

Management of FBSS Pain

FBSS can be a challenging, difficult and frustrating syndrome to treat. Most of these FBSS patients have had pain for a longer duration, have had multiple interventions, and often have financial and psychosocial difficulties and they travel for long distances which complicates the logistics of long-term follow-up. On top of this, many pain physicians avoid FBSS patients.[6]

Percutaneous Procedures under Image Intensifier

In FBSS patients, an increasing number of blocks are being performed under image intensifier. The commonest one is Facet (or Zygapophyseal) joint block. The facet joint form an articulation between the inferior articular process of the vertebra above and the superior articular process of the vertebra below. The joint is enclosed by a capsule and it is an under-appreciated cause of low back pain and of pain radiating to the buttocks or upper legs. Patients with pain of facet origin usually present with axial and proximal radicular type pain, worsened by lumbar extension and not associated with sciatic tension signs. Because these joints are innervated by terminal twigs of the medial branch of the posterior primary ramus, it is presumed that these "non-anatomic" sensations are due to convergence upon second order sensory neurons within the spinal cord. In FBSS patients, facet block determines that whether facet arthropathy is contributing to their low back pain.

Epidural Steroids in FBSS

In FBSS patients, it is true that optimal response to epidural steroids is achieved when the drug is placed in closest proximity to the pain source. The use of fluoroscopy in the management of FBSS patients is found to be most valuable not in locating the epidural space, but rather in verifying the inaccessibility of the target tissue.

Following epidural methyl prednisolone, improvement in cognitive functions and pain relief go hand in hand but the relief may last for only 3–9 months.

Physical Therapy / Acupuncture / Relaxation / Biofeedback

Acupuncture is effective, satisfactory results are achieved in 10–12 sittings, applied daily or on alternate days. Subsequently a combination of stretching and strengthening with endurance exercises and proper body mechanics speed up patient's return to work.

Relaxation techniques like meditation and hypnosis can also ease chronic pain. They appear to blunt body's sensitivity to pain. Following meditation, a decrease in the activity of right parietal lobe (on functional MRI) has been noticed after half an hour of meditation.

EMG biofeedback allows the patient to become aware of the degree of muscle contraction and the patient can then see, or here, the results of attempts to achieve muscle relaxation by thoughts of pleasant experiences or sensations.

Once the conservative approach fails, invasive procedures that can be followed, include:

★ **Surgical approach:** It is essential to realize that the favourable outcome after reoperation are less likely than for primary surgeries,[3] and the American Association of Neurological Surgeons has published criteria for patients' selection for lumbosacral spine surgery for FBSS patients as well as patients without prior surgery. They include the following:

1. Failure of an extended programme of conservative therapy.
2. An abnormal myelogram, CT, MRI showing nerve route or cauda equine compression and / or signs of segmental instability consistent with the patient's presenting symptoms and physical findings.
3. In patients with radicular pain, conformity to physiologic dermatomal patterns and one or more of the following:

Corresponding (*a*) segmental sensory loss, (*b*) motor loss in the appropriate segments or (*c*) abnormal deep tendon reflexes in appropriate segment(s).

Outcome of Repeated Surgery

Among decompression reoperations, repeat microdiskectomy has been successful and within one large reoperation series, previous diskectomy was a favourable prognostic factor.[3] Central or lateral recess stenosis might have been overlooked at the initial surgery.

Ablative Procedures

Ablative procedures have had a relatively poor outcome and significant morbidity in FBSS patients.

Spinal Cord Stimulation (SCS)

FBSS has been the most common indication for SCS; SCS is a reversible "neuro augmentive" technique that has been successful in a majority of FBSS patients, for upto 20 years. It compares favourably with reoperation as assessed retrospectively and also by a prospective, randomized study[7] and transcutaneous electric nerve stimulation (TENS) has been used to screen patients for implanted stimulation techniques. It uses external electrodes and follows the same rationale. Its prognostic value is limited, but it gives patients useful experience and it's itself therapy in some. Therefore, it is commonly prescribed before considering an implant.

Implantable, Programmable Drug Infusion System

The use of implanted pumps for subarachnoid infusion to deliver opiates intrathecally (and it is hoped to minimize systemic complications) has been reported in small number of patients with FBSS.

There are four choices of programmable infusion modes including continuous, complex-continuous, single bolus and periodic bolus, for therapeutic flexibility.

Other Neuro Augmentive Methods

FBSS is also one of the most common indications for implantation of chronic electrodes into various locations in the brain. In contrast to other augmentive procedures, this is one of the more invasive techniques and so it is usually used only when many other treatment options have failed.

Conclusion

FBSS presents a biggest challenge to the "**pain physician**" as well as the patients. Inappropriate primary surgery is the commonest cause. The majority of patients will not need reoperations and those who do will have a worse outcome. Thus the onus is on the "**pain physician**" to diagnose and treat these patients skillfully and with compassion, while acknowledging the limitation of conventional pain therapy and appreciating the genuine benefits of techniques like spinal cord stimulation which prove to be much more cost effective in the long run.

REFERENCES

1. Wilkinson HA. The failed back syndrome: etiology and therapy, 2nd edi.: Philadelphia, Harper and Row, 1991.
2. Wilkinson HA. The failed back syndrome: etiology and therapy. Philadelphia, Harper and Row,1983.
3. North RB, Campbell JN. Neuro surgery 1991; 28:685–691.
4. Woolf CJ. Hyperalgesia and allodynia. New York: Raven Press. 1992:221–243.
5. Kostuik JP. The adult spine. New York: Raven Press, 1991; 2027–2068.
6. American Association of Neurological Surgeons. AANS, 1989;17:957–960.
7. North RB, et al. Pain 1996-An Updated Review 1996;453–466.

•••

SECTION–X

Acute Pain in Medical Conditions

MUSCLE CONTRACTION HEADACHE AND ABDOMINAL MIGRAINE

61

Of the headache patients seen by either the family physician or the generalist, 80% suffer from muscle contraction or tension headaches. There are two types of muscle contraction, episodic and chronic.

A person suffering with episodic tension headaches will usually seek relief with over-the-counter analgesics, and consult a physician in the event that the headaches do not respond to simple analgesics or increase in frequency and severity and the patient is faced with diminished functioning in either an occupational or social setting. The pain specialist or neurologist will rarely treat an episodic tension headache, but will usually be confronted by the patient with chronic, daily, or almost daily, muscle contraction headache or the mixed headache syndrome.

Muscle contraction headache can manifest itself in relationship to stress, depression, anxiety, emotional conflicts, fatigue, repressed hostility, or by simply creating an environment too great to handle. Muscle contraction headaches can occur at any age but are usually present in adulthood, as life's frustrations become dominant. Friedman and his colleagues[1] reviewed 2000 cases of muscle contraction headaches, and noted that most of the patients were female. Only 40% reported family history of headaches in contrast to 70% of migraine sufferers. The majority of their subjects reported the onset of the headaches occurred between the age of 20 and 40 years. Daily pain was reported by many of the patients and 20% had persistent pain occurring at least four times weekly.

Muscle contraction headaches are generally described as bilateral steady, and a nonpulsatile ache. Other descriptions include "vicelike" pressure, drawing, soreness, bitemporal or occipital tightness, and bandlike sensations about the head, often termed as "hatband" effect. Patients may also complain of distinct cramping sensations, as if the neck and upper back were in a cast.

The site of the headache varies, frequently occurring in the forehead and temples, or at the back of the head and neck. The pain may be unilateral or bilateral, and involve the frontal, temporal, occipital, or parietal regions, or any combination of these sites. Other complaints include soreness and combing or brushing the hair or putting on a hat. Although this headache may undergo frequent changes in severity and site, the pain will usually localize in one region and may continue with varying intensity for weeks, months, or years. Sharply localized "nodules" may be administered when the tender areas of the neck, head, and upper back are palpated. During physical examination, pressure on contracted, tender muscles may increase the intensity of the headache.

A discussion of muscle contraction headaches would be incomplete without a review of the diagnosis and treatment of the mixed headache syndrome. The mixed headache patient usually presents to a neurologist or headache specialist. This type of headache is composed of the following symptomatology: (1) daily, continuous headache; (2) a "hard" or "sick" migrainous headache occurring 1 to 10 times monthly; and (3) easy susceptibility to habituation to over-the-counter or prescribed analgesics and/or ergotamine tartrate.

Mechanism of Muscle Contraction Headache

Emotional factors are of primary significance in provoking muscle contraction headaches. Chronic muscle contraction headaches may conceal a serious emotional disorder, such as depression. The patient will complain of a persistent and vague headache, for which no organic cause can be determined. For the patient, the physical symptoms of headache are more socially acceptable than the anxiety of depressive symptoms. Also, many patients must be cognizant of other signs of depression, such as early morning fatigue, irritability, loss of energy or spontaneity, lack of interest, insomnia, or early morning awakening.

The mechanism of this type of headache is similar to that of chronic muscle contraction in any other part of the body. Local pathologic processes and their central influences are related to muscle spasm. This involves three independent reflex arcs and four consecutive steps:

1. Muscle spasm is usually initiated by a multisynaptic reflex of withdrawal. The stimulation of nerve fibres is caused by a local pathologic process, with the impulse transmitted directly to

the spinal cord and then to the ventral roots. The stimulus then passes over the efferent nerves to the neuromuscular junction, that in turn causes the muscle to contract acutely and to spread the painful stimulus.

2. Via the polysynaptic spinal pathways and the lemniscal system, that are also stimulated, the initial impulse is conducted up the spinal cord to the thalamic and central levels. At these areas, the stimulus is perceived as painful.
3. At this point, the brain will transmit impulses through the reticulospinal system to activate the gamma-efferent neurons that contract the muscle spindle.
4. During the contraction of the muscle spindle, a monosynaptic stimulus is evoked, that travels directly to the ventral horn. The discharge in the efferent nerve is augmented and, more important, muscle contraction is augmented.

It should be noted that the contraction of the muscle spindle itself (the third reflex arc) is a monosynaptic pathway, related to the simple tendon stretch reflexes demonstrated in neurologic examination. Normally, the contracting muscle inhibits firing of the muscle spindle and terminates the third arc stretch reflex, thus providing relaxation of the muscle. The state of activity of the gamma motor system determines the degree of muscle tone. If cortical influences or local or systemic disease causes the gamma-efferent system to continue to fire, the muscle spindle will remain tight. The muscle continually contracts until the contraction itself becomes painful. The cycle of pain evolves as spasm, anxiety, and pain, or a muscle contraction headache.

Many modern researchers[2] have observed that chronic muscle contraction headache may not result from disorders of the blood vessels and muscles. Instead, the headaches may be affected by a chronic or intermittent disturbance of the monoaminergic, serotonergic, and endorphin systems of the central nervous system involving the hypothalamus, brain stem, and spinal cord. This occurrence may be due to referral or a central pain phenomenon from the intermingling of major circuits of the brain and spinal cord.

Depression and Chronic Muscle Contraction Headache

The depressed patient often presents with a wide variety of complaints that can be categorized as physical, emotional, and psychic.

Table 61.1 : Physical complaints

Complaints	Percentage of patients
Sleep disturbances	97
Early awakening	87
Headache	84
Dyspnea	76
Loss of weight	74
Trouble getting to sleep	73
Weakness and fatigue	70
Urinary frequency	70
"Spells"—dizziness	70
Appetite disturbances	70
Decreased libido	63
Cardiovascular disturbances	60
Sexual disturbances	60
Palpitations	59
Paresthesias	53
Nausea	48
Menstrual changes	41

Table 61.2 : Emotional complaints

Complaint	Percentage of patients
blue: low spirits; sadness	90
crying	80
feelings of guilt, hopelessness, unworthiness, unreality	65
anxiousness or irritability	65
anxiety	60
fear of insanity, physical disease, death, rumination past, present, future	50

Table 61.3 : Psychic complaints

Complaint	Percentage of patients
"morning is the worst time of day"	95
poor concentration	91
no interest, no ambition	75
indecisiveness	75
poor memory	71
suicidal thoughts, death wishes	35

A headache, secondary to depression, is usually attributed to muscle contraction. They are capricious, bizarre, and follow no definite pattern as to location, although the occipital portion of the skull is frequently affected. The duration is a distinguishing feature. A depressed person will describe his headache as lasting for years or throughout his life. The patient will also describe a headache that is usually dull and generalized, characteristically worse in the morning and evening. This diurnal variation is the most distinctive feature of the headache, thus facilitating a correct diagnosis of severe depression, although other symptoms have been inconspicuous.

Certain features of the headache may indicate an underlying depression. These headaches usually occur at regular intervals, consistent with daily life, such as occurring on weekends, holidays, on the first days of vacation, or after a stressful period, such as at the end of examinations. The greatest incidence of "nervous type" of headache occurs from 4:00 p.m. to 8:00 p.m. and from 4:00 a.m. to 8:00 a.m. these are usually the periods of the greatest and, sometimes, the most silent family crises.

These headaches may occur early in the morning, when the depressed patient awakens and fantasies of conflict with family members or at work are manifested. The depressed patient often relates the headaches as occurring when the patient leaves the relatively quiet atmosphere of the office for a weekend at home. These headaches often coincide with the interpersonal situations in which the sufferer feels compelled to appear comfortable, relaxed, and agreeable, while struggling to repress resentment toward someone they are expected to love and respect.

People with depressive illness may develop bodily symptoms, and conversely people with painful organic diseases tend to become depressed. It should be noted that too little attention is given to the depressive aspects of chronic pain and its treatment. The physical complaints dominate the situation so that the underlying depression tends to be overlooked.

Treatment of Muscle Contraction Headache

Episodic Muscle Contraction Headache

The headache is due to anxiety, stress, tension or pyschogenic determinants. As part of the medical history, a carefully detailed psychiatric inventory should be obtained. This should include details of the patient's marital relations, occupation, social relationships, life stresses, personality traits, habits, methods of coping with stressful situations, and sexual difficulties.

Chronic Muscle Contraction Headaches With and Without Depression

The success of antidepressant drugs in pain control results from their effects on the synthesis and metabolism of serotonin (5-hydroxytryptamine) and norepinephrine. It has been found that neurons containing serotonin and norepinephrine are part of the brain's analgesic system.[3,4] A descending serotonin pathway in the dorsal spine cord, originating in the raphe nucleus, and an interlacing of norepinephrine and opioid neurons in the locus ceruleus, are of particular interest to pain researchers.[3] Drugs that alter the synthesis or uptake of serotonin and/or norepinephrine, that includes virtually all antidepressant agents, would be expected to play a role in the brain's regulation of pain.

demethylated neuroleptic and thus carries a potential for extrapyramidal side effects, particularly with long-term use. Its effects are somewhat milder than those produced by tricyclics. In some patients, amoxapine may cause galactorrhea, seizures, and cardiac problems and has not been consistently effective.

Trazodone is a triazolopyradine derivative that selectively blocks serotonin uptake and has some alpha adrenergic profiles and very low and the most frequently reported adverse effect is drowsiness. Trazodone's antidepressant effect is comparable to that of the tricyclics. Its onset of action is relatively rapid.

Table 61.4 : Effects of tricyclic antidepressants[5]

Drug	Serotonin inhibition	Norepinephrine inhibition	Dopamine inhibition	Sedative effects	Anticholinergic effects
Amitriptyline	Moderate	Weak	Inactive	Strong	Strong
Desipramine	Weak	Potent	Inactive	Mild	Moderate
Doxepin	Moderate	Moderate	Inactive	Strong	Strong
Imipramine	Fairly potent	Moderate	Inactive	Moderate	Strong
Nortriptyline	Weak	Fairly potent	Inactive	Mild	Moderate
Protriptyline	Weak	Fairly potent	Inactive	None	Moderate

Tricyclic antidepressants are the drugs of choice in the treatment of muscle contraction headache. This group includes amitriptyline, imipramine, desipramine, nortriptyline, doxepin and protriptyline. The tricyclics are considered more effective in endogenous depression and less beneficial when the depressed patient has many accompanying neurotic traits. The choice of tricyclic is not simple because each drug has unique characteristics and shown in Table 61.4.

MAoxidase inhibitors (MAOIs) are generally considered the second line of drugs for depression, although not considered as efficacious as the tricyclics and known to have more drug interactions. A patient on an MAOI must follow a special diet and avoid foods with tyramine. The most frequently used MAOI is phenelzine sulphate (Nardil). These drugs block the oxidative deamination of numerous monoamines, including epinephrine, norepinephrine, serotonin and dopamine. According to the brain and other tissues, and the depression created by their deficiency is ameliorated or cured. Despite the precautions and fears with monoamine oxidase inhibitors, they are often found effective when the tricyclics fail.

Fluoxetine and zimelidine are bicyclic agents that have not been marketed in the United States. Their action is similar to amitriptyline. It is difficult to determine whether the relative capacity for inhibiting serotonin uptake is a major factors in their analgesic effect or that the majority of antidepressant drugs evaluated for analgesia are simply potent blockers of serotonin uptake.

Amoxapine, another new antidepressant, inhibits both serotonin and norepinephrine uptake and also blocks dopamine receptor activity. The agent is a

Several other new antidepressants are being tested and will become available over the next few years. When pain is the predominant presenting symptom of depression, and for those cases in which depression cannot be the definitive diagnosis and no organic cause for the pain, antidepressant therapy should be considered as the initial therapy.

Treatment of Mixed Headache Syndrome

If the mixed headache syndrome is presented, the physician should avoid the use of sedation, tranquilizers, habituating analgesics, and narcotics, in order to prevent addiction, which thereby perpetuates the problem. To prevent the rebound phenomenon, the use of ergotamine should be restricted to relief of the "hard" or "sick" headache, and never be prescribed on a daily basis.

The tricyclic antidepressants or the MAOIs are the drugs of choice in the prophylactic treatment of the mixed headache syndrome. For refractive cases, combination therapy with a tricyclic antidepressant and an MAOI may be indicated. However, this treatment should be cautiously selected with regard to individual patients and pharmaceutical agents. The cautious addition of propranolol (Inderal) in the long-acting form may be considered in daily doses of 80,120, and 160 mg. Occasionally, the addition of a nonsteroidal anti-inflammatory agent to the therapeutic regimen may be helpful.

The patient with the mixed headache syndrome may require a co-pharmacy approach with several agents. To ensure the successful treatment of chronic muscle contraction headaches, the mixed headache syndrome, the patient must receive continuity of care and habituating analgesics must be avoided.

Table 61.5 : Classification of headache according to the International Headache Society

A.	*Migraine*		
	1.1	Migraine without aura	
	1.2	Migraine with aura	
			Migraine with typical aura
			Migraine with prolonged aura
			Familial hemiplegic migraine
			Basilar migraine
			Migraine aura without headache
			Migraine with acute onset aura
	1.3	Ophthalmoplegic migraine	
	1.4	Retinal migraine	
	1.5	Childhood periodic syndromes that may be precursors to or associated with migraine	
	1.6	Complications of migraine	
			Status migrainosus
			Migrainous infarction
	1.7	Migrainous disorder not fulfilling above criteria	
B.	*Tension-type Headache*		
	2.1	Episodic tension-type headache	
			Episodic tension-type headache associated with disorder of pericranial muscles
			Episodic tension-type headache unassociated with disorder of pericranial muscles
	2.2	Chronic tension-type headache	
			Chronic tension-type headache associated with disorder of pericranial muscles
			Chronic tension-type headache unassociated with disorder of pericranial muscles
	2.3	Headache of the tension-type not fulfilling above criteria	
C.	*Cluster Headache and Chronic Paroxysmal Hemicrania*		
	3.1	Cluster headache	
			Cluster headache periodicity undetermined
			Episodic cluster headache
			Chronic cluster headache *e.g.,*
			Unremitting from onset
			Evolved from episode
	3.2	Chronic paroxysmal hemicrania	
	3.3	Cluster headache-like disorder not fulfilling above criteria	

Abdominal Migraine

Aetiology, symptoms and signs. Occurs in children and adults[6]. It is called as periodic syndrome of children, cyclic vomiting, recurrent abdominal pain and headache and navel colic, symptoms include attacks of paraumbilical pain, nausea, vomiting, headache, pallor, perspiration, bradycardia, fever, occasionally diarrhea and limb pains. Attacks last for 6 hours with a history of migraine in parents. Children having recurrent abdominal pain (crises) develop migraine during adult life.

Diagnosis and treatment: Bruyn[7] advised history, association of abdominal attacks with migraine, family history. Ergotamine reduces or even cause cessation of the attacks altogether. Exclusion of appendicitis, biliary colic, pancreatitis, lead intoxication should be excluded. The normal results of routine investigations, normal ECG. A presence of nausea, vomiting, perspiration, fever.

The headache associated with gastric infection is a common complaint in the general population. Patients having dyspepsia, bacterial or amoebic colitis similar to other pneumococcal, coliform infection in malabsorption syndrome, gastroenteritis.[8] The history of recurrent gastritis, constipation, faulty food and water, gaseous distension is the most common problem in India. The associated bacterial infection due to constipation or small intestine mucosal infection leads to gastric symptoms alongwith headache which at times is the presenting symptom in most of the patients. The analgesics like paracetamol have little effect while ibuprofen may be effective in some patients. Often these patients have a nervous disposition associated gastritis and may respond to carbamazepine. The headache reappears after the effect of analgesic is over, so an antibiotic like norfloxacin, metrogyl relieves gastrointestinal symptoms. This scenario is true for India with polluted drinking water and unhygienic food. The author has included history of gastrointestinal symptoms for all migrainous headaches. Majority of the cases in the present day setup clearly shows constipation and colon infection to be the most common cause of headache in general and can be successfully treated with ibuprofen and paracetamol combination, ranitidine and norfloxacin and laxatives. The absence of much literature on this headache leads to unsuccessful use of various drugs for migraine as advised in the textbooks of medicine. However, ayurvedic practitioners are more successful since they tend to treat constipation and poor digestion in majority of their patients. Even the widely used "churan" preparations claim treatment of headache along with constipation and dyspepsia.

REFERENCES

1. Friedman AP, Von Storch TJC, Merritt HH. Migraine and tension headaches. A clinical study: 2000 cases. Neurology, 1964; 4:773.
2. Lance JW, Lambert GA, Goadsby OJ, Duckworth JW. Brainstem influence on the cephalic circulation: experimental data from cat and monkey of relevance to the mechanism of migraine, headache, 1983; 23: 258–265.
3. Diamond S. Depression and headache, Headache, 1983; 23: 122–126.
4. Messing RB, Phebus L., Fisher LA, et al. Analgesic effect of fluoxetine HCl (Lilly 110140), a specific uptake inhibitor for serotonergic neurons, Psychopharmacol. Comm 1975; 1:511-521.
5. Diamond S. Nine experts review a FP's depression regimen. Patient Care. 1977; 11: 42–47.
6. Santoro G, Curzio M, Venco A. Abdominal migraine in adults. Funct. Neurol. 1990; 5:61–64.
7. Bruyn GW. Migraine equivalents. In handbook of clinical neurology. Rose PC (Ed) Vol 4 headaches. Amsterdam, Elsevier; 1986:158.
8. Davidson S, Macleod J. The principles and practice of medicine: A textbook for students and doctors. 10 Ed. Edinburg. Churchill-Livingstone; 1971.

FIBROMYALGIA AND MYOFACIAL PAIN SYNDROMES

62

Fibromyalgia (FM) is a multisymptomatic syndrome defined by the core feature of chronic wide spread pain.[1] Many FM patients also have severe fatigue and associated symptoms related to visceral hyperalgesia, such as irritable bowel and blader. This population accounts for about 20% of patients consulting rheumatologists in North America.[2] Contemporary research implicates abnormalities of sensory processing and neuroendocrine dysfunction as being related to the symptomatology of these patients.

Any tissue generated cause of pain (peripheral pain generators) can accentuate and /or perpetuate central pain mechanisms. Focal loci of muscle pain are referred to as myofascial trigger points. These are hyperalgesic zones in muscle that often feel indurated on palpation. Prolonged pressure over these areas may cause a pattern of pain that is referred distally, hence the name of "trigger points".

Central Pain Mechanisms in Fibromyalgia

Patients with severe FM have clinical features commonly observed in states of central sensitization, namely a reduced pain threshold (allodynia), an increased response of painful stimuli (hyperalgesia), and an increase in the duration of pain after nociceptors stimulation (persistent pain). In 1965 Mendell and colleagues noted that repetitious stimulation of a peripheral nerve at sufficient intensity to activate C fibres caused a progressive build-up in amplitude of the electrical response recorded in the corresponding dorsal horn neurons of the spinal cord.[3] Interestingly, this phenomenon was more marked when muscle nerves were stimulated than when skin nerves were stimulated, which is in keeping with the notion that muscle pain may be a potent, but nonspecific, peripheral generator. The authors termed this phenomenon "wind-up". It is now appreciated that wind-up is crucial to understanding central sensitization. Furthermore, the biochemical basis for this neuro physiological phenomenon is now being unravelled at a molecular level in terms of the activation of N-methyl-D-aspartate (NMDA) receptors. Good evidence indicates that central sensitization is relevant to the pain experience in FM patients.[4]

Deficient Pain Modulation in Response to Repeated Thermal Stimuli

An up regulation of pain threshold can be demonstrated in normal individuals subjected repeated non-noxious skin stimulation. This finding is the basis for the use of transcutaneous nerve stimulators (TENS) to manage chronic pain states. The physiological basis for this effect is the inhibitions of dorsal horn neuron excitability by persistent stimulation of type-A myelinated axons. This effect known as diffuse noxious inhibitory control, is defective in FM subjects, thus supporting the notion that they have a defective descending inhibitory pain system.[5]

Hyper Responsive Somatosensory Induced Potentials

Somatosensory induced potentials refer to the electrophysiological activity in the brain that can be measured by skull electrodes in response to peripheral sensory stimulation. Gibson et al. (1994)[6] reported an increased late nociceptive somatosensory response evoked by CO_2 laser stimulation of the skin in 10 FM patients compared to 10 matched controls. Lorenz et al. (1996), reported increased amplitude of the N170 and P390 brain somatosensory potentials in FM patients compared to controls evoked by laser stimulation of the skin. Furthermore, they observed a response in both hemispheres, whereas in controls, the response was localized to one side of the brain. These two studies provide objective evidence that FM patients have an altered processing of nociceptive stimuli in comparison to pain-free controls.[7]

Secondary Hyperalgesia on Electrocutaneous Stimulation

Primary hyperalgesia is the normal perception of pain from nociceptors stimulation in an injured tissue. Secondary hyperalgesia refers to pain elicited from uninjured tissues. Arroyo and colleagues (1993), while attempting to treat FM patients with electrical nerve stimulation, reported sensory phenomena characteristic of secondary hyperalgesia[8].

Abnormalities on SPECT imaging

Pain-induced changes in brain blood flow or metabolism can now be visualized by several different imaging techniques. Reports describe reduced thalamic blood flow in FM subjects.[9] It is interesting that chronic pain states have been associated with reduced thalamic blood flow, whereas acute pain increases it. The reason for this difference is postulated to be a disinhibition of the medial thalamus, which results in activation of a limbic network.[10]

Elevated Levels of Substance-P in the CSF

Substance-P is an important nociceptive neurotransmitter. Studies have shown a threefold increase of substance-P in the CSF of FM patients compared to controls.[11] Animal models of hyperalgesia and hypoalgesia have implicated substance-P as a major aetiological factor in central sensitization and have highlighted its relevance in human pain states.[12]

intravenous ketamine (an NMDA-receptor antagonist) attenuates pain and increase pain threshold, as well as improving muscle endurance, in FM patients.[14]

Clinical Features

- ★ **Pain:** The core symptom of FM syndrome is chronic widespread pain. The pain is usually perceived as arising from muscle, although many FM patients also report joint pain.[15] Stiffness, worse in the early morning, is a prominent symptom of most FM patients; along with the perception of articular pain, this may reinforce the impression of an arthritic condition.
- ★ **Fatigue:** Easy fatiguability from physical exertion, mental exertion, and psychological stressors is typical of FM. The aetiology of fatigue in FM is multifaceted and is thought to include non-restorative sleep, deconditioning, dysautonomia, depression, poor coping mechanisms, and secondary endocrine dysfunction involving the hypothalamic-pituitary-adrenal axis and growth hormone deficiency[16].
- ★ **Disordered sleep:** Fibromyalgia patients usually report disturbed sleep. Even if they sleep continuously for 8-10 hours they awake feeling tired; this is referred to as nonrestorative sleep and is fully described below in the section "sleep".
- ★ **Cognitive problems:** Cognitive dysfunction is a major problem, according to self-reports, for many FM patients. Patients commonly describe difficulties with short-term memory, concentration, logical analysis and motivation as described in "cognitive dysfunction" below.[17]

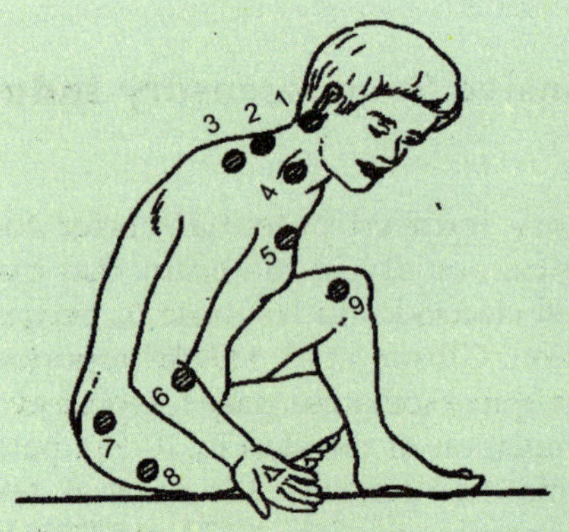

Tender points of fibromyalgia:
1. Insertion of nuchal muscles into occiput;
2. upper border of trapezius-mild-portion;
3. muscle attachments to upper medial border of scapula;
4. anterior aspects of the C5, C7 intertransverse spaces;
5. 2nd rib space – about 3 cm lateral to the sternal border;
6. muscle attachments to lateral epicondyle;
7. upper outer quadrant of gluteal muscles;
8. muscle attachments just posterior to greater trochanter;
9. medial fat pad of knee proximal to joint line.

Fig. 62.1 : A total of eleven or more tender points in conjunction with a history of widespread pain is characteristic of the fibromyalgia syndrome

Elevated Levels of Nerve Growth Factor

Nerve growth factor (NGF) is required for the normal development of sympathetic and sensory neurons. The intravenous administration of recombinant NGF in humans results in a muscle pain syndrome resembling FM that lasts for up to a week after the initial injection. The mechanism whereby NGF causes hyperalgesia may be related to its stimulation of protein synthesis in the central nervous system (CNS).[13]

Beneficial Response to an NMDA Receptor Antagonist

The excitatory amino acid glutamine reacting with NMDA receptors plays a central role in the generation of non-nociceptive pain. Studies have reported that

- ★ **Associated disorders:** It is not unusual for FM patients to have an array of somatic complaints other than musculoskeletal pain.[18] It is now thought that these symptoms are in part a result of the abnormal sensory processing as well as the neuroendocrine effects of chronic stress.
- ★ **Psychological distress:** As in many chronic conditions, the prevalence of psychological diagnoses is increased in FM patients. Depression is more common in FM patients than in healthy controls.[2] Importantly FM is not common in patients with major depression; even depressed individuals who complain of pain do not have multiple tender points. Although psychiatric disorders are more prevalent in FM patients than in FM nonpatients, they do not seem to be intrinsically related to the patho-physiology of the FM syndrome, but rather appear to depend on symptom severity.[19]
- ★ **Prognosis and impact:** Fibromyalgia symptomatology often persist over many years. Chronic musculoskeletal pain often severely affects a patient's quality of life. An analysis of 1604 FM patients followed in academic centres reported that pain, fatigue, sleep disturbance, functional status, anxiety, depression, and health status were essentially unchanged after 7 years of follow-up. The consequences of pain and fatiguability influence motor performance; everyday activities take longer in FM patients, they need more time to get started in the morning, and they often require extra rest periods during the day. They have difficulty with repetitive sustained motor tasks, unless frequent time-outs are taken. Tasks may be well tolerated for short periods of time, but when carried out for prolonged periods they become aggravating factors. Prolonged muscular activity, especially under stress or in uncomfortable climatic conditions, worsens the symptoms of FM.[21] The adaptation that FM patients have to make in order to minimize their pain experience often have a negative impact on both vocational and avocational activities.

Management

A structured multidisciplinary approach to managing FM patients requires an appreciation of the parts that make up the whole. One cannot successfully manage FM patients if one treats the diagnosis of FM as a unified entity. Twelve separate management issues usually require attention in most FM patients seeking medical help:

1. diagnosis and evaluation
2. education
3. pain
4. fatigue
5. sleep
6. psychological disorders
7. endocrine dysfunction
8. dysautonomia
9. deconditioning
10. cognitive dysfunction
11. the existential crisis
12. associated syndromes.

Diagnosis and Evaluation: The diagnosis of FM is usually based on the 1990 American College of Rheumatology (ACR) classification criteria.[22] First; these patients have widespread body pain-defined as pain in at least three quadrants of the body that has persisted for at least 3 months. Patients describe their pain in different ways, but commonly they use adjectives such as aching, stabbing, knife-like, or lancinating. There is usually an associated feeling of stiffness in the muscles and an increase in pain after exertion. These symptoms are seldom found in any other medical condition, with the exception of polymyalgia rheumatica in elderly patients, severe hypothyroidism, and widespread bone pain due to neoplasia or osteomalacia. Other pain states, such as widespread arthritis have symptoms predominantly referred to joints. Most primary muscle diseases, such as the muscular dystrophies and polymyositis, have weakness, not pain, as the predominant symptom. Having the patient fill out a pain diagram is simple and effective way of screening for a history of widespread pain.

The second step in making a diagnosis of FM is to systematically palpate the muscles for "tender points". This is done with a pressure of about 4 kg – enough to blanch a thumbnail. In general, tender points are located toward one end of a muscle where it is narrowing to join a tendon or bone. For instance, common tender point locations are the insertion of the extensor muscles of the hand at the lateral epicondyles of the elbow, the insertion of the nuchal muscles into the occiput, the origin of the gluteus medius muscle from the pelvic brim, and its insertion into the greater trochanter. The ACR criteria recommend palpation of nine paired tender-point areas (18 points in all)(Fig. 62.1). A diagnosis of FM demands the finding of 11 or more tender points. However, it is increasingly evident that many patients with widespread pain have fewer than the recommended 11 out of 18 tender points. If patients have widespread pain and tenderness in many other areas, they are unlikely to have a different neurophysiological basis for their pain than patients with strictly ACR-defined FM. Thus it is important to look at other sites that commonly harbour myofascial trigger points. The reason for this more extensive evaluation is two fold: (1) to establish a probable diagnosis of FM in patients with fewer than 11 tender points, and (2) to find relevant myofascial pain generators that would benefit from trigger point therapy.

Fibromyalgia is not a diagnosis of exclusion, and thus laboratory tests and imaging studies play no role in establishing the diagnosis according to the 1990 ACR criteria. However, FM patients may have concomitant conditions that are relevant to overall management in terms of peripheral pain generators that can accentuate and maintain central sensitization. In many cases these concomitant problems require an investigational approach to diagnosis. An FM-focused history and examination are an important requisite in obtaining data for an effective management programme. The history and examination will probably suggest certain problems that need further evaluation in terms of specialist referral or investigations.

Pain: Opioids are effective in most acute and chronic pain states. Although opioids are fairly commonly used in the treatment of FM, there have been no controlled clinical trials.

Tramadol is proving to be a useful drug to treat pain in chronic conditions, including FM. Tramadol has a dual mechanism of action, being a weak opioid agonist as well as inhibiting the re-uptake of serotonin and norepinephrine at the level of the dorsal horn. A double-blinded study demonstrated its efficacy and tolerability in the management of FM pain at an average dose of 200 mg/day.[23]

Antagonists of the serotonin 5-HT_3 receptor have been the subject of several encouraging short-term trials in FM patients.[24] These receptors are found only in neuronal tissues, both central and peripheral. The complex biochemistry of 5-HT_3 receptors suggests that antagonists would have nociceptive and antinociceptive actions under different circumstances.

Fatigue: Recent studies using the 5-HT_3 receptor antagonist tropisetron reported benefits both in FM-related fatigue and in chronic fatigue syndrome.[25]

Sleep: Important non-pharmacological aspect of sleep management includes ensuring an adherence to the basic rules of sleep hygiene and regular low-grade exercise. The use of low dose tricyclic antidepressants has been the main stay of sleep pharmacotherapy in FM patients.[26] Many FM patients cannot tolerate tricyclic antidepressants due to unacceptable levels of daytime drowsiness or weight gain. In these patients benzodiazepine-like medications such as alprazolam was beneficial. A subset of FM patients suffers from a primary sleep disorder, which requires specialized management. About 25% of male and 15% of female FM patients have sleep apnea, which usually requires treatment with positive airway pressure or surgery. By far the commonest sleep disorder in FM patients is restless leg syndrome/periodic limb movement disorder.

Psychological distress: Psychological intervention in terms of improving the internal locus of control and more effective problem solving is important in such patients. Techniques of cognitive-behavioural therapy seem particularly well suited to effect positive changes and may be enhanced when introduced as a part of group therapy.[26]

Dysautonomia: Abnormalities of autonomic function appear to be associated with both FM and chronic fatigue syndrome. These patients have an exaggerated increase in their heart rate, rather than a pronounced fall in blood pressure, in response to standing and exercise.[26] Treatment involves education as to the triggering factors and their avoidance, increasing plasma volume (increased salt intake, prescription of fludrocortisone), avoidance of drugs that aggravate hypotension (*e.g.*, tricyclic antidepressants, antihypertensive), preventing the ventricle-baroreceptor reflex (alpha-adrenergic antagonists or disopyramide) and minimizing the efferent limb of the baroreceptor reflex (alpha-adrenergic agonists or anticholinergic agents).

Deconditioning: Most FM patients are aerobically unfit, with suboptimal strength and poor flexibility. The notion that exercise is good for FM patients is an accepted contemporary truth. Acute exercise is associated with reduced pain perception and a lowered pain threshold. Although endorphins are secreted in response to acute exercise, they probably are not the sole mechanism of exercise induced analgesia. During graded exercise, endorphins only start to increase at the anaerobic threshold (*i.e.*, lactate production), and in moderate steady-state exercise they do not increase until exercise duration exceeds one hour.[27] The benefits of exercise are based on reasonable scientific evidence, but exercise may also be deleterious.[28] Whether it is good or bad for FM patients probably depends upon many variables, such as age, current level of conditioning, rate of increase of exercise intensity, frequency of exercise, ratio of eccentric to concentric muscle use, hormonal anabolic status, and negative factors such as obesity, arthritis and concomitant muscle disease.

Cognitive dysfunction: Cognitive dysfunction is a major problem, according to self-reports, for many FM patients. Patients commonly describe difficulties with short-term memory, concentration, logical analysis and motivation. Problems with cognitive function are being increasingly recognized in FM patients and are the subject of increasing research efforts. Currently, defects have been described in terms of working memory, episodic memory, and verbal fluency. These decreases in cognitive performance have been estimated to be equivalent to 20 years of ageing.[29]

Associated disorders: Recognition and treatment of problems that are commonly associated with FM are important in the overall management scheme.

1. **Restless leg syndrome:** Treatment is simple and very effective : carbidopa / levodopa in an early evening dose of 10/100 mg or clonazepam

(0.5 mg or 1.0 mg at bedtime). More recently other dopamine agonists such as pergolide, ropinirole, and pramipexole have been proven effective[30]. Some patients respond to gabapentin. Recalcitrant cases are often helped by low-dose opioid therapy.

2. **Irritable bowel syndrome:** Treatment involves (*a*) eliminating foods that aggravate symptoms; (*b*) minimizing psychological distress; (*c*) adhering to basic rules for maintaining a regular bowel habit; and (*d*) prescribing medications for specific symptoms such as constipation (stool softener, fibre supplementation, and gentle laxatives such as bisacodyl), diarrhoea (loperamide or diphenoxylate), and antispasmodics (dicyclomine or anticholinergic/sedative preparations).
3. **Irritable bladder syndrome:** Treatment involves (a) increasing intake of water, (b) avoiding bladder irritants such as fruit juices (especially cranberry), (c) pelvic floor exercises (*e.g.*, Kegel exercises), (d) antispasmodic medications (*e.g.*, oxybutynin, flavoxate, or hyoscyamine).
4. **Cold intolerance:** Treatment involves (a) keeping warm, (b) low-grade aerobic exercise (which improves peripheral circulation), (c) treatment of neurally mediated hypotension, (d) the prescription of vasodilators, such as the calcium channel blockers.
5. **Multiple sensitivities:** Treatment involves being aware that sensitivity to medications is an FM-related problem and employing avoidance tactics. Medications often need to be started at half the usual doses.
6. **Dizziness:** Treatable causes related to FM include (*a*) proprioceptive dysfunction secondary to muscle deconditioning, (*b*) proprioceptive dysfunction secondary to myofascial trigger points in the sternocleidomastoid and other neck muscles, (*c*) neurally mediated hypotension, and (*d*) medication side effects. Treatment is dependent on making an accurate diagnosis.

Myofascial Pain Syndromes

It is one of the most common types of neck pain in the pain clinic. It is necessary to rule out radioculopathy, disc disease, malignancies of the vertebrae and visceral referred pain before reaching out to make a diagnosis of myofascial pain syndrome. Myofascial syndromes are characterized by presence of trigger point.[31]

Clinical Features

There is a history of prolonged sitting posture in reading and writing. The use of an improper pillow or bed, sleeping in lateral position and accidental rupture (microtrauma) of muscle fibres during exercises or sports may lead later to a chronic pain referred to the other areas. Apart from movement of the patients.

The trigger points have been described to be located in the body, in the sternomastoid muscle (pain in the face behind the eye and the neck), in the splenius capitis muscle (pain in the top of the head, subocciput, upper part of the neck), levator scapulae muscle (neck, shoulder) and posterior cervical trigger point region (over the trapezius muscle). There are other trigger points in other areas (Figs. 62.2, 63.3 A and B). It is important to know the location of fairly constant trigger points in the individual muscles. With experience it is very easy to locate these points and feel the subtle changes such as nodules, knots or bands in the involved muscle. If injection of local anaesthetic relieves the pain, confirmation of diagnosis is made.

Aetiopathology

There is a fracture to myofascial structures and acute overload of muscles. After injury small and hypersensitive regions develop in the muscles and connective tissues. They are known as trigger points. Impulses from these points arise and bombard the central nervous system. There is a nerve injury/neuropathy which responds with hyperactivity or supersensitivity of the normal function.[32]

The muscle fibres hosting the tender point are contracted for a long time and fatigue develops, local ischaemia leads to release of histamine, kinin, bradykinins and prostaglandins,[33] leading to increase in motor and sympathetic activity and pain with TP as a focus of distress signals to CNS. The painful event later sustains itself. (Fig. 62.1).

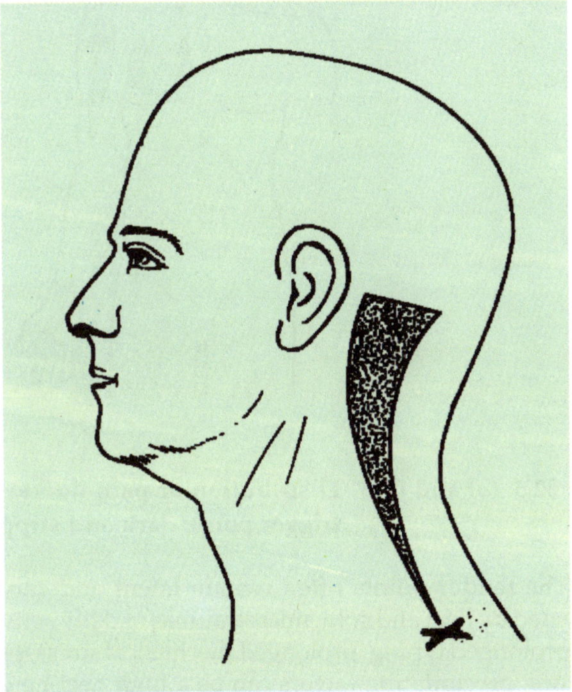

Fig. 62.2 : Distribution of pain due to myofascial pain affecting the trapezius muscle. X indicates trigger point; shaded and stippled areas indicate radiation of pain

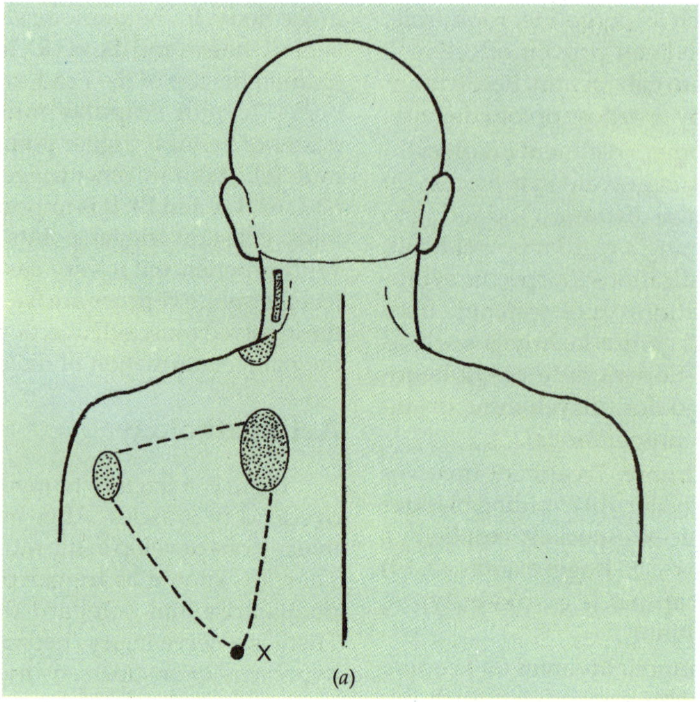

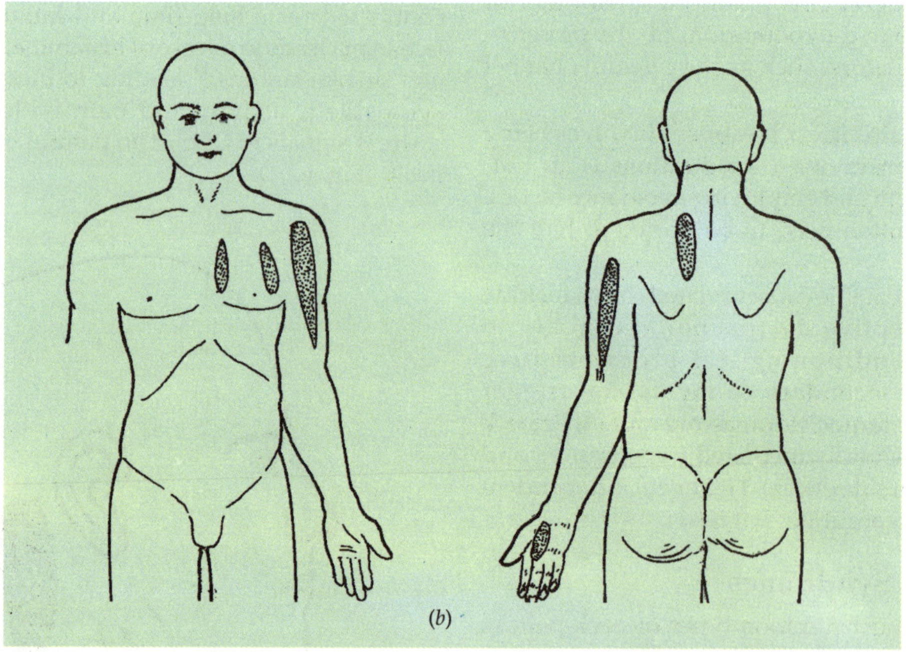

Fig. 62.3. (*a*) and (*b*) : Distribution of pain due to myofascial pain affecting the leavator scapulae. X indicates trigger point; dark and stippled areas indicate radiation of pain

The tender points often remain latent and can be activated by heat and cold, microtraumas of daily activity *e.g.*, prolonged typing, prolonged mechanical stress, poor posture, precipitating factors can be a high heel height, too low table for working, highly polished floors.

Management

Injection and stretching of muscles is the effective treatment. The muscle is injected with a local anesthetic/ saline and steroid. It is important to reproduce patient's pain by injecting right into the band or nodule. Lignocaine 1%, 5 mL alone or with other local anesthetics *e.g.*, bupivacaine 0.5% or etidocaine can be used along with hydrocortisone acetate (150 mg) methyl prednisolone depot 40–80 mg, after the injection, patient is advised to keep the muscle in a relaxed state for 4 days by avoiding driving, and strain on neck muscles. Application of heat over involved area, ultrasound and interferential current for 15 minutes, followed by exercises after 4 days, is very useful. Many patients develop recurrent spasm during stress and need relaxation therapy, antispasmodics and analgesics.

REFERENCES

1. Yunus MB. Psychological aspects of fibromyalgia syndrome: a component of the dysfunctional spectrum syndrome. Baillieres Clin Rheumatol 1994; 8:811–837.
2. White KP, Speechley M, Harth M, Ostbye T. Fibromyalgia in rheumatology practice: a survey of Canadian rheumatologists. J Rheumatol 1995;22:722–726.
3. Mendell LM, Wall PD. Response of single dorsal cord cell to peripheral cutaneous unmyelinated fibers. Nature 1965;206:97–99.
4. Bennett RM. Emerging concepts in the neurobiology of chronic pain: evidence of abnormal sensory processing in fibromyalgia. Mayo Clin Proc 1999;74:385–398.
5. Mense S. Neurobiological concepts of fibromyalgia- the possible role of descending spinal tracts. Scand J Rheumatol Suppl 2000;113:24–29.
6. Gibson SJ, Littlejohn GO, Gorman MM, Helme RD, Granges G. Altered heat pain threshold and cerebral event-related potentials following painful CO_2 laser stimulation in subjects with fibromyalgia syndrome. Pain 1994;58:185–193.
7. Lorenze J, Grasedyck K, Bromm B. Middle and long latency somato sensory evoked potentials after painful laser stimulation in patients with fibromyalgia syndrome. Electoencephalogr Clin Neurophysiol 1996;100:165–168.
8. Arroyo JF, Cohen ML. Abnormal responses to electro cutaneous stimulation in fibromyalgia. J Rheumatol 1993;20:1925–1931.1.
9. Kwiatek R, Branden L, Tedman R, et al. Regional cerebral blood flow in fibromyalgia: SPECT evidence of reduction in the pontine tegmentum and thalami. Arthritis Rheum 2000;43:2823–2833.
10. Craig AD. A new version of the thalamic disinhibition hypothesis of central pain. Pain Forum 1998;7:1–14.
11. Liu Z, Welin M, Bragee B, Nyberg F. A high recovery extraction procedure for quantitative analysis of substance P and opioid peptides in human CSF. Peptides 2000;21:853–860.
12. Abbadie C, Brown JL, Mantyh PW, Basbaum AI. Spinal cord substance P receptor immunoreactivity increase in both inflammatory and nerve injury models of persistent pain. Neuroscience 1996;70:201–209.
13. Bennett DL. Neurotrophic factors: important regulators of nociceptive function. Neuroscientist 2001;7:13–17.
14. Sorenson J, Graven-Nielsen T, Henriksson KG, Bengtsson M, Arendt-Nielsen L. Hyper excitability in fibromyalgia. J Rheumatol 1998;25:152–155.
15. Reilly PA, Littlejohn GO. Peripheral arthralgic presentation of fibrositis/fibromyalgia syndrome. J Rheumatol 1992;19:281–283.
16. Pillemer SR, Bradley LA, Crofford LJ, Moldofsky H, Chrousos GP. The neuroscience and endocrinology of fibromyalgia. Arthritis Rheum 1997;40:1928–1939.
17. Park DC, Glass JM, Minear M, Crofford LJ. Cognitive function in fibromyalgia patients. Arthritis Rheum 2001; 44:2125–2133.
18. Clauw DJ. Fibromyalgia: more than just a musculoskeletal disease. Am Fam Physicians 1995;52:843–851, 853–853.
19. Aaron LA, Bradley LA, Alarcon GS, et al. Psychiatric diagnoses in patients with fibromyalgia is related to health care seeking behavior rather than to illness. Arthritis Rheum 1996;39:436-445.
20. Wolfe F, Anderson J, Harkness D, et al. Health status and disease severity in fibromyalgia: results of six center longitudinal study. Arthritis Rheum 1997; 40:1571–1579.
21. Waylonis GW, Ronan PG, Gordon C. A profile of fibromyalgia in occupational environments. Am J Phys Med Rehabil 1994;73:112–115.
22. Wolfe F, Smythe HA, Yunus MB, et al. The American College of Rheumatology 1990 criteria for the classification of fibromyalgia: report of the multicenter criteria committee. Arthritis rheum 1990;33:160–172.
23. Russell IJ, Kamin M, Sager D, et al. Efficacy of Ultram™(Tramadol HCl) treatment of fibromyalgia syndrome: preliminary analysis of a multi center randomized, placebo controlled study. Arthritis Rheum 1997;40:S214.

24. Farber L, Startz T, Bruckle W, et al. Efficacy and tolerability of tropisetron in primary fibromyalgia – a highly selective and competitive 5-H_3T_3 receptor antagonist. German Fibromyalgia Study Group. Scnd J Rheumatol Suppl 2000;113:49–54.

25. Spath M, Welzed D, Farber L. Treatment of chronic fatigue syndrome with 5-HT_3 receptor antagonists-preliminary results. Scand J Rheumatol suppl 2000; 113:72–77.

26. Sandroni P, Opfer-Gehrking TL, McPhee BR, Low PA. Postural tachycardia syndrome : clinical features and follow up study. Mayo Clin Proc 1999;74(11): 1106–1110.

27. Schwartz L, Kindermann W. Changes in beta-endorphin levels in response to aerobic and anaerobic exercise. Sports Med 1992;13:25–36.

28. Mengshoel AM, Vollestad NK, Forre O. Pain and farigue induced by exercise in fibromyalgia patients and sedentary healthy subjects. Clin Exp Rheumatol 1995;13:477–482.

29. Glass JM, Park DC. Cognitive dysfunction in fibromyalgia. Curr Rheumatol Rep 2001;3:123;127.

30. Montplaisir J, Nicolas A, Denesle R, Gomez-Mancilla B. Restless legs syndrome improved by pramipexole: a double blind randomized trial. Neurology 1999:52:938–943.

31. Sola AE, Bonica JJ., Myofascial pain syndromes. In Bonica's management of pain. Loeser J. (ed) Philadelphia, Lippincott-Williams and Wilkins, 2001;530–542.

32. Cannon WB, Rosenblueth A. A supersensitivity of denervated structures. New York: Macmillian, 1949.

33. Zimmerman M. Peripheral and central nervous mechanisms of nociception, pain and pain therapy: facts and hypotheses. In: Bonica JJ, Liebeskind JC, Albe-Fessard DC, (eds) advances in pain research and therapy. Vol 3, New York, Raven press, 1979:3–32.

•••

RHEUMATOID ARTHRITIS

63

The WHO classifies common rheumatic complaints under four headings including inflammatory arthropathies, osteoarthritis and related disorders, regional periarticular or soft tissue disorders, and back pain. A more detailed classification is given below.

Classification of the Rheumatic Diseases

1. Immune based joint diseases: Rheumatoid arthritis, juvenile chronic arthritis, spondylarthritis (includes ankylosing spondylitis, reactive, psoriatic and enteropathic arthritis.
2. Connective tissue disorders: SLE, scleroderma, polymyositis, polyarteritis nodosa, Chug Strauss syndrome, Wagener's granulomatosis, Giant cell arteritis, Takayasu's disease.
3. Infectious arthritis: Bacterial, viral, fungal
4. Crystal deposition diseases: Gout, chondrocalcinosis.
5. Osteo arthritis
6. Soft tissue rheumatism: Tendonitis, capsulitis, enteritis, bursitis, fasciitis.
7. Disorder of bone: Osteoporosis, osteomalacia, Paget's disease.
8. Miscellaneous: Bechet syndrome, Whipple's disease, fibromyalgia syndrome.

Irrespective of the diagnosis, pain remains the most disabling feature of musculoskeletal disease. This chapter aims to provide the non-specialist with the overview of the clinical feature of the rheumatoid arthritis, a description of the neurobiological mechanisms underlying rheumatic pain and evidence based discussion of the current therapeutic strategies for the disorder.

Rheumatoid Arthritis

Rheumatoid arthritis is a chronic systemic inflammatory disease of unknown aetiology. Population studies suggest that 1 in 2000 adults will develop the disorder each year. Rheumatoid arthritis has an overall prevalence of 0.5–1.5% and affects more women than men in a ratio of 2.5:1. It can occur at any age but is most common between the ages of 40 and 70 years.[1] The disorder can present in many ways but the onset is usually insidious with a symmetrical polyarthritis affecting the small joints of the hands and feet. In rare cases it present as a mono arthritis in which case infection or crystal arthritis must be excluded. In elderly patients the onset of the disease may be indistinguishable from polymyalgia rheumatica, a relatively rare condition characterized by myalgia, morning stiffness and a mostly transient arthritis lasting a few hours to days. Classification criteria have been proposed (Table 63.1) and are now widely used in both research and clinical practice.[2]

Clinical Features

The cardinal features are pain and swelling involving many joints. Other symptoms and signs of inflammation include warmth, erythema and loss of function. The pain is usually more prominent and more persistent than in osteoarthritis, occurring at rest, at night, and on activity. Synovial fluid may accumulate causing an effusion.

Table 63.1 : Summary of 1998 revised American Rheumatism Association Criteria for classification of rheumatoid arthritis

1.	Morning stiffness more than 6 weeks.
2.	Arthritis of 3 or more joint areas for more than 6 weeks.
3.	Arthritis of hand joints more than 6 weeks.
4.	Symmetric arthritis more than 6 weeks.
5.	Rheumatoid nodules.
6.	Positive rheumatoid factor.
7.	Radiographic changes.

Uncontrolled disease eventually results in inflammation spreading beyond joint to other nearby structures including the tenosynovium of tendons, ligaments, other soft tissue structures and bone. Extra articular features are common and may involve multiple organ systems.[3]

Pathophysiology

Family studies demonstrate a modest genetic predisposition to the development of rheumatoid arthritis with the concordance rate for mono zygotic twins being in the order of 12–15 % and the rate for dizygotic twins being 2–5 %. First degree relatives of patients with rheumatoid arthritis have a 4 fold risk of developing the disorder compared to the general population.[4] The central pathophysiological feature of rheumatoid arthritis is inflammed synovial tissue characterized by angiogenesis, cellular hyperplasia and influx of inflammatory leucocytes and change in the expression of cell surface adhesion molecules, proteinases and proteinase inhibitors and many cytokines.[3] Uncontrolled and locally invasive synovium (pannus) is responsible for many of the clinical features including joint erosions and other destructive changes. The molecular pathogenic mechanisms driving pannus formation and the joint destruction remain poorly understood, although experimental and clinical observation suggest a central role for the proinflammatory cytokines TNF-alpha and IL-1.

Investigations

The laboratory features in rheumatoid arthritis reflect the acute phase response and chronic inflammation of the joints. Anaemia and abnormal liver function tests may also be caused by drug toxicity. The earliest radiographic changes are seen in the hands and feet in the form of soft tissue swelling and periarticular osteoporosis, but these are non specific signs. Erosion typical of rheumatoid arthritis develop in bare areas of bone (*i.e.*, areas lacking articular cartilage) within 3 years of onset in 90% of those patients who ultimately develop erosive disease.[5] Bone Scintigraphy is helpful in confirming synovitis, in determining the distribution of joint involvement and in assessing disease activity.[6] The use of MRI is still being evaluated in rheumatoid arthritis but it may detect bone erosion earlier than conventional approaches.

Prognosis

It is difficult to predict the prognosis of rheumatoid arthritis in individual patients, but it is usually a persistent disease with a progressively disabling course. Biopsy studies of clinically asymptomatic joints in patients with early arthritis have shown active synovitis, and there is a relatively poor correlation between clinical assessment and disease progression.[7] Nearly half of all patients will be disabled or unable to work within 10 years and after 20 years approximately 25% of patients will have undergone joint replacement surgeries.[8] Rheumatoid arthritis also shortens life expectancy and in the most severely affected patients mortality increase to a degree comparable to that seen in triple vessel coronary artery disease.[9]

Neurobiology of Arthritic Pain

★ Pain classification: Measurement of pain is far from straight forward, and responses to even simple inquires can be influenced by a range of cultural, social, demographic and environmental factors and by current psychological state, previous history and physical pathology.[10] Clinical instruments to measure pain in adult patients with rheumatoid arthritis have recently been proposed.[10] Although pain is the most common symptom of rheumatoid arthritis, it is not always present and the correlation between symptoms and disease progression is relatively poor. A graphic example is provided by rheumatoid patients who present with "arthritis robustus" which is characterized by a proliferative synovitis that appears to cause little pain and even less disability.[11]

★ Pain in Rheumatoid arthritis, as in other disorder, can arise either in response to injury to non-neuronal tissues (nociceptive pain) or to the nerves themselves (neuropathic pain) (Table 63.2). This division has clinical relevance in so far as nociceptive pain tends to be more responsive to NSAIDs and opioids, whereas neuropathic pain syndromes are less responsive. Clinical observations from other musculoskeletal disorders indicate that pain may also arise in the absence of either tissue or nerve pathology and under these circumstances it is apparent that psychosocial factors are the dominant influence on nociceptive pathways (psychogenic pain).

Table 63.2 : Potential causes of pain in rheumatoid arthritis

Aetiology	Neurophysiological Mechanisms
Tissue injury (nociceptive pain)	Peripheral sensitization
Nerve injury (neuropathic pain)	Peripheral ectopia
Psychological stress (psychogenic pain)	Central disinhibition
	Central sensitization

★ **Neurophysiological mechanisms:** Minor incidence experienced as part of everyday life produce short lived excitation of specialized high threshold nociceptors with brief spatially localized pain. Mediators released in response to tissue injury or inflammation on the other hand serve to modify the response properties of nociceptors to subsequent stimuli (peripheral sensitization).[12] This mechanism results in a decreased threshold for a response to a given stimulus, leading to increased stimulus or activity related pain. In some situations, unprovoked activity occurs leading to spontaneous pain.

★ While pain hypersensitivity following nerve or tissue injury is contingent to a large degree on peripheral mechanisms, other processes are also involved. Sustained or repetitive activity within peripheral fibres leads to substantial changes to the function and activity of central nociceptive pathways (central sensitization).[13] In neurophysiological terms, central sensitization causes exaggerated responses to normal stimuli and expanded receptive field size, producing tenderness and referred pain in areas away from the site of injury. The threshold for activation by novel inputs is reduced such that non-nociceptive fibres can activate central nociceptive pathways, causing pain in response to trivial non injurious stimuli.

★ In contrast to mechanisms that enhance neural activity, others act to reduce plasticity within nociceptive pathways. Normally these pathways are subject to powerful internal controls that operate at all levels to reduce activity. Suppression or dysfunction of these inhibitory systems may lead to abnormal nociceptive activity and hence pain in some chronic pain conditions (central disinhibition).[14]

Joint Innervation

The musculoskeletal system is abundantly supplied with both encapsulated receptors and free nerve endings. These receptors are associated with rapidly conducting A-beta fibres (with conduction velocity > 30 m/sec) and are found mainly in fibrous periarticular structures including ligaments, tendons and joint capsule. They are activated by non-noxious stimuli and for the most part are mechanoreceptors. In contrast to encapsulated receptors, free nerve endings are more widely distributed in fibrous capsules, adipose tissues, ligaments, menisci and periosteum. They are associated with small diameter fibres including A-delta fibres (with conduction velocities of 2.5–30 m/sec) and C fibres (with conduction velocities < 2.5 m/s) and respond to noxious stimuli.[15]

Under normal circumstances, structures in the immediate vicinity of the intra-articular cavity are relatively insensitive and can be mechanically stimulated in various ways without causing pain. These findings accord with neurophysiological studies performed largely in Cat Knee showing the joint nerves contain a significant proportion of fibres that are usually unresponsive to strong pressure or either benign or noxious movements.[13] This "silent" or "sleeping" nociceptor was first described in joints but has subsequently been characterized in other tissues.

Peripheral Sensitization

Peripheral sensitization undoubtedly makes a significant contribution to pain sensation experienced by patients with rheumatoid arthritis. In the joint responses of previously high threshold and silent nociceptors are lowered such that they become responsive to benign mechanical stimuli. In patients with rheumatoid arthritis, neurogenically mediated skin flares are selectively increased over inflamed joints, but not at control sites, which provide support for the enhanced peripheral responsiveness of sensory fibres in this disorder.

Within the joint experimental application of PGE-2 sensitizes nociceptors to mechanical and chemical stimuli with a time course that matches the development of pain related behaviour in awake animal. In acute situations, proinflammatory cytokines such as IL-1 and TNF appear to induce nociceptor sensitization via receptor associated kinases and phosphorylation of ion channels, whereas in chronic inflammation transcriptional up regulation of receptors and secondary signaling become more important. Long-term changes to nociceptor sensitivity also involve neurotrophin growth factors including NGF which exert a global influence on nociceptor activity by regulating the activity of neuropeptides, receptors and ion channels. Other mediators on the other hands such as endogenous opioids and canabinoids act at peripheral sites to reduce nociceptor activity. It is, therefore, clear that in rheumatoid arthritis as in other inflammatory situations there is a critical balance between various mediators that act to augment or inhibit the sensitivity of nociceptors in a number of complex and often unpredictable ways.

Central Sensitization

The clinical observation that pain may be referred away from rheumatic joint and reports of increase tenderness over apparently normal tissues have led to speculation that changes in central modulation of nociceptive input might contribute to symptoms in rheumatoid arthritis. Consistent with this idea, quantitative sensory testing in patients with rheumatoid arthritis has shown enhanced responsiveness to repetitive painful stimuli compare to healthy matched control subjects. The finding of increased areas of punctate hyperalgesia in rheumatoid patients at controlled sites over normal tissues following topical applications of capsaicin is also in accord with this idea.

The clinical consequences of central sensitization include enhanced pain perception at the site of injury and development of pain and tenderness in normal tissues both adjacent to and removed from the primary sites. A further consequence of central sensitization is that sensory input from joint proprioceptors and other specialized nerve endings in and around joint now gains access to nociceptive pathways, such that innocuous mechanical stimuli from movement within the normal range now produce pain.

Management of Rheumatoid Arthritis

★ Pharmacological therapies: The aims of treatment for rheumatoid arthritis are listed in Table 63.3. Pain continues to be treated accordingly to standard WHO guidelines using a stepwise approach involving simple analgesics, NSAIDs, weak opioids and adjunctive therapy. The major change in the management of rheumatoid arthritis has been a much earlier use of disease modifying anti rheumatic drugs (DMARDs) in an attempt to suppress joint inflammation and ultimately reduce joint damage. Most rheumatologists no longer find it sensible or acceptable to delay DMARD therapy.

★ Analgesic agents, including acetaminophen with or without dextropropoxyphen, codeine, dihydro codeine and tramadol, are all effective for symptom control. They may also be used singularly or in combination with each other or with NSAIDs, but they tend to be less effective than NSAIDs in reducing morning stiffness. The general principles for the use of analgesic agents in rheumatoid arthritis and other arthropathies are the same as for other disorders.

★ NSAIDs are widely used in the treatment of rheumatoid arthritis for their anti-inflammatory and analgesic properties. They reduce morning stiffness and the pain and swelling of inflammed joints. Currently used NSAIDs do not influence the acute phase response or radiological progression. No individual NSAID has been shown to have a clear advantage over other NSAIDs with respective efficacy, although selective COX-2 inhibitor such as rofecoxib, celecoxib reportedly have less GI toxicity compared to classical NSAIDs.

Table 63.3 : Aims of therapy for rheumatoid arthritis

★ Halting of the disease process.
★ Relief of symptoms especially pain.
★ Improvement in functional and vocational capabilities.
★ Prevention of deformity by joint protection and splintage.
★ Correction of existing deformity using surgery.

The Role of Antidepressants

The role in relieving pain and depression in rheumatoid arthritis is not clear. A randomized double blind placebo controlled study of 48 female outpatients with rheumatoid arthritis and depression/anxiety reported that dothiepine in doses of up to 150 mg/day relieved pain and disability and reduced the duration of early morning stiffness but further studies are awaited.

DMARD Therapy

It is effective in alleviating the short-term signs and symptoms of joint inflammation as well as improving long-term clinical and radiological outcome scores. The newer DMARD, which include sulphasalazine, methotrexate and leflunomide work relatively quickly. Although efficacy cannot be predicted for an individual patient, upto 2/3 of patients may respond. Each drug has a specific toxicity that requires individual monitoring. Novel therapies with agents that modify the biological response to key cytokines including TNF and IL-1 are now widely available, although optimism for the use of these agents have been tampered by the potential for long- term side effects and toxicities.

Corticosteroids

These are often used for prompt relief of symptoms of inflammation. In practice they are frequently given for acute exacerbation of the disease or as a bridge therapy until DMARDs become effective. They may be given directly into joints or as intramuscular/intravenous depot injections. The long-term use of oral steroids as a DMARD remains controversial because of the fear of side effects.

Non Pharmacological Therapy

Rest has long been recommended for patients with rheumatoid arthritis, specially during periods of active joint inflammation, but such recommendation have been based largely on empirical observations. Controlled studies of the effects of hospitalization and bed rest have found no benefit unless the patient is seriously ill with active disease. The effect of joint immobilization in rheumatoid arthritis have been examined in several studies that indicate that joint splintage may have short-term effects that are not maintained in the longer-term.

Studies of the effects of exercise in rheumatoid arthritis have tended to focus on changes in strength and aerobic conditioning rather than changes in range of motion. Available evidence suggests that range of motion; strengthening and aerobic conditioning exercises are safe for patients with rheumatoid arthritis and improve muscle strength, cardiovascular fitness and probably physical functions. They do not seem to exacerbate joint symptoms.

Dietary advice should include recommendation to maintain a reasonable weight and consume a diet containing high amounts of PUFA and adequate calcium, vitamins and minerals. Food allergies may be a factor in rheumatoid arthritis in a very small number of patients. Controlled studies have shown that Omega-3 fatty acids (present in pacific herring, king mackerel, salmon and mullet) may reduce fatigue and joint tenderness in patients with rheumatoid arthritis. Patients with rheumatoid arthritis may be deficient in zinc, copper and magnesium probably as a result of chronic inflammation, but there is no evidence that wearing copper bracelets or taking zinc supplements improves symptoms.

REFERENCES

1. Wile N, Symmons D, Harrison B, et al. Estimating the incidence of rheumatoid arthritis: trying to hit a moving target? Arthritis Rheum. 1999;42:1339–1346.
2. Arnett F, Edworthy S, Bloch D, et al. The American Rheumatism Association 1987 Revised criteria for the classification of rheumatoid arthritis. Arthritis Rheum 1988:31:315–324.
3. Levine J, Reichling D. Peripheral mechanism of inflammatory pain. In : Wall PD, Melzack R (ed) Textbook of pain. Edinburgh: Churchill Livingstone 1999; 59–84.
4. Macgregor A, Sneider H, Rigby A, et al. Characterizing the quantitative genetic contribution to rheumatoid arthritis using data from twins. Arthritis Rheum 2000;32:903–907.
5. Resnick D. Rheumatoid arthritis in: Resnick D (ed). Bone and joint imaging. Philadelphia. WB Saunders: 1996;195–209.
6. Weissberg D, Resnick D, Taylor A et al. Rheumatoid arthritis and its variance. Analysis of scinti photographic, radiographic and clinical examination. Am J Radiol 1978;131:665–673.
7. Soden M, Rooney M, Cullen A, et al. Immuno histological features in the synovium obtained from clinically uninvolved knee joint of patients with rheumatoid arthritis. Br J Rheumatol 1989;28:287–292.
8. Wolfe F, et al.The long-term outcome of rheumatoid arthritis. Arthritis Rheum 1998;41:1072–1082.
9. Pincus T. The underestimated long-term medical and economic consequences of rheumatoid arthritis. Drugs 1995;50:1–14.
10. Anderson DL. Development of an instrument to measure pain in rheumatoid arthritis. Rheumatoid arthritis pain scale. Arthritis Rheum. 2001;45:317–323.
11. Haas W, Boor W, Griffioen F, Oosten-elst P. Rheumatoid arthritis of the robust reaction type. Ann Rheum Dis. 1974;33:81–85.
12. Kidd BL, Urban LA. Mechanism of inflammatory pain. Br J Anaesth 2001;87:1–9.
13. Schaible HG, Grubb BD. Afferents and spinal mechanisms of joint pain. Pain 1993;55:5–54.
14. Kosek E, Ordeberg G. Lack of pressure pain modulation by heterotrophic noxious conditioning stimulation in patients with painful osteo arthritis before, but not following, surgical pain relief. Pain 2000;88:69–78.
15. Grigg P, Schaible HG, Schmidt RF. Mechanical sensitivity of group-III and IV afferents from posterior articular nerve in normal and inflammed cat knee. J Neuro Physiol 1986;55:635–643.

•••

64

OSTEOARTHRITIS

Osteoarthritis (OA) is by far the most prevalent joint disorder. It strongly associates with ageing and is a major cause of pain and disability in the elderly. The knee is the principal large joint to be targeted by OA, resulting in disabling knee symptoms in 10% of the U.K. population over age 55, one quarter of who is severely disabled.[1]

The Pathology of OA

The morphological and biochemical changes of OA are characteristic and distinct from those of ageing alone.[2] There is a combination of both tissue attrition and synthesis. Although there is focal thinning, fibrillation and loss of hyaline cartilage, the cartilage cells increase their production of matrix components and increase their numbers to form clones of cells. New fibro cartilage is produced at the joint margins and transforms to new bone of osteophyte by the process of endochondral ossification. The turnover of subchondral bone also increases and is associated with trabecular thickening, "cyst" formation (focal osteonecrosis), reduced venous drainage in bone, and intraosseous hypertension. The synovium undergoes hyperplasia and its outer layer, the capsule, thickens; the changes in the synovium, though less extensive, are qualitatively often indistinguishable from those of inflammatory rheumatoid disease. Osteochondral "loose bodies" embedded in synovium are common. These arise from synoviocytes that have undergone chondroid metaplasia, or by uptake and subsequent growth of cartilage fragments within the synovium. Other changes include reappearance of immature cartilage epitopes and an increased tendency for calcium pyrophosphate and basic calcium phosphate crystals to form within cartilage (chondrocalcinosis). Such changes, together with the increased vascularity of the tissues, almost suggest that the joint is reverting to the situation of an immature joint that is geared up to produce new tissue, further supporting the concept of OA as a potential repair process.[2]

Clinical Features and Physiological Associations

The physical signs evident in an OA joint are variable but may include the following:

1. Bony swelling (osteophyte) at the joint margins
2. Restriction in range of movement.
3. Coarse crepitus or crunching, initially reflecting the roughened cartilage surfaces and later reflecting bone grating on bone
4. Soft tissue swelling and effusion, usually only modest (cf. inflammatory arthropathy)
5. Joint laxity, reflecting loss of cartilage and relative slackening of ligament/capsule
6. Joint deformity with malalignment across the joint, a later feature

There are no nerves in cartilage. Pain, however, could potentially arise from any structure that contains nociceptors, including the synovium and capsule, the underlying bone and periosteum, or periarticular tissues such as ligament, muscle, tendon, and bursa.

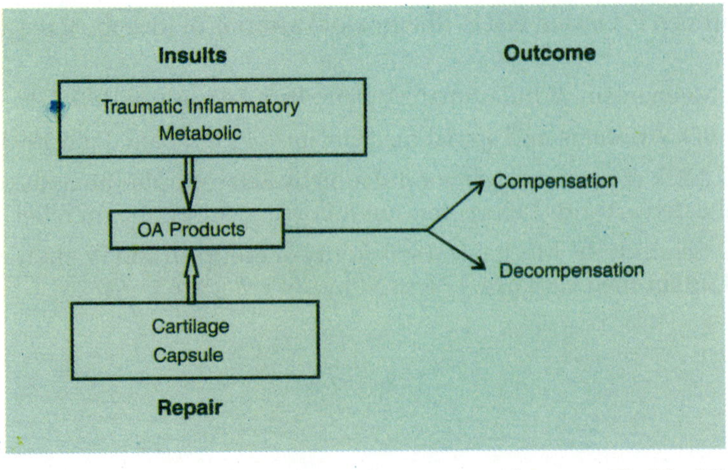

Fig. 64.1 : Model of the dynamic process of osteoarthritis (OA)

Management of OA

Evidence based interventions that should be considered in all LJOA patients include:[3]

- ★ **Education:** Although the mechanisms are unclear, information access and therapist contact both reduce the pain and disability of LJOA, improve self-efficacy, and reduce health care costs. Such benefits are modest but long-lasting and safe.
- ★ **Exercise:** Aerobic fitness training gives long-term reduction of pain and disability of LJOA, improves well-being, encourages restorative sleep, and benefits comorbidity such as obesity. Local strengthening exercise also reduces pain and disability from LJOA, with accompanying improvements in the reduced muscle strength, proprioception, and balance that are associated with knee OA.
- ★ **Reduction of Adverse Mechanical Factors:** Simple pacing of activities throughout the day and use of shock absorbing footwear and walking aids can be of benefit.
- ★ **Advice on Weight Loss for Obese Patients:** Epidemiological data and some recent trial data show that reduction of obesity improves symptoms of LJOA and may retard further structural progression.
- ★ **Simple Analgesia :** Acetaminophen (paracetamol) is the agreed oral drug of first choice and, if successful, is the preferred long-term analgesic. This recommendation is because of its efficacy, lack of contraindications or drug interactions, long-term safety, ready availability and low cost.

Various other interventions may be considered, additional options to be added, as required, to these core interventions. These include:

1. Other oral agents - combined analgesics, NSAIDs, opioid analgesics, amitriptyline, and "nutripharmaceuticals" such as glucosamine and chondroitin sulphate.
2. Topical NSAIDs and capsaicin.
3. Intra-articular injection of long-acting steroids or hyaluronan and joint lavage.
4. Environmental modifications such as a raised toilet seat and other household aids.
5. Other local physical treatments including heat, cold, acupuncture, ultrasound, spa baths, patellar taping, and knee braces.
6. Surgical realignment (osteotomy) and joint replacement.

REFERENCES

1. Peat G, McCarney R, Croft P. Knee Pain and osteoarthritis in older adults: a review of community burden and current use of health care. Ann Rheum Dis 2001;60:91–97.
2. Pritzker KPH. Pathology of osteoarthritis. In: Brandt KD, Doherty M, Loohmander LS (Eds). Osteoarthritis. Oxford: Oxford University Press,1998;pp50–61.
3. American College of Rheumatology Subcommittee on Osteoarthritis Guidelines. Recommendations for the medical management of osteoarthritis of the hip and knee: 2000 update. Arthritis Rheum 2000;43:1905–1951.

FROZEN SHOULDER AND CARPAL TUNNEL SYNDROME

65

In upper limb pain syndromes, the most common problem encountered in clinical practice by pain physician are (1) adhesive capsulitis of shoulder (frozen shoulder) and (2) carpal tunnel syndrome. In our scenario, patients hardly come directly to us, but most of the time referred by other specialists. Diagnosis is almost certain many times and most of the therapies already tried. The treatment left to us is nerve blocks and/or trigger point injections and reassurance.

Adhesive Capsulitis of Shoulder (Frozen Shoulder)

The Clinical Syndrome

It affects the gleno humeral joint. Adhesions form as a result of an inflammatory response, which produces saturation with sero fibrinous exudates. The actual cause is unknown, but the blamed one are: heavy use, immobilization, injury, tendonitis, tenosynovitis, fractures about the shoulder, infections, neoplasm, general surgery and heart attacks. Mc Laughlin (1961)[1] mentioned that a shoulder which is put through the full range of movement a few times daily will not develop adhesive capsulitis, indicating that prolonged dependency is the initiating factor. It is unusual under 40 years of age.

Signs / Symptoms

★ Patient may report pain with a gradual onset without any known injury.

★ Often seen in sedentary person who has recently begun to participate in an activity involving upper extremities such as golf, tennis or bowling.

★ Difficulty putting on a shirt, combing hair or placing the hand in a back pocket.

★ Little pain of palpation but it will be aggravated by both external and internal rotation.

★ Pain may seem to localize in the deltoid, particularly at its insertion and frequently causes suffering at night.

Diagnosis

Confirmation with arthrography:

★ Differentiate a simple stiff shoulder from the inflammatory condition.

★ Neviaser[3] (1975) classified patients according to how much of the injected dye is accepted into the capsule and what the patient's range of passive abduction indicates.

Mild — Abduction to more than 90° and dye acceptance of more than 10 mL.

Moderate — Dye acceptance 5–10 mL and abduction not over 90°.

Severe — Severe capsulitis, usually seen only after proximal humerus fracture or following severe shoulder dislocation.

★ AP X-ray often gives false impression of a normal gleno humeral relationship owing to super imposition, a lateral view is mandatory.

Treatment Course and Prognosis

★ Primary aim of treatment: prevention with regular, daily range of movement exercises.

★ Many cases respond to a conservative treatment programme, mainly of steroid therapy and pain management in conjunction with an aggressive physical therapy.

★ The judicious use of steroids injected into the rotator cuff and intra-articular space may be helpful when applied in combination with intensive physical therapy" (Sheon et al, 1987).[4]

NSAIDs and Muscle Relaxants Helpful

★ Trigger points can be injected to reduce the possibility of a pain cycle.

★ Manipulation is frequently used.

★ In severe form, manipulation may require general anaesthesia.

★ The arm may be positioned in 90° abduction during a period of 2 weeks bed rest, followed by a 3–6 months therapy programme usually leading to a full recovery.

- ★ Use of narcotics is not recommended over an extended period of time.
- ★ In recalcitrant cases, patients may benefit from a supra clavicular nerve block just before physical therapy session. It contains sensory fibre to joint and surrounding structures. It is a fairly superficial nerve and can be blocked easily.
- ★ Depression is not uncommon; it should be recognized and treated as necessary.

Shoulder Joint Injection

Intra-articular injection of the shoulder is extremely effective in the treatment of shoulder pain. Coexistent bursitis, tendonitis, or rotator cuff tear may also contribute to shoulder pain and may require additional treatment with more localized injection of local anaesthetic and methyl prednisolone acetate steroid. Care must be taken to use sterile technique to avoid infection. The incidence of ecchymosis and haematoma formation can be decreased if pressure is placed on the injection site immediately after injection.

Carpal Tunnel Syndrome

"Tingling sensation and decrease functioning in the wrist, hand and fingers resulting from compression of the median nerve within the tunnel".

Causes and Incidence

- ★ Second most common industrial injury in the US surpassed only by low back pain, 5 times more common in women.
- ★ The exact cause is unknown, but highly repetitive flexing motions of the wrist are strongly implicated.
- ★ Workers at risk are: data entry operators, grocery checkers, pipe fitters, tool workers, carpenters, secretaries and pianists.
- ★ Conditions that cause oedema and synovial hypertrophy like rheumatoid arthritis, gout, hypothyroidism, diabetes, ganglion tumours, lipomas, pregnancy or trauma also have been suggested as causes.
- ★ One theory links to a vitamin B-6 deficiency in conjunction with repetitive movements.
- ★ Malaligned Colle's fracture is also one of the causes.
- ★ Exacerbates by psychological stressors, boredom, insecurity, or the stress of other painful procedures.

Disease Process

The median nerve in the volar aspect of the wrist is compressed between the longitudinal tendons of the forearm muscles that flex the hand and transverse superficial carpal ligament. This causes parasthesia in the thumb, forefinger and middle finger and half of the ring finger.

Signs and Symptoms

- ★ Paraesthesia and dysesthesia along the median nerve into the hand and wrist.
- ★ Pain may be localized at the wrist and may show retrograde spread to the elbow or shoulder.
- ★ Associated weakness in the hand and wrist that radiates to the thumb, index finger, middle finger and radial half of ring finger.
- ★ Causes the patient to awaken several hours after getting to sleep with burning and numbness of the hands that is relieved by exercise.
- ★ Shaking or moving the hand may relieve symptoms, a pressure gradient involving the lymphatic or circulatory system.
- ★ If shaking increases pain, cervical radiculitis should be suspected. Thenar atrophy may be present.
- ★ Untreated, progressive motor deficit and ultimately, flexion contracture of the affected fingers can result.

Testing

- ★ Clinical evaluation with characteristic signs, inability to make a fist.
- ★ Positive Tinel's sign: tingling and burning produced by light tapping over the tendon sheath on the ventral surface of the wrist.
- ★ Positive Phalen's sign: pain or numbness after 30 seconds of wrist flexion.

  Electromyography : distinguish cervical radioculopathy and diabetic polyneuropathy from carpal tunnel syndrome.
- ★ Plain X-ray to rule out occult bone pathology.
- ★ MRI of the wrist for space occupying lesion.
- ★ Application of a BP cuff on the upper arm sufficient to produce venous distension may initiate the symptoms.

Treatment Course and Prognosis

- ★ General: Restriction of repetitive wrist flexion, splinting to reduce nerve pressure and relieving pain, rest and/or change in activities, occupational or physical therapy to develop strength and endurance.

  Drugs : Simple analgesics, NSAIDs or cyclo-oxygenase inhibitors, cortisone injection into tendon sheath to reduce inflammation, trigger point injection in the fore arm, shoulder, neck may help relieving both pain and dystrophy like symptoms.

★ Surgery: Release of carpal ligament for decompression of nerve if conservative measures fail.

Carpal Funnel Injection

Carpal tunnel syndrome should always be differentiated from cervical radioculopathy involving the cervical nerve roots, which may at times mimic median nerve compression. It should be remembered that cervical radioculopathy and median nerve entrapment may co-exist in the Double Crush Syndrome.

Carpal tunnel injection is a simple and safe technique in the evaluation and treatment of these painful conditions. Careful neurological examination to identify pre-existing neurological deficits that may later be attributed to the nerve block should be performed on all patients before beginning median nerve block at the wrist, specially in those patients with clinical symptoms of diabetes or clinically significant carpal tunnel syndrome.

Care should be taken to place a needle just beyond the flexor retinaculum and to inject slowly to allow the solution to flow easily into the carpal tunnel without further compromising the median nerve.

REFERENCES

1. McLaughlin HL .The frozen shoulder. Clinical Orthopedics 1989; 20:126–131.
2. Neer CS, Welsh RP. The shoulder in sport. Orthopedic Clinic of North America 1977; 8:583–891.
3. Neviaser JS. Arthrography of the shoulder, the diagnosis and management of the lesions visualized. CC Thomas, Springfield 1975.
4. Sheon RP. Soft tissue rheumatic pain, 2nd edition , Lea and Fabiger, Philadelphia 1987.
5. Bleecker ML. Medical surveillance for carpal tunnel syndrome and workers. J of Hand surgery.1987; 12A:845.
6. Rosenbaum, Ochoa. Carpal tunnel syndrome and other disorders of the median nerve. Butterworth-Heinemann, New York 1993.

•••

SECTION–XI

Diagnostic Modalities in Pain

PAIN IMAGING

66

Spinal Cord Central Pain

64–94% of patients with spinal cord injury have central pain. Aetiology includes trauma (65%), iatrogenic (12%) inflammatory neoplasm, skeletal or vascular and congenital lesions.

Brain Central Pain

98.6% incidence caused by brain lesions are more intractable than those arising from spinal cord. It is caused by vascular causes, iatrogenic trauma, infra temporal infection, syringo bulbia and degenerative diseases. Right side lesions are involved in stroke induced pain having thalamus involvement.[1]

Treatment

Surgical: The pain can disappear after removal of the tumour. Trauma pain can be relieved by exploring and excising the patient's atrophic cortex. Thalamic pain syndrome relieved by resection of post central gyrus. Cordotomy, trigeminal dorsal root entry zone, PVG stimulation relieves pain.

Features of central brain pain: Central pain is of burning, cold, numb, tingle, sting, or itchy or aching bruise, sore, throbbing, cramping, tight or tearing.

Pathophysiology is similar to peripheral neuropathic pain. The pain delays from a few weeks to months.[1]

Pattern of sensory loss: Hemi body sensory loss-46.5%, associated sensory–20.5%, hyperpathy, allodynia or both–6.8%, touch, position, vibration, sensory loss–5.5%

Functional Imaging in Brain

Functional imaging is a promising tool for investigating the mechanism of central pain. It has been found that stimulating the affected half of body, so as to produce hyperpathia in patients with stroke induced hyperpathic pain, produced thalamic hyperactivity in the SPECT scans, but this was not seen after stimulation of the unaffected side.[2] Patients without hyperpathia did not show this hypersensitivity to stimulation. It was hypothesized that loss of function of inhibitory thalamic neurons after a stroke result in disinhibition of medial thalamic nucleus and possibly pain. There was a reduced perfusion in parietal lobe further reduced by induced allodynia attributed to cortical inhibition. The injection of propofol reduced brain central pain for 5 minutes during which cerebral hypoperfusion improved.[3]

In stroke patients studied with SPECT scans, found that patients with thalamic lesions tend to have superficial pain, while those without it tend to have deep pain. In the former there was reduced background neural activity and reduced O_2 consumption in thalamus.[4] The central pain resulted from a chemical imbalance between glutaminergic and GABAergic mechanisms in transmission between sensory thalamus and cortex, which opposing glutaminergic and potentiating GABAergic transmission, by administering ketamine or propofol respectively.

Spinal cord pain functional imaging– An associated spinal cord injury, peripheral neuropathic or cancer pain, diminished perfusion of the human contralateral thalamus in SPECT and PET. These changes could be normalized by relief of the pain by resection of syrinx in case of spinal cord or by cordotomy in cancer pain.[2]

Imaging the Brain during Pain

The large volume of the human forebrain in relation to the spinal cord suggests that descending modulatory influences are more important in humans than in other species. In humans the forebrain occupies 85% and the spinal cord 2% of the volume of the central nervous system,[1] but in rats the corresponding percentages are 44% and 35%, respectively. The human corticospinal tract contains almost a million fibres, but the spinothalamic tract contains only a few thousand. Consequently, descending forebrain influences are likely to play a uniquely important role in humans. Brain imaging depicts the activity of multiple supraspinal structures ranging from the brainstem to the forebrain. Supraspinal processing of nociceptive information activates somatic and autonomic reflexes, neuroendocrine responses, attention, arousal, evaluation of the spatiotemporal and physical features of the stimulus, hedonic experience, mnemonic functions, cognitive processes, and the ascending and descending control systems that mediate and modulate these activities and their interactions. To understand how multiple neuronal populations contribute to distinct nociceptive responses, and how they unite to produce integrated responses, requires conjoint analysis of conscious behaviour and the activity of multiple synaptic populations.

Imaging Pathological Pain

Most acute pain subsides with wound healing, but unfortunately, sometimes pain from injuries may persist, as in chronic complex regional pain syndromes (CRPS).[2] In animal models, continuing afferent activity originates spontaneously from damaged nerve fibres and from their cell bodies in the dorsal root ganglion. Evidence also suggests long-term changes in the physiology of spinal and supraspinal neurons, perhaps exaggerated by abnormal inputs from damaged peripheral nerves. Functional reorganization of sensory neurons in the spinal cord, thalamus, and cerebral cortex of animals occurs after peripheral injury with or without nerve damage. It was demonstrated that the intensity of phantom limb pain experienced by amputees correlates with the extent of functional reorganization of the somatosensory cortex. Patients with central pain provide evidence that central lesions alone may produce chronic pain in the absence of any nociceptive input.[3] These examples emphasize the need for information about supraspinal systems, including the forebrain, to better understand pathological pain of peripheral or central origin.

Types of Functional Imaging

Functional imaging includes single photon emission computerized tomography (SPECT), positron emission tomographic (PET) studies of glucose metabolism or receptor binding, and electrophysiological methods such as magnetoencephalography (MEG) and high-density electroencephalography (EEG) with equivalent current dipole analysis (ECD). This brief review will concentrate on PET and functional magnetic resonance imaging (fMRI) methods to detect changes in regional cerebral blood flow (rCBF).

Physiological Basis for SPECT, PET, and MRI

Imaged brain events correspond to activity in populations of synapses. The energy demand of synaptic activity requires rapid increases in local blood flow to deliver glucose and oxygen. Several experiments have demonstrated the close coupling of synaptic neurotransmitter release, recycling, and glucose utilization,[4] the global cerebral blood flow increased during brain activity. The, special optical sensors can monitor the reflectance of different wavelengths of light by synaptic populations as they respond to specific stimuli. Signals detected by this optical imaging originate within a few hundred microns of evoked synaptic activity and are thus capable of defining anatomical boundaries within the synaptic neuropil. In PET activation, radiolabelled water or CO_2 is used, and the accumulated count of radioactivity provides an estimate of the regional cerebral perfusion during the scan (about 1 minute). This value is compared across conditions (*e.g.*, pain or no pain) to obtain estimates of task-related or stimulus-specific changes in rCBF. When a population of active synapses uses oxygen, oxyhaemoglobin is changed locally to deoxyhaemoglobin. The different magnetic resonance signals of these two forms of haemoglobin make fMRI possible. The amplitude of the signal is proportional to the rCBF, which (as in PET) correlates with functional measures of neuronal activity. Among the advantages of fMRI is the lack of radiation, which offers the opportunity to repeat individual studies frequently. fMRI provides better spatial resolution than PET or SPECT. A disadvantage of fMRI is that ferromagnetic materials, present in most electronic devices and recording instruments, cannot be brought near the scanner magnet. Subjects with implanted ferromagnetic metal prostheses or other devices thus cannot be studied with fMRI. Another disadvantage of fMRI is that the imaging of resting (unstimulated) activity and the statistical analysis of the responses of the whole brain are less well established than for PET.

What PET and fMRI Reveal about Pain

Many discrete brain structures are active during pain. Although for many years multiple brain structures and pathways were known to participate in the processing of nociceptive information activity with the perception of pain which correlates specifically with synaptic activity in the primary and secondary somatosensory cortex (S1 and S2) and the anterior cingulate cortex. PET and fMRI studies have confirmed that activation of a network of interactive subsystems consistently occurs during perception of pain. Pain-related activity is found most frequently within the medial midbrain, thalamus, lentiform nucleus, cerebellum, and the insular, prefrontal, parietal (including S1 and S2), and anterior cingulate cortices. Thus, sensory, motor, association, and limbic systems combine to mediate the multiple components of the pain experience and response.[6]

Normal group differences in pain perception are associated with differences in brain activation. There are differences in the spatial pattern and intensity of synaptically induced rCBF during different forms and intensities of innocuous and noxious thermal stimuli, the perceived differences between acute skin and acute muscle pain reflect differences in the intensity and spatiotemporal pattern of neuronal activity within overlapping sets of forebrain structures.

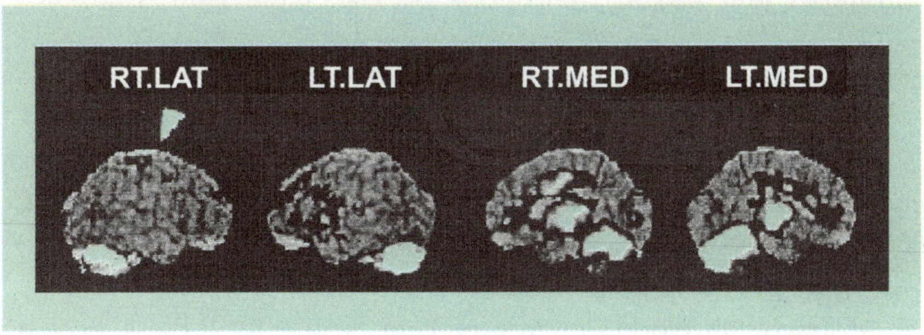

Fig. 66.1 : Regional cerebral blood flow. (rCBF) increases during cold water immersion of left hand

Significant pooled rCBF increases (averaged across 11 normal subjects) during immersion of the left hand in painfully cold (1°C), compared to mildly cool (29°C) water. Responses significantly ($P < 0.05$) above global blood flow are shown in gray scale (white corresponds to $P < 0.0001$). Arrow indicates a response in the right (contralateral) sensorimotor cortex. Note strong responses in the cerebellum, bilateral thalamus, and anterior cingulate gyrus (mid-anterior and perigenual regions).[7] Both male and female subjects rated 40° C contact heat stimuli as warm and 50°C stimuli as painful, and activation of the contralateral prefrontal cortex, insula, and thalamus overlapped completely in males and females. However, females rated the 50° C stimuli as more intense than did males, and showed significantly more intense activation of the responding areas, [7] perception and brain activation were similar (Fig. 66.1).

The functional specificity of pain-activated brain regions can be identified in imaging experiments intensity in normal subjects, pain unpleasantness correlated with the intensity of rCBF response in a far anterior (dorsal perigenual) region of the anterior cingulate cortex, but not in the S1 cortex. The information about pain intensity was widely distributed among many, but not all, pain-activated regions, including the cerebellum, these brain structures are highly heterogeneous in function. In fMRI experiments designed to separate the perception of pain from the anticipation of pain, the activation of certain regions is better correlated with anticipation of pain than with pain perception.

Unique patterns of forebrain activation occur in neuropathic pain. Imaging studies of pain caused by damage to the peripheral or central nervous system reveal that there is a thalamic hypoactivity at rest in patients with central neuropathic pain.[8] Painful dysaesthesia of the left hemibody and face following a lacunar infarction at the lateral edge of the right ventral posterior lateral thalamus on sensory examination revealed deep pressure allodynia on the left and symmetrical cutaneous heat pain thresholds. At rest, rCBF was less in the right thalamus than the left. The noxious heat stimulation (55°C) as equally painful on either side. During noxious heat stimulation of the right (normal) side, there was a slight reduction in rCBF in the left thalamus compared to its value at rest. When noxious heat was applied to the patient's left (abnormal) side, there was a strong rCBF increase in the right (contralateral) thalamus compared to the left. These results suggest that pathological hypoactivity in the resting hemithalamus masks an underlying hyper-responsiveness to noxious stimulation. This pathological hyper-responsiveness may be due to a loss of resting inhibitory activity within the thalamus.

Therapeutic Implications of Pain Imaging

Understanding the pathophysiology of chronic, severely painful conditions could suggest preventive measures and physical or pharmacological methods targeted specifically against maladaptive central adaptations. Researchers must first distinguish between adaptive, neutral, and maladaptive reorganization. Anatomical and physiological differences among patients may require new, genetically based technology. Therapy may include local delivery of growth factors or specific suppressors, neurosurgical stimulation, or ablative procedures. Ultimately, defining each patient's pathophysiology will allow effective interventions to target specific sites and pathways based on information obtained through imaging that patient's pain.

REFERENCES

1. Blinkov SM, Glezer II. The Human Brain in Figures and Tables. New York: Plenum Press, 1968.
2. Merskey H, Bogduk N. Classification of Chronic Pain: Descriptions of Chronic Pain Syndromes and Definitions of Pain Terms. Seattle: IASP Press, 1994.

3. Casey KLE. Pain and Central Nervous System Disease: The Central Pain Syndromes. New York: Raven Press, 1991.
4. Sokoloff L. In: Lassen NA, et al. (Eds). Brain Work and Mental Activity. Copenhagen: Munksgaard, 1991; 52–64.
5. Casey KL, et al. In: Bromm B (Ed). From Nociception to Pain. New York: Raven Press, 1994.
6. Casey KL, Minoshima S. In: Jensen TS, et al. (Eds). Proceedings of the 8th World Congress on Pain. Seattle: IASP Press, 1997; pp 855–866.
7. Paulson PE. Pain perception and brain stimulation. Pain. 1998;76:223–229.
8. Casey KL, et al. Abstracts: 9th World Congress on Pain. Seattle: IASP Press, 1999; pp 435–436.

•••

67

PERIPHERAL NERVE STIMULATORS

The use of a nerve stimulator to assist in the location for peripheral neural blockade of peripheral nerves with motor fibres has been advocated for peripheral neural blockade procedures on the basis of efficacy, efficiency, and patient safety. The peripheral nerve stimulator allows for localization of a peripheral nerve without the need for elicitation of a paraesthesia; thus peripheral neural blockade can be performed in patients who are sedated, unconscious, or otherwise unable to understand or cooperate or in circumstances where the nerve is difficult to localize due to anatomic variability.

The technique of peripheral nerve stimulator was originally described in 1912. The stimulating current was transmitted to the nerve using a pure nickel needle insulated with lacquer down to the tip. Needle localization of nerves with motor responses was described in 1955. In 1962 the construction and use of a portable needle nerve stimulator-locator as an instrument to assist in locating of nerves of neural transistorized stimulator provided variable, pulsed output of between 0.3 and 30 V and utilized a plastic coating as insulation of all but the tip of the needle.

In 1973, the use of a nerve stimulator with standard, unsheathed (uninsulated) needles commonly used for neural blockade procedures was reported. The nerve stimulator output was attached to the stimulating needle with a standard alligator clamp. The reported advantages of the use of uninsulated needles included better feel of the tissue planes, fewer complications resulting from problems with insulating materials, and less dependence on special equipment. While the use of uninsulated needles may result in stimulation of needle other than the tip, experimental investigation demonstrated greater current density at the tip of unsheathed hypodermic needles than at the shaft. In a study using peripheral nerve stimulator in cancer patients as a block aid monitor, better localisation of a nerve was observed during neurolytic blocks.[2]

In a study of the electrical characteristics of peripheral nerve stimulators that contributed to the localization of peripheral nerves, the following characteristics were found to be important.

1. High and low output ranges which allow the use of higher output when the needle is distant from the nerve and a wide range of low output control when the needle is close to the nerve.
2. Clearly marked polarity of the output extending to the ends of the connecting cables. It is important to attach the cathode (–) to the stimulating needle and the anode (+) to the surface of the patient.

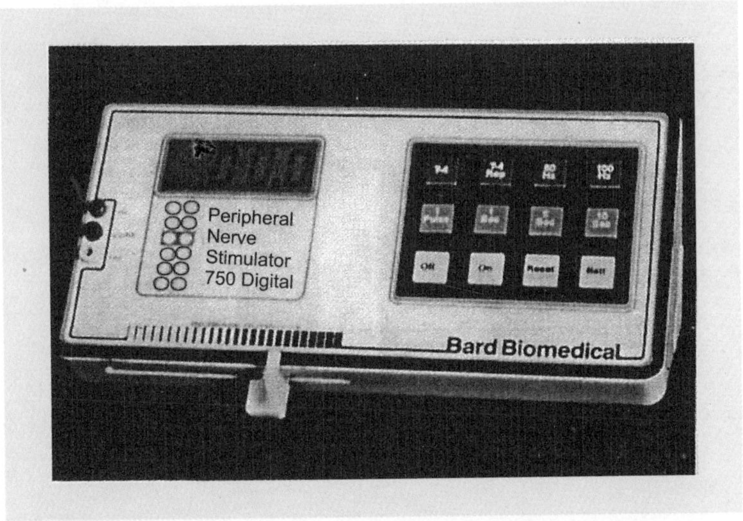

Fig. 67.1 : Bard Biomedical 750 digital peripheral nerve stimulator

On some stimulators, it is difficult to determine which is the cathode by colour in that on some models the anode is red, and on others the cathode is red.

3. Constant current output, that is, current output remains the same regardless of different resistance applied to the output; in contrast, a constant voltage output instrument will decrease current output as resistance increases.
4. A short stimulation pulse. The shorter the stimulation pulse, the greater the ratio of the current required to stimulate the nerve when the needle is 1 cm away from the nerve compared to when the needle is on the nerve. For example, for a pulse width of 40 msec, this ratio is 11, whereas for a pulse width of 1000 msec the ratio is only 5.
5. Design features, including a large, easily turned current output dial, a digital current output meter, and a battery check.

Technical Considerations

1. The anode (+) terminal of the stimulator is connected to an electrode on the patient's skin clear of the prepped site of the block.
2. The cathode (–) terminal of the stimulator is connected to the stimulating needle. The needle is inserted and advanced near the nerve. The stimulator is set to an output of 1 to 2 mA. Local muscle contraction should be minimal at this setting.
3. Stimulation of the nerve to be blocked should be measured by observing or feeling for muscle contractions within the motor distribution of the nerve. When using an insulated (sheathed) needle, stimulation will increase as the needle tip approaches the nerve and then decrease as the needle tip passes the nerve. The current output of the stimulator is decreased, as the needle approaches the nerve, to the lowest output which results in nerve stimulation and muscle contraction. At the point of maximum stimulation

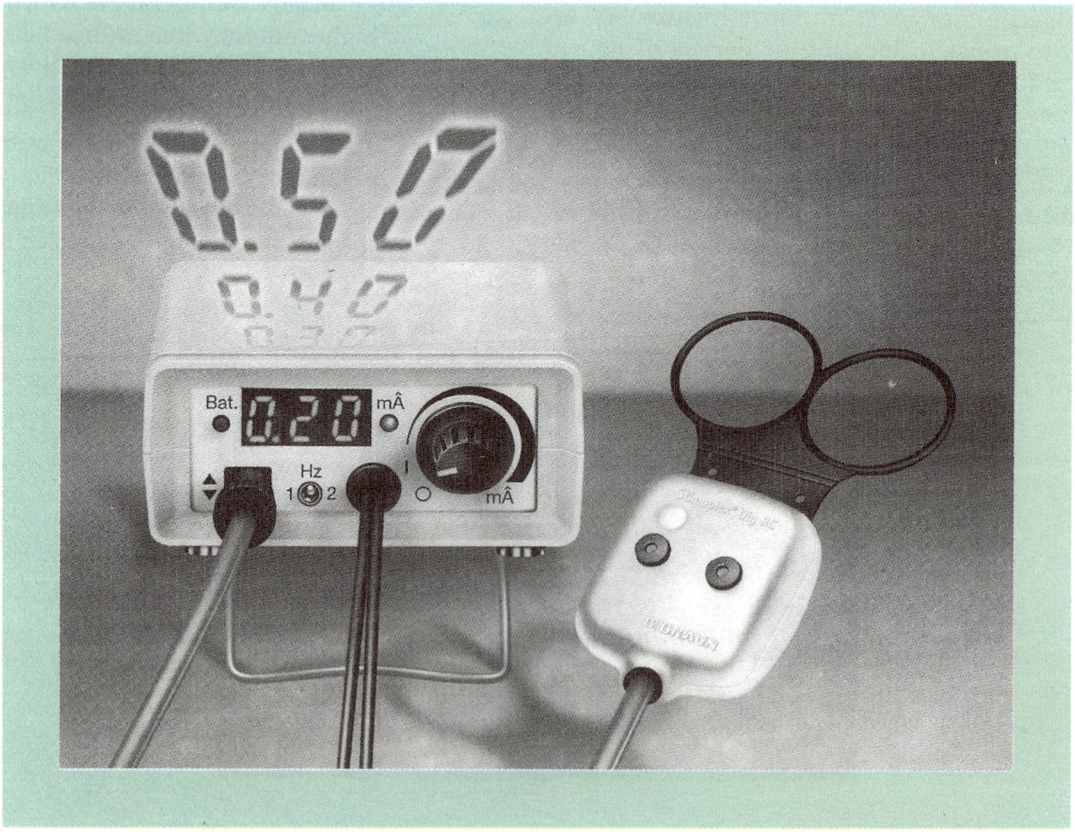

Fig. 67.2 : Stimuplex® Dig RC (B-Braun) Nerve Stimulator for Regional Anaesthesia

with the minimum stimulator output the needle tip should be proximate to the nerve and the local anaesthetic solution may be injected. When using an uninsulated needle, care must be taken to determine that the nerve stimulation is resulting from proximity of the needle tip to the nerve rather than from the needle shaft. This may be determined by systematically advancing and withdrawing the needle to the point of maximum nerve stimulation with minimum stimulator output.

4. Injection of 1 to 2 mL of local anaesthetic will immediately abolish nerve stimulation and muscle contraction, if the tip of the needle is at the site of the nerve. If this does not occur the needle should be withdrawn slightly and the process repeated. A further test is to increase the output of the stimulator after the test dose. It should still be possible to elicit some muscle response at the higher output. After a successful test dose, the full dose of local anesthetic required for the nerve block may be injected.

REFERENCES

1. Raj PP. Practical management of pain, 3rd ed, St louis, Mosby year books, 1998.
2. Rastogi V, Kumar P. Use of peripheral nerve stimulator as a blockaid monitor alcohol block. Anaesthesia, 1983; 38: 163–164.

•••

THERMOGRAPHY

68

Thermography is a harmless noninvasive, non-ionizing accurate method of measuring body surface (infrared radiation) temperature, reflecting dysfunction in the microcirculation from autonomic response to the disease. *e.g.*, cancer, tender areas of myofascial pains, discogenic diseases, headache, neurology, trauma.

Scientific Basis

There are two dermal circulations present in the body, one for thermal regulation, another for nutritive support of skin. The skin controls temperature through specific sensory nerve endings through arterio capillary system in the papillae, supplied through transverse subdermal vessels and arteriovenous shunts.

Technique

Patient takes a bath but not use talcum powder or deodorants, exercises, avoid sun, medications to prevent temperature changes in the skin. The environmental temperature of the procedure room is kept at 20° C ± 1. Thermography is done for regional areas or neurological deficits, spinal nerves and peripheral nerves. The thermographic equipment involves liquid crystal using flexible detector screens each having a temperature window of 3° to 5° C. Thermogram of hands with computerized telethermography and liquid crystal thermography is seen in Fig. 68.1. The contralateral side was evaluated for comparison and correlation of the thermogram.[2]

The most easily recognizable pattern is the asymmetry of the thermotome or peripheral cutaneous nerves due to vasodilatation or vasoconstriction and localized hypothermia. (musculoskeletal or visceral pains) autonomic function can be assessed in the former. Test for ANS function by cold or hot bath (immersion), ischaemic, test for blood pressure and diagnosing efficacy of sympathetic ganglion and epidural block other

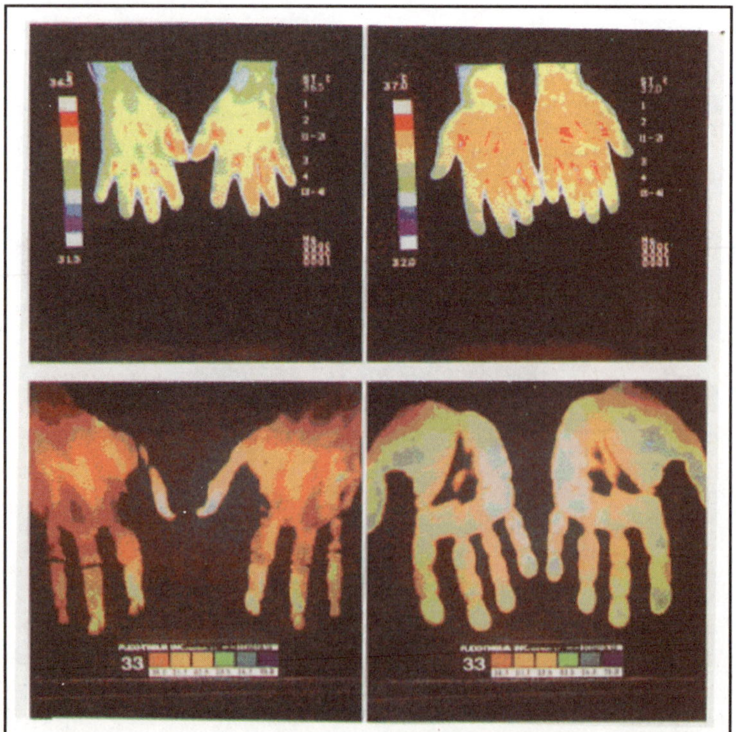

Fig. 68.1 : Thermographs of Hand. Computerized telethermography

applications are diagnosing carpal tunnel syndrome, nerve root irritation due to neurosurgery and chronic pain, spinal cord lesions and acute geniculate neuralgia.

This diagnostic technique is not much in use now-a-days, but can be a useful tool, if further work is done on it.

REFERENCES

1. WD Inbaums, Jiji JM, Lemmons DE. Theory and experiment for the effects of vascular microstructure on surface of tissue heat transfer. J. Biomed. Eng.; 1984;106:386.
2. Raj PP. Practical management of pain St. Louis, Mosby year books; 1992.

•••

SECTION–XII

Peripheral Nerve Blocks

PERIPHERAL NERVE BLOCKS GENERAL CONSIDERATIONS

69

Local and Regional analgesia achieved by injecting a local anaesthetic into the tissues or in the proximity to peripheral nervous system, has been used since a century to relieve pain. Initially these techniques were empirical resulting in failures and complications. Fortunately in the last 3-4 decades the new scientific knowledge about pain and new modalities for its treatment helped to clarify their role as diagnostic and therapeutic tools in acute and chronic pain management. There is an initial illustration showing dermatomes of the skin of the whole body which later is narrowed down by illustrations of the supply of upper and lower limb. For the sake of Post Graduates of Anaesthesiology, spinal intrathecal and epidural blocks are also described. The material is presented in the following order:

(1) Head and Neck (2) Upper extremity (3) Trunk and (4) Lower Limb. The techniques are not described in detail as it requires personal instructions by experienced teachers, but useful for those with interest in pain relief modalities available in the form of peripheral nerve blocks.

Basis for Use of Peripheral Nerve Blocks

To interrupt the nociceptive input at its very source or blocking the nociceptive impulses coursing in the peripheral nerves. This also interrupts abnormal reflex mechanisms contributing towards path physiology of some pain syndromes and blocking sympathetic hyperactivity. Low concentrations of local analgesics block unmyelinated C and B fibres and small unmyelinated delta C fibres with only a minor interruption of somatic motor functions. The neurolytics also acts in the same way on unmyelinated fibres sparing the other sensations *e.g.*, touch, temperature and motor functions for a prolonged period.

Indications for Nerve Blocks

1. Diagnostic Blocks
   - (*a*) Ascertain specific nociceptive pathways.
   - (*b*) Help determine mechanism of chronic pain syndromes.
   - (*c*) Aid differential diagnosis of the site and cause of pain.
   - (*d*) Determine patient's reaction to the pain relief.
2. Prognostic Block
   - (*a*) Predict the effects of neurolytic block/surgery.
   - (*b*) Afford the patient to experience the numbness and other side effects and help patient to decide whether or not to have it done.
3. Therapeutic Blocks
   - (*a*) Control acute post operative and traumatic pain.
   - (*b*) Breaking of vicious circle involved in the pain syndrome.
   - (*c*) Provide temporary relief to permit other therapies of development of accessory muscle functions providing mobility.

Causes of Failures

1. Inadequate knowledge of pain syndromes.
2. Inadequate evaluation of patients.
3. Inadequate management of patients before and after the block.
4. Lack of appreciation of specific indications, limitations and possible complications of these procedures.

Basic Principles of Application of Nerve Block

1. Ample knowledge of pain syndromes and therapeutic measures.
2. Devoting adequate time and effort to evaluate the patient through history, examination and assessment of pain syndromes.

3. High skill with the knowledge of anatomy, pharmacology and side effects.
4. Patients must be fully informed about the procedure.

Diagnostic / Prognostic Blocks require

(*a*) Precise localization of nerves to be blocked with X-ray image intensifier.

(*b*) Injection of small volumes (2–4 mL) of local analgesics, avoiding spillage to adjacent nerves.

(*c*) No decisions made till 2-3 blocks produce consistent results.

6. Local anaesthetic vial.
7. Neurolytic solution vial or ampoule (phenol, alcohol).

Side Effects and Complications of Regional Analgesia

1. Systemic Toxic reactions – excessive close infection, intravenous infections.
2. A very high or total spinal anaesthesia due to dural puncture accidentally.
3. Pneumothorax – brachial, caeliac, intercostal and para vertebral blocks.

Clinical Characters and Doses of Local Analgesics[1]

Character	Lignocaine	Bupivacaine	Prilocaine	Etidocaine
Latency (speed of onset)	Fast	Fast	Moderate	Very Fast
Penetration	Marked	Moderate	Moderate	Moderate
Duration	45 min	90-120 min	1 hr	> 90 min
Optimal concentration-				
infiltration	0.25	0.05	0.25	0.1
spinal nerve and plexuses	0.5-1.0	0.25-0.5	0.5-1.0	0.5-1.0
Maximum concentration (mg/kg)	3-5	2	6	2

Careful Assessment of Patients by Physician for Results

(*a*) Reaction of patient to needle insertion to evaluate pain threshold.

(*b*) Ascertain if intended nerve has been blocked.

(*c*) Evaluate efficacy of block in relieving pain, pathophysiology and duration of pain relief.

(*d*) Record results in detail in patient's chart.

Equipments for Peripheral Nerve Blocks

1. Needles – 22 SG – 15 cm, 12 cm, 8 cm. 25 SG – 4 cm, 3 cm, disposable needles.
2. Ring forceps.
3. Syringes – 1 mL, 2 mL, 5 mL, and 10 mL (preferably leur lock).
4. Bowls for antiseptic and spirit.
5. Gauze pieces 5–10 pieces.

4. Neurological complications – neuropathy, dysfunction.
5. Other systemic reactions – psychogenic responses to local analgesics, anxiety, allergic reactions, idiosyncratic reactions. Prevented by aspiration, treatment by oxygenation and artificial ventilation, vasopressors,I/V fluids.

Neurolytic Agents[2]

1. Absolute alcohol – 95% hypobaric, causes burning sensation for 2-5 minutes. Side effects – neuritis.
2. Aqueous phenol – 5% hyperbaric, no initial burning sensation. Selective analgesic action (?), ease of injection. Less neuritis.
3. Phenol in glycerol – 5–8% solution. Not used now-a-days. Difficult to inject.
4. Chlorocresol – 4–6% solution, hyperbaric, selective analgesia.

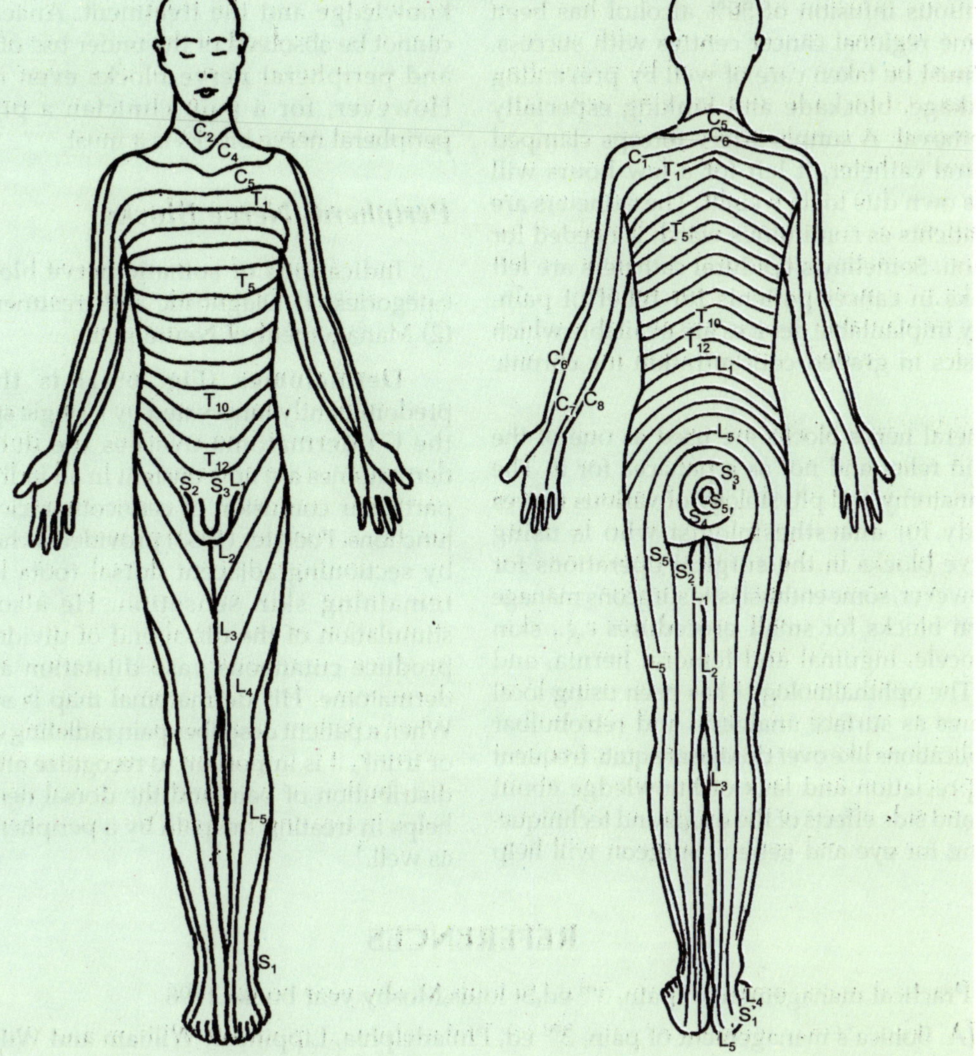

Fig. 69.1 : Dermatomes[4]

Premedication

A barbiturate or anxiolytic drug is must for successful regional and peripheral nerve block.

Monitoring and Resuscitation Equipments[3]

A careful monitoring of pulse, BP, twitching of eye muscles is needed for early local analgesic toxicity or sympathetic block. In the patients having cardiac diseases an ECG monitor is applied. Watch of respiration and Spo2 (pulse Oxymeter) may be needed. The X-ray or image intensifier is useful guide for nerve block.

The cardiac respiratory resuscitation instruments must be at hand. ECG defibrillator monitor, and i/v line with a pint of 5% dextrose / saline running, a tilting table, ambu-bag or anaesthesia machine with facilities for endotracheal intubation. The oxygen can be supplied by ventimask, nasal mask or by anaesthetic machine.

Drugs

For emergency cardiac support: Atropine, adrenaline, antiemetics, midazolam, vasopressors, antierrythmics etc., must be available in nearby tray.

Oral Analgesics used along with Peripheral Nerve Blocks

Aspirin, non steroidal anti-inflammatory drugs, opioids, tricyclic antidepressants, antiemetics.

The peripheral nerve blocks are used in combination with oral analgesics. Sometimes, catheters are placed for continuous/bolus injections of local analgesics. In cancer patients continuous infusion of 50% alcohol has been reported in some regional cancer centres with success. The catheters must be taken care of well by preventing infection, breakage, blockade and kinking especially during their removal. A simple artery forceps clamped over the epidural catheter, if left for a few hours will remove it on its own due to its weight. The catheters are put in the in patients as continuous watch is needed for any complication. Sometimes epidural catheters are left for many weeks in cancer patients for relief of pain. Currently many implantable devices are available which deliver analgesics in graded concentration for chronic pain relief.

The peripheral nerve blocks are used as one of the tools of the pain relief and not as a panacea for it. The knowledge of anatomy and physiology of various nerves comes in handy for anaesthesiologist who is using peripheral nerve blocks in the surgical operations for anaesthesia. However, some enthusiastic surgeons manage local infiltration blocks for small procedures *e.g.*, skin grafting, hydrocele, inguinal and femoral hernia, and caudal blocks. The ophthalmologist has been using local anaesthetic drugs as surface analgesia and retrobulbar block, but complications like over dosage are quite frequent due to less appreciation and lack of knowledge about pharmacology and side effects of the drugs and technique. A better training for eye and general surgeon will help them performing many operative procedures in the field areas or nowadays fashionable medical eye camps. However, there is no replacement of the adequate knowledge and the treatment. Anaesthesiologist also cannot be absolved of the under use of regional epidural and peripheral nerve blocks even in major centres. However, for a pain clinician a proper training of peripheral nerve blocks is a must.

Peripheral Nerve Blocks

Indications of somatic nerve blocks fall into two categories (1) Diagnostic and treatment of cancer pain. (2) Management of Neuralgias.

Dermatomes (Fig. 69.1) is the area of skin predominantly innervated by a single spinal segment *e.g.*, the C5 dermatome overlies the deltoid region. The dermatomes are not constant in all individuals. There is a particular confusion of cervicothoracic and lumbosacral junctions. Foerster (1933) provided a chart of dermatomes by sectioning adjacent dorsal roots leaving a zone of remaining skin sensation. He also used electrical stimulation of the distal end of divided dorsal roots to produce cutaneous vaso dilatation approximating its dermatome. His dermatomal map is still in clinical use. When a patient describes pain radiating down an extremity or trunk, it is important to recognize and record the exact distribution of pain and the dorsal nerve involved. This helps in treating the pain by a peripheral nerve blockade as well.[5]

REFERENCES

1. Raj PP. Practical management of pain, 3rd ed,St louis,Mosby year books,1998.
2. Loeser JA. Bonica's management of pain, 3rd ed, Philadelphia, Lippincott-William and Wilkins, 2001.
3. Wall PD and Melzack R. Textbook of pain (3rd) ed Edinburg: Churchill, Livingstone,1994.
4. Kumar Pramod. Atlas on peripheral nerve blocks, Jamnagar ISSP Con 2002.
5. Foerster O. The dermatomes in man. Brain. 1933;56:1–39.

NERVE BLOCKS OF HEAD AND NECK

70

Trigeminal Block

The Trigeminal nerve (V cranial nerve) originates from Gasserian ganglion on the ventral surface of brain stem. These rootlets pass forward within the posterior cranial fossa and across the superior border of petrous temporal bone to enter Meckel's cave. From anterior border of Gasserian ganglion the three division of trigeminal nerve leave the skull to innervate the head. The ophthalmic nerve leaves through superior cervical fissure, the Mandibular division through foramen rotundum and maxillary nerve through foramen ovale. These nerves further subdivides into various tributaries supplying face and occiput. [1]

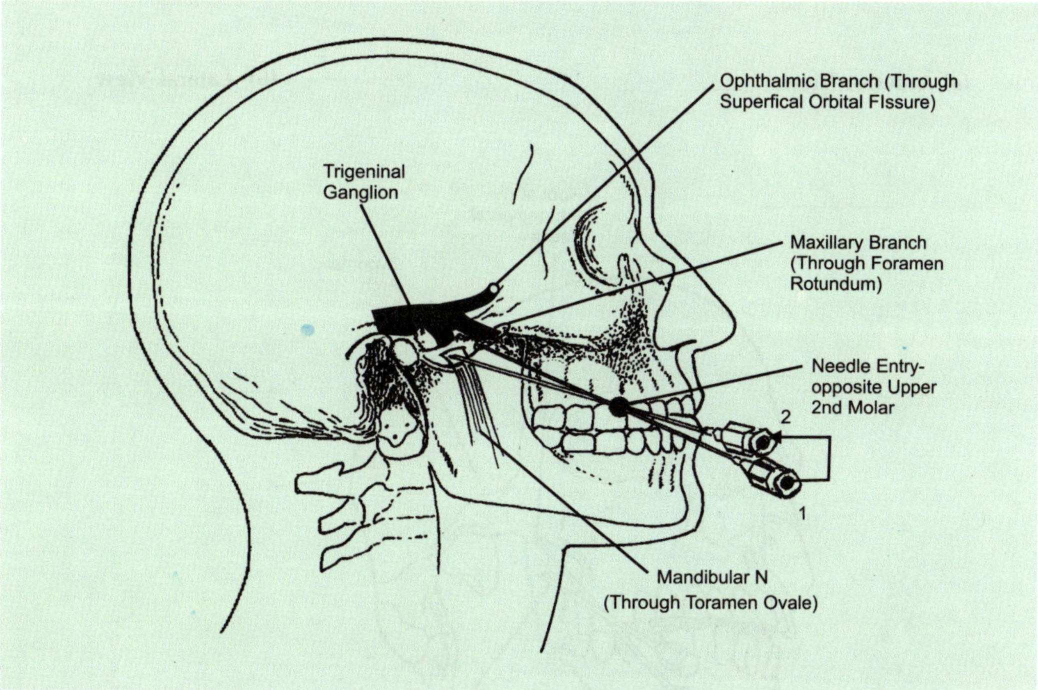

Fig. 70.1 : Gasserian ganglion, branches and technique of block

Gasserian Ganglion Block (Anterolateral Approach)

The needle is inserted through a skin wheal on the skin overlying the second upper molar tooth. It is advanced in a direction so that viewed from side, its point is directed to the mid point of zygomatic arch and viewed from the front, it is directed to the pupil of infratemporal plate just anterior to the foramen ovale. The depth marker is set 1.5 cm from the skin surface and the needle withdrawn until its point is in the subcutaneous tissue, then reinserted so that its point enters foramen ovale 1 cm farther than the previous point of insertion. Eliciting paraesthesia and CSF drop over the hub of needle confirms the successful block. After a negative insertion 1-1.5 mL of aqueous phenol 5% or absolute alcohol is injected. This block can be done through a CT guided technique as well.[2]

Indications – Trigeminal neuralgia.

Maxillary and Mandibular Nerve Blocks

Figure 70.2 on the right rectangle at the top indicates point of entrance into the skin just below the mid point

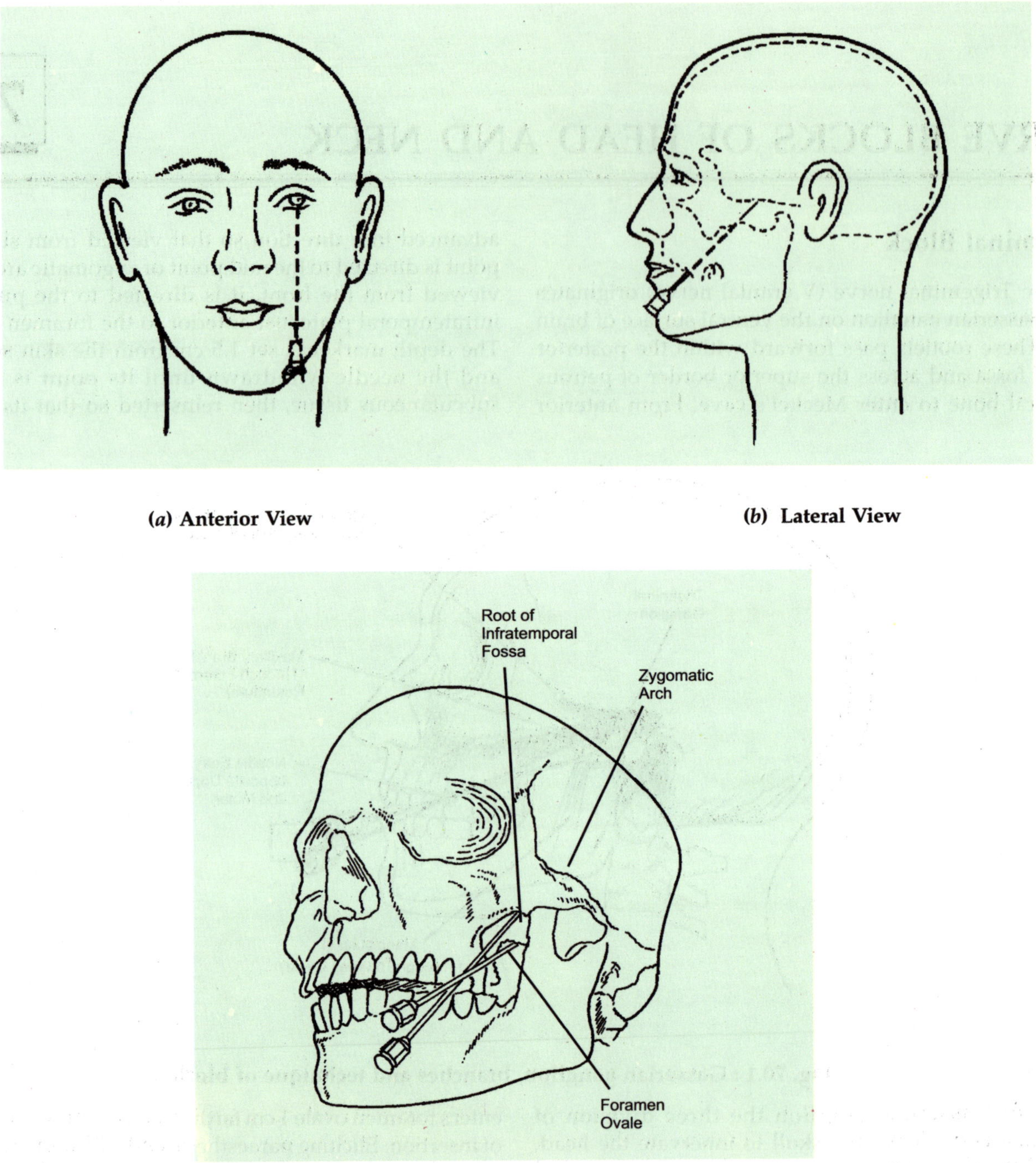

Fig. 70.2 : Techniques of Gasserian ganglion block

of the zygomatic arch. The needle is inserted straight perpendicular to the skin and impinges on the lateral pterygoid plate. To carry out the Maxillary nerve block the needle is withdrawn until its point is in the subcutaneous region and then reinserted so that it will pass 1 cm anterior and superior till it enters the pterygopalatine fossa and contacts the maxillary nerve eliciting paraesthesia or electrical sensations, if a block aid monitor is used.[2]

For Mandibular nerve block, needle 1 is withdrawn and reinserted 1 cm posterior and superior. It is advanced till its point contacts the Mandibular nerve just below foramen Ovale[3] eliciting paraesthesia with or without the help of a nerve block aid monitor. 2-3 mL of solution of local analgesic or neurolytic is injected.

Indications: 1. Pain in the distribution of maxillary and Mandibular nerves.

2. Trigeminal neuralgia.

Terminal Branches of Trigeminal Nerve Blockade

Supraorbital, Infraorbital and mental nerves are blocked at their exits from their respective foraminae which are in the same plane as the pupil. A line drawn perpendicular to the centre of pupil passes through these three foraminae. Further a small tubercle can be felt just lateral to these foraminae giving indication of their presence and acts as a surface landmark. These foraminae are easy to block, safe without injury to any deeper structure and the needle hits to bone superficially. About 2-4 drops of neurolytic solution is injected after eliciting paraesthesia with a nerve block aid monitor.

Indication : Leftover pain after maxillary, Mandibular, Gasserian block.

Spenopalatine ganglion block has been modified by the author in left over pain after maxillary nerve block in neuralgia when a pain in the region of an area above the centre of upper lip, just below the tip of nose is present. This block can also be indicated in hyperhydrosis. A small cotton wick 4-5 cm long is winded down as in a oil lamp wick and inserted into the nares involved. This is a non-invasive method for the tough leftover pain, in maxillary neuralgia. Alternatively anaesthetist can put a small cotton pledget on the middle turbinate under vision through a nasal speculum. The local analgesic instillation break the cycle of pain which disappears after 3-4 days. The wick method used by the author has the simplicity of removal of the wick and again putting another wick by the patient him/herself at home.

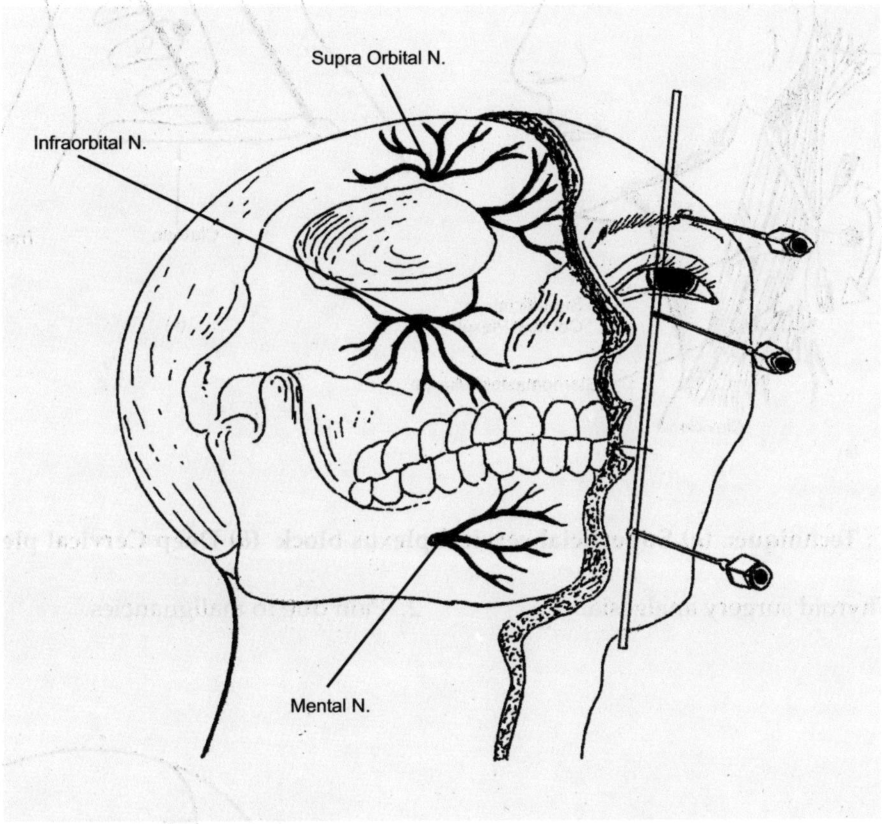

Fig. 70.3 : Terminal branches of Trigeminal N

Deep Cervical Plexus Block

The local analgesic solution (2-5 mL) is deposited along the line drawn on the posterior border of the sterno-mastoid muscle. These wheals are raised with local analgesic just below the mastoid process, second to one finger breadth below wheal one and third wheal is drawn one finger breadth below the second wheal. These wheals corresponds to second, third and fourth cervical vertebrae. The fairly easily palpable tubercle of Chassaignac of C6 on transverse process is a useful landmark. A 5 cm needle is inserted transversely about 2-4 cm deep till it reaches transverse process. After a negative aspiration test local analgesic or neurolytic is deposited.

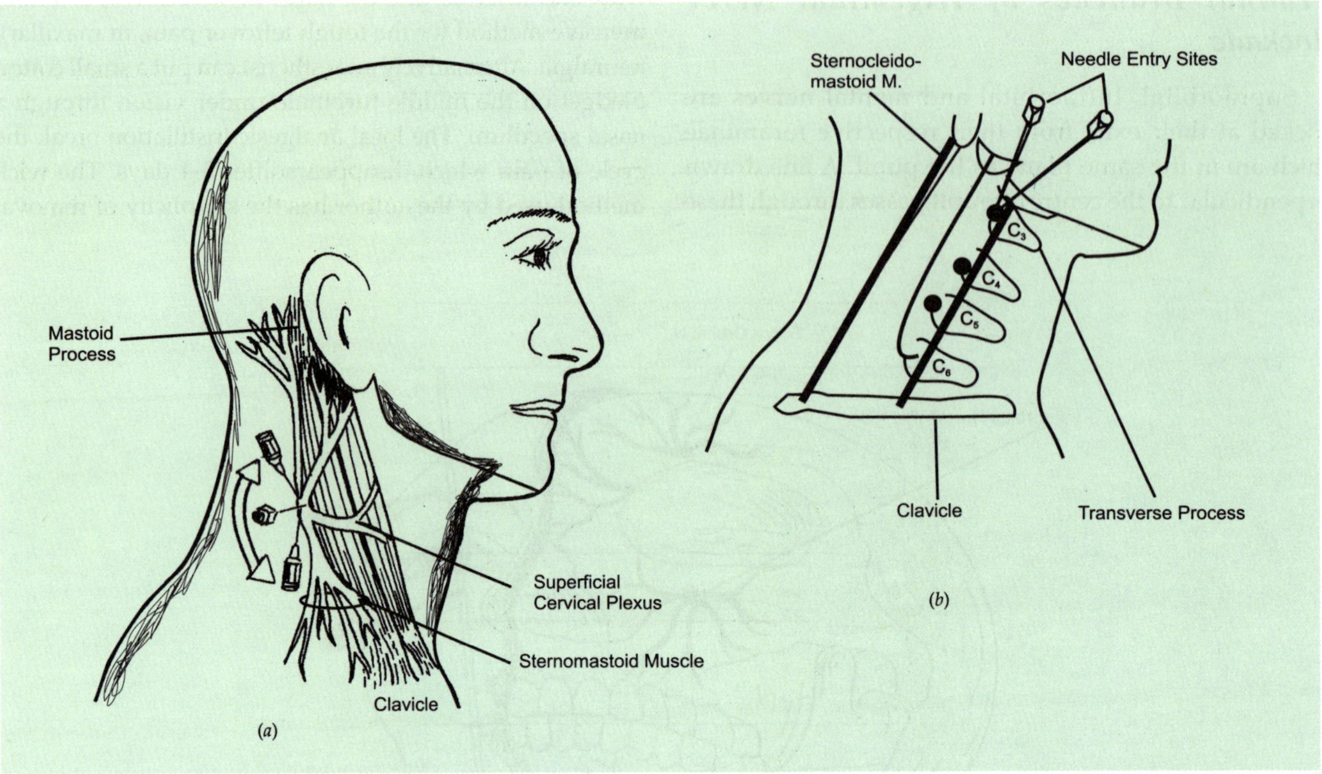

Fig. 70.4 : Technique: (*a*) Superficial cervical plexus block (*b*) Deep Cervical plexus block

Indications: 1. Thyroid surgery analgesia, 2. Pain due to malignancies.

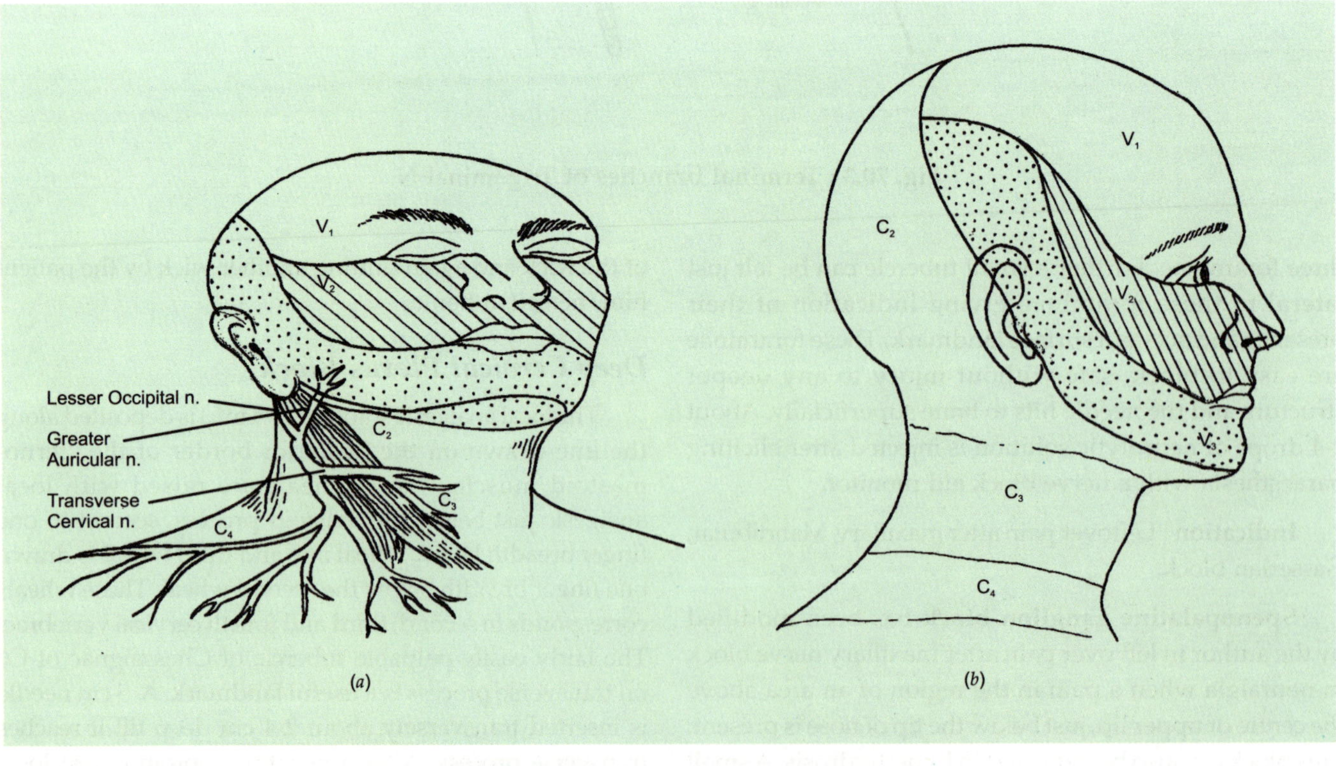

Fig. 70.5 : Innervation of head and neck

Stellate Ganglion Block

Patient lying supine with neck extended without a pillow. Wheal is raised two-finger breadth lateral to jugular notch and similar distance above clavicle, which is on the medial border of the sternomastoid overlying 7th cervical vertebra transverse process. The position is confirmed by palpating tubercle of Chassaignac (C7) transverse process. A 5 cm needle is directed backwards till it reaches bone. Needle is withdrawn 0.5 cm and after careful aspiration 10 mL of local analgesic or neurolytic agent is injected. This technique produces Horner's syndrome which is temporarily requiring neosporin eye ointment for lacrimation and red eye.[2]

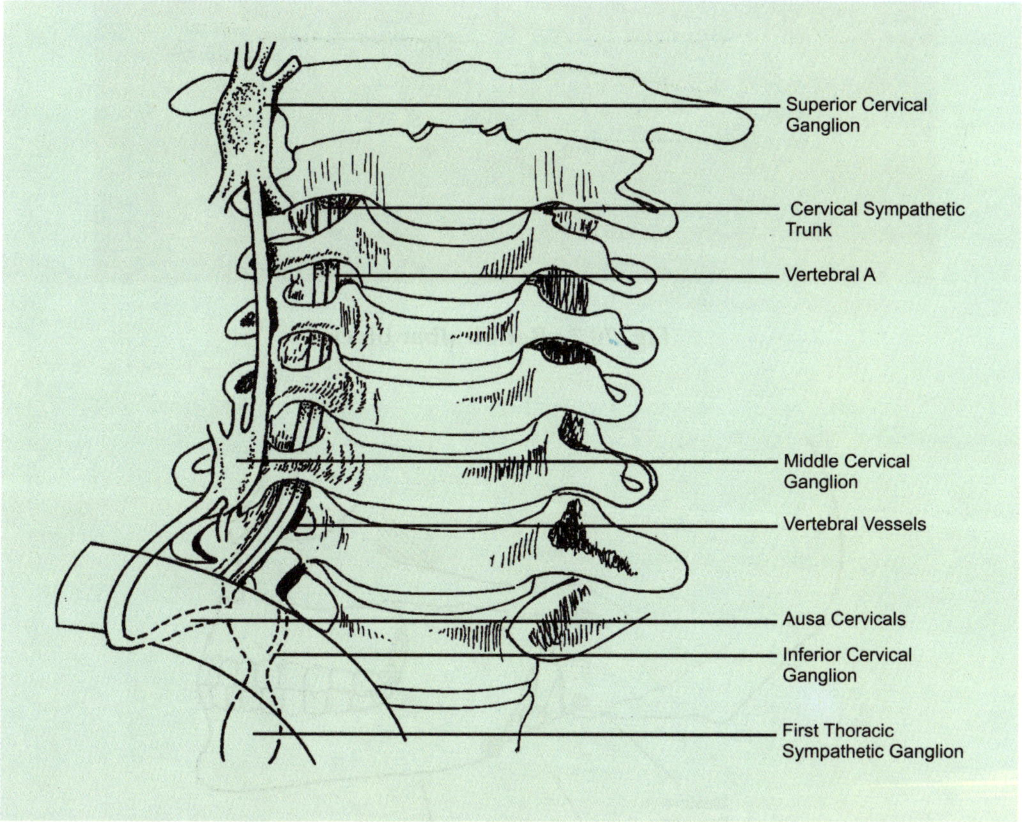

Fig. 70.6 : Stellate ganglion

Indications : Hyperhydrosis, causalgia of upper limb, thromboembolism, headache, spastic pain of upper limb.

Retrobulbar Injections

(a) **Infero Lateral Approach** : A wheal is raised at the infero lateral margin of orbit. A 5 cm needle is inserted backwards along the floor of orbit till its tip is posterior to the eye at the apex of the orbit. Local analgesic 1-2 mL is injected after negative aspiration. A trans conjunctival approach may also be used. Deposition of a little solution in superior rectus is necessary. This block dilates pupil, reduces intraocular pressure and exophthalmia (Fig. 70.7).

(b) **Superior approach:** Through superior rectus with patient looking downwards, from a wheal raised just above the middle of the tarsal plate with a needle direction inwards and downwards.

Indications: Operation over the globe of the eye.

Disadvantage: Haemorrhage.

Glossopharyngeal nerve – IX cranial nerve supplies posterior part of tongue and oropharynx. It arises from the jugular foramen receiving communicant branches from vagus and tympanic nerve and lesser petrosal nerve (Fig. 70.9). Blockade of the Glossopharyngeal nerve alone or in combination with vagus nerve is indicated in diagnostic / prognostic procedures in patients with glosssopharyngeal neuralgia, severe cancer pain of throat or other painful conditions in the areas supplied by it.

The blockade of both vagus and glossopharyngeal nerve is done at the base of skull just below jugular foramen.[3]

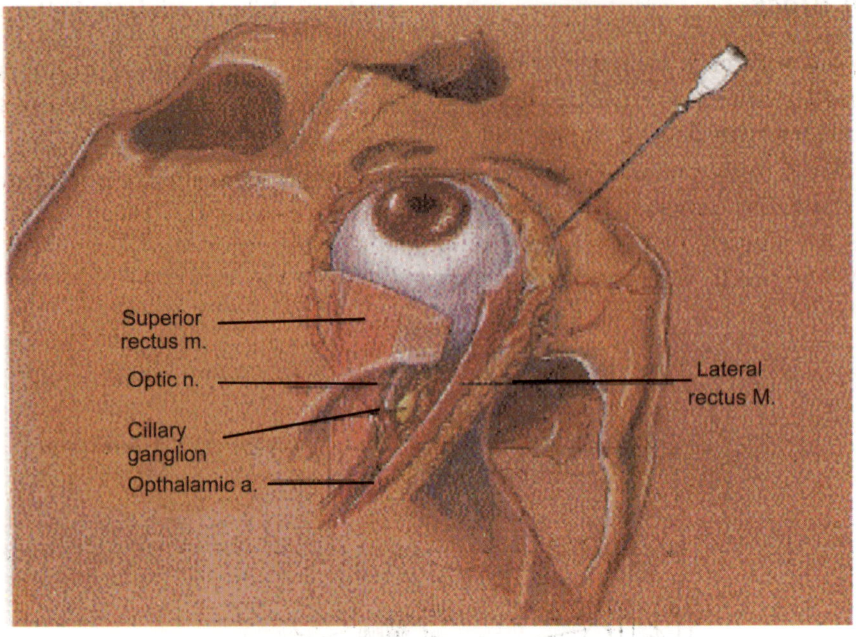

Fig. 70.7 : Retrobulbar block

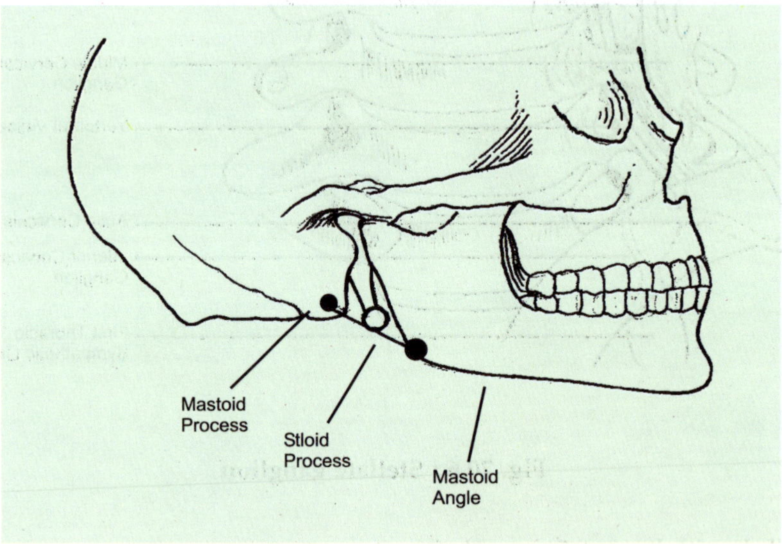

Fig. 70.8 : Glossopharyngeal N. block

With patient in supine position with head lying rotated to opposite side, a line is drawn joining tip of mastoid process and the angel of jaw (Fig. 70.8). A wheal is raised on the mid point of this line and the needle is inserted perpendicularly till it strikes the tip of the mastoid process 2-4 cm deep. The needle is withdrawn and reinserted anterior to the Styloid process 0.5 cm deeper till it reaches Glossopharyngeal nerve (II). The Vagus nerve is blocked by the needle posterior to the styloid process advancing it 1 cm deeper than the first injection. (Fig. 70.10).

Indications: Glossopharyngeal neuralgia, carcinoma posterior third of tongue.

Larynx

Larynx is the organ of voice, connecting the pharynx with trachea, opposite C3 to C6 vertebrae, higher in children and females. It is covered by the depressor muscles of hyoid bone, thyroid gland and cricothyroid muscles. It is composed of thyroid, cricoid, 2 aretenoids, 2 corniculates, 2 cuneiforms and epiglottis cartilages. The cavity of larynx joins pharynx

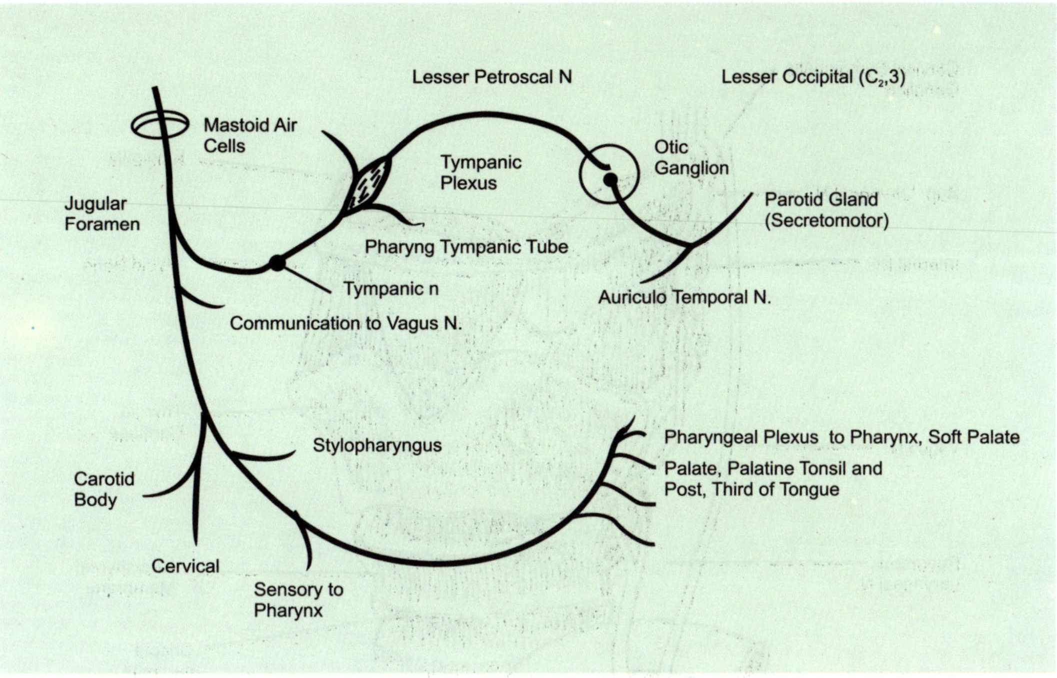

Fig. 70.9 : Branches of Glossopharyngeal nerve

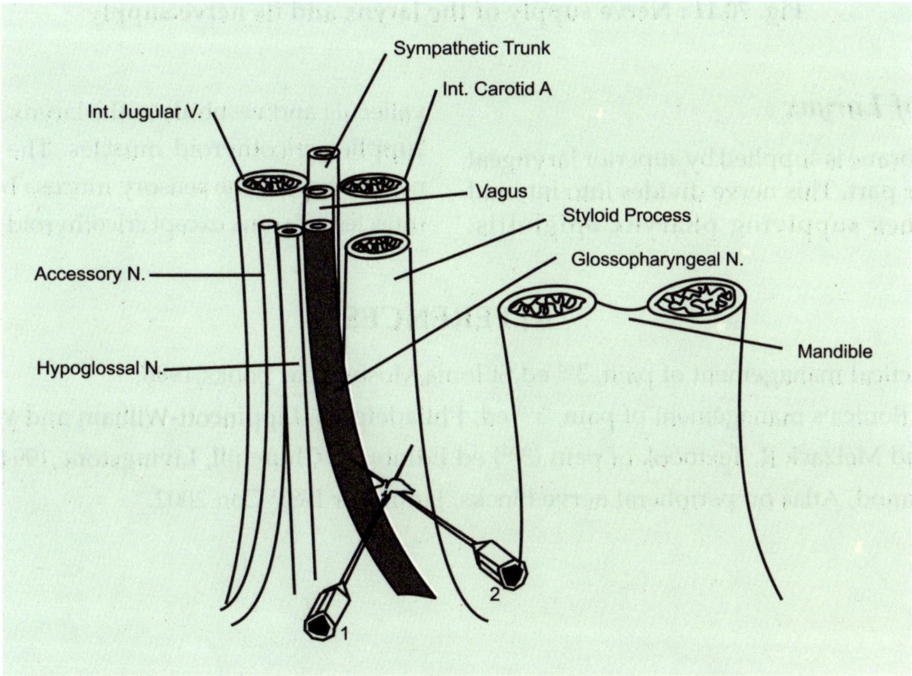

Fig. 70.10 : Technique of Glossopharyngeal Relations and block

with the trachea. Internal laryngeal branch lies beneath its mucosa and blocked near pyriform fossae. Muscles-extrinsic, muscles-thyrohyoid, sternothyroid, and inferior constrictor of pharynx, which elevate, depress or constricts the larynx. Intrinsic muscles which open and close the glottis *e.g.*, cricoarytenoids and interarytenoids. Tensors of the cords are cricothyroids and areyenoids while ary and thyroepiglotticus control the inlet of the cord. Local anaesthesia can be provided by spray of vocal cord and transtracheal route (Fig. 70.11).

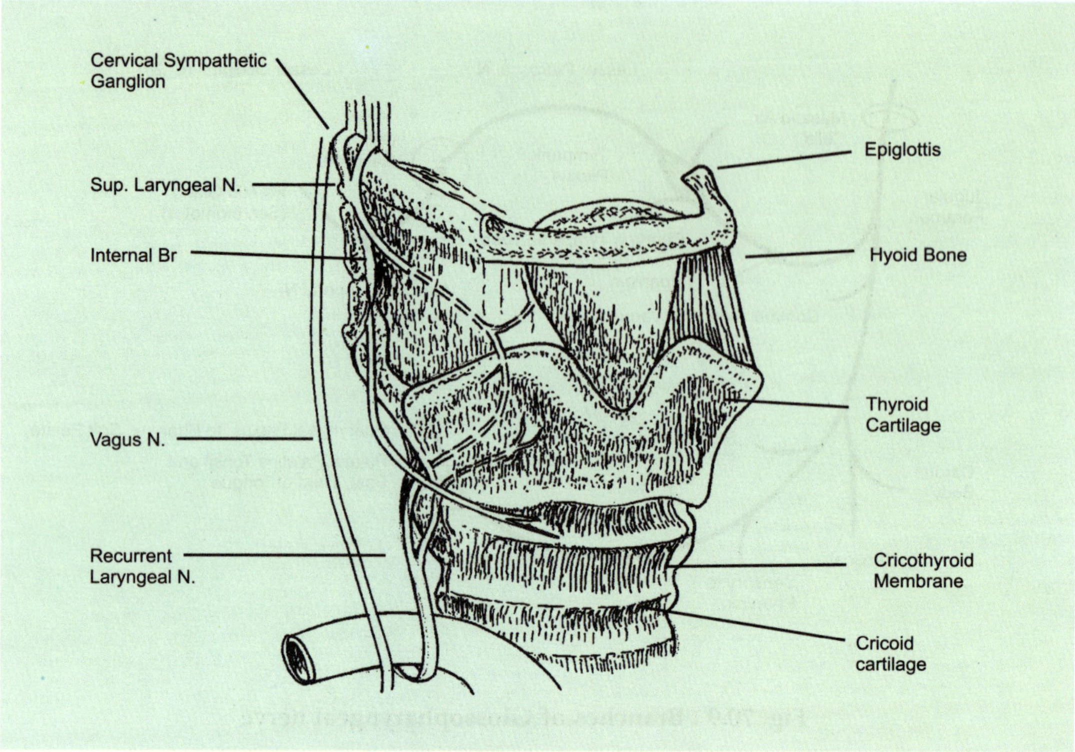

Fig. 70.11 : Nerve supply of the larynx and its nerve supply

Nerve Supply of Larynx

Mucous membrane is supplied by superior laryngeal nerve in the upper part. This nerve divides into internal laryngeal branches supplying pharynx epiglottis, vallecula and vestibule of the larynx. The external branch supplies cricothyroid muscles. The recurrent laryngeal nerve supplies the sensory mucosa below vocal cord and muscles of larynx except cricothyroid and aretenoid partly.

REFERENCES

1. Raj PP. Practical management of pain, 3rd ed,St louis,Mosby year books,1998.
2. Loeser JA, Bonica's management of pain, 3rd ed, Philadelphia, Lippincott-William and Wilkins,2001.
3. Wall PD and Melzack R. Textbook of pain (3rd) ed Edinburg: Churchill, Livingstone,1994.
4. Kumar Pramod, Atlas on peripheral nerve blocks, Jamnagar ISSP Con 2002.

•••

71

UPPER LIMB BLOCKS

Anatomy of Brachial Plexus

Brachial plexus is formed from anterior primary divisions of C5 to C8 and T1 and supplies motor and sensory nerve to the arm. It receives communicating twigs

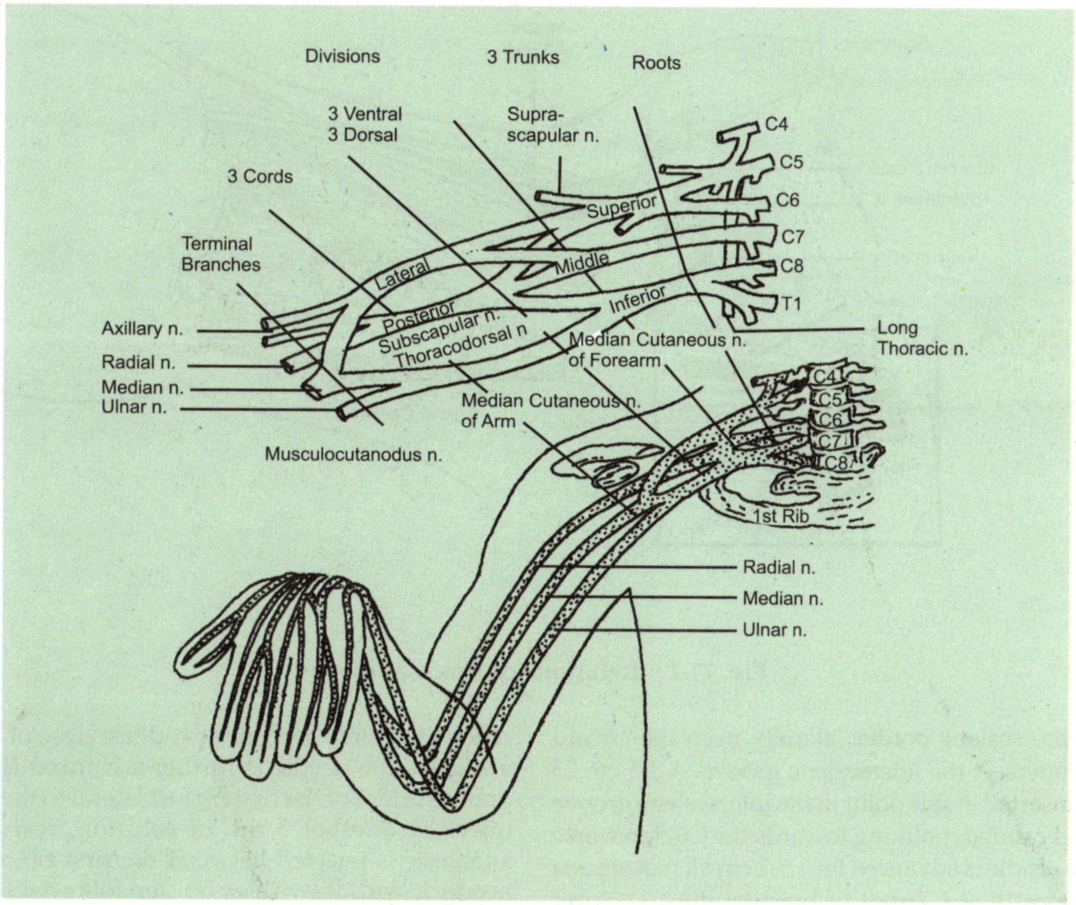

Fig. 71.1 : Anatomy of brachial plexus

from C4 and T2. These nerves unite to form 3 trunks in the neck above the clavicle. Each trunk divides into anterior and posterior division behind the clavicle which unite in the axilla to form cords (Fig. 71.1).

Relations

ANTERIOR – Skin, superficial fascia, platysma, supraclavicular branches of cervical plexus, the deep fascia and the external jugular vein with scalenus anterior and clavicle. POSTERIOR – scalenus medius and long thoracic nerve. INFERIOR—first rib, subclavian artery anteriorly and scalenus medius behind (Fig. 71.2).

Branches

FROM THE ROOTS – Nerve to serratus anterior (C5,C6, C7), dorsalis scapulae nerve, a muscular branches to longus cervices, the three scalene, rhomboids and a twig to phrenic (C5). FROM TRUNKS – suprascapular and subclavius. FROM CORDS : lateral cord : lateral pectoral, lateral head of median, musculocutaneous. Posterior cord : radial (C5-C8,T1), circumflex, lattismus dorsi, subscapular nerves. Median cord : medial head of median, medial pectoral, ulnar, medial cutaneous nerve of forearm, medial cutaneous nerve of arm. (Fig. 71.1).

Indications – (1) For surgical anaesthesia of arm. (2) Causalgia, phantom limb pain, post amputation pain, traumatic and spastic pain.

Interscalene Brachial Plexus Block

The patient lies in supine, with head down on a pillow and rotated to opposite side. Identify the interscalene groove by asking the patient to lift the head causing a tension of scalene muscles (Fig. 71.2). Draw a line along the scalene border laterally from the cricoid cartilage to intersect the interscalene groove. A 3-5 cm 25 G needle is inserted at this point in the interscalene groove medially and caudad, pointing towards the C6 transverse process. The needle is advanced for 1.5-2 cm till paresthesia is elicited (mostly at C7 root of brachial plexus). After negative aspiration inject 20-30 mL of local anaesthetic drug. A 18-20 SG intravenous catheter can also be placed and tapped securely for a continuous technique, using 15-25 mL of 0.25-0.37 % Bupivacaine every 6 hours or a continuous infusion of 0.25 % of Bupivacaine at the rate of 6-12 mL /hr. Avoid–pneumothorax, over dosage of local analgesics and phrenic nerve block.

Indications : (1) Diagnostic or prognostic measure in causalgia, phantom limb and sympathetic pain. (2) For operation of the upper limb especially near the shoulder joint.(3) Accidental dural puncture.

In children : Interscalene groove is easily palpable. Peripheral nerve stimulator is used in lieu of paraesthesia.

Supraclavicular Technique

The relation of brachial plexus with various structures of neck are shown. After identifying two ends of clavicle and subclavian artery is palpated. A skin wheal is raised 1 cm above the mid point of clavicle just postero lateral to the pulsation of the artery. A 22 SG, 5-8 cm needle attached to a syringe filled with a local analgesic in a caudad, slightly posteriorly until paraesthesia is elicited. After a negative aspiration and test dose of 3-4 mL local analgesic the needle is further advanced till it contacts upper surface of the first rib just lateral to the artery. After injecting another 5 mL of solution, rest of the local analgesic is injected between the first rib and fascia as needle is withdrawn step by step followed by a negative aspiration (Fig. 71.3). Some of the workers prefer to create a wall of anaesthesia by repeated 3 injections as above, each 0.5 cm posterolateral to the previous injection.

However, present author prefers to deposit 10 mL of local analgesic at the site of paraesthesia, another 10 mL on the rib and rest infiltrating in a posterolateral plane between the rib and the skin fascia. This has never resulted in a failure since it can cover most of the lateral divisions of the cord.

Side effects : (1) Pneumothorax more on left side.(2) Horner's syndrome. (3) Phrenic nerve block. (4) Haemorrhage due to arterial puncture.

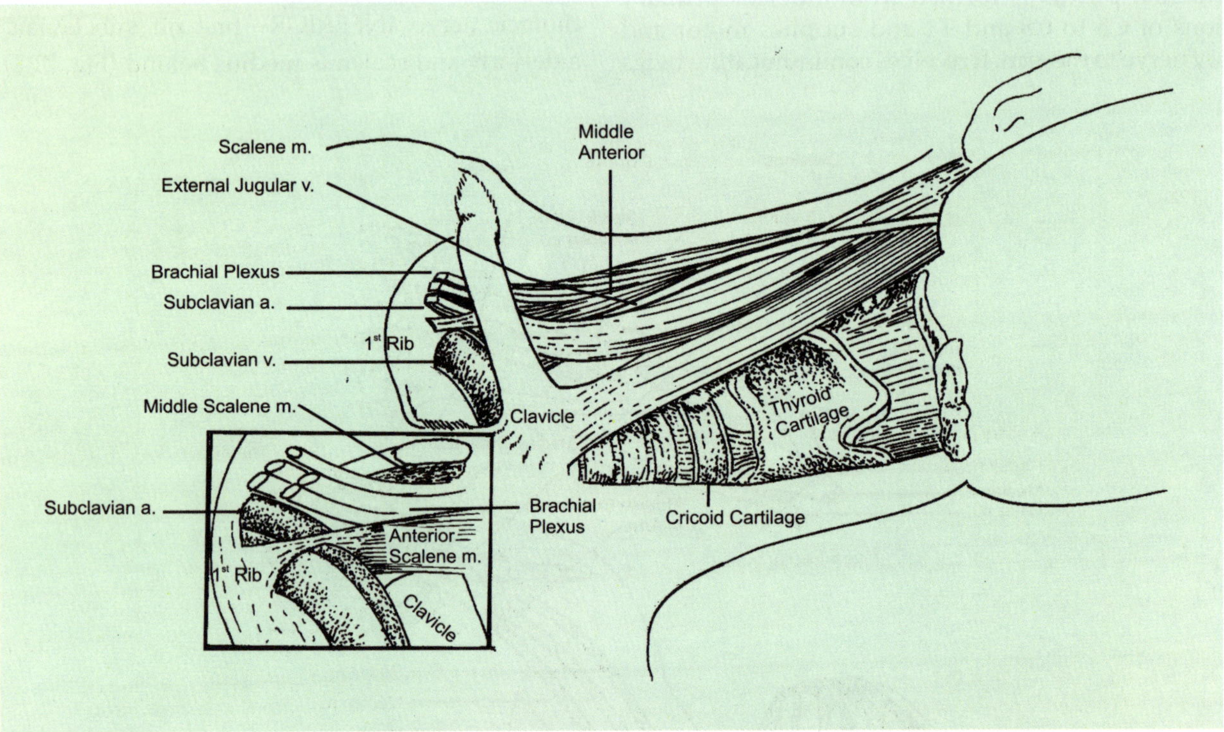

Fig. 71.2 : Relations of brachial plexus

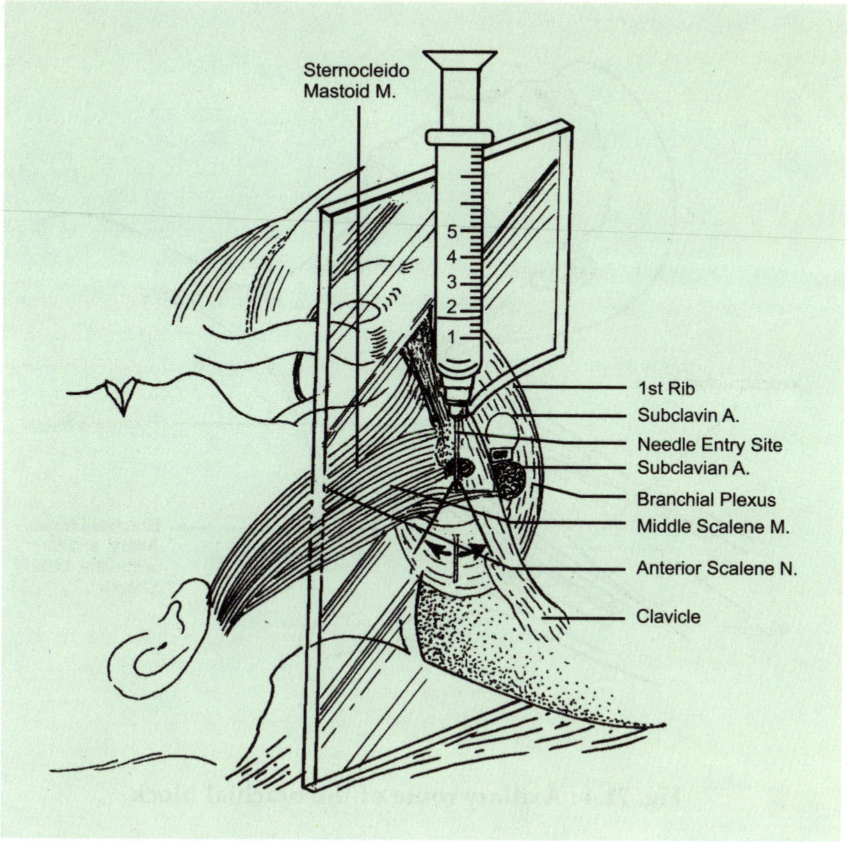

Fig. 71.3 : Supraclavicular block

Axillary approach of Brachial Plexus

The patient is supine with arm abducted to 90°, rotated externally. Axillary artery is palpated and traced as far as upwards in the axilla (B) (Fig. 71.4). A skin wheal is formed over this point and a 3-5 cm 25 SG needle over a local analgesic filled syringe is inserted at angle of 45° with the medial aspect of arm in a cephalad direction towards the apex of axilla. When the needle is felt to penetrate the sheath containing axillary artery, and 3 major cords of brachial plexus. A click is felt as the needle penetrate the sheath, advancing it a further 1-2 mm inside till paraesthesia are felt (Fig. 71.5). Local analgesic drug 30 mL is injected here after negative aspiration for arterial puncture. An 18 SG intravenous catheter can be introduced for continuous infusion for prolong surgery or pain relief. This technique spares brachial nerves leaving the shoulder above clavicle. There are other techniques described such as parascalene and suprascapular. The later can produce a transient disability due to paralysis of supra-and infraspinatus muscles. In children it is safe and easy to perform but nerves are superficial, so deep injections lead to failure. Musculocutaneous block is more frequent.

Anatomy and Technique of Elbow Block

Interdermal and subcutaneous circles of infiltrations are made just proximal to the internal epicondyle.[1]

Median Block

A skin wheal is raised mid way between the outer side of the tendon of biceps and the medial epicondyle or from a wheal 1cm medial to the brachial artery at the bend of the elbow. The needle is directed upwards, paraesthesia is elicited with 5 mL of local analgesic injected. The median nerve supplies lateral part of the palm and fingers.

Radial Block

A wheal is raised 1 cm lateral to the tendon of biceps at the line of bend of the elbow and the needle is inserted

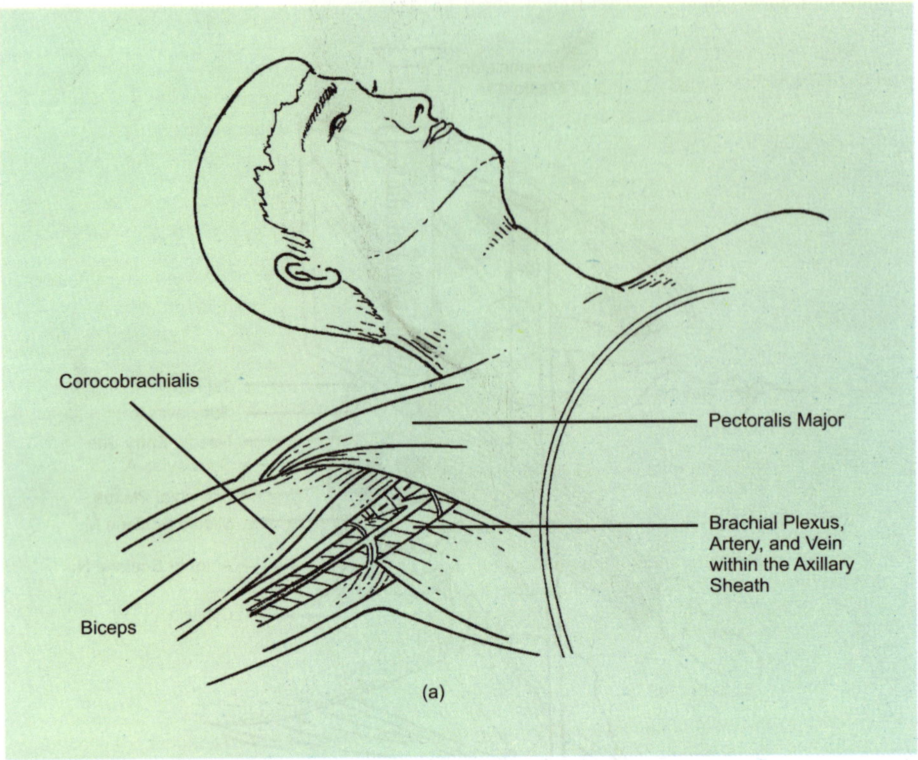

Fig. 71.4 : Axillary route of the brachial block

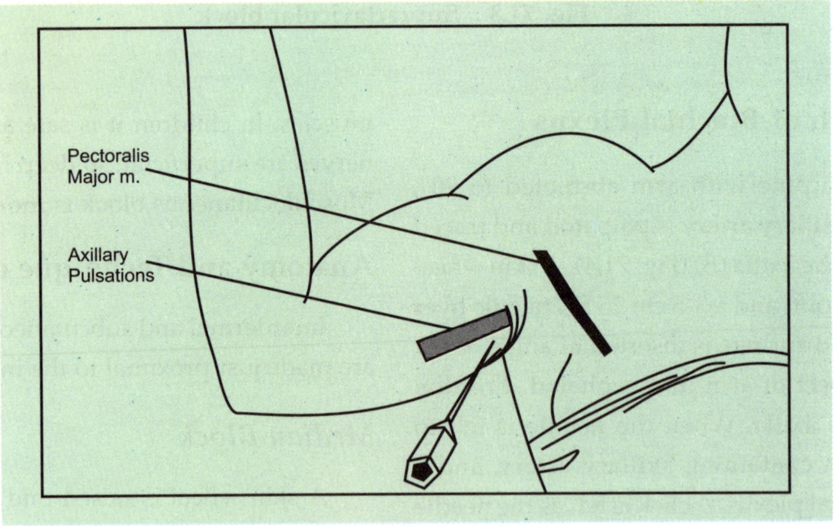

Fig. 71 : Technique of Axillary route of brachial plexus block

upwards to reach the front of the outer surface of the lateral epicondyle and solution deposited between skin and bone. (Fig. 71.6)

Alternatively, a wheal is raised 4-finger breadth proximal to the lateral epicondyle of the humerus, near its exit from intermuscular septum and is close to the bone. A 10 mL local anaesthetic solution can be injected.

Ulnar block is performed 2-3 cm proximal to the point where the nerve can be palpated behind the medial epicondyle, using 2-4 mL of 2% lignocaine or 0.5% bupivacaine. The ulnar nerve supplies skin on the medial side of the palmar and dorsal aspects of the hand and fingers (Fig. 71.7).

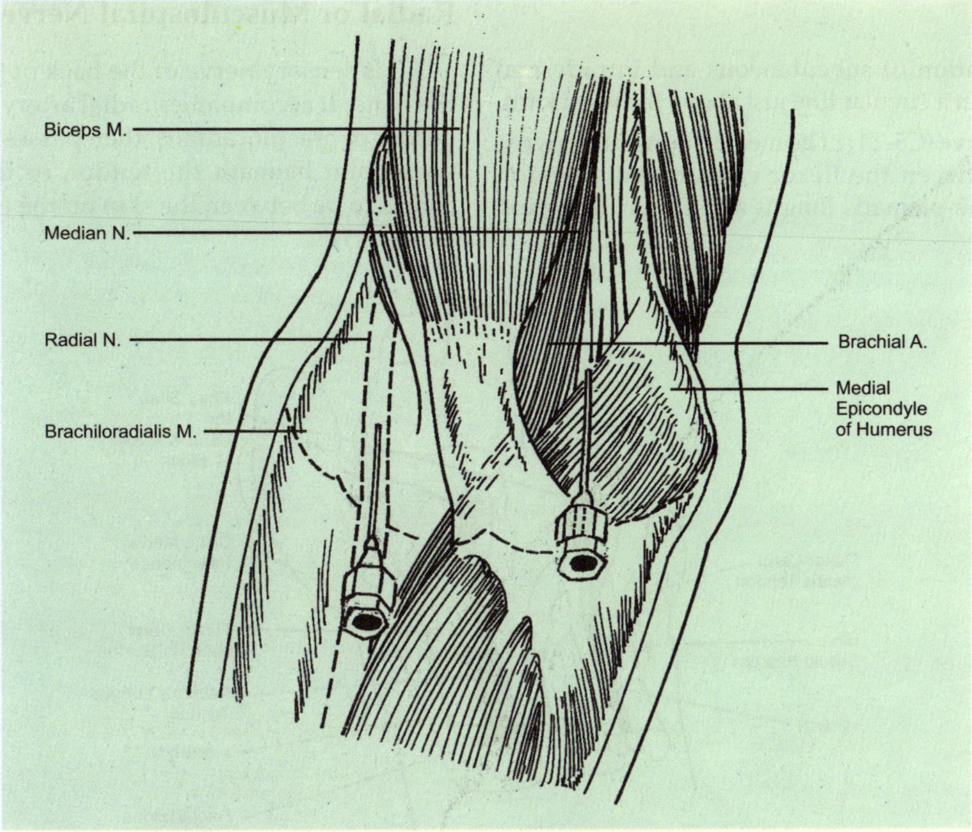

Fig. 71.6 : Elbow nerve blocks–median and radial n

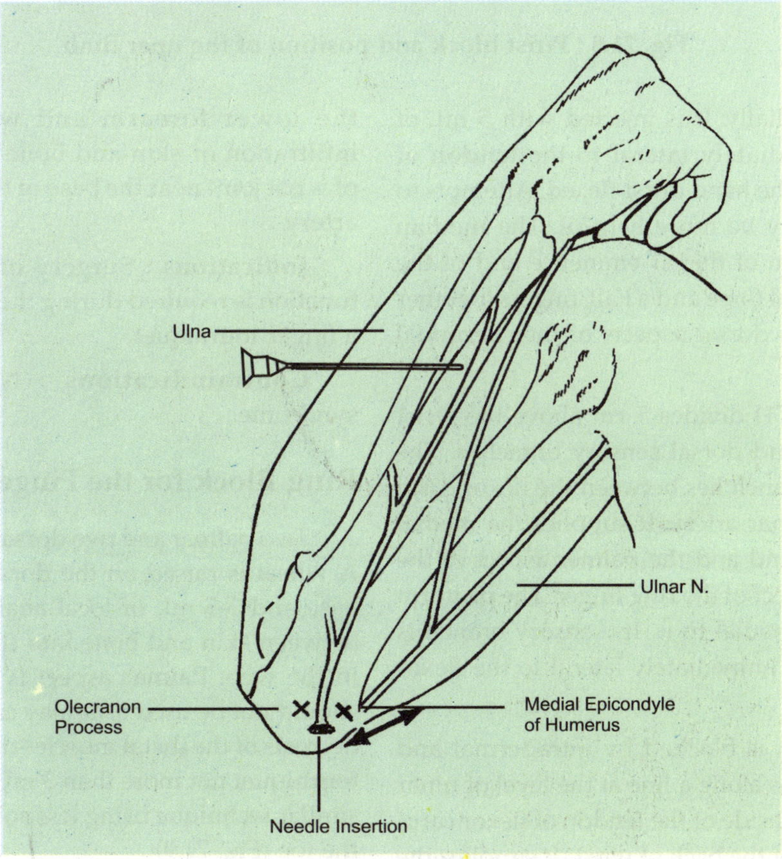

Fig. 71.7 : Ulnar Nerve block

Wrist Block

The infiltration of subcutaneous and intradermal tissues is done in a circular line just above the wrist joint.

Median nerve (C5-T1) : The median nerve at the wrist lies deeply between the flexor carpi radialis tendon laterally and the palmaris longus and flexor digitorum sublimes tendons medially. It is injected with 5 mL of local analgesic immediately lateral to the tendon of palmaris longus with the hand dorsi-flexed. Attempts to elicit paraesthesia may be more helpful. The median nerve supplies the skin of thenar eminence and of the anterior aspect of lateral three and a half-fingers together with the skin over the dorsal aspects of their terminal phalanges (Fig. 71.8).

Ulnar nerve (C7-T1) divides 5 cm above the wrist joint into superficial and dorsal sensory branches. The superficial terminal branch lies between the flexor carpi ulnaris tendon and ulnar artery. It supplies the medial part of the palm of hand and the palmer aspect of the fifth and the radial aspect of the ring finger. The pisiform bone is immediately medial to it. Its sensory branch is blocked from a wheal immediately lateral to the flexor carpi ulnaris.

The dorsal branch is blocked by intradermal and subcutaneous injections along a line at the level of ulnar styloid from the medial side of the tendon of flexor carpi ulnaris to the middle of the back of wrist. It supplies the ulnar border of the dorsum of the hand.

Radial or Musculospiral Nerve (C5-T1)

It is sensory nerve of the back of the lateral part of the hand. It accompanies radial artery along the medial border of brachioradialis, then passes 6-7 cm above the wrist joint beneath the tendon of that muscles and comes to lie between the skin on the extensor aspect of the lower forearm and wrist. It is blocked by infiltration of skin and bone on posterolateral aspect of wrist joint near the base of thumb lateral to the radial artery.

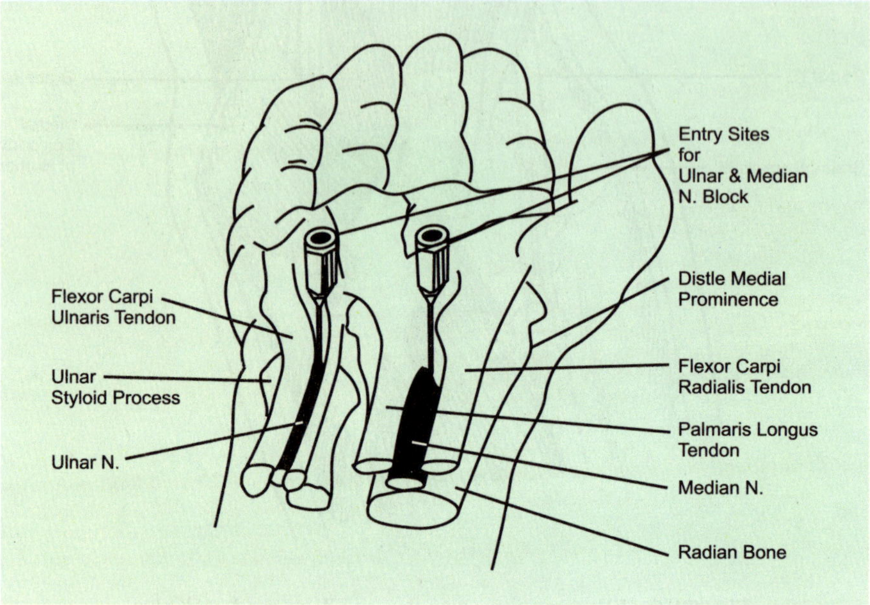

Fig. 71.8 : Wrist block and position of the uper limb

Indications : Surgery of hand especially motor function is required during the operation. It is used with a finger tourniquet.

Contraindications : Neuritis, carpal tunnel syndrome.

Ring Block for the Finger[3]

Two palmar and two dorsal nerves supply each digit. A wheal is raised on the dorsum of the finger near its base and 3-5 mL of local analgesic solution is injected between skin and bone into the substance of the finger in the web. Palmar aspect is not injected. Adrenaline should not be used as it may cause vasoconstriction and necrosis of the distal muscles of the fingers. With a finger tourniquet not more than 3 mL solution of LA is used. A similar technique using less solution can be employed in the toe (Fig. 71.9).

Contraindications : Raynaud's disease.

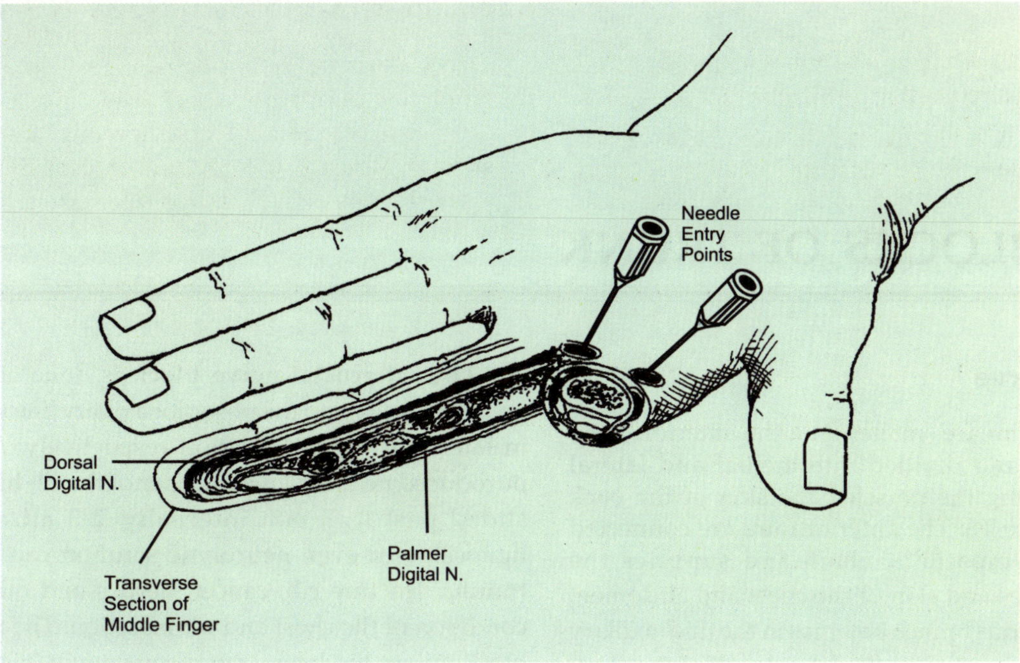

Fig. 71.9 : Ring block for fingers[4]

REFERENCES

1. Raj PP. Practical management of pain, 3rd ed,St louis,Mosby year books,1998.
2. Loeser JA, Bonica's management of pain, 3rd ed, Philadelphia, Lippincott-William and Wilkins,2001.
3. Wall PD and Melzack R. Textbook of pain (3rd) ed Edinburg: Churchill, Livingstone,1994.
4. Kumar Pramod, Atlas on peripheral nerve blocks, Jamnagar ISSP Con 2002.

•••

NERVE BLOCKS OF TRUNK

72

Intercostal Nerve [1]

The dorsal rami are smaller than the anterior. They turn backwards and divided into medial and lateral branches supplying the muscles, the skin of the back respectively above T6. The anterior rami are connected to the lateral sympathetic chain and supplies the intercostal muscles and skin of the chest and abdomen. The lateral cutaneous branch emerges in the mid-axillary line and supplies the skin on the lateral wall of the chest as far as the nipple line. The anterior cutaneous branch supplies skin in front of chain internal to the nipple. There are variations in this at 1st and 12th thoracic nerve level (Fig. 72.1).

The intercostal nerve block is done either at the angle of the rib or in the posterior axillary line with patient in lateral or supine position respectively. A needle is introduced near the lower border of the rib hitting it and slided past it, 3 mm internally. 2-3 mL of 1.5-2 % lignocaine or even neurolytic solution can be used in trauma, fracture rib, cancer, herpes and other painful condition of the chest and rib resection. The midaxillary block misses the lateral cutaneous nerve (Fig. 72.2).

Side effects : Pleural irritation or puncture.

Geriatric patients : The spines are fused so lateral approach is easier.

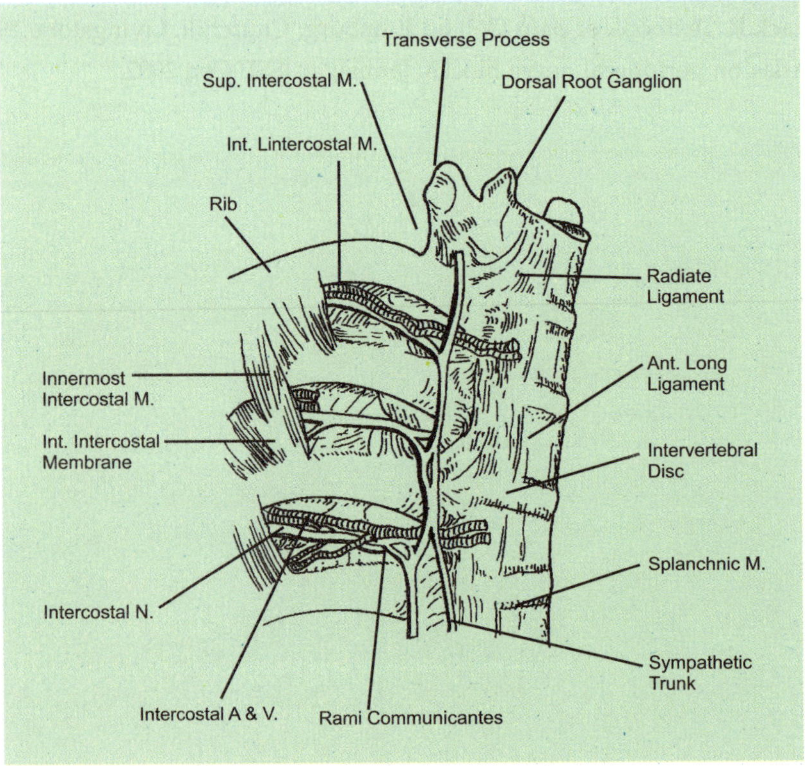

Fig. 72.1 : Anatomy and technique of intercostal nerve block

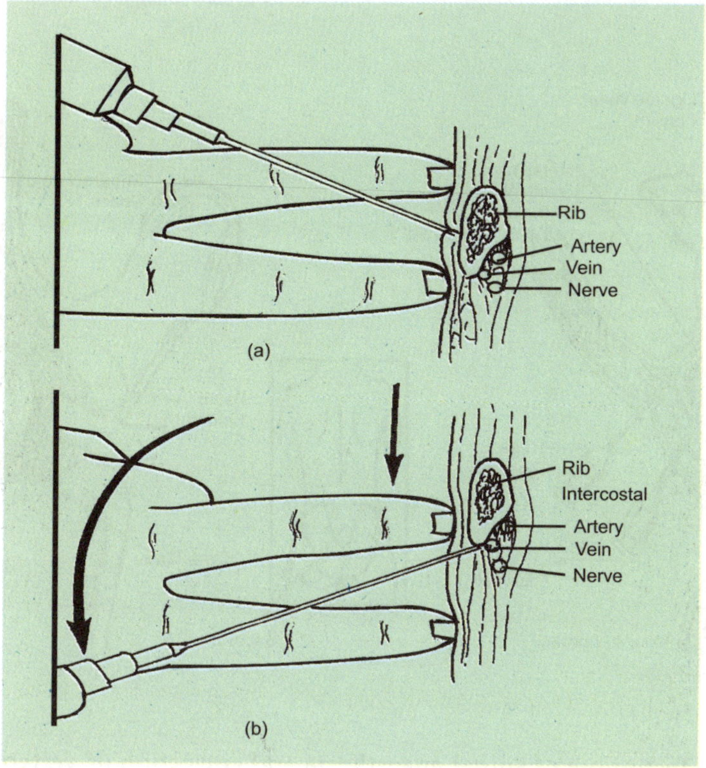

Fig. 72.2 : Cut section of the rib with the position of the needle in the mid axillary position (*a*) striking the rib (*b*) walking the rib

Techniques of Spinal Anaesthesia

Intrathecal injection: The patient in sitting or lateral position is painted and draped. A 25-27 SG lumbar puncture needle is introduced through an already formed wheal near the midpoint of lumbar vertebral spinous space. The needle punctures skin, subcutaneous tissue, supraspinous, interspinous ligaments and ligamentum flavum. There is loss of resistance to the needle which marks crossing the ligamentum flavum. In the lateral approach only ligamentum flavum is pierced. There is a click feeling as soon as the dura is punctured which is confirmed by a free flow of cerebro spinal fluid. Local analgesic 3-4 mL of bupivacaine 0.5% is injected through the needle and patient is made to lie supine with slight head up tilt to prevent reduction in blood pressure (Fig. 72.3).

Side effects : Hypotension, tachycardia, bradycardia, nausea, regurgitation, headache, respiratory depression, neurological problems, backache at the site of puncture. Later is due to trauma to the tissues and multiple punctures. It is a very common complaint especially in females which remains for many years, increase on bending and with change of weather. It responds to analgesics orally. The author has used epidural hydrocortisone and methyl prednisolone along with local analgesic and buprenorphine with limited success.

Epidural block is given using an 18 SG Touhy's needle which allows an epidural catheterization for prolonged analgesia and anaesthesia. The procedure is same except dura is not punctured as in spinal intrathecal injection. This block has the advantage of no headache and more controlled segmental analgesia. Its use in trained hand is better and safer.

Side effects : Same as intrathecal injections except headache. An occasional total/ high spinal due to accidental puncture which is treated by endotracheal intubation, IPPV with vasopressor if needed. Surgery should be continued as planned as the patient regains consciousness and respiration as the local anaesthetic effect wears off.

Vertebral column (cut section)[2] shows structure of a typical vertebral body, transverse process and spine. The ligaments coming across, along with intrathecal and epidural spaces are shown in the diagram. The piercing needle enters parallel to the spinous process through these ligaments, epidural space consisting of fatty areolar tissue, punctures the layers of dura into the subarachnoid space where CSF circulates. The cross section of H-shaped spinal cord is shown in the centre (Fig. 72.3, b).

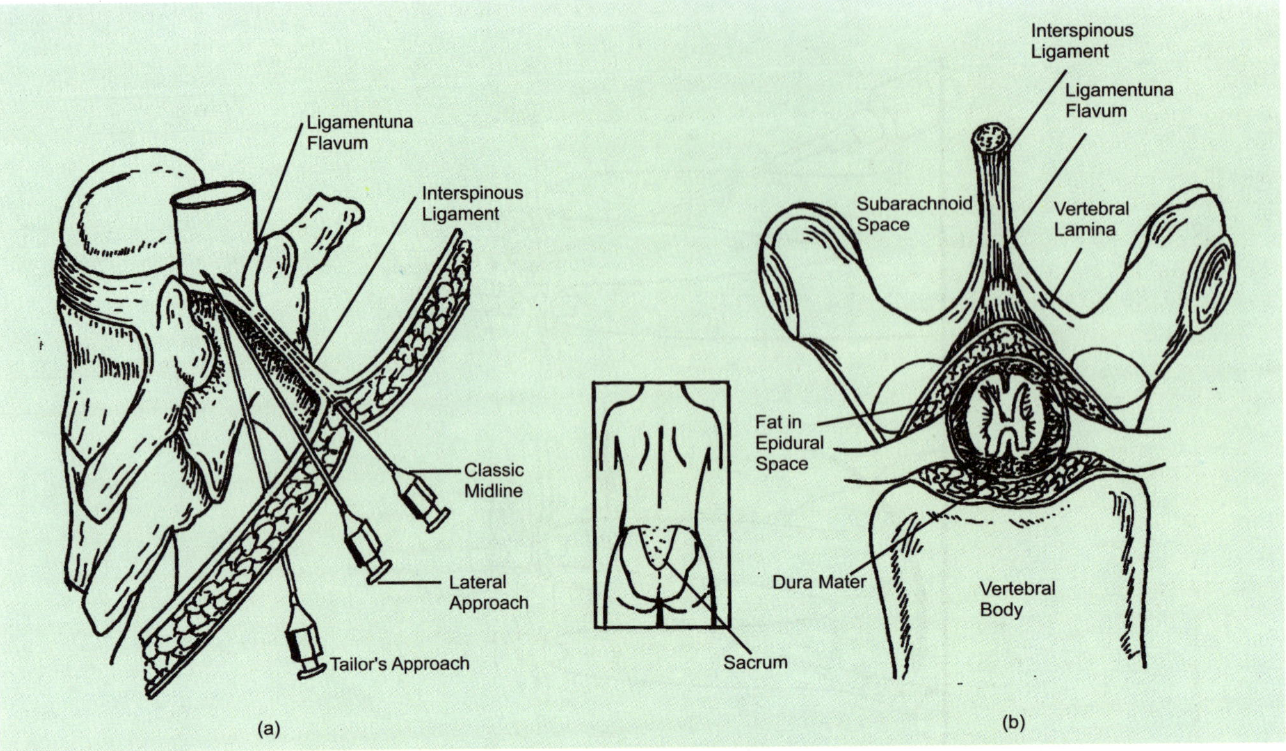

Fig. 72.3 : Technique of spinal anaesthesia and cutsection of vertebral column

Spinal Anaesthesia in Children

Children vary in size and anatomy. Dura and spinal cord are at lower levels in infants and epidural space is shallow. The epidural fat is looser, more areolar, so easy catheterization. The nerves are thin and incompletely myelinated, so onset of analgesia is faster with decreased concentration of local anaesthetic drug.

Anatomical Difference

Lower end of spinal cord is at L3 level in neonate, which moves upto L1 after 1 year of age. Dura is at the lower level S4 and moves upto S2 level after 1 year. The amount of CSF is 4mL /kg in neonate which reduces to 3 mL/kg in small child and 2 mL/kg in an adult. Skin to subarachnoid depth is 1.5 cm. Psychological fear is to be taken care in children.

Low plasma protein binding enables more of the drug to remain in the active form upto 2 years of age, so danger of LA drug toxicity which can be masked by general anaesthesia.

A 22 SG Quincke needle (3.75 cm) is used in children with 3 mg/kg of lignocaine. Spinal opioids can lead to respiratory depression, nausea and vomiting.

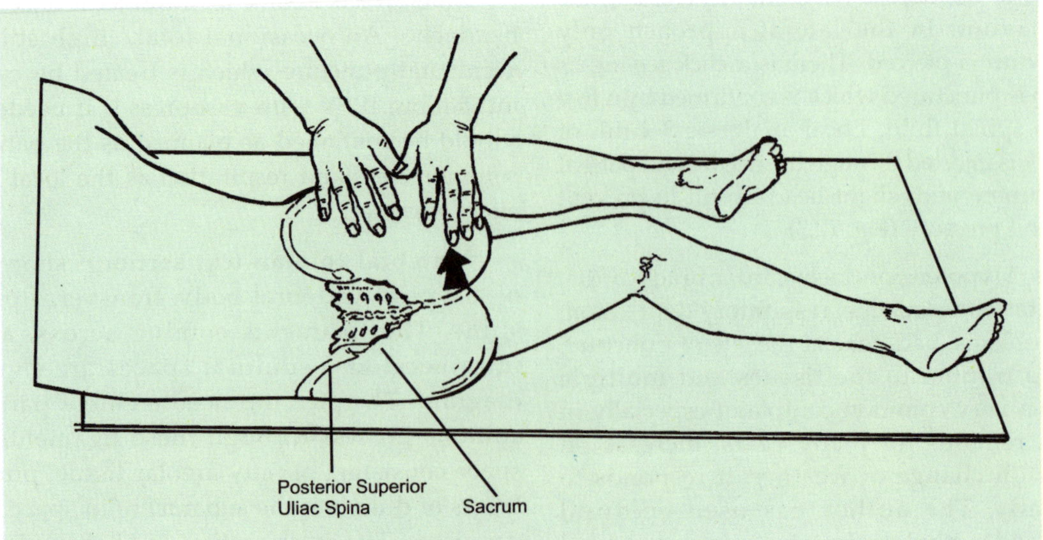

Fig. 72.4 : Caudal epidural block–lateral position

Caudal Epidural Block

Sacrum is formed by fusion of 5 sacral vertebrae articulating above with L5 and below with coccyx. Sacral canal runs through the length of the bone and terminates at the sacral hiatus which is covered by posterior sacrococcygeal membrane. The sacral hiatus is a triangular opening, caused by the failure of the fifth laminar arch to fuse. It has its apex upwards and sacral cornua on each side below and laterally. It is about 3.5 cm above the tip of coccyx directly beneath the upper limit of inter gluteal cleft. The average capacity of the sacral canal is 34 mL with a length of 10-15 cm. The local analgesic spreads upwards and some may leak through 8 sacral foramina (Fig. 72.4).

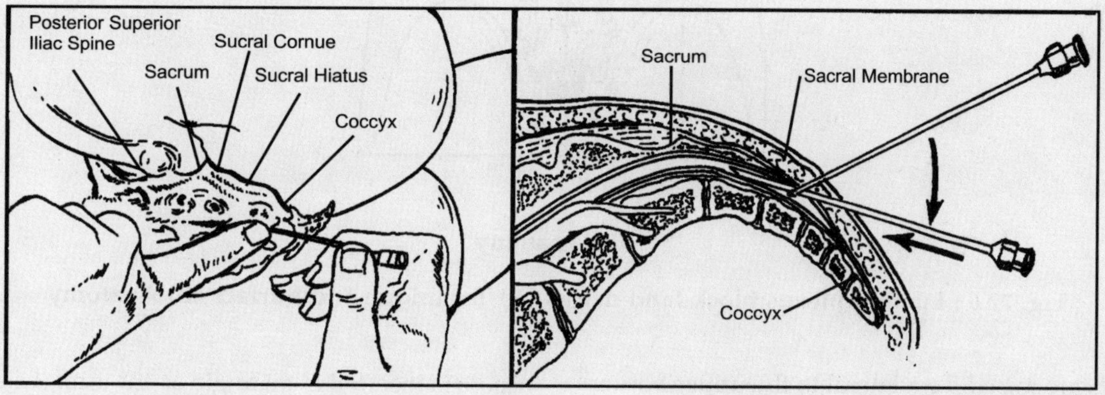

Fig. 72.5 : Technique of caudal block [3]

Technique of Block

With patient in supine or lateral position a wheal is raised over the sacral hiatus and entering the sacro-coccygeal membrane at angle of 45° to the skin (Fig. 72.5). Once the membrane is punctured the needle is depressed at an angle of 30° entering the sacral canal for 2-3 cm. After aspiration and feeling of crepitus, after air injection in the canal, after a test dose of 8 mL, the local analgesic solution is injected (upto 30 mL).

Indications : Surgery in lower pelvis, gynaecology, forceps delivery, orthopaedic operations, low back pain, pelvic pain.

Disadvantages : (1) Anatomical variations (40%), (2) lack of control of height of analgesia, (3) intrathecal injection (4) hypotension and (5) infection.

Lumbar Plexus Block [4]

Patient is in prone position with pillows flexing the lumbar spine or in lateral position with affected side up.

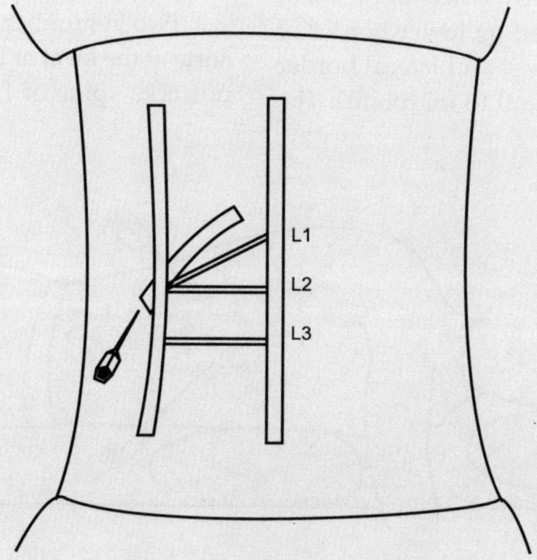

(A) Surface landmarks and Technique

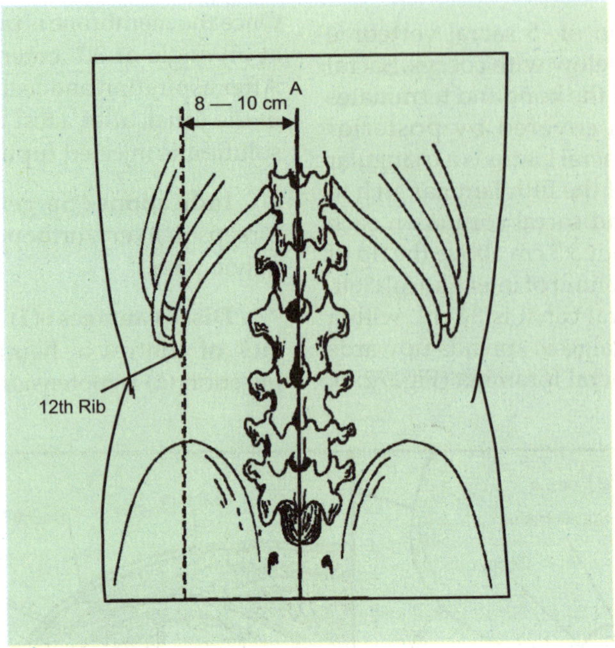

(B) Anatomy

Fig. 72.6 : Lumbar plexus block land marks (A) Technique and Surface (B) Anatomy

Skin wheals are raised 5 cm lateral to the upper borders of the spinous processes of L2, L3, L4 vertebrae just anterior to transverse process. A 15 cm needle is introduced through each wheal at right angle to the skin for 4-5 cm till it reaches transverse process. The needle is slightly withdrawn and directed upwards and inwards to pass in between transverse processes for 3-4 cm deep, to strike anterolateral aspect of the body of vertebrae. After careful aspiration, 10 mL of 1% lignocaine is injected at each side. In the lateral approach, wheal is raised at the apex of lumbar triangle formed by lower border of 12th rib, superior border of iliac crest and lateral border of paravertebral muscle (8 cm lateral to midpoint). The needle is inserted at an angle of 15° until it strikes body of vertebrae (Figs 72.6 and 72.7).

Indications : Raynaud's disease, Burger's disease, traumatic vasospasm, thrombophlebitis, delayed healing of fractures, causalgias, labour pain, renal colic.

Side effects : Intradural puncture, intravascular injection, shock, haemorrhage.

Caeliac Plexus Block

Two in number lying on each side of midline, on the aorta at the level of L1 vertebra. With the patient in prone position, spine of L1 vertebra is identified. Wheals are

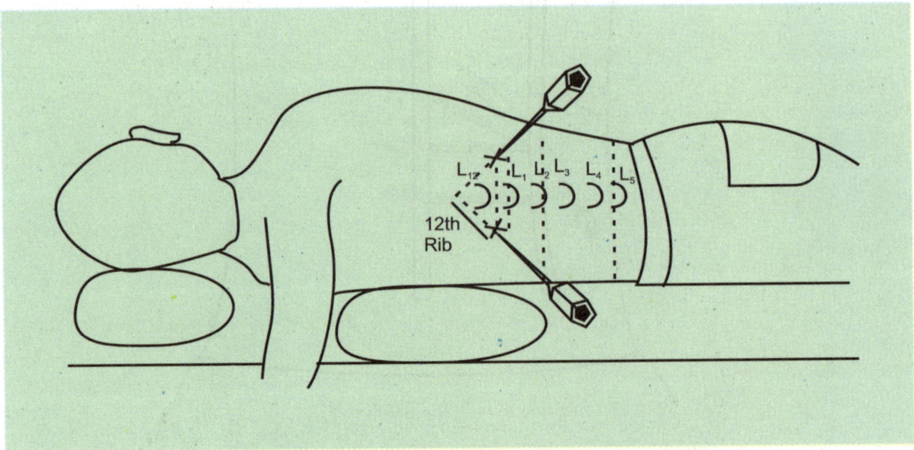

Fig. 72.7 : (A) Caeliac plexus block : The position of the patient and skin markings for needle entries

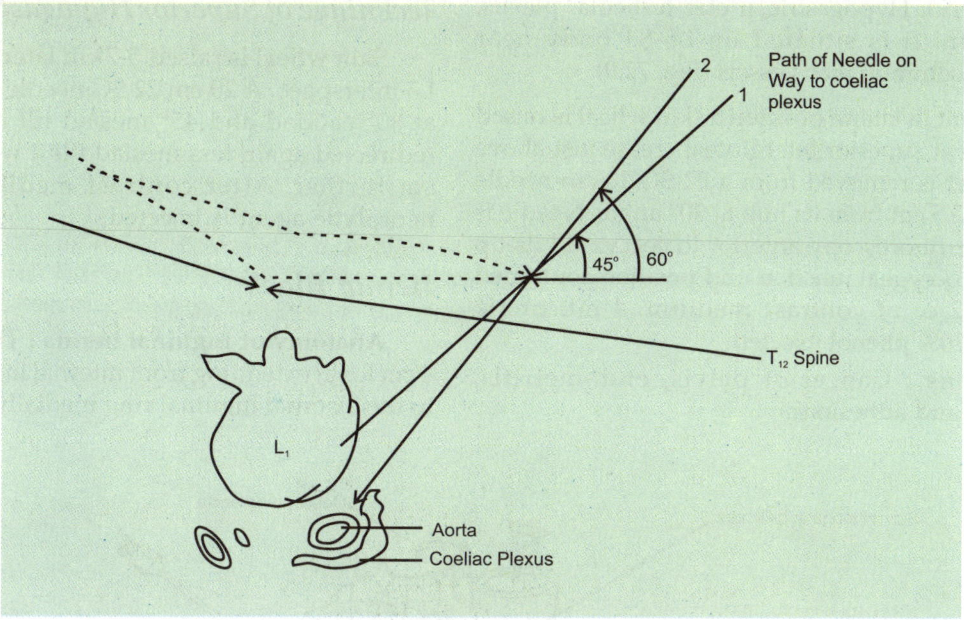

Fig. 72.7 : (B) Caeliac plexus block : Oblique section to show the path of the needle

raised four finger breadth from the spine on each side below the 12th rib. A 20 cm needle is inserted at 45° to the median plane, facing inwards and upwards. It strikes body of L1 vertebra, partially withdrawn and directed more laterally until its bevel glances past the L1 body for a further 1 cm for 7 cm. After a careful aspiration 10-20 mL solution of absolute alcohol (50%) or local analgesic is injected on each side. This block is given under sedation (Fig. 72.7, 8).

Indications : Acute pancreatitis, abdominal cancer.

Side effects : Hypotension, puncture of aorta, renal vessels.

Superior Hypogastric Plexus Block

This plexus is formed by joining of lumbar sympathetic chain, branches of aortic plexus, nervi erigentes (S2–S4). It divides into left and right branches

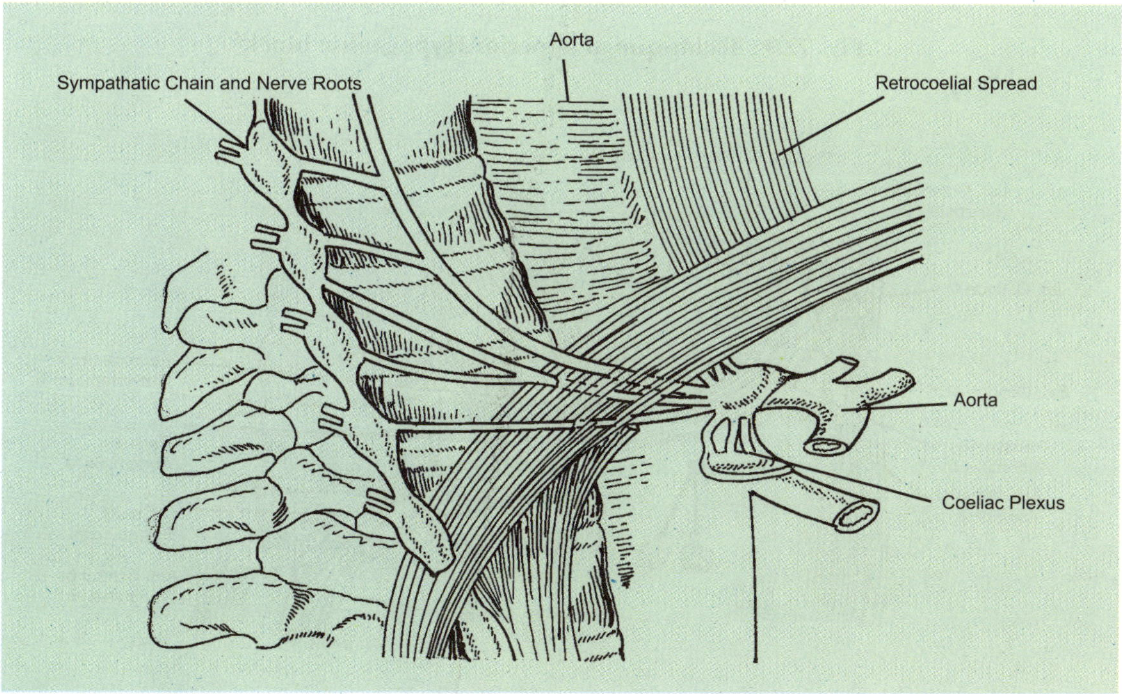

Fig. 72.8 : Anatomy of celiac plexus[4]

supplying inferior Hypogastric, ureter, testicular plexus, sigmoid colon. It is situated on L5-S1 body near bifurcation of common iliac vessels (Fig. 72.9).

With patient in lateral position a skin wheal is raised in the midline at superior intergluteal crease just above the anus. Stylet is removed from a 22 SG 10 cm needle which is bent 2.5 cm from its hub at 30° angle. Needle is inserted under fluoroscopy anterior to coccyx till its tip reaches sacrococcygeal junction and position continued by injecting 2 cc of contrast medium. 4 mL of 1% lignocaine or 10% phenol injected.

Indications : Cancer of pelvis, endometritis, inflammation and adhesions.

Technique of Superior Hypogastric Plexus Block

Skin wheal is raised 5-7 cm lateral to midline at L4-L5 interspace. A 20 cm 22 SG needle is directed midline at 30° caudad and 45° mesiad till it reaches L5 body, redirected again less mesiad till it walks off the body 1 cm further. After contrast medium confirmation, neurolytic agent is injected.

Hernia Block

Anatomy of inguinal hernia : The inguinal canal is 4 cm long, extending from internal inguinal ring laterally to the external inguinal ring medially. Former lies above

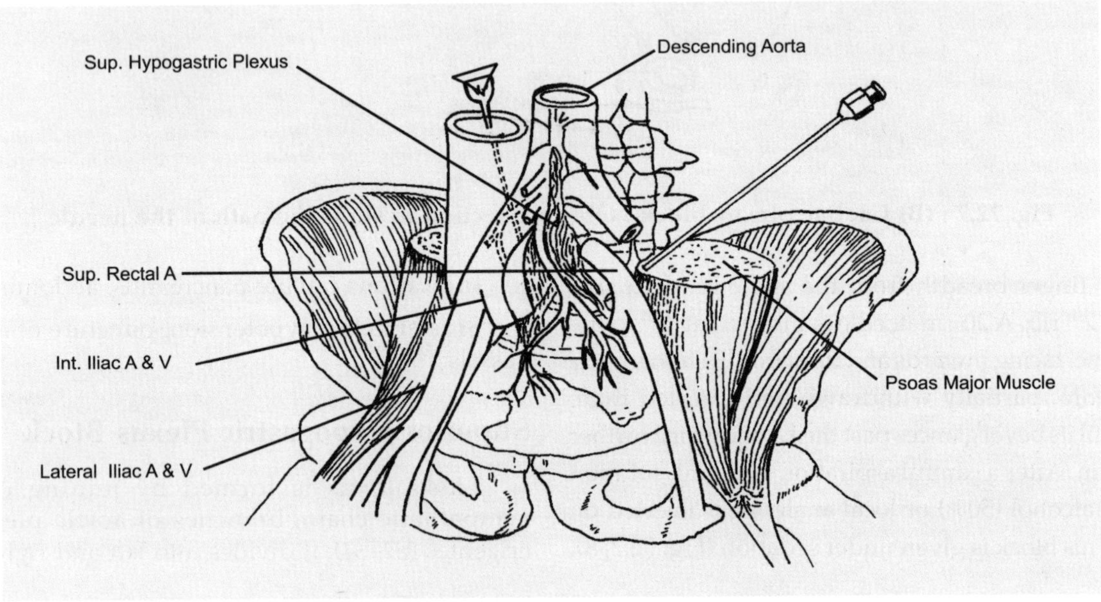

Fig. 72.9 : Technique of superior Hypogastric block[4]

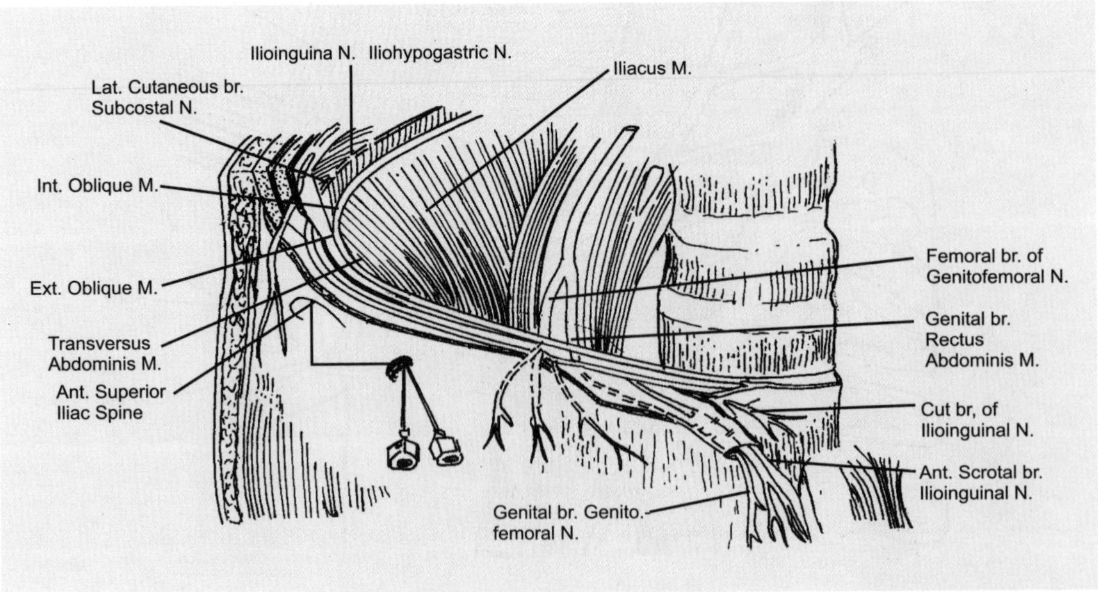

Fig. 72.10 : Inguinal hernia block [4]

the inner half of the inguinal ligament while the later lies above and lateral to pubic crest and through it passes the spermatic cord or round ligament (Fig. 72.10).

Boundaries

Anterior wall : external oblique, internal oblique laterally.

Posterior wall : fascia transversalis, conjoint tendon and reflected part of inguinal ligament medially.

Floor : inguinal ligament.

Roof : arching fibre of the conjoint tendon.

Contents : Ilioinguinal nerve, spermatic cord, round ligament and contents.

A hernia is indirect – congenital or direct through Hassalbach's triangle.

Nerve supply : Last two thoracic, first two lumbar nerves via Ilioinguinal, Iliohypogastric and genito-femoral nerves.

Technique

Three wheals are raised (1) a finger breadth medial to anterior superior iliac spine. (2) Over the pubic spine. (3) 1.5 cm above the midpoint of inguinal ligament. Through the first wheal the needle is introduced vertically backwards till it pierces aponeurosis of external oblique with a click and 10-20 mL solution is given to surround both Ilioinguinal and Iliohypogastric nerves. Through wheal 2 a needle deposits solution in the intradermal and subcutaneous layers in the direction of umbilicus. Through wheal 3, a needle is introduced perpendicular to skin until it pierces external oblique aponeurosis to block genital branch of genitofemoral nerve (Figs. 72.10, 11).

Indications : Inguinal hernia operations difficult in obesity, hernia mesh.

Femoral Hernia Block

Anatomy : A femoral hernia passes through the femoral canal and the saphenous opening in the deep fascia of the thigh, 3.8 cm below and lateral to the pubic tubercle. Femoral canal is the most medial of the three compartments, the most lateral containing the femoral artery and the intermediate containing the femoral vein. The femoral canal is 1.2 cm long and at its mouth is the femoral ring. The femoral ring is bounded in front by the inguinal ligament and behind by pectineus, laterally by femoral vein and medially by the lacunar ligament of Gimbernat, the pelvic brim is bounded by Ashley Cooper's ligaments. The ring contains the femoral septum or fatty pad (Fig. 72.12).

The coverings of femoral hernia are from within outwards – the fat from femoral septum, the prolongation of the fascia transversalis forming the anterior wall of femoral sheath, the cribriform fascia of the fascia ovalis.

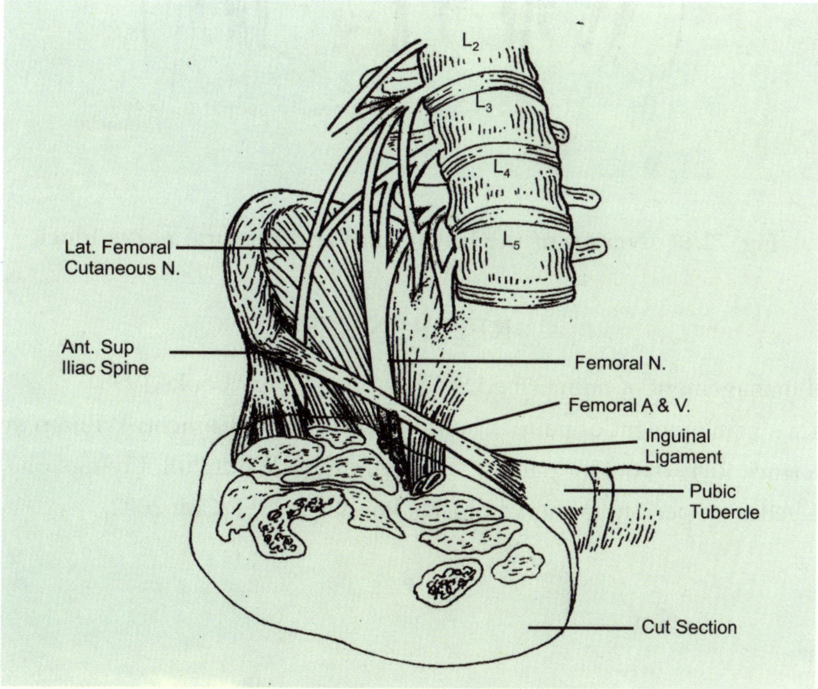

Fig. 72.11 : Inguinal hernia block [4]

Technique : The technique is similar to that repair of inguinal hernia, with addition that the lump in the thigh is surrounded by subcutaneous and intradermal wheals.

Paravertebral block from T10 to L3 may be carried out.

Indications : Strangulated herniae, both inguinal and femoral.

Femoral nerve block : A wheal is raised one-finger breadth in the outer ring of femoral artery, just below the inguinal ligament. A needle is inserted for 3-4 cm till the pulsations of the artery are transferred to the needle and 20 mL of 2% lignocaine is injected. The nerve lies beneath the deep fascia.

Indications : (1) Operations 5 cm below the patella and on lower femur when femoral nerve block is combined with sciatic nerve block.(2) For operation above the knee, lateral femoral cutaneous or obturator block.

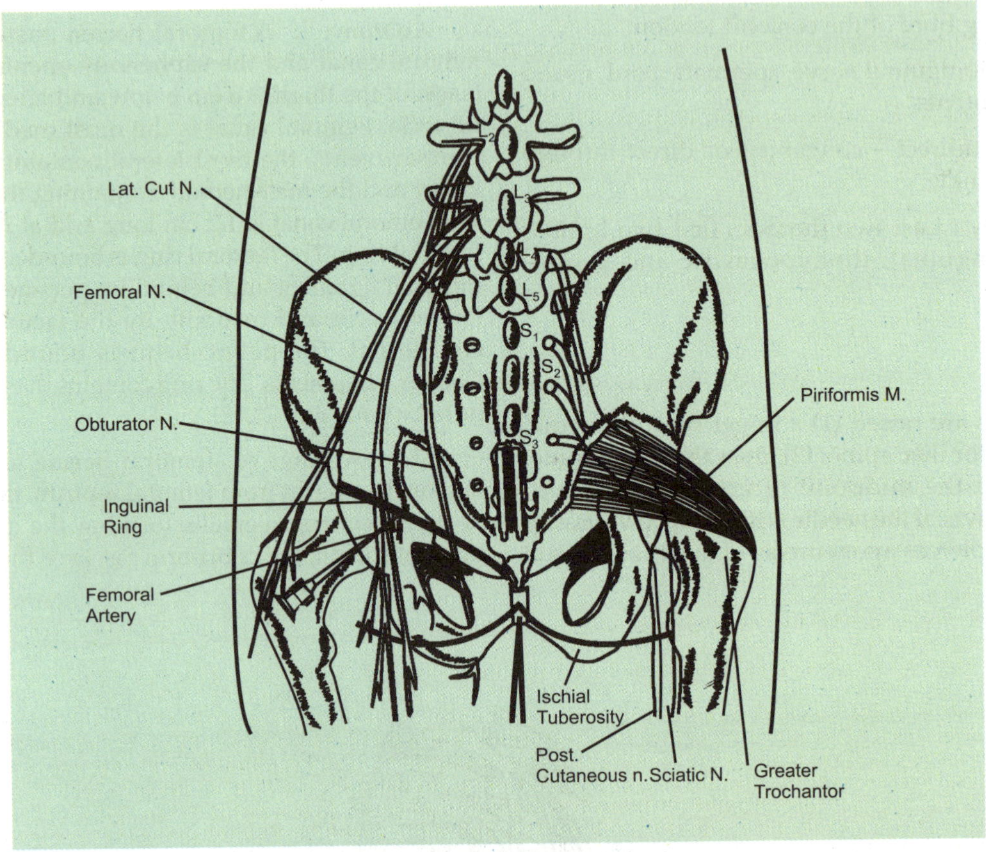

Fig. 72.12 : Nerves of the lower limb and Femoral nerve block

REFERENCES

1. Raj PP. Practical management of pain, 3rd ed,St louis,Mosby year books,1998.
2. Loeser JA, Bonica's management of pain, 3rd ed, Philadelphia, Lippincott-William and Wilkins, 2001.
3. Wall PD and Melzack R. Textbook of pain (3rd) ed Edinburg: Churchill, Livingstone,1994.
4. Kumar Pramod, Atlas on peripheral nerve blocks, Jamnagar ISSP Con 2002.

NERVE BLOCKS OF LOWER LIMB

73

Sciatic Nerve [1]

Leaves the pelvis through greater sciatic foramen under the pyriform muscle and lying between the ischial tuberosity and the greater trochanter. It is a nerve arising from sacral plexus. This nerve supplies the skin of the back of leg and the sole of the foot, after dividing into lateral and medial popliteal nerves in the popliteal fossa apex.

Pudendal Nerve

Also leaves pelvis through greater sciatic foramen, crosses the ischial spine and enters lesser sciatic foramen along with pudendal vessels. It gives branches to anus, rectum, clitoris and scrotum and its block is useful during labour.

Sciatic Nerve Block[2]

Anterior Approach (B) : In supine position the line of inguinal ligament is trisected into equal parts. A line is drawn parallel to above from the greater trochanter. From the junction of inner and middle third of inguinal ligament a line is drawn perpendicular to the lower line and a wheal is raised at this point. A 10-15 cm needle is inserted backwards and outwards till it meets the femur. A marker is placed 5 cm from the skin, needle partly withdrawn, redirected slightly medially just beyond the point where needle touched the needle, 20-30 mL of 1.5% of lignocaine / bupivacaine is injected in the area around the neurovascular space around the sciatic nerve (Fig. 73.2).

Posterior Approach (A) : Patient on lateral position with hip slightly flexed.(1) A line drawn connecting sacral hiatus with most prominent part of greater trochanter. A wheal raised at its mid point and needle inserted and 10-15 mL solution injected after eliciting paraesthesia. (2) A line is drawn between the upper part of greater trochanter and posterior superior iliac spine from the midpoint of this line, a perpendicular is dropped 3-5 cm long and a wheal raised at its end. A needle is introduced at right angle to the skin until it reaches the ischial spine, 5-7 cm from the skin surface. Paraesthesiae are elicited and local analgesic is given (Fig. 73.3).

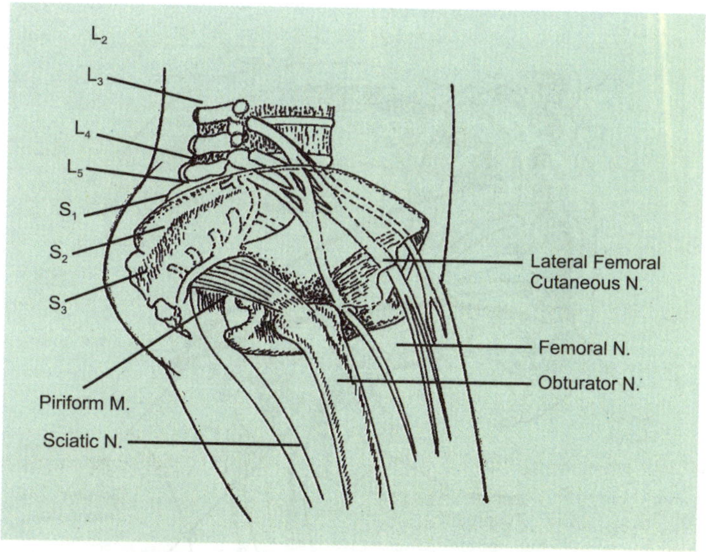

Fig. 73.1 : Origin of nerves of lower limb

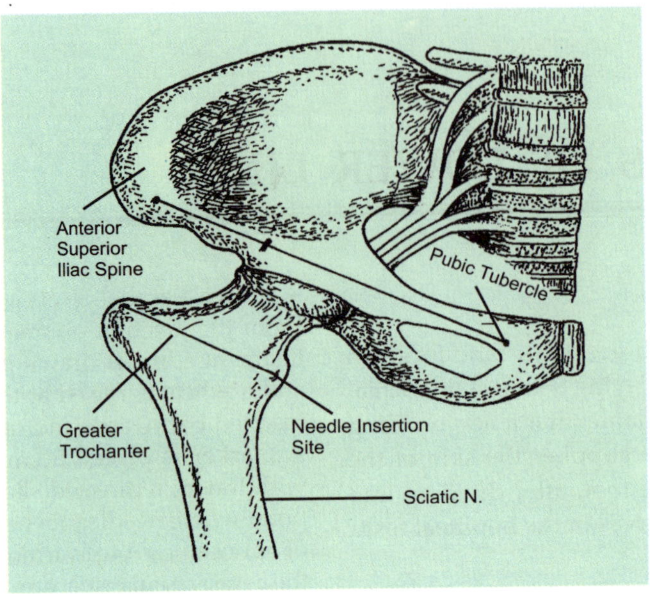

Fig. 73.2 (*a*) : Sciatic nerve block–Anterior approach

Indications : Fractures around the ankle, skin grafting, ligation of varicose vein in combination with femoral block.

Obturator Nerve Block

A wheal is raised 1 cm below and lateral to the pubic tubercle and a 5 cm needle introduced backwards until it strikes bone. As it is withdrawn 10 mL of solution is injected. An 8 cm needle is now inserted in the track of first one and moved laterally until it enters obturator foramen (2) where 10 mL of solution is injected. An additional 10 mL is injected while withdrawing the needle (Fig. 73.3).

Indications: Analgesia of lower extremity below the level of pubic symphysis when combined with sciatic nerve block, for fracture of femur, skin graft.

Lateral Cutaneous Nerve of Thigh Block

A wheal is raised 1-finger breadth below and medial to the anterior superior iliac spine. A needle is inserted perpendicularly to the skin and local analgesic (10 mL)

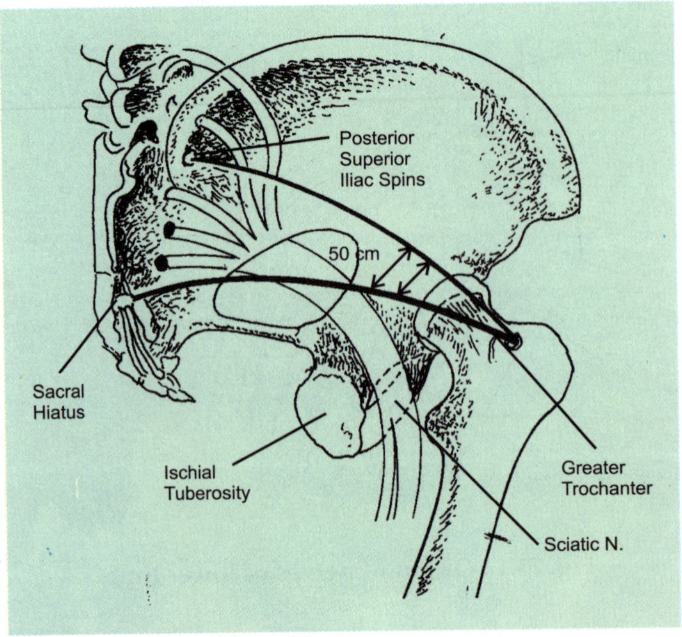

Fig. 73.2 (*b*) : Sciatic nerve block–Posterior approach

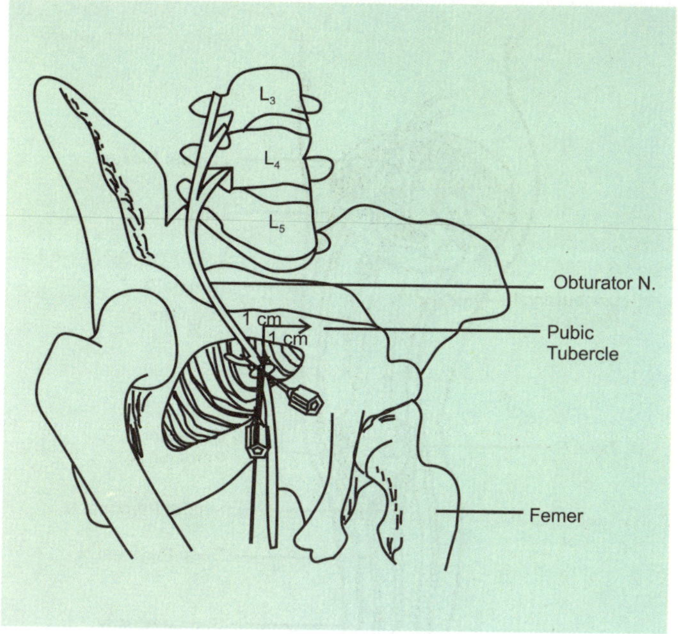

Fig. 73.3 : Obturator nerve block[3]

deposited between skin and iliac bone and along the pelvic brim for 2-finger breadth internally to the anterior superior iliac spine. The nerve lies deeper to the fascia lata of the thigh (Fig. 73.4).

Indications : Skin grafts of thigh when used with femoral nerve block.[4]

Nerves of the Lower Limb

The nerves of the lumbar plexus, (1) lateral cutaneous nerve (L2-3), (2) femoral nerve (L3-4) with twigs from L2 and L3, (3) femoral nerve with twig from L2, (4) obturator nerve (L2-3-4) (Fig. 78.1).

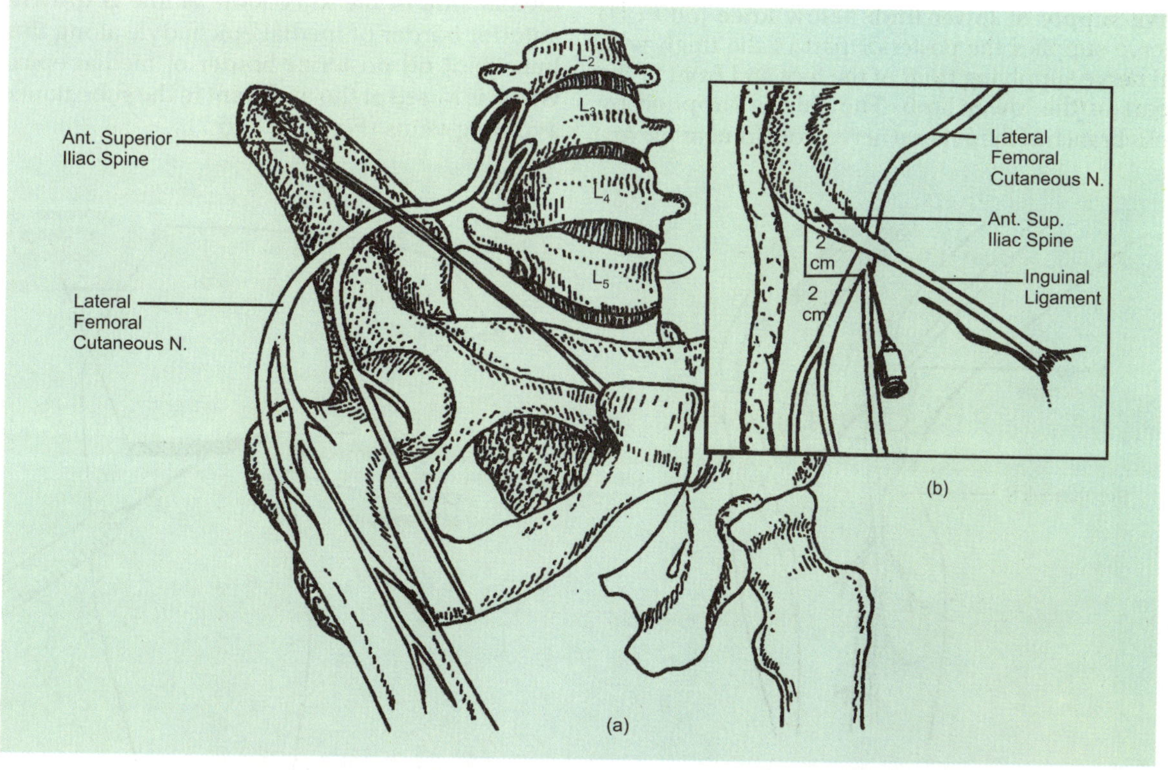

Fig. 73.4 : Lateral cutaneous nerve of Thigh (*a*) Anatomy (*b*) Block

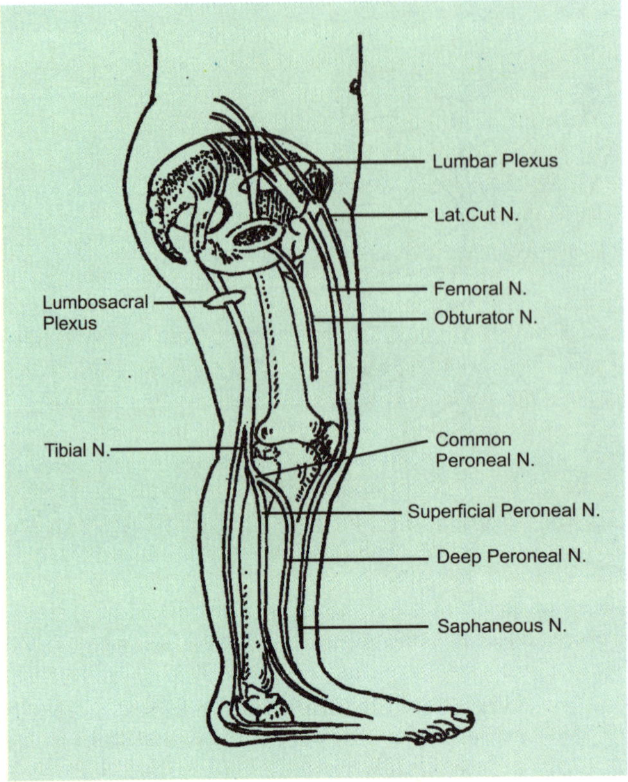

Fig. 73.5 : Lower Limb nerves

Nerve of sacral plexus (S1-3) : The nerves of sacral plexus are (1) sciatic nerve and (2) posterior cutaneous nerve of thigh. Showing the skin supply of the lower limb, the upper thigh by lateral cutaneous nerve of the thigh and obturator nerve (Fig. 73.5).

Nerve supply of lower limb below knee joint : (1) Tibial nerve supplies the posterior part of the thigh with peroneal nerve supplying front of the foot and front of the lower part of the lower limb. The shin is supplied by saphenous branch of the femoral nerve from lumbar plexus.

Saphenous Nerve Block at the Knee (with the patient in sitting position)

This is a terminal branch of the femoral nerve which becomes subcutaneous below the sartorius muscle at the medial side of the knee joint. A line is drawn from the anterior border of medial epicondyle along the crease of knee joint till posterior border of medial epicondyle. A wheal is raised at the midpoint in the subcutaneous tissue avoiding veins (Fig. 73.6 and 7).

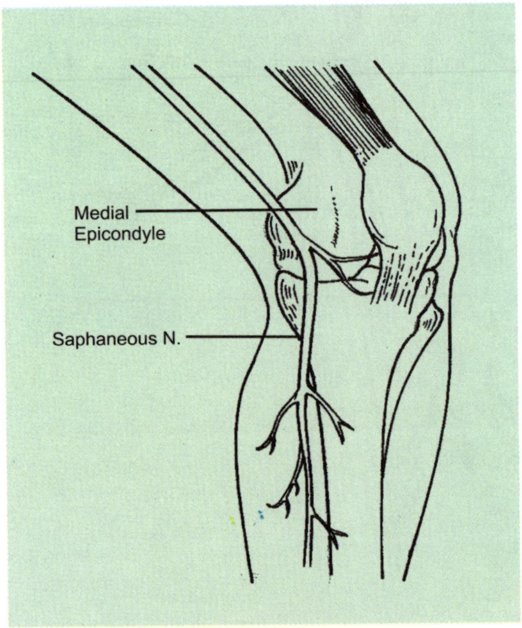

Fig. 73.6 : Saphaneous N

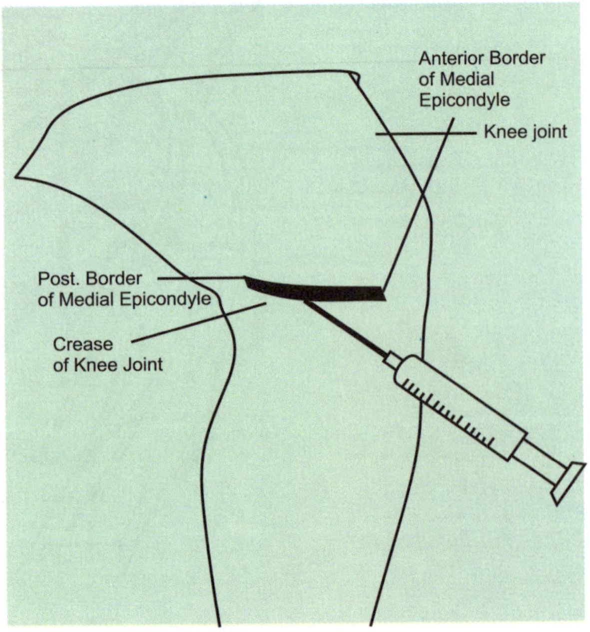

Fig. 73.7 : Saphaneous nerve block

Popliteal Fossa Anatomy

Popliteal fossa is a diamond shaped structure with sciatic nerve at the lateral border of the apex. The common peroneal nerve of the tibial nerve runs along the lateral border of the lower apex and is blocked there. The tibial nerve runs lateral to the Popliteal vein and artery and is blocked at the crease of the knee joint (Fig. 73.8).

the sole is supplied by the sural nerve, as shown in the (Fig. 73.9).

Ankle block : A subcutaneous and intradermal wheal is raised circumferentially around the ankle just above the medial malleolus.

Sural nerve is blocked on line joining medial and lateral malleolus. The sural nerve is blocked below and posterior to the lateral malleolus (Fig. 73.10).

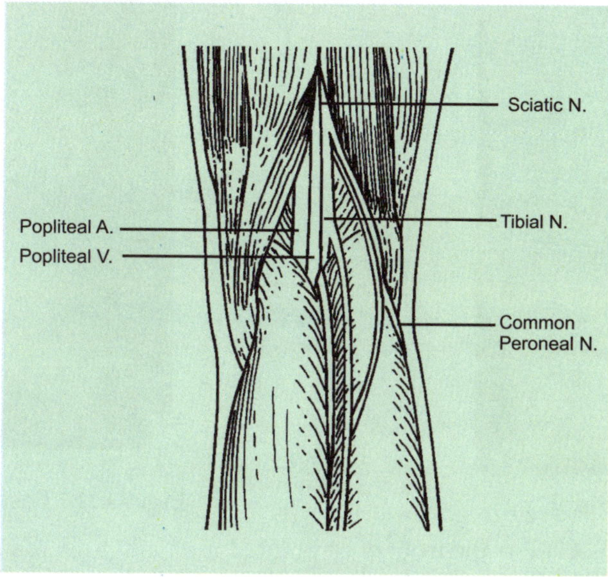

Fig. 73.8 : Popliteal Fossa Anatomy

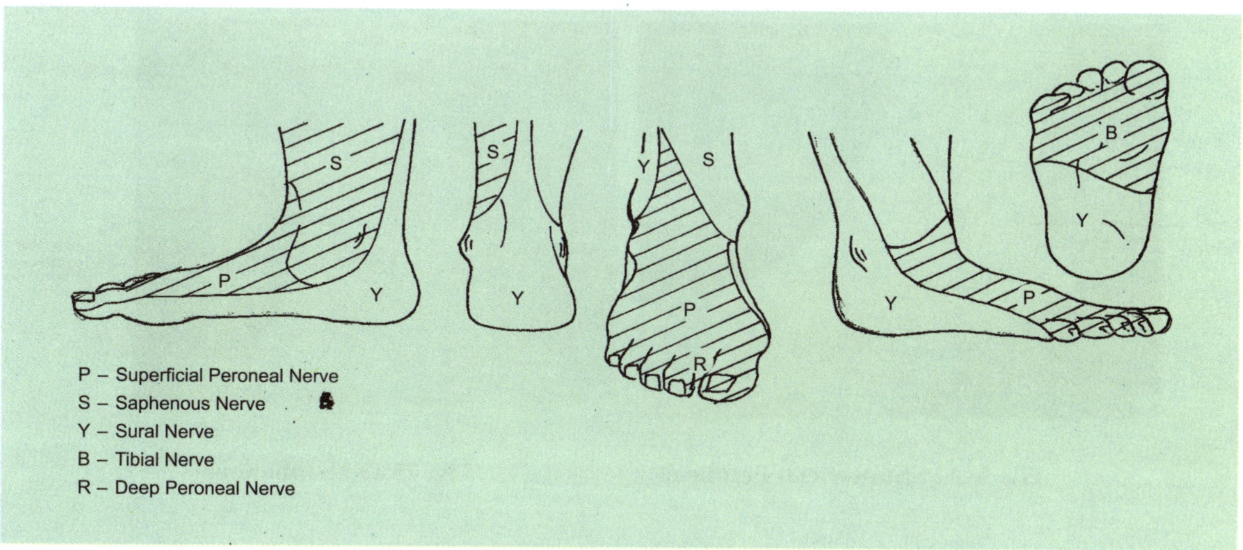

Fig. 73.9 : Cutaneous distribution of nerve of the foot

Cutaneous Nerve Distribution of the Ankle

The front of the ankle joint is supplied by deep peroneal and superficial peroneal nerve. The back of the ankle joint upto heel and the posterior sole of the foot is supplied by sural nerve. The anterior part of

Posterior tibial nerve is blocked through a point on the circular wheal just internal to the tendo achillis, deep to the flexor retinaculum near the palpable posterior tibial artery, with the patient lying in prone position. The nerve is blocked behind the medial malleolus near the bone using 10 mL of solution (Fig. 73.11).

The anterior nerve of the ankle joint is blocked with patient in supine position.

Saphenous nerve is blocked anterior to the medial malleolus using 10 mL of solution. It blocks the skin just below and above the internal malleolus (Fig. 73.13).

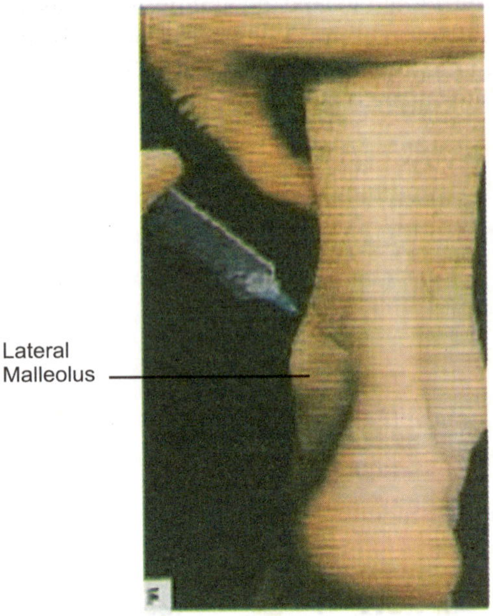

Fig. 73. 10 : Sural

Superficial peroneal nerve is blocked in the front of tibia above the ankle joint by a subcutaneous wheal extending from the front of the tibia to lateral malleolus. It supplies front of the foot (Fig. 73.12).

Anterior tibial nerve is blocked by inserting a needle midway between the most prominent points of the medial and lateral malleoli on the circular line of infiltration in front of the ankle joint. The needle is

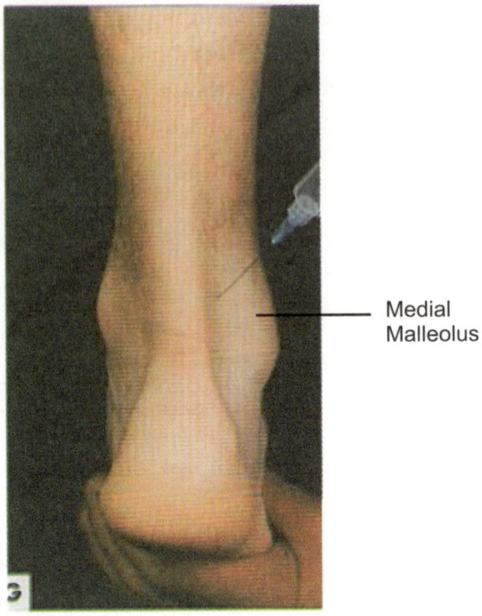

Fig. 73.11 : Posterior Tibial

pointed medially towards the anterior border of medial malleolus and the solution is injected between the skin and bone.

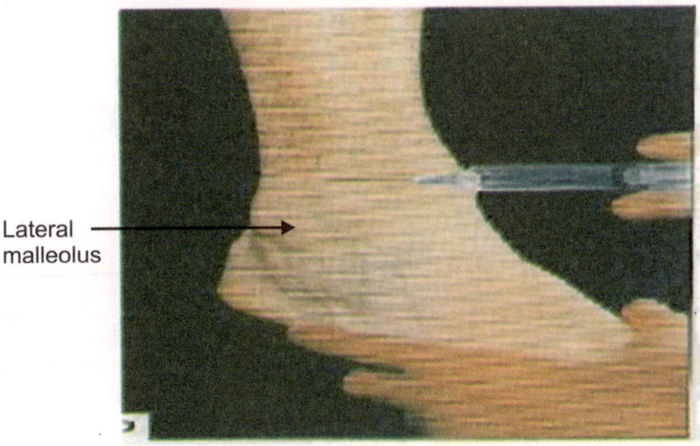

Fig. 73.12 : Superficial Peroneal

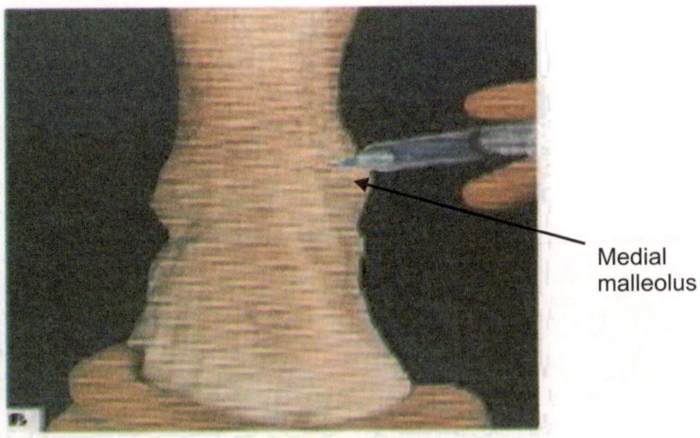

Fig. 73.13 : Saphenous

REFERENCES

1. Raj PP. Practical management of pain, 3rd ed,St louis,Mosby year books,1998.
2. Loeser JA, Bonica's management of pain, 3rd ed, Philadelphia, Lippincott-William and Wilkins,2001.
3. Wall PD and Melzack R. Textbook of pain (3rd) ed, Edinburg Churchill, Livingstone,1994.
4. Kumar Pramod, Atlas on peripheral nerve blocks, Jamnagar ISSP Con 2002.

•••

NEUROLYTIC NERVE BLOCKS

74

Management Consists of

i. Reassurance

ii. Pharmacological support

- Antidepressants (amitryptyline) in gradually increasing evening dose.

  It will reduce unpleasant anticholinergic, hypotensive and sedative effects.

- Tranquilizers – If muscle switching, anxiety are too much (given thrice daily).
- Analgesics – start with milder smaller doses.

iii. Referral to Pain Clinic – when moderately strong oral analgesics *e.g.*, codiene phosphate, have ceased to be effective. It may be due to increased intensity of pain, tolerance to analgesics or distressing side effects.

iv. Reassessement – once the patient has become physically dependent on a powerful opioid, it is difficult to assess the efficacy of the nerve block. Neurolytic block may not be satisfactory as the disease might have spread beyond the anatomic limits of the nerve block.

Primary aim of the neurolytic block is to keep the patient ambulant, maintain on oral mild analgesics, and maintain high moral, physical and mental well being of the patient and relatives.

Myths surrounding neurolytic block are:

- Neurolytic blocks are permanent, so answers all the pain problems.
- Neurolytic blocks are indicated as a last resort.
- Neurolytic blocks involve no side effects.

Indications for the use of neurolytic nerve block techniques to control cancer pain are:

- Pathological indications – Localised pain, absence of coagulopathies.
- Presuming that anticipated unexpected cardiovascular instability will not cause an increased risk.
- Tumour directed therapy failed to control pain.
- Pain poorly controlled with opioid analgesics.
- Increasing untoward side effects of oral therapy.
- Patient's behavioural and functional status will not be compromised.
- Patients and family members understand and accept the risk/benefit ratio of the procedure.

Types of Nerve block Procedures

- Non destructive procedures.
- Epidural or intrathecal use of opioids.
- Central neuraxial– epidural.
- Peripheral – somatic, intercoastal, sympathetic (stellate) block.
- Visceral – coeliac plexus nerve block.
- Destructive Procedure.
- Chemical neurolysis (alcohol, phenol) central, peripheral, sympathetic agents.
- Freezing by cryoprobe for Stump neuroma, Facet nerve.

Neurolytic Agents

Persistent chronic pain of malignant origin warrants nerve destruction with neurolytic agents. The commonly used destructive neurolysis is achieved by:

1. *Alcohol*

It is the classic neurolytic agent, used extensively in 50-95% concentration. It is hypobaric (sp gr 0.80) with respect to CSF (sp gr 1.1). Administered in dose of 0.5-10 mL depending on the site of injection. Very painful immediately after injection, but for short duration till neurolysis is achieved. Onset of pain relief achieved in days and duration of pain relief varies from weeks to months. Duration of analgesia over the distributed nerve involved lasts 6 weeks to 6 months but may be permanent.

Ethyl alcohol acts on the nervous system by extraction of cholesterol, phospholipid and precipitation of lipoprotein and mucoprotein. It scleroses the nerve tissue by its dehydrating action – typical Wallerian degeneration may occur. Myelinated nerve regenerates but small unmyelinated nerve fibres may be permanently destroyed.

Because of hypobaric property, the patient is positioned semi-prone during intradural block so that the affected segment is placed uppermost.

2. *Phenol*

Its primary effect is to coagulate protein.

Subarachnoid injection of 5-8% phenol produces mild meningeal irritation. Both segmental demyelination and Wallerian degeneration can occur. Used as anaqueous form of a solution in glycerine because glycerine diffuses more rapidly to achieve higher neurolytic concentrations and delays the release of active constituent phenol.

Dose 0.5-1 mL. Duration of analgesia varies between 1 week–3 months. It is hyperbaric to CSF so the patient is positioned semi-supine during intra dual posterior root back. Phenol in glycerine is prepared immediately before the block by dissolving phenol crystals in 10% glycerine, warming the crystals makes the solution easier to use. Being viscid a wider bore needle is used.

Aqueous solution is most commonely used with predictable effects.

3. *Glycerol*

Neurolytic property discovered accidently and rapidly led to use of the agent in treating facial pain specially percutaneous retrogasserian glycerol rhizotomy for the treatment of tic douloureux. 50% solution produces extensive myelin swelling and axonolysis.

4. *Ammonium Salts*

Action of ammonium chloride or hydroxide produces obliteration of C-fibres potential with only a small effect on A-fibres. Upto 10% concentration produces neither weakness nor loss of touch, pressure, pin prick and temperature sensibility. In man 0.5-1% solution is used. After injection there is an increased intensity of pain which subsides during the first 30 minutes. The neuralgic pain is relieved, zone of hyeperaesthesia contracts and disappears.

5. *Chlorocresol*

2% in glycerine (solution 1:40 or 1:50 chlorocresol in 0.5-1mL dose) used intradurally. Duration of analgesia lasts weeks to months. It does not produce any pain on injection, so anaesthetist must wait till pain disappears or for the onset of numbness to confirm the correct position of the needle.

6. *Hypertonic cold saline*

Osmotic swelling of the nerve bundle adding to the freezing action of lower temperature (<5°C) produce neurolysis. It selectively blocks C-fibres. The action lasts for few weeks. Very painful during subarachnoid administration, so GA has to be supplemented.

Subarachnoid Neurolytic Block

It is an effective method of pain control and is restricted ideally to patients with advanced malignancy with unilateral pain limited to few segments only. The aim is to produce chemical posterior rhizotomy and interrupt the pain pathways from the affected area.

Commonly used agents are Alcohol or Phenol.

Positioning of the patient places the affected side up or down, so that the neurolytic solution bathes the effected posterior nerve roots only.

Alcohol effect depends on

- Lateral oblique, semi prone (Fig. 74.1).
- Injection at spinal cord/vertebral level.
- Affected segment/volume/rate.

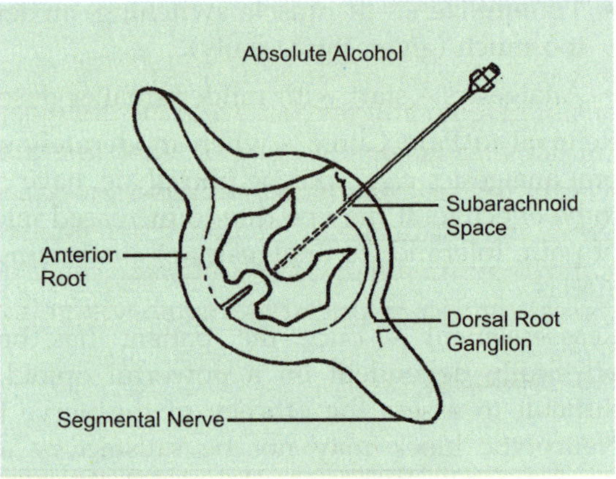

Fig. 74.1 : Subarachnoid alcohol injection

Phenol in glycerine hyperbaric used as

- 5-6% solution in glycerine;
- lateral oblique/semi supine (Fig. 74.2).
- acts on nerve roots just before right pierces the dura;
- vertebral level;
- initial local anaesthetic action - warmth, tingling, pricking sensation.

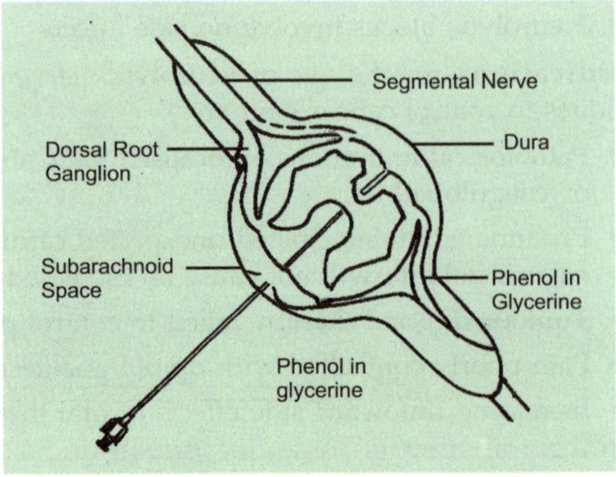

Fig. 74.2 : Subarachnoid phenol injection

Success of subarachnoid neurolytic block depends on

- Precise placement of solution.
- Correct use of posture.
- Minimum effective dose.

Epidural Neurolytic Nerve Block

Not commonly used, however, epidural injection of 5-10% phenol in saline has been used in chronic cancer pain, specially in patients with bilatral pain without major motor weakness.

Complications

Complications of intrathecal neuroloysis are primarily bladder, bowel involvement and motor paresis. So if the bladder and bowel functions are intact, epidural or intrathecal morphine or percutaneous cordotomy may be preferred. Commonly seen complications are:

- Failed block.
- Sphincter disturbances.
- Retention of urine with overflow, incontinence.
- Alcohol neuritis.

Concentration of Neurolytic Blocks

Long acting local anaesthetical bupivacaine blocks can be useful in progonosticating the results of the neurolytic blocks planned. This will enable the patient to feel the sensation of numbness that will be associated with subsequent neurolysis and also prognosticate dysfunction.

Injection of various concentrations of neurolytic agents intrathecally or epidurally or into the ganglia and peripheral nerves have been used for more than six decades.

Drugs most commonly administered are – alcohol, phenol, glycerol. Concentration and the volume needed for nerve block will depend on the site of injection. Nociceptive pain must be differentiated from deafferentated pain by neurologic examination and difference in chemcial neuroloysis (Table 74.1).

Table 74.1 : Concentrations of alcohol and phenol used in neurolytic blocks

Type of Neurolytic block	Concentration (%)	
	Alcohol	Phenol
Intrathecal	100	4-15 in glycerol
Epidural	30	10 in 10% glycerol, 7 in water
Coeliac plexus	50	
Sympathetic ganglion	50	10 in 10% glycerol
Pituitary	100	7 % in water

The type of neurolytic blocks performed will depend on the site of injection as well as the pathophysiology of pain.

1. **Neurosurgical procedures** for the management of cancer pain are reserved for those patients unresponsive to other less invasive procedure.

These can be:

- Neuro ablative procedures – Interrupt pain transmission along the nerve pathway.
- Cordotomy – Open and percutaneous interruption of spinothalamic tract in the spinal cord.
- Treatment of unilateral pain involving upper or lower extremity or thoracic region.
- Few patients with limited life expectancy.
- Percutaneous route better with 6% perioperative morbidity or mortality.

Table 74.2 : Various types of nerve blocks used in the body

Region	Nociceptic pain	Deafferentation pain
Head and neck	Somatic block of peripheral nerves	Upper and middle cervical ganglion block
Upper extermity	Cervical epidural or intrathecal	Stellate ganglion block
Chest wall/Pleura	Intercostal nerve/thoracic epidural/ intrathecal	Thoracic epidural/ intrathecal
Abdomen/Viscera	Coeliac plexus block intercostal nerve/thoracic epidural/intrathecal	Coeliac plexus block
Lower extremities	Intrathecal phenol epidural/ intrathecal morphine	Lumbar sympathetic
Perineum	Intrathecal phenol/alcohol epidural/ intrathecal morphine,	Caudal block caudal block

– **Dorsal Rhizotomy**

Interruption of the sensory nerve roots (open or by a neurolytic agent).
Localised pain to a specific dermatome level.

2. **Neuro stimulatory procedure neuropathway**

Operations during which electrodes are placed for electrical stimulation of portion of CNS.

REFERENCES

1. Raj PP. Practical management of pain, 3rd ed,St Louis,Mosby Year Books.1998.
2. Loesser JA, Bonica's management of pain, 3rd ed, Philadelphia, Lippincott-William and Wilkins, 2001.
3. Wall PD and Melzack R. Textbook of pain (3rded), Edinburg Churchill-Livingstone, 1994.

•••

REGIONAL ANAESTHESIA AND ANALGESIA IN CHILDREN AND NEONATES

75

Introduction

Bier in 1899 used spinal anaesthesia in a 11-year old. The reasons for under utilization of regional block are lack of experience, fear of adverse effects and lack of patient co-operation. By 1990 there was an increased awareness about regional blocks due to better postoperative analegsia, faster ambulation and less side effects. The use of general anaesthesia before regional block takes care of patient's cooperation.

The paediatric regional anaesthesia have the advantages of early ambulation, longer lasting pain relief and less intra-operative anaesthetic requirements.

Perception of Pain

C-fibres are fully functional since early foetal life so motivational-directive pain (slow or true pain) is perceived well. However, cognitive evaluative component is not fully developed due to thinly myelinated a delta-fibres. This is influenced by environmental, socio-cultural, and individual past experiences of pain. Apart from communication, a major difficulty is assessment and identification of pain in early age.

General Considerations

Children vary in size and anatomy. Dura and spinal cord reach lower level in infants and epidural space is shallow. The fat in the epidural space is looser, more areolar, so easy catheterization. The ligaments and fasciae offer less resistance to the needle tip. The nerves are thin and incompletely myelinated, so onset is faster with decreased concentration of LA. Parental acceptance is high (90%) but child appears to be restless (40%).

Physiological and Psychological Considerations

Stress response to surgery is depressed. Central nerve blocks are well tolerated with little haemodynamic change. So preloading with saline is not advised in children.

Children are frightened by new environment, and cannot distinguish between adjacent parts of their body *e.g.*, forearm with arm, there is no concept of paraesthesia and that of differential block, so localization of a nerve is achieved with a nerve stimulator.

A pain free post-operative period helps the psychology of the patient, parents and medical team. Occasionally persistence of motor or sensory block may prove frightening to some children, which can be taken care of by a careful explanation.

Table 75.1 : Anatomical Difference in Children from Adults

Anatomy variable	Neonate	Small child	Adult
Lower end of spinal cord	L3	L1	L1
Dura	S4	S2	S2
CSF/Kg	4 mL	3 mL	2 mL
Epidural fat	Loose	Loose	Firmly packed

Toxicity of LA in Children

Low plasma protein binding enables more of the drug to remain active (till 1 year of age). Neurological toxicity occurs at lower concentration. Reduced metabolism due to decreased plasma pseudo cholinesterase and decreased hepatic microsomal activity. Larger cardiac output leading to increased concentration and shorter duration. General anaesthesia may mask the signs of LA toxicity.

Indications of Sole Regional Anaesthetic

- Premature infants requiring surgery below umbilicus.
- Risk of post-operative apnea–Neuromascular disease.
- Chronic airway or pulmonary diseases *e.g.*, tracheomalacia, asthma.

- Malignant hyperthermia.
- Post-operative, malignant and vascular spastic pain.

Contraindications

Infection, bleeding disorders, allergy, uncorrected hypovolemia, vertebral anomalies, degenerative compressive neuronal disorders and parents' refusal. The medicolegal aspects must be taken care of in paediatric patients and complications, if any, must be immediately treated. Monitoring with precordial stethoscope, blood pressure, ECG and SaO_2 etc. is mandatory.

Specific Blocks in Children–Caudal Analgesia[2]

Easy to perform and reliable upto 10 kg BW. More cardiovascular stability. Rare but serious complications as with any regional block. In awake patients psychological trauma and restlessness present.

Anatomy : Sacrum is formed by the fusion of five vertebrae. Sacral hiatus is the result of non-fusion of 5th vertebral arch. Large bony prominences on either side are sacral cornua. Sacral hiatus more cephalad, dural sac nearer.

Technique : In lateral position identify the hiatus by finger between cornua. Taking antiseptic precautions a 23 G, 2.5 cm long needle over syringe filled with LA, is placed midline at 60 degree to coronal plane. Needle is advanced ventrally till sacrococcygeal membrane is punctured. Then lower the needle to a 20 degree angle and advance 2–3 minutes. After negative aspiration 0.5-0.75 mL/kg LA is injected. Analgesics used are buprenorphine and clonidine.

Continuous Caudal in Children

Easier cephalad access than lumbar epidural and is less traumatic to spinal cord. 20 G Tuohy needle or Crawford needle (3.75-5 cm) with 24 G catheter or 22 g IV catheter over needle is used.

Lumbar Epidural Block

Used as an adjunct to general anaesthesia (GA) for post-operative (P.O.) analgesia. Less chances of faeco-urinary contamination as in caudal. Depth of epidural space from skin increases with age (10–18 mm). Loss of resistance technique can lead to air embolism. Intravenous micro infusion with air bubble technique. Bupivacaine infusion-loading 2 mg/kg, infusion 0.2-0.4 mg/kg/bw. Analgesics – morphine, fentanyl, sufentanil, butorphanol, if used, can cause respiratory depression, nausea, vomiting.

Spinal Anaesthesia

It is used in infants for high risk of P.O. apnea following GA. Lumber puncture is perfomed at L4/L5 interspace. Skin to subarachnoid space depth is 1 to 1.5 cm. A 22 G, 3.75 cm Quincke needle is used. Less distinct pop of ligaments at dural puncture. There is a shorter duration of LA in younger age. Respiratory depression negates sedation in infants. Lignocaine dose – 3 mg/kg of 5% solution (7.5% with adrenaline). Incidence of post spinal headache is small as compared to adults. Spinal opioids leads to respiratory depression, nausea, vomiting.

Intravenous Regional Anaesthesia

Butterfly needle is inserted into a vein after that the extremity is exsanguinated by gravity. Tourniquet pressures of 180-240 mm Hg for lower limbs are applied for 20 minutes. Dose of lignocaine is 3 mg/kg (0.5%).

Extremity Blocks in Children

Bony landmarks are easily palpable. Children are less cooperative to needle placement. They have no concept of paraesthesia. A peripheral nerve stimulater (PNS) is helpful. Propofol 1-1.5 mg/kg bolus then infusion of 100-150 microgram/kg/min. Bupivacaine (0.25%) 0.25 mg/kg, lignocaline (0.25-0.50%) 5 mg/kg is used. Radial, median and ulnar nerves blocked at wrist.

Axillary Block : It is safe and easy to perform. Nerves are superficial so deep injection leads to failure. Technique is same as in adults. Musculocutaneous nerve block is more frequent. Catheters can be employed for continuous infusions.

Interscalene/Parascalene Block : Best for shoulder and upper arm involvement. PNS is used in lieu of paraesthesia. Interscalene groove is easily palpable. Parascalene block is softer than interscalene block.

Sciatic Nerve Block : It is employed in combination with femoral or lumbar plexus block.

Anterior Approach (McNicol and Salens) : A line is drawn from anterior superior iliac spine (ASIS) to pubic tubercle. A second line is drawn parallel and medial from greater trochanter. A perpendicular line is drawn from middle and medial parts of first and second line. Loss of resistance after sciatic neurovascular compartment is entered. PNS elicits dorsiflexion (tibial) or plantar flexion (common peroneal) of foot.

Posterior Approach (Lateral Position) : Labat's line a perpendicular line from midpoint of line drawn between superior border of greater trochanter and posterior superior iliac spine (PSIS) Winnie's modification for height: line between greater trochanter and sacral hiatus. Sciatic nerves are entered at the intersection of these lines.

Illioinguinal/Illiohypogastric Nerve Block : It is used in hernia repair, hydrocele, orchldopexy and PO analgesia. Simple infiltration of abdominal wall medial to ASIS. A 25 G needle 1.5 cm medial and inferior to ASIS punctures skin, external and internal oblique fascias. 3

to 5 mL of 0.25% bupivacaine is injected. Wound edge infiltration also provides analgesia.

Penile Block (Dorsal Nerve of Penis) : It is used in hypospadias repair and circumcision. At the base of penis 0.5 cm on either side of midline 0.25% bupivacaine is used through a 25 G needle.

Ring Block : Subcutaneous infiltration at the base of the penis. Topical lignocaine can also provide analgesia.

Intercostal Nerve Block : Used for analgesia for rib fractures and PO analgesia. Distance between rib margin and pleura is 2 mm. Bupivacaine 0.25% 2-5 mg/kg with or without adrenaline is used. A 25 G needle enters lower margin of rib and made to walk past the edge for 1-2 mm posteriorly.

Inter-pleural Block : Used in analgesia for thoracotomy or upper abdominal surgery and trauma. Continuous injection with 0.25% bupivacaine 0.25 mL/kg./hr. Caution–high doses, posture dependent analgesia and pneumothorax.

Paravertebral Block : Used in PO analgesia following thoracotomy. In lateral position skin puncture is made 1–2 cm lateral spinous processes of T7-9. Superior border of transverse is walked past till a loss of resistance is felt after costo-transverse ligment is pierced. Catheterization using 0.25 mL/kg/hr can also be done. Caution to be taken as there are chances of pneumothorax, vessel injury and high dose toxicity.

Epidural/Spinal Analgesics used in Children [2]

1. **Morphine :** Antinociception of morphine epidurally/intrathecally potentiated by magnesium sulphate decreasing post-operative requirements as compared to intra-venous route. A dose of 0.8-1.6 n mol has a peak effect in 15 minutes. It has ED 50 of 2.5/nmol–0.7/n mol.
2. **Fentanyl :** 50–75 mcg or 25–100 mcg followed by 10–20 mcg/hr provides analgesia for duration of 24 minutes.
3. **Sufentanil:** 5–30 mcg used epidurally has a quick onset. It has sedative action, increased Et CO_2, pupillary constriction, pruritis, nausea and vomiting. Intrathecal dose is 7.5 mcg for 24 minutes.
4. Alfentanil: 100 mcg with a loading dose of mL. Increase pain relief, less sedation, less plasma concentration, a rapid and maximum analgesia for 15 minutes, side effects are pruritis, supraspinal sedation and respiratory depression.

Commonly used Regional Nerve Blocks in Children.[2]

A better understanding of local anaesthetic drugs along fascial planes and compartments have allowed regional analgesia to be used in children, which previously were considered unsuitable, leading to discovery of old infiltration blockes *e.g.*

1. Para-umblical or rectus sheath block for umblical hernia repair.
2. Pudendal nerve block for incision of scrotum as a complementary block in undescended festes undertaken under ilio-hypogastric and ilio-inguinal nerve block.
3. Iliohypogastric and iliohypogastric nerve block for inguinal hernia and post-operative pain.
4. Penile block via subpubic space for glans and foreskin of penis.
5. Thoracic paravertebral space block for thoracic surgery and avoiding epidural block.
6. Incisional infiltrations and field blocks with ropivacaine with rapid and longer pain relief.
7. Combined spinal epidural allows rapid and improved emergence.
8. Plexus blocks have useful haemodynamic effects.
9. Study of continuous infusion of 0.11 mcg/kg/hr bupivacaine showed greater plasma concentration in children with ECG signs of epileptic activity. This may be due to high unbound bupivacaine in children. A safer dose in 2 mg/kg in 3–4 minutes.
10. In plexes blocks – proximal blocks to be preferred via median and saphanous nerve blocks.
11. Post dural puncture headache is less in children.The headache may be due to large boro, there may be low backache transient radicular irritation apnoea and respiratory depression.
12. Ropivacaine 0.25%, 1 mg/kg has less prolonged duration.
13. Opioide, ketamine and elonidine also has been used epidurally.
14. Pre emptive analgesia: Still debatable. Used in infiltration of local anaesthetics and opioids. Perception of side effects by patients family changed with better post-operative pain management. Adequate analgesia alone is not sufficient for a satisfactory technique. In children nausea, vomiting and motor blockade are less tolerated.

REFERENCES

1. Kumar. P. Regional Anaesthesia Paediatric Patients. Proceedings of U.P. ISA CON 2002. Varanasi.
2. Kumar P. Regional Anaethesia and Analgesia in children. Proceedings of South Asian Congress of Anaesthesiology. (SACA). Dhaka, Bangladesh, 2003.
3. Kumar P. Recent Advances in Regional Anaesthesia. AAAR. XXX, 126, 2005.

●●●

SECTION–XIII

Other Treatment Modalities

PRACTICAL ASPECTS OF TRANSCUTANEOUS ELECTRICAL NERVE STIMULATION THERAPY

76

Physiological Background

The interest in TENS (transcutaneous electrical nerve stimulation) as a therapy for pain can be traced back to at least four main reasons:

1. The inadequate long-term results of surgical and anaesthesiological techniques to alleviate chronic mainly neurogenic pain.
2. Gastrointestinal and mental side effects of pharmacological analgesic agents in general as well as the relative absence of such agents for the relief of neurogenic pain.
3. The increased knowledge of inhibitory mechanisms in the central nervous system that might be utilized to produce analgesia (symbolized by the gate theory).
4. The development of microelectronic circuitry.

The gate theory[1] and subsequent therapeutic attempts with the nerve stimulation to relieve pain[2] was, therefore, received with great enthusiasm.

According to the gate theory (Fig. 76.1) activity in coarse afferent fibres increases the segmental pre and postsynaptic inhibition of all afferent inputs, whereas activity in the thin fibres would decrease that inhibition. Since the coarse afferents are mainly mechanoceptive and thin afferents are mainly nociceptive, rubbing or massage would tend to decrease a nociceptive input, which is also common experience.

Interestingly, it is possible to selectively activate the coarse afferent fibres by graded electrical stimulation, since the threshold criterion of a nerve fibre is dependent upon its inner longitudinal resistance, being the lowest in these fibres. Therefore, by placing two conductive rubber electrodes on the skin overlying the nerve bundles from a painful area and attaching the electrodes to a signal generator with adjustable output, it is possible to evoke an intense artificial barrage of impulses in mainly mechanoceptive afferents. This stimulation technique is called conventional TENS (Figs. 76.2A, 2B). An alternative working hypothesis for the analgesia from such stimulation has been that fatigue in nociceptive fibres would be elicited by the stimulation. This is, however, unlikely since the stimulation as such is not painful *i.e.*, it does not activate nociceptive nerve fibres. Furthermore, experimental evidence speaks against this hypothesis.[3]

A complementary form of TENS is acupuncture like TENS, where muscle nerves are stimulated transcutaneously with trains of stimuli given at a low repetition rate to induce muscle twitches in myotomes segmentally related to the painful area. The development of this technique was inspired by the reports that classical

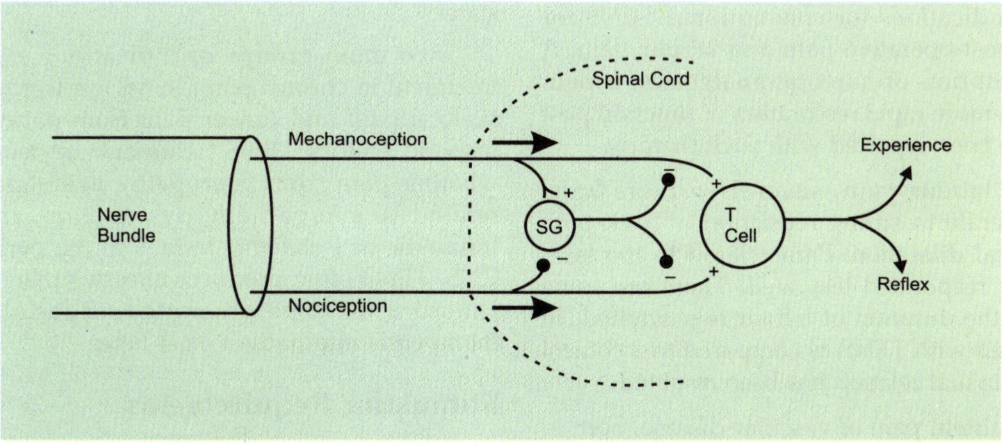

Fig. 76.1 : The gate theory (modified from [15]). SG = inhibitory interneuron in the substantia gelatinosa; T Cell = transmission neuron to higher centres

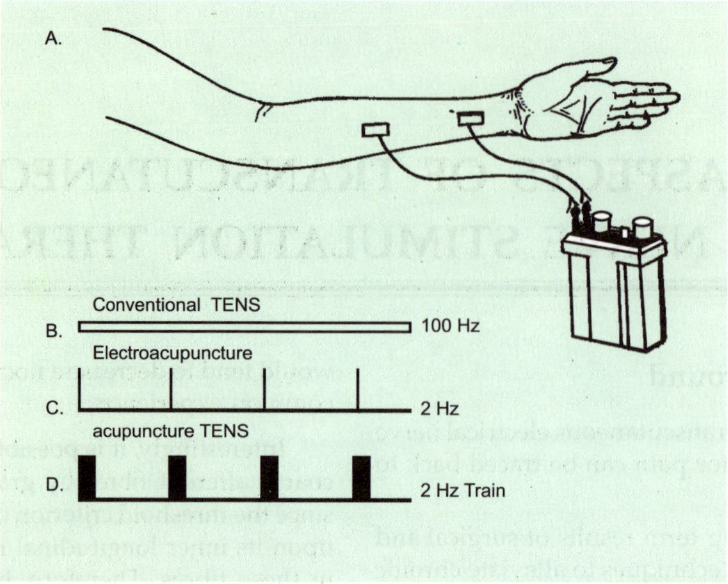

Fig. 76.2. A : TENS stimulator with dials for stimulation frequency and amplitude and connected to electrodes placed over the median nerve. B-D, Stimulus patterns explained in the text.

needle acupuncture as well as electro acupuncture can produce pain threshold increases in humans and that the development of such pain threshold.[4] By substituting the single pulses given via electrodes inserted into the tissue in electro acupuncture (Fig. 76. 2C) for short trains of stimuli (with an internal frequency above the fusion frequency of mammalian skeletal muscle), it was possible to evoke forceful muscle contractions by transcutaneous stimuli in patients with chronic pain.[5] This stimulation may produce analgesia when conventional TENS is without effect and is probably elicited via release of endorphins, whereas that from conventional TENS is not.[5]

Indications

Acute Pain

Important indications for conventional TENS for acute pain are post-operative pain and labour pain. A reduced consumption of narcotic analgesics, a pain experience and a more rapid restoration of function post operatively have been reported with such therapy.

As regards labour pain, several workers have reported a moderate to strong reduction of back pain related to cervical dilatation. Pain related to the later stages of labour responded less well. There are some indications that the duration of labour is shortened. In primiparae treated with TENS as compared to a control group.[6] But this casual relation has been doubted.

In the intermittent pain of vascular disease, both in peripheral vascular disease and in angina pectoris, interesting treatment results have recently been published. As regards peripheral vascular disease, acupuncture like TENS has been reported to diminish the exercise related pain and also to decrease and even heal ulceration. In angina pectoris, conventional TENS treatment has been directed toward the pain referred to chest.[7] Interestingly, all patients tested showed an increased working capacity, a decreased ST segment depression as well as an increased tolerance to pacing and an improved lactate metabolism. Indirect evidence was obtained that the coronary blood flow to ischaemic areas in the myocardium was increased.

Chronic Pain

As seems to be the case with acute pain, TENS in chronic pain influences significantly only those pain states referred to parietal structure of the body. True visceral pain does not seem to be influenced by TENS. This is the case also with psychogenic or functional pain states.[8]

Two main groups of indications exist for TENS treatment in chronic pain. In nociceptive pain musculoskeletal pain and cancer pain from parietal structures respond well to TENS treatment. In neurogenic pain, whether pain from neuropathy neuralgia, pain states related to sympathetic dysfunction, rhizopathy or traumatic or ischaemic lesions to the peripheral of the CNS, TENS often produces effective relief. The therapy should always be attempted, especially since few therapeutic alternatives exist here.

Stimulator Requirements

Most stimulators manufactured today are of constant current design, *i.e.,* they deliver the current set on the amplitude dial in spite of impedance variations in the electrode patient circuit. It is important, however, that the maximal output is not less than 50 mA into 1500–2000 ohms, since this is a common load with present electrode designs. The stimulus modes available should include both conventional TENS and acupuncture like TENS.

Choice of Stimulation Mode and Parameters

Conventional TENS should be tried first in naturopathic pain, neuralgia, causalgia and nociceptive pain from bone and joints. A suitable stimulation frequency is 80 – 100 Hz and the stimulation intensity should be 2-3 times that at the sensory threshold. To be effective the stimulation should always evoke electrical paraesthesiae in the painful area.[9]

In some patients, the underlying pathology or previous treatment has destroyed the afferent nerve fibres to the extent that electrical paraesthesiae cannot be evoked. Acupuncture like TENS should then be tried. This mode is further the primary choice in irradiating pain such as in sciatica and in deep myogenic pain. Here, short trains of 8-16 stimuli are given at a low repetition rate of 1-2 Hz. The intensity should be 3-5 times that at the sensory threshold to evoke visible muscle contractions in myotomes segmentally related to the painful area. The patient may feel muscle fatigue the first few days of treatment, but this does not present a problem in the long run.

Placement of Electrodes

A careful placement of electrodes is an essential element of TENS therapy. In conventional TENS, the electrodes should be put in or around the painful area, if on the trunk and over relevant nerve bundles, if in pain of the extremities (Fig. 76. 3). The stimulation should always be segmentally related to and include the painful area. Rarely stimulation of the contralateral dermatome may be effective. The active electrode should usually be placed proximally.

In acupuncture like TENS, the electrodes should be put over nerves supplying muscles in the myotomes segmentally related to the painful area. The cathode should usually be placed distally, since the stimulation is intended to evoke muscle contractions and indirectly a deep afferent inflow.

Several electrode designs are available. Conductive rubber electrodes, coated with a thin layer of conductive

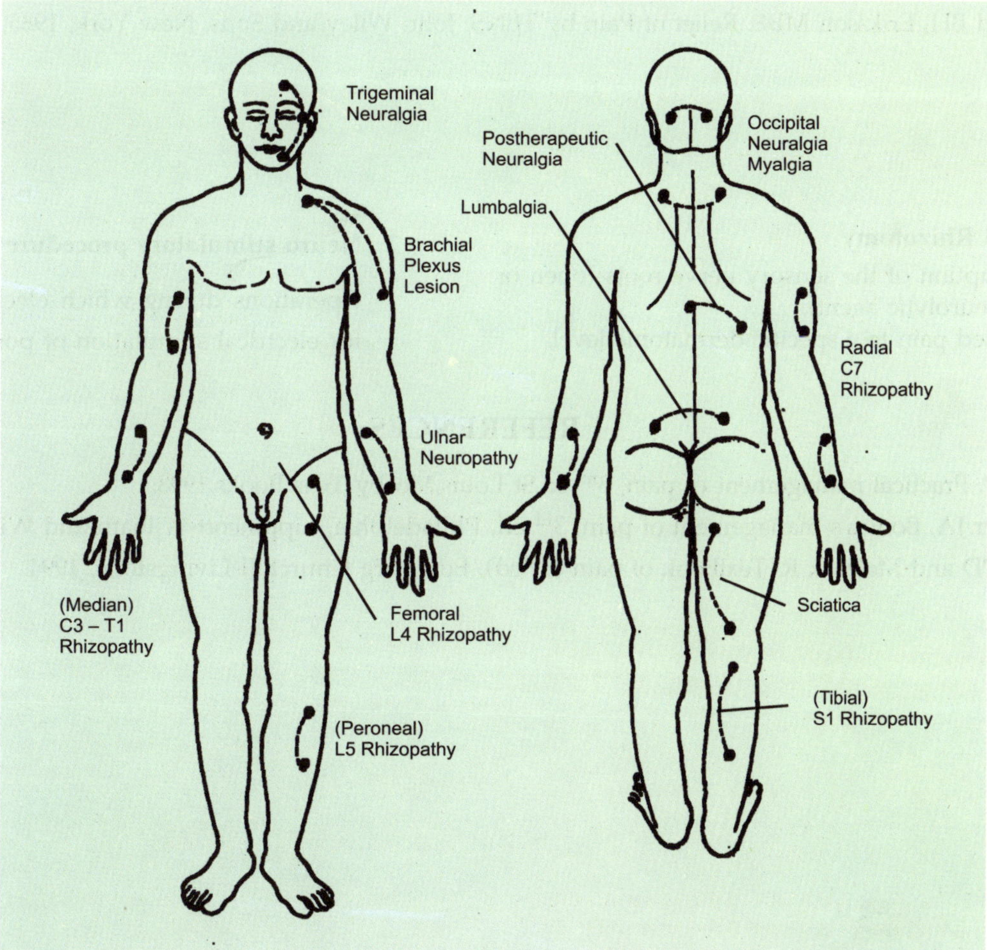

Fig. 76.3 : Examples of electrode placements for conventional and acupuncture like TENS

gel and attached to the skin by hypoallergenic tape are the most commonly used alternative. More handy but also more expensive are self-adhesive electrodes, coated with a karaka rubber material that increases its adhesion to the skin when moistened. Such electrodes seldom last more than 2-3 weeks of regular use, whereas rubber electrodes can be used for 4-6 months before losing their conductive properties. An interesting new alternative is a self-adhesive conductive gel to be used with ordinary rubber electrodes.

REFERENCES

1. Melzack R, Wall PD. Pain mechanisms: a new theory. Science, 1965; 150: 972-979.
2. Meyer GA, Fields HL. Causalgia treated by selective large fibre stimulation of peripheral nerve. Brain, 1972; 95: 163-168.
3. Swett JE, Law JD. Analgesia with peripheral nerve stimulation: absence of a peripheral mechanism, Pain, 1983; 15: 55-62.
4. Andersson SA, Ericson T, Holmgren E, Lindqvist G. Electro-acupuncture: effect on pain threshold measured with electrical stimulation of teeth. Brain Res., 1973; 63: 393-396.
5. Eriksson MBE, Sjolund BH. Acupunture like electro analgesia in TNS-resistant chronic pain. In Zotterman Y., ed., Sensory Functions of the skin, Pergamon, Oxford, 1976; pp. 575-581.
6. Bundsen P, Ericson K, Peterson LE, Thringer K. Pain relief in labor by transcutaneous electrical nerve stimulation. Acta Obstet, Gynecol, Scand., 1982; 61: 129-136.
7. Mannheimer C, Carlsson CA, Vendin A, Wilhelmsson C. Transcutaneous electrical nerve stimulation (TENS) in angina pectoris. Pain, 1986; 26: 291-300.
8. Neilzen S, Sjolund BH, Eriksson M,BE. Psychiatric factors influencing the treatment of pain with peripheral conditioning stimulation. Pain, 1982; 136: 365-371.
9. Sjolund BH, Eriksson MBE. Relief of Pain by TENS. John Wiley and Sons, New York, 1985;116pp.

●●●

- **Dorsal Rhizotomy**

  Interruption of the sensory nerve roots (open or by a neurolytic agent).
  Localised pain to a specific dermatome level.

2. **Neuro stimulatory procedure neuropathway**

   Operations during which electrodes are placed for electrical stimulation of portion of CNS.

REFERENCES

1. Raj PP. Practical management of pain, 3rd ed,St Louis,Mosby Year Books.1998.
2. Loesser JA, Bonica's management of pain, 3rd ed, Philadelphia, Lippincott-William and Wilkins, 2001.
3. Wall PD and Melzack R. Textbook of pain (3rded), Edinburg Churchill-Livingstone, 1994.

●●●

PERCUTANEOUS AND STEREOTACTIC ABLATION AND PITUITARY ADENOLYSIS

77

In many cancer patients pain is most distressing, disabling, affecting their quality of life. When other therapies fail neurosurgical interventions can be considered. The stereotactic percutaneous techniques are quiet safe and effective providing pain relief in various cancer pain syndromes for rest of the patient's life for upto 2 years. Otherwise deep brain stimulation or intrathecal, epidural implants are considered.

Contraindications to neurosurgical techniques are of very short life, coagulopathy, generalized sepsis, poor general condition and lung infection.

1. Percutaneous stereotactic ablations for head and neck are:

- R.F. thermal rhizotomy of 5th, 9th cranial nerves and C_2, C_3.
- Stereotactic trigeminal tractotomy (medullary, mesencephalon), extremities, trunk and pelvis.
- R.F. thermal spinal rhizotomy, intercostal.
- Percutaneous C $_{1\text{-}2}$ or lower cervical cordotomy, extrameniscal myelotomy.

2. **Osseous, visceral pain** – Stereotactic hypophysectomy, stereotactic cingulotomy.

Percutaneous stereotactic radiofrequency lesioning of afferent nerves, ascending tracts in the brain stem, thalamus have success upto 78% in a 25 months follow-up[2] along with RF thermocoagulation of $C_{2\text{-}3}$, 5th and 9th cranial nerves. There is reported permanent dysphagia vocal cord paralysis (20%), numbness and decreased secretions on the affected side.

The percutaneous rhizotomy of cranial nerves is performed under fluoroscopy under local analgesia with monitoring of vital signs during foramen ovale penetration and thermocoagulation. The needle points towards medial pupillary line (frontal view) and towards a point 3 cm anterior to ear canal in lateral view. The needle is then reinserted 40° from infraorbital meatal line in same mediolateral plane under fluoroscopy, electrical stimulation within trigeminal ganglion should elicit low threshold (0.5 V, 1 msec pulse duration, 50-100 Hz), paraesthesias in the painful division. Stimulation of IXth nerve (0.1 to 0.3 V, 1 ms pulse duration, 10-75 Hz) should evoke deep pain in ear or throat accompanied by increase in heart rate (10-20 beats/min) and blood pressure (20-40 mmHg). Bradycardia and hypotension indicate vagal effects, indicating repositioning of the needle. Temperature monitored RF coagulation at 60° C for 60 seconds and increased by steps of 5° C is continued until desired level of analgesia is reached.[3]

Spinothalamic Tractotomy (Mesencepholotomy)

Have a success rate of 80 to 100% in cancer patients till death. The pain relief of face, head[4] the operation is performed under local anaesthesia and mild sedation. A CT scan or MRI performed with patients head in stereotactic frame. The trigeminothalamic tract lies 4-7 mm lateral to the midline at the level of superior colliculus, 5 mm below the posterior commissure. The PAG and reticulothalamic fibres lie medial to these fibres. Thrust a burr hole 1.5 cm lateral to the midline, 1-2 cm anterior to coronal suture. The stereotactic probe trajectory is put in, electric stimulation at the target site elicits warm, cold or burning sensations in contralateral head, face or upper body. Incremental temperature monitored R.F. thermocoagulation is done at 44° C for 30-60 seconds, final lesioning done at 60-70° C for 30-60 seconds. Probe removed only after its temperature reduces to 37° C to prevent damage to surrounding structures.

Thalamotomy

For cancer of head, face and neck is effective in 70-75% patients. Targets include ventroposterior – medial nucleus, centromedian, pulvinar and dorsomedial nucleus.[5]

A mild sedation is used with local anaesthesia with a physiological localization and CT and MRI imaging. The spinothalamic responses referred to the face region by low threshold electrical stimulation obtained 0-10 mm above intercommissure line, 13-15 mm lateral to the midline and 0-10 mm posterior to mid commissural point. An R.F. lesion at 44° is made and patient examined closely for side effects before final coagulation at 60-70° C. A sensory loss over contralateral face and body occurs immediately, later contracting to the distribution of evoked spinothalamic responses elicite target points.

Open Surgical Ablation

Open operations or midbrain and thalamus are no more performed after interventricular morphine injections. The access to lower cranial nerve and upper cervical roots require a unilateral craniectomy and laminectomy of C_{1-3} through an inverted "hockey stick" incision in sitting or lateral position. The spinomedullary junction required a small suboccipital craniectomy and a pain relief of 75% has been reported with 20% mortality. However, these operations are now rarely performed as mentioned earlier.[6]

Percutaneous Rhizotomy

For cancer pain below neck limited to 1-4 dermatomes in trunk, percutaneous RF coagulation of spinal, intercostal or peripheral nerves is performed. Operation is performed under local anaesthesia under fluoroscopy in supine (cervical), or prone position. A 12 gauze 1.1 mm diameter temperature monitored electrodes are introduced to the rostral, dorsal portion of the desired neural foramina. Stimulation with 1 ms pulses at 0.2-0.8 V should induce a motor response at 2-5 Hz, dermatomal pain at 20-25 Hz and dermatomal paraesthesias at 50-100 Hz. The needle tip is extradural in all cases except at S_1. Thermocoagulation at 50-60° for 60-120 seconds is performed.[7] There is a relief of pain in 75-80% patients.

Electrical Stimulation

Of peripheral nerves; dorsal column – lemniscal system of spinothalamic pathways can be performed for chronic non cancer pain. For cancer patients deep brain electrical stimulation of PAG, PVG has 60-100% success rate. A CT or MRI guided transfrontal trajectory via a precoronal burr hole is employed. The distal pole of 4 contact DBS electrode is placed 3 mm lateral to the wall of 3rd ventricle 3-5 mm below the posterior commissure under local or general anaesthesia.

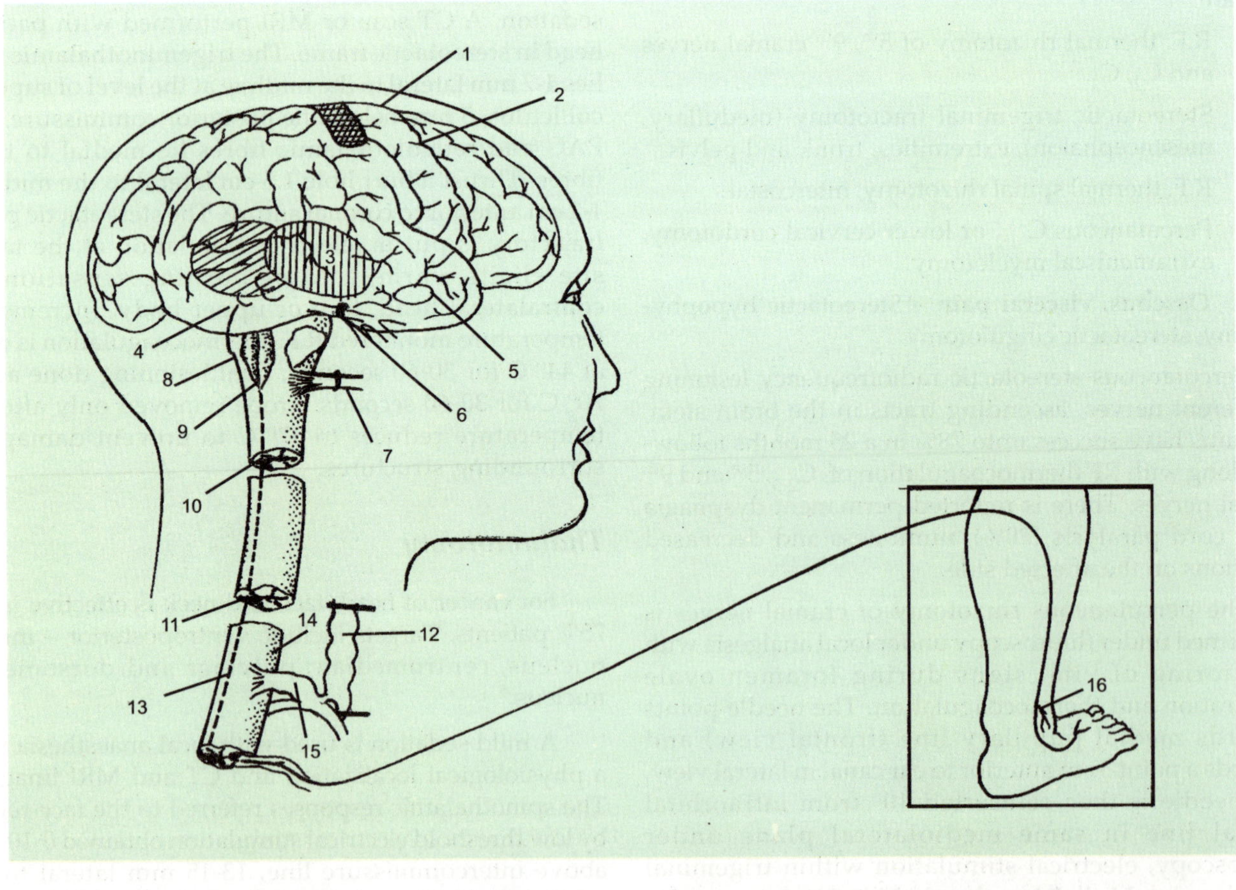

Fig. 77.1 : Schematic illustration of the various sites for ablative neurosurgical operations to relieve pain

1. Postcentral gyrectomy; 2. Prefrontal lobotomy (leukotomy); 3. Thalamotomy; 4. Mesencephalotomy (spinothalamic mesencephalic tractotomy); 5. Hypophysectomy, 6. Trigeminal rhizotomy; 7. Glossopharyngeal rhizotomy; 8. Medullary tractotomy; 9. Trigeminal tractrotomy; 10. CJ-2 anterolateral cordotomy; 11. Thoracic cordotomy; 12. Sympathectomy; 13. Commissural myetotomy; 14. Lissauer tractotomy, 15. Dorsal rhiozotomy; 16. Peripheral neurectomy

Spinal Cord Stimulation

Patient in left lateral position under fluoroscopy., the needle through which stimulating electrode is inserted is placed in low thoracic or upper lumbar region. A steep paramedian insertion is done using 15-16 SG needle. The stylet is removed before epidural space is entered using loss of resistance technique. The electrode catheter is then inserted and placed posteriorly, verified by fluoroscopy. The negative electrode is connected to wire extension of the catheter tip while positive electrode is connected to a Medtronic (3623) stimulating box using 75 pulses/second, pulse width 400 ìsec and 2 volt amplitude. Pulse width can be adjusted by turning a screw located inside the box. The needle is carefully removed after surgical dissection; the electrode is anchored to skin. Surgical implantation of the electrode anchor, leads that cannot the stimulation pack to the electrode and the stimulation pack is completed under local anaesthesia. There is a success rate of 75% with 13% failure rate. There can be a severe back pain after spinal cord stimulation.[8]

Intraspinal and Interventricular Morphine

Chronic administration of morphine into the ventricular or spinal CSF via fully implantable access systems has been a major advance in the treatment of regional or cancer pain. The direct delivery of small drug doses to spinal or cerebral receptor sites provides effective analgesia without side effects. Even in the tolerant intraspinal patients, the intraventricular delivery system recaptured the analgesic effect. Fully implantable pumps have been developed to deliver morphine to either site. Each manipulation of the device delivered a precise volume of the drug is concentration which is predetermined. A success rate of 73-94% good relief was reported.[9] Tolerance has been reported with an infection of the device site.

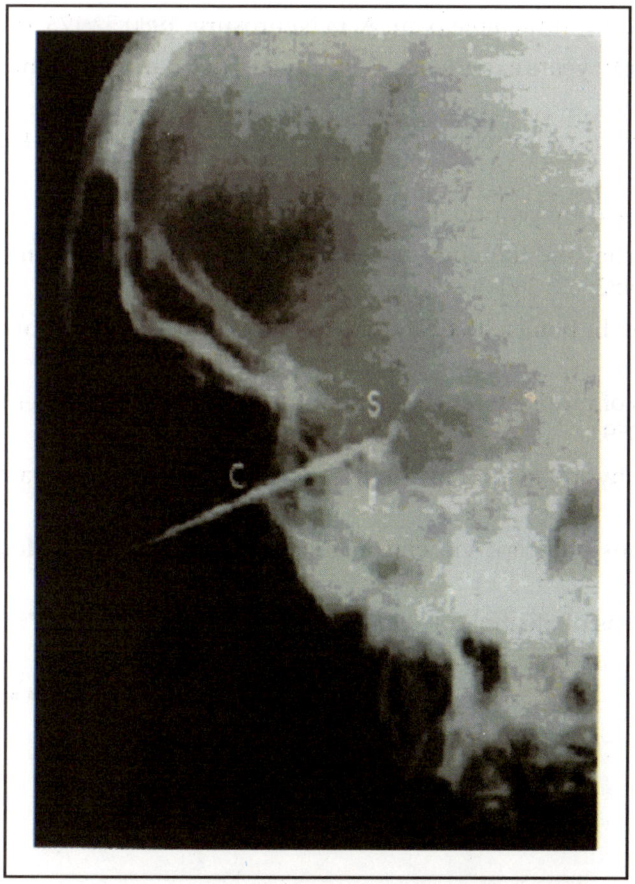

Fig. 77.2 : Contrast being injected through a cannula and tracking up the pituitary stalk C, Cannula, S. Pituitary stalk

Pituitary Adenolysis

Anatomy: Pituitary gland has oval shape and transverse axis lying in the pituitary fossa, covered by dura mater through which pituitary infundibulum towards tuber cinerium (Fig. 77.3).

The pain relief following secretion of pituitary stalk, alcohol injection into the sella is well described but mechanism is not explained.[10] There may be removal of mechanism that sensitizes pain by inhibiting the tumour tissue or by reduction of pressure infiltration. After pituitary ablation there is slight increase in ACTH, beta endorphin an beta lipotrophin[11] along with altered electrolyte levels low BP.

There is another view that some of the neurolytic enters hypothalamus producing pain relief (Fig. 77.2).[12]

Thirdly, there is an endorphine mechanism which can be attributed to large amounts of a endorphin in

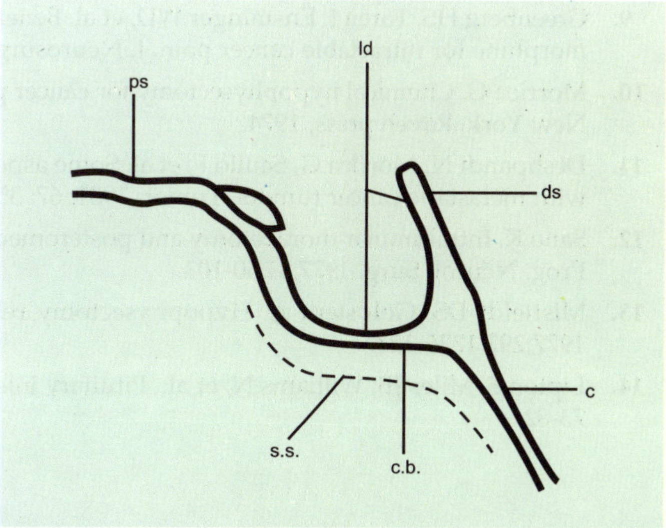

Fig. 77.3 : Detailed drawing of later X-ray view of pituitary fossa. cb, cortical bone lining stalk; ds. dorsum sellae; c, clivus; ld, lamina dura (cortical bone lining sella turcica); ps, planum sphenoidal; ss, sphenoid sinus

anterior pituitary gland. Naloxone, however, failed to reproduce pain relieved by hyphophysectomy.[13]

A stress induced analgesia has also been proposed and stimulation of gland with an electric current also has the same effect.

When mucosa shrank and sphenoid stoma is wide, cannula drops into the sphenoid sinus and when tapped with small blows with the lightest hammer. The trocar and cannula are advanced in midline since pituitary gland and sella are midline structures. The image intensifier is then changed to lateral towards sella. Then it is changed to AP view till needle impinges on the anterior wall of the sella in its lower one third. CSF rhinorrhea occurs lasting for a few hours to days. Then removal of trocar is done and a 20 SG needle is inserted to penetrate posterior pituitary. After injection of 1 mL of air, radiocontrast (myodil) solution 1 mL in small 0.25 mL increments is injected,which is seen trickling to third ventricle. Incremental injections for 2 mL pure (100%) alcohol are made, noticing the pupil size, reaction to light and accommodation, checking blood pressure. The pupil dilatation responds to hydrocortisone. There is a relief of upto 60% with this technique, higher than surgery for hormone dependent tumours. There can be high mortality following this procedure due to pituitary insufficiency and circulating failure.[14] The diabetes insipidus is produced in almost all patients responding to steroids, oral drinks, desmopression in snuff into the nose. Rhinorrhea lasts for a few days to months, along with visual field defects.

REFERENCES

1. Long DM. Relief of cancer pain by surgical and nerve blocking procedures. JAMA, 1980; 244 (24): 2759-2761.
2. Giorgi C, Broggi G. Surgical treatment of Glossopharyngeal neuralgia and pain for cancer of nasopharynx: 20 yrs experience J. Neurosurg. 1984;61:952-955.
3. Schvarcz JR, Stereotactic. Trigeminal Tractotomy, contin. Neurol. 1975;37:73-77.
4. Amino K, Kawabatake H, Tani kawa T, et al. Long term follow up study of Stereotactic rostral mesencephalic reticulotomy in patients with intractable pain. Appl. Neuro-physiol. ; 1986; 49:105-111.
5. Steinor L, Forster D, Laksell L, et al. Gamma thalamotomy intractable pain. Acta Neurosurg. 1980;52:173-184.
6. White JC, Sweet WH. Pain and the neurosurgeon : a forty years experience. Springfield, III, Charls C Thomas. 1969.
7. Uematsu S, Udvarhelyi G, Benson DW, et al. Percutaneous radiofrequency rhizotomuy. Surg. Neurol. 1974; 2: 319-324.
8. Raj PP. Practical management of pain III ed. St. louis, Mosby year book, 1992.
9. Greenberg HS, Taren J, Ensminger WD, et al. Benefit from and tolerance to continuous intrathecal infusion of morphine for intractable cancer pain. J. Neurosurg. 1982; 57: 360-364.
10. Morrica G. Chemical hypophysectomy for cancer pain. In Bonica J.J. et al (ed) Advances in neurology. Vol 4, New York, Raven press, 1974.
11. Deshpandi N, Morrica G, Saullo F, et al. Some aspects of pituitary function after neuro adenolysis in patients with metastatic cancer tumors. Tumor, 1981; 67: 355-359.
12. Sano K. Intraluminar thoracotomy and posteromedial hypothalamotomy in the treatment of intractable pain. Prog. Neurol. Surg. 1977;81:50-103.
13. Misfieldt DS, Goldstein A. Hypophysectomy relieves pain not via endorphins. Letter N. Engl. J. Med. 1977;297:1236-1237.
14. Lipton S, Miles JB, Williams N, et al. Pituitary injections of alcohol for widespread cancer pain. Pain 1978;5: 73-82.

CHEMONUCLEOLYSIS VERTEBROPLASTY, BOTULINUM TOXIN AND SPINAL ENDOSCOPY

78

Chymopapain is a proteolytic enzyme, affects proteoglycan water aggression in the nucleosus pulposus of the disc. Chromonucleolysis is indicated for patients not responding to adequate conversative care for more than 60 days in proven disc disease[1] requiring laminectomy and disc excision. These patients with disc prolapse difficulty in straight leg raising, motor weakness, asymmetric reflex and sensory deficit.[2]

Investigation – X-ray may show narrowing of the intervertebral disc space, CT and myelogram confirm the disc prolapse.

Contraindications[3] – Neurologic deficit, previous surgery, pregnancy, history of allergy to palpate, chymopapain, ankylosing spondylitis, rheumatoid arthritis, diabetes, cancer, cervical and thoracic discs, stenosis, complete block in myelography and psychogenic pain disturbances.

Technique

Chemonucleosis is done at least 3 days after myelography. Patient should be fasting overnight with preoperative diphen-hydramine (100 mg) and hydro-cortisone (100 mg) intramuscularly. With patient in lateral or prone position. The iliac crest and the posterior superior iliac spine are marked and a point just over these, 10 cm lateral to the tip of spinous process of L_3. After local infiltration a 5 cm, 18 SG needle with stylet is inserted at 45° to sagittal plane and 30° to the transverse plane, under fluoroscopy. The needle is advanced to superior posterolateral corner of the disc space then further advanced 1 cm impacting near the superior facet of the vertebra on which the disc rests, when a localized or referred pain is felt in the buttocks. If a rubbery resistance is felt the tip of needle is advanced further 2 cm (Fig. 78.1) into the disc.[4] If there is difficulty with 18 SG needle a two needle technique is used, inserting a 22 SG needle in the 18 SG needle used, after withdrawing the stylet. As the needle reaches nucleus pulposus the bevel is turned superiorly confirming the position with conray 60(2-5 mL) under lateral and AP X-ray and fluoroscopy. Afterwards injection of 1000 units of 1 ml of chymodiactin is slowly injected.[1] Apart from neurological complications, haemorrhage a careful watch for systemic allergic reaction *e.g.*, anxiety, tingling, cardiovascular collapse, paraesthesia, goose flesh, wheeze or stridor is kept[3] and treated by IV fluid infusions; 1:10000 adrenaline (1 mL), aminophylline 250 mg 15 minutes, diphenhydramine and hydrocortisone 100 – 200 mg IV. Success rate is 70-90%.

Vetebroplasty

The use of bone cement into a crack or fissure of a fractured vertebra through a injector is a currently popular noninvasive method. The advantage of avoidence of an operation is possible in case of fracture of vertebrae. However, extensive trauma to the vertebrae may not be a suitable indication for vertebroplasty. The technique is done under deep sedation or light general anaesthesia with a danger of anaphylactic reaction due to the injected cement.

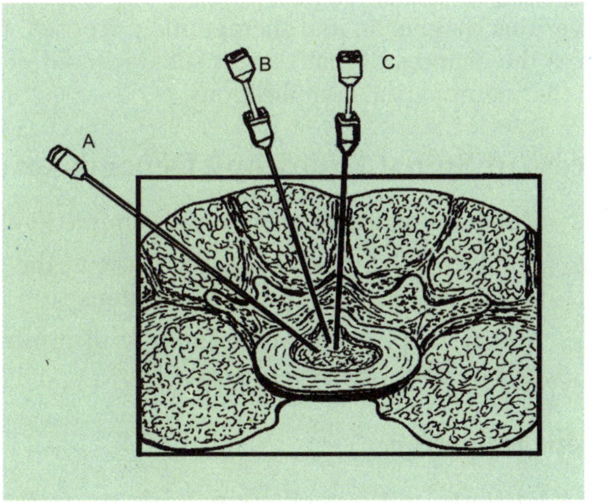

Fig. 78.1 : Cross section of the lumbosacral disk with the two-needle technique. A. Lateral approach; B. Posterolateral approach C. Median approach. Only the lateral approach is recommended. (From Brown MD: Intradiscal therapy; chymo-papain or collagenase, Chicago, 1983, Year Book Publishers, Inc.)

Botulinium Toxin Injection

Randomized, double blond; controlled trials have delivered positive results for injection of botulinum toxin type A as an effective treatment for primary axillary hyperbidrosis and migraine prevention[5], This fact was however, not confirmed in some other studies. Further a single dose treatment may not be effective for chronic neck pain. Injections of botulinum toxin A has been suggested for prostatic pain, whiplash, myofascial pain syndrome and chronic facial pain associated with temperomandibular dysfunction.

Spinal Endoscopy (SE)

Introduction

Endoscopic surgical procedures are one of the most significant advances in modern medicine.

The components of miniature endoscopic instrument has made as a better insight into the contents of the epidural space and helps to treat various diseases of spinal canal.

It also allows to diagnose and treat the patient while awake and without the need for surgical incision. This results in reduced risk and trauma, shorter recovery time and reduced cost.

History

Micheal and Barman used spinal endoscopy in 1951 in Cadavers. More recently in 1995, Saberski in USA, popularised the caudal approach for spinal endoscopy. The various diagnostic and therapeutic purposes, this reduces the chances of inadvertent subarachnoid entry and other neurological complications.

Success of Spinal Endoscopy Depends on

1. Miniature instruments which are simple to use.
2. Ability to perform the procedures with the patients awake and under light sedation.
3. Ability to perform procedures with minimal trauma (day care procedures).

Patient Selection

1. Patients with back pain with or without radiculopathy with surgically incorrectable pathology or imaging.
2. Backpain with history of previous unsuccessful spine surgery.
3. Backpain not responding to physiotherapy, transcutaneous electrical nerve stimulation, pharmacological treatment, neural blockade such as epidural steroids.
4. Backpain with filling defect on caudal epidurogram.

Contraindications

1. Lack of consent.
2. Local infection at the sacral entry site.
3. Use of anticoagulants/bleeding tendencies.
4. Hypersensitivity to amide local anaesthetic or contrast media.
5. Pregnancy.
6. Obesity.
7. Uncontrolled hypertensin.

Mechanism of Action

Pathology of Backache

Radicular pain is caused by inflammation and/or nerve trauma. Phospholipase A_2 and other irritant chemicals can leak from damaged intervertebral discs and can irritate the nerve roots.

Also, application of nucleus pulposus material to the nerve roots, slows down nerve conduction and impairs neve function.

Synovial cytokines from the damaged facet joints can leak and cause nerve irritation.[1]

By dilution of and washing out phospholipase A_2 and other irritant material from the intervertebral disc and other facet joints, spinal endoscopy helps to reliev backpain. Spinal endoscopy also improves nerve roots nutrition by improving vascularity by breaking down adhesions. This is done by the saline flush which helps in hydrostatic adhesionolysis (neuroplasty) and by mechanical adhesionolysis by the tip of the spinal endoscope. Also, placement of medications like local anaesthesia, steroids, clonidine and hyaluronidase provides pain relief.

Failed Back Surgery Syndrome (FBSS)

It is the term used for patients who continues to have persistent back or leg pain even after surgery. As spinal endoscopy can mobilise adhesions by mechanical or hydrostatic neuroplasty, it may have a specific role to play for these patients without causing any further major trauma.

Requirements

This procedure requires non-traumatised instruments because the patient is awake or under light sedation during this procedure.

The requirements are:

1. Patient's cooperation

2. High quality optics
3. Bold light source
4. Flexibility of the endoscope and system for constant administration of a distending medium of saline.

Procedure

I. Aim

It is used for visualisation and treatment of spinal canal.

Approach: It is commonly performed via the caudal approach, but the epidural space can also be visualised by carefully passing the spinal endoscope through a Touhy needle at any level of spine.

II. Position

For spinal endoscopy, patients are placed in prone position with their feet inverted, as this improves access to the caudal epidural space. Soft pillows are placed under the patient. The lumbar, sacral and caudal area is cleared with betadine and draped.[2]

III. Epidural Access Kit

Needles and syringes to inject local anaesthetic into the skin, 18 G. Tuohy needle, guidewire, dilator, epidural sheath.

The procedure is carried out under midazolam sedation but a sensible verbal contact must be maintained with the patient during the entire procedure. Lignocaine 1% is injected into the skin over the sacrococcygeal area and the caudal epidural space is entered with an 18G. Tuohy's needle. Once the caudal epidural space is identified, radio-contrast dye is injected to obtain a baseline epidurogram. This will identify the areas of filling defect that may correspond to patient's symptom. A guidewire is then advance into the epidural space through the Tuohy needle under fluoroscopy. The Tuohy needle is removed and a bold incision made.

The entry point of the guidewire to facilitate smooth entry of the dilator along with the epidural sheath into the caudal epidural space. Adequate care is taken to prevent the guidewire become kinked.2

Video Guided Catheter (VGC)

This is radioopaque and guides the flexible fibre-optic endoscope in the epidural space. It has 3 mm external diameter and two 1.3 mm working channel with a 2-way steering mechanism, a radio-opaque tip. The 2 working channel can be used. One for the fibrescope and other for saline flush/instrumentation.

Two Side Ports

Use

2. To monitor epidural space pressure. The other part is left open to air to act as a vent for excess saline, thus preventing excessive rise in epidural pressure.

Flexible Fibre-optic Endoscope

1. It works in conjunction with the VGC to provide direct visualisation of the targeted pathology. The fibre-optic scope is 0.8 mm in external diameter. It has a micro-lens at the tip.
2. Length: 125 cm, magnification 40X, Eyepiece standard 32 mm.
3. The scope is connected to a cold light source and further connected to a video staking system to obtain images on the screen.
4. The flexible fibreopticscope is passed through one of the lumens of the VGC and threaded to projects about 1 mm beyond the tip of the VGC. The side part of the VGC is connected to saline flush which is about 1 m above the level of the patient.
5. It is important to keep the epidural pressure as low as possible and at least below the mean atmospheric pressure.
6. **Side-effects** like headache, paraesthesia and backache are directly proportional to epidural space pressure.
7. **Saline** is necessary for visibility and helps in hydrostatic adhesionolysis (Neuroplasty).
8. The tip of the VGC is guided towards the suspected sites of nerve root pathology under fluoroscopy.
9. The hydrostatic pressure and movement of the tip of the VGC helps in releasing the epidural adhesions and improved visibility and further spread of saline.
10. With time, the epidural space clears and it may be possible to identify structures such as nerve roots and blood vessels.
11. When the nerve root responsible for the patient's symptom is touched, it produces exactly the same type and pattern of the patient's pain.
12. At the end of the procedure, an epidurogram is performed and can be compared with the pre-procedure image.
13. At the end, a steroid containing solution is injected at the site through the one of the side parts of VGC.

14. Now, GC along with the fibreoptic endoscope and epidural sheath is removed.
15. Wound covered with dressing.
16. Patient is kept supine for next 1 hour and then discharged.

Sterilisation

1. Ethylene oxide
2. Nucidere 5-10 min contain 3500 ppm peracetic acid.

4. Chances of dural puncture.
5. Meningitis, arachnoiditis, paralysis.

Various Operations that can Be Performed

1. Drainage of an epidural abscess.
2. Neurofibroma excision.
3. Pediculectomy.
4. Saminectomy and de-compression.

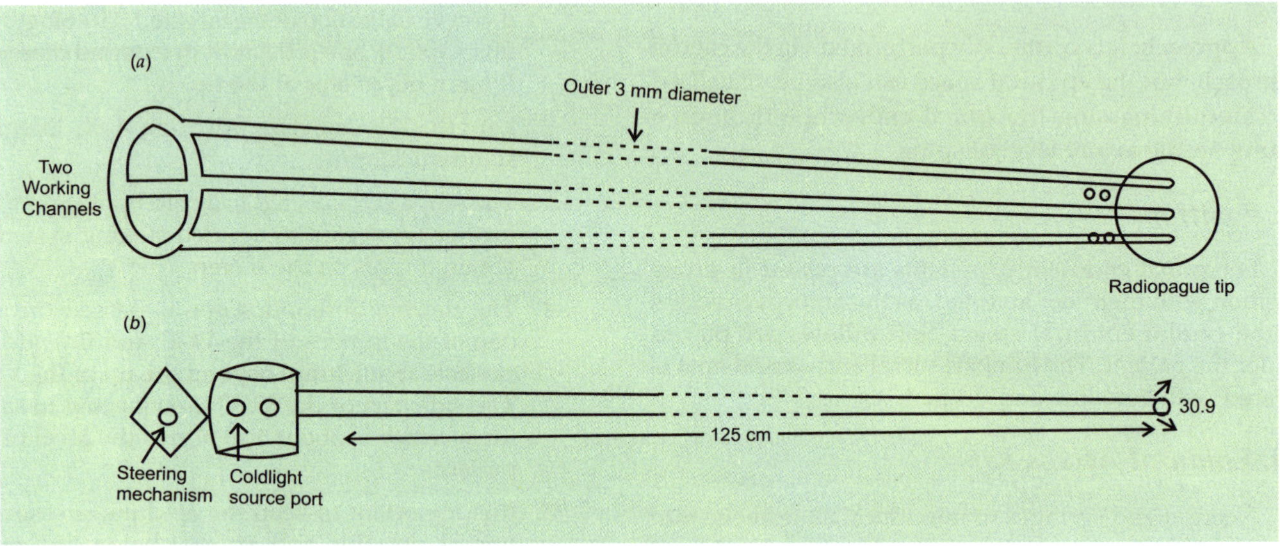

Fig. 78.2 (*a*) : Video guided catheter (*b*) Flexible fibreoptic endoscope

Safety Features

1. Patient must be awake, as they serve as their own monitor.
2. Epidural space pressure due to saline infusion should not exceed mean arterial pressure.
3. If patient reports pain, paraesthesia or complains headache, during the procedure, ear pain, neck or shoulder pain, stop the procedure.

Side Effects

1. Pain at insertion site.
2. Headache during/after the procedure.
3. Paraesthesia during the procedure.
4. Small amounts of drainage from the insertion site.

Complications

1. Epidural infection/abscess.
2. Numbness/tingling paraesthesia.
3. Nerve root injury.

SE is better than MRI in identifying

1. Nerve root vascularity.
2. Nerve root inflammation.
3. Nerve root sensitivity.
4. Identification of fibrous tissue.
5. Diagnostic localisation of pain.
6. Therapeutic aspect of pain management.

SE is better than MRI in delineating nerve root anatomy, identifying disk prolapses, assessment of canal size and exclusion of serious pathology.

Place of Spinal Endoscopy in Pain Management

Treatment Algorithm

Conservative treatment-medication, physiotherapy, psychological.

Pain relief with conservative therapy.

If no pain relief–Epidural steroid injection–If relief–give medication.

If no relief with steroid epidurally–spinal endoscopy is done.

If SE successful–continue conservative therapy.

If SE unsuccessful–Advanced therapy.

SE Out come Studies

Gupta S. studied pain using VAS, assessing ability to perform different function at the twice of SE and 2, 6 and 12 months after the procedure using Waddell and main patient function score. This consists of nine parameters with one point awarded to each. A score of zero represented a severe functional restriction and a score of nine represents good function. Ability to fit about 15-18 kgs, ability to sit, stand, walk and travel in a bus, car for half an hour were assisted two point each. Lack of sleep disturbances, social life restriction, sex life restriction due to low backpain and ability to wear foot wear without any help were awarded one point each. This study used 100 mL epidural saline without any respiratory or CNS effect.

Results: Thirty-eight patient were recruited and there were 21 male and 17 female patients and man age of 46 years with duration of pain of 10.9 years. 50% patients had one or more surgery and were termed failed back syndrome. Overall improved was stability significant using with improvement in pain and function score at 2 months sustained at 6 and 12 months.

In another report there was probable outcome after 50 but with medullar irritation, seizures, bradycardia, respiratory depression requiring emergency treatment and controlled ventilation. It may be due to large volume of epidural fluid (12 00 mL) and sedation.

REFERENCES

1. Raj PP and Nordby EJ. Chemonucleolysis: In: Practical management of pain. II nd ed. St. louis. Mosby yearbook, 1992; 856-867.
2. Shoning B, Lorenz W, Doenicke A. Prophylaxis of anaphylactic reactions to a polypeptidal plasma substitute by H_1 plus H receptor antagonists : synopsis of three randomized controlled trials. Klin Wochernschr, 1982; 60;:1048.
3. Mcculloch JA. Discometry. In: Sciatica and Chymopapain. Mcculloch JA, Macnab J. Ed. Baltimore, Waverly press, 1983.
4. Brown MD. Intradiscal therapy, Chymopapaine or Collagen are, Chicago, 1983, Year Book Publishers Inc.
5. Silber Stein S. Mathew N, Saper J et al. Botulinum toxic type A as a migraine preventine treatment. Headache. 2000; 40: 445-450.
6. Gupta S et al. Study of SE in chronic low back pain with associated radiculopathy. Anaesthesia 2001;56:454-460.

•••

PATIENT CONTROLLED ANALGESIA

79

The concept of patient controlled analgesia (PCA) is not new. Oral analgesics medication has been widely used under patient control for many centuries. Patients are best managers of their own pain, since they can best detect when they need relief. Before the advent of PCA pumps, post-operative patients had limited ability to control their pain. Oral route is frequently not available. Although patients may be able to request medications on the PRN basis, this is not an adequate mode of therapy because:

1. They may face a busy nurse that does not attend the call when needed.
2. There may be a delay in preparing the dose.
3. Inadequate doses may be provided.
4. Inappropriate time schedule may be used.
5. But more importantly, this is not adequate pharmacological method: somnolence-pain

Today PCA pumps microprocessors avoid this problems by[1]:

1. Allowing programming of a continuous infusion.
2. Permitting the patient to have a rescue dose at a set interval of time at a push of a button.
3. Enabling patients to have full control over their pain management without the risk of overdosing.

PCA pumps have become very popular and are extensively used in hospitals because[1]:

1. Patients like the security of knowing that they can achieve pain control quickly and reliably without involving a nurse.
2. Nurses find the machines easy to use and time saving.
3. Doctors have found that they are safe and make pharmacological sense: peaks and throughs in the medication are avoided [(1)]

Patient Satisfaction

★ *Positive aspect* :

- control over pain relief
- not having to wait for pain relief
- not having injection
- not having to bother nurses.

★ *Negative aspect* :

- inadequate analgesia
- presence of side effects
- not trusting PCA machine
- fearing overdose
- fearing addiction.

In fact, with appropriate liberal dose regimens and lockout intervals, patients using PCA may compensate for any difference in the pharmacokinetics and pharmacodynamics of the opiods prescribed until satisfactory analgesia is attained[2]. PCA techniques may be used for IV and epidural therapy.

IV-PCA versus IM opioids

The vast majority of studies have documented that IV-PCA is superior to IM intermittent opioid therapy (Fig 79.1). More recently, meta-analysis has been used to evaluate the results of these studies–Meta-analysis is a statistical method used to integrate and interpret the results of separate investigations. It is defined as the quantitative synthesis of data from multiple clinical experiences.

It is particularly useful when the numbers of patients in individual trials are small, and it may help identify a trend if the results of individual trials do not display a clear direction. A recent meta-analysis of IV-PCA Vs IM opioids showed that:

1. There was a greater analgesic efficacy with IV-PCA.
2. There was a significant trend towards reduced opioid used with IV-PCA.
3. A 42% difference in the proportion of patients expressing satisfaction over dissatisfaction.
4. IV-PCA was the strongly preferred technique by patients.
5. A non-significant trend towards shortening of hospital stay.
6. No significant difference in the incidence of side effects.[3]

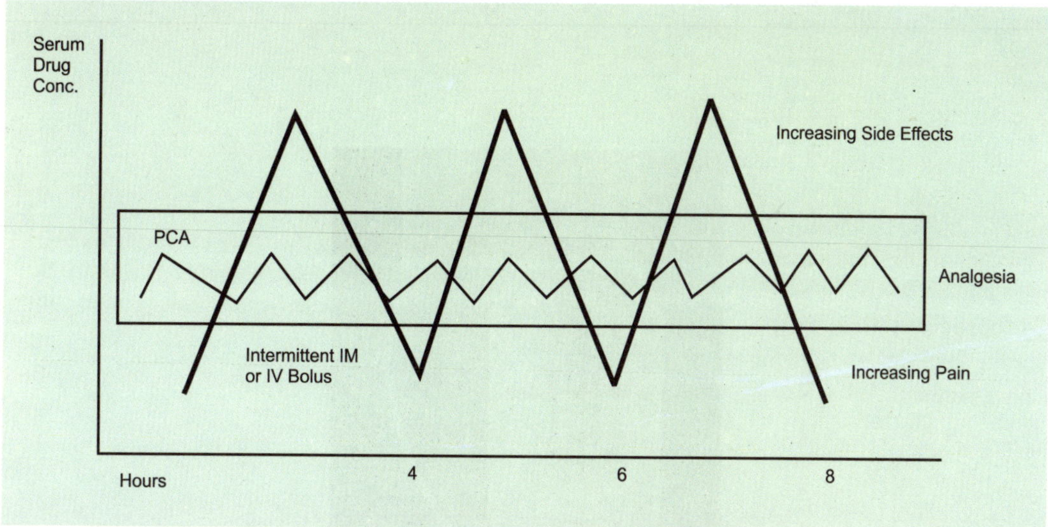

Fig. 79.1 : Difference between PCA and bolus

Problems that may occur during PCA use:

★ Operator errors:

1. Misprogramming PCA device
   1.1 Inappropriate drug, dose or concentration
   1.2 Inappropriate lockout period.
   1.3 Inadvertent addition or deletion of a basal infusion.
2. Failure to clamp or unclamp tubing while loading or unloading the drug reservoir.
3. Improperly loading the cartridge.
4. Inability to respond to safety alarms.
5. Misplacing PCA pump key.

★ Patient errors:

1. Failure to understand PCA therapy.
2. Alterations in negative-feedback loop.
3. Misunderstanding PCA device.
4. Intentional analgesic abuse.

★ Mechanical errors:

1. Failure to deliver on demand.
2. Cracked drug reservoir.
3. Defective one-way valve at Y-connector.
4. Faulty alarm system.
5. Malfunctions (*e.g.*, block).
6. Block or kink in the intravenous catheter or tubing, leak, or disconnect.

Inappropriate Use of PCA

Oversedation with PCA by

- repeated use at end of every lockout period;
- mistaking PCA handset for nurse-call button;
- family, visitor, unauthorized nurse-activated demands.

Device designs

★ Malfunction

- absence of 'O' ring;
- 'fail safe' electrical corruption;
- uncontrolled siphoning of syringe contents.

Loading Dose:

- PCA is essentially a maintenance therapy that should begin with a loading dose.
- Before initiating PCA, titrate the analgesic medication to achieve adequate analgesia.
- The loading dose is typically administered in the PACU once the patient has recovered from anesthesia- If the patient has received an adequate dose of opioid intraoperatively and he/she is not experiencing pain then a loading dose is not necessary.

Demand (Bolus) Dose:

- This is the amount of drug that the patient receives every time the PCA device is activated.
- If the demand dose is too small, patients will be unable to achieve adequate pain relief.
- Because of operant conditioning with PCA, the patient will loose faith in the form of therapy.
- If the demand dose is too high, side effects may appear.

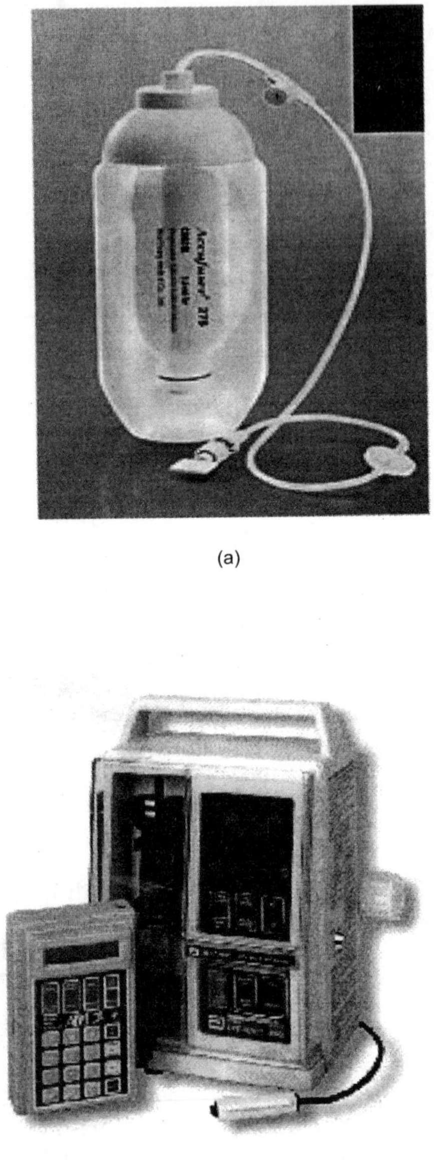

(a)

(b)

Fig. 79.2 : PCA-related consumables

Thus, patients must be followed closely after the first two hours of therapy to optimize the bolus dose. Due to wide variability of the MEAC for all the opioids, it is not possible to make rigid recommendations for the size of the bolus dose. However, frequent evaluations of the level of pain and the number of attempts in a PCA during an hour period will determine the need to increase or decrease the size of the bolus dose. Most patients will require at least one adjustment in the size of the bolus dose during the course of therapy.

Table 79.1 : Guidelines for Bolus Doses and Lockout Intervals for IV Use

Drug	Bolus Dose	Lockout Interval (min)
Morphine	0.5–3.0 mg	5–20
Methadone	0.5–3.0 mg	10–20
Butarphanol	0.1–0.5 mg	5–15
Oxymorphone	0.2–0.8 mg	5–15
Pethidine	5–15 mg	5–15
Fentanyl	15–75 ug	5–10
Sufentanyl	2–15 ug	5–10
Pentazocine	5–20 mg	5–15
Nalbuphine	1–5 mg	5–15
Buprenorphine	30–200 ug	10–20

Lockout (Delay) Interval[(1)]

- This is the interval of time between two demand (bolus) doses.
- The lockout interval is set to avoid overdosing (boluses too frequent) and inadequate analgesia (boluses interval time too long)
- The lockout interval depends on the size of the bolus dose (Table 79.1)
- The ratio between boluses delivered and boluses demanded by the patient should be one. If the number of demands is significantly greater that the number of boluses delivered then the lockout interval is too long, the bolus dose is too small, or the patient fails to understand PCA.

Basal Infusion [3]

Theoretical advantages for a basal infusion during PCA therapy are:

1. Need for improved analgesia during sleep and when they wake up.
2. Better analgesia during movement.

However, controlled studies have failed to validate these theoretical advantages.

In fact studies have shown no clinical advantages in using continuous infusions. Moreover, the incidence of side effects and complications may be increased.

Adjuvant Therapy

- The use of NSAIDs will decrease opioid consumption and improve analgesia.
- Studies have evaluated parenteral ketoralac, diclofenac, and paracetamol with good results.
- Oral clonidine (300 ug) has also been used but bradycardia and sedation may occur. Local anaesthetic perfusion at the site of surgery has also been used successfully.
- Metoclopramide (10 mg) has also been proven to reduce pain and morphine requirements.

Epidural PCA

- Epidural opioids have the advantage of producing analgesia without motor or sympathetic blockade.
- Studies have determined differences among the frequently utilized opioids for epidural analgesia.
- Onset of analgesia is more rapid with the highly lipid soluble opioids.
- Conversely, lipid insoluble opioids, such as morphine, are retained in the CSF. This provides a reservoir to the spinal cord and is consequently associated with a slower onset.
- Lipophilicity, as assessed by octanol:buffer distribution coefficient, does correlate with the meningeal permeability coefficient but in a nonlinear fashion.
- The optimal octanol:buffer distribution coefficient that results in maximal meningeal permeability is between 129 (alfentanil) and 560 (bupivacaine).
- This biphasic relationship between lipophilicity and a drug's meningeal permeability coefficient,

Table 79.2 : Epidural Opioids Administered by Continuous Infusion[1]

Drug	Solution	Bolus Dose	Basal Infusion	Breakthrough Doses	Increments in Breakthrough
Morphine	0.01% (0.1 mg/mL)	4-6 mg	0.5-0.8 mg/hr	0.2-0.3 mg q 10-15 min	0.1 mg
Hydro-morphone	0.005% (0.05 mg/mL)	0.8-1.5 mg	0.15-0.3 mg/hr	0.15-0.3 mg q 10-15 min	0.05 mg
Fentanyl	0.001% (10 ug/mL)	0.5-1.5 ug/kg	0.5-1 ug/kg/hr	10-15 ug q 10-15 min	10 ug
Sufentanil	0.0001% (1 ug/mL)	0.3-0.7 ug/kg	0.1-0.2 ug/kg/hr	5-7 ug q 10-15 min	5 ug
Alfentanil	0.025% (0.25 mg/mL)	10-15 ug/kg	10-18 ug/kg/hr	250 ug q 10 min	250 ug

may be explained by the dual nature of the arachnoid membrane which is the main barrier. After a drug is deposited in the epidural space, but before it reaches the spinal cord, it must first 1. Cross a hydrophilic zone (extracellular and intracellular fluids) and then 2. Cross a hydrophobic zone (cell membrane lipids) of the arachnoid membrane. Thus, before diffusion through these two areas occur, the drug must first dissolve in those environments.

- Opioids with high octanol/buffer distribution coefficients, such as fentanyl and sufentanil move more easily to the intravascular compartment than to the subarachnoid compartment. Thus, spinal cord concentrations of an opioid following epidural administration are the result of the net difference between the rate of uptake and distribution to the vascular and subarachnoid spaces.
- These differences explain why morphine, despite having a meningeal permeability coefficient similar to fentanyl and sufentanil is a useful agent for epidural analgesia.

REFERENCES

1. Raj PP. Practical management of pain, 3rd ed, St. Louis, Mosby year books,1998.
2. Loeser JA, Bonica's management of pain, 3rd ed, Philadelphia,Lippincott-William and Wilkins,2001.
3. Wall PD and Melzack R. Textbook of pain (3rd) ed Edinburgh Churchill, Livingstone, 1994.
4. Kumar P. Patient controlled Analgesia (PROS). Proceedings of ISACON 2004. Bhubeneshwar, 2004.

•••

SPECIFIC THERAPEUTIC TECHNIQUES IN PAIN MANAGEMENT

80

There are several kinds of psychotherapeutic approaches to the management of chronic pain. Of those which have a sufficient literature to permit description and evaluation, we may distinguish five: (1) individual psychodynamic psychotherapy, (2) group psychodynamic psychotherapy, (3) operant behaviour therapy, (4) cognitive behaviour therapy and (5) a group of related therapies which include relaxation training, biofeedback treatment, and hypnotherapy.

Individual Psychodynamic Psychotherapy

This is the oldest of the traditional psychotherapies and derives from Freudian psychoanalytic principles. The application to chronic pain was made by Engel.[1] The assumption is that those with chronic pain may have certain personality characteristics predisposing them to this condition. Such patients are called "pain-prone" and tend to have more frequent incidents of pain in their lives than do others, to be relatively intolerant of success, and to have a developmental history which makes the acquisition and retention of the pain state a coping process.[2]

The patients are those whom we could now characterize as having "psychogenic" pain as a result of a conversion or other somatization mechanism. The psychological features of such patients may not be applicable to those whose chronic pain state is due to a physical disease or injury. However, some authors have attempted to extend the concept of "pain-prone" to those whose pain is "somatogenic," describing a much lengthier check-list of features of the pain-prone patient.[2] Chronic pain is seen as a form of masked depression, and may be a consequence of denial of inner psychological conflict and the repression of anger.

Sifneos[3] has characterized such somatizing patients as lacking a vocabulary for their feelings. Pain (or other medical symptoms) may come to stand for affects which are unrecognized and, therefore, not appropriately expressed. He describes the problems of psychotherapy with such "alexithymic" patients.

Those with psychogenic pain or whose somatogenic pain is due to "pain-proneness" are thought by some to require individual psychotherapy, based on psychoanalytic principles, in order to help resolve the inner conflicts, repressed affects, and alexithymia causing the pain problem.

Group Psychodynamic Psychotherapy

Finsky[4] has written eloquently of the rationale for group psychotherapy for those with the disorder he refers to as a "chronic intractable benign pain syndrome." Since the first characteristic of this syndrome is that it "cannot be shown to be causally related to the her-and-now with any active pathophysiological or patho-anatomic process," he seems to be describing a similar patient to those characterized above as "psychogenic" or "somatizing" or "pain-prone" and excluding those who, with peripheral neuropathies, thalamic pain, etc., have ongoing somatogenic pain generators.

For such patients, therapy in a group setting is said to offer significant advantages over individual treatment. Group support by others with similar problems makes the patient more tolerant of and responsive to suggestions and persuasion, patients can learn modelling techniques from those more successful in coping with pain, and the alexithymic patients have more opportunity to identify their feelings and emotional responses in an affect-evocative group setting.

As with individual therapy, the group treatment will vary in its dynamic emphasis according to the orientation of the therapist. Some may be more didactic, and focus on immediate pain coping-skills, while others may be more permissive and attempt to evoke fantasies and associated affects and relate these to past significant events. The former approach is also more likely to occur in a setting of a short-term treatment programme of 3-4 weeks, the latter emphasis may be found in longer programmes of 6 to 8 weeks' duration, with the opportunity of 60 or more hours of group therapy.

The effectiveness of this treatment approach seems not to have been reported in an outcome study. Group treatment tends to occur in a setting of a multidisciplinary, multimodality pain programme, in which it is not possible to assess the effectiveness of each treatment element separately.

Operant Behaviour Therapy

Operant behaviour therapy has been reported by a number of centres for the treatment of pain. This approach deals primarily with such observable pain behaviours as medication overuse, verbal complaints, grimacing, limping, decreasing physical activity, etc. There is no concern for whether pain is psychogenic or somatogenic, but only with such pain behaviours as comprise excess disability and which may be maintained by environmental reinforcers.[5]

Patients are enrolled in a physical therapy/ occupational therapy rehabilitation programme, in which they perform a comprehensive series of exercises and tasks in a graduated, progressive stepwise fashion, so that they become "extinguished" by eliminating the environmental reinforcers which are said to maintain them, and the more adaptive or normal behaviours are reinforced by staff praise and compliments and display of graphs which show the patient's progress.

Operant behaviour therapy for pain succeeds in the desired rehabilitation goals of making the patients more functional, that this improvement is maintained at follow-up, and that there is some improvement in subjective pain intensity rating by patients, although many such programmes do not obtain this information.[6]

Cognitive Behaviour Therapy

This approach is based on the assumption that, just as psychogenic pain, anxiety, and depression result from negative thoughts and distorted concepts, so maladaptive adjustment to chronic somatogenic pain may have similar causes. Like the operant approach, the cognitive therapeutic approach does not attempt directly to eliminate the patient's pain, but rather to so modify the perception of and reaction to the pain that the patient can live a more satisfying and effective life.

As described by Turk et al.[7] the cognitive-behavioural programme is as specific, detailed and organized as is the operant-behavioural approach. Patients' ways of thinking about their pain and other areas of their lives are identified, and these are "reconceptualized" so that more effective coping strategies can be developed. Cognitive and behavioural coping skills are taught, rehearsed with "homework" assignments, and generalization, maintenance, and relapse-prevention techniques are also reviewed and practiced.

In so far as this approach also uses graduated and progressive physical conditioning techniques, drug reduction, behavioral rehearsal and other behavioural techniques, there is considerable overlap with the operant approach.

Relaxation, Biofeedback, Hypnosis

Among the concomitants of chronic pain are muscular tension, nervousness, irritability, anxiousness, and other signs of sympathetic or adrenergic arousal. A variety of relaxation training techniques has been employed to reverse these responses. The assumption is that such arousal and tension states, elicited by pain, serve to perpetuate or potentiate the pain, and that relaxation can end or reduce the pain. Almost without exception, reviews of studies on the effectiveness of relaxation training have shown that such treatment is significantly effective in pain reduction, and that improvement is maintained at follow-up.[6] There does not seem to be any particular advantage of one method over another, and quite mechanical (demystified) meditative and relaxation techniques seem to serve equally well.

Biofeedback as a treatment was initially thought to be an application of operant conditioning to physiologic responses. It was thought that specific muscle or vasomotor or other responses could be modified, so that the pain intensity could be reduced or abolished. In fact, studies have shown that training in scalp muscle contraction is as effective as scalp

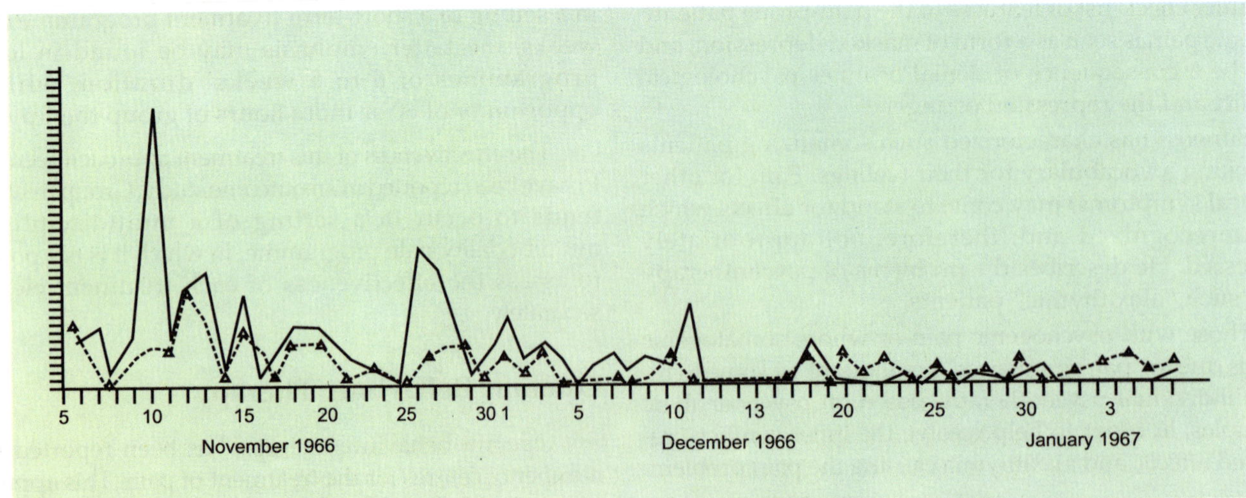

Fig. 80.1 : Change in the frequency of vomiting episodes and headache (H.A.S) in a child undergoing relaxation and biofeedback treatment for a migraine equivalent syndrome

muscle relaxation in the treatment of tension headache (Fig. 80.1) that digital temperature reduction is as effective as digital warming in migraine treatment, etc. Several reviews have concluded that biofeedback has been an effective modality for pain treatment, and that the effectiveness is due to a nonspecific relaxation rather than to a conditioning of specific physiologic responses.[6]

Hypnosis has an ancient history, and many well-documented case studies exist on its effectiveness as a means of pain treatment. Recently there have been more systematic studies performed, and hypnosis has been shown to be as effective as other relaxation techniques, but not necessarily more so. Some claims have been made for special mental effects induced by hypnosis belong general relaxation, but this may occur only in subjects that are highly hypnotizable.[8] This effect may be obscured in experimental designs which randomly assign subjects to treatments and do not examine whether degree of hypnotization has a special effect on outcome.

Table 80.1 : Cognitive and behavioural pain-relieving strategies

Strategy	Description	Mechanism
Breathing techniques	For younger children, simple breathing techniques: use party blowers and bubble blowing. Bubble blowing combines regulated breathing with the visual distraction of watching the bubbles. For older children, breathing techniques incorporate consistent, slow, and rhythmical breathing patterns.	Combines the physiological benefits of deep regulated inhalations/exhalations with distraction to produce relaxation, thus reducing pain and anxiety.
Distraction	Sometimes referred to as cognitive refocusing. Focusing the child's attention and concentration away from the pain onto more enjoyable things. Parents can play an important role in distracting the child through activities such as reading, watching television, playing, walking and talking.	Mechanisms are unclear but may be related to the resources of limited capacity model of attention where an individual's capacity to process information is limited.Allocation of attention to one task limits the attention to another (*e.g.* pain) .
Progressive muscle relaxation (PMR)	The child is coached to focus on relaxing specific muscle groups in a stepwise fashion. Can be used in combination with breathing techniques to produce relaxation.	PMR is thought to decrease oxygen consumption, muscle tension, metabolic rate, heart rate, and respiratory rates and to increase alpha brain waves.
Imagery/ guided imagery	Imagery is used to reduce tension from stress, access unconscious meaningful thoughts and emotions, identify internal resources, and reinforce positive emotions and coping. When a coach is used, the process is referred to as guided imagery. Particulary successful with children as vivid imagination is natural and allows the child to conjure up the image of situations and places that are pleasant. More effective with repeated use.	In acute pain, imagery appear to function primarily as a distraction. In chronic pain, transformation may function to reduce negative evaluation of the situation.
Massage	Passive form of relaxation. Most common areas to massage are the back and shoulders. Described as soothing and relaxing from both a physical and emotional perspective.	Same as relaxation. May have a positive effect on cardiovascular parameters such as blood pressure.
Music	Involves the controlled use of music to decrease pain through its influence on physiological and psychological responses to stress. Requires a quiet environment, a comfortable position, a passive attitude, and focused concentration on the music.	Form of distraction to focus attention on stimuli other than the pain and a method of promoting relaxation and general well-being.

Selection of treatment

The several reviews of psychologic treatment for chronic pain suggest that a pattern of specificity may be emerging. Although there does seem to be a great deal of overlap of nonspecific treatment effects, there may also be some specific effects among the therapies.

If the pain problem is primary psychogenic or a somatization effect resulting from inner conflicts or denial of affect, the treatment of choice may be psychodynamic group therapy.

If the problem is one of excess disability associated with chronic pain, the patient may most likely benefit from an operant behavioural programme specifically designed to normalize levels of function.

If the patient's functioning is not the primary problem, but subjective distress and psychologic inability to cope with pain is the major complaint, then a cognitive-behavioural approach may be the most appropriate intervention. Hypnotherapeutic techniques for pain control are much the same as those taught in cognitive-behavioural treatment, but the latter does not require a trance state and emphasized patient responsibility for coping with pain.

Whenever tension states and arousal are factors contributing to pain, relaxation or biofeedback can be effective in correcting this, and such treatment can be a part of operant- or cognitive-behavioural therapy programmes.

REFERENCES

1. Engel GL."Psychogenic" pain and the pain-prone patient. Am. J. Med., 1959; 26: 899-918.
2. Blumer D, Heilbronn M. Chronic pain as a variant of depressive disease. The pain-prone disorder. J. Nerv. Ment. Dis., 1982; 170: 381-392.
3. Sifneos P. Problems of psychotherapy of patients with alexithymic characteristics and physical disease. Psychother. Psychosom., 1975; 26: 65-70.
4. Pinsky JJ, Cure BL. Intensive group psychotherapy. In: Wall P.D., Melzack R., Eds., Textbook of Pain, Churchill Livingstone, Edinburgh, 1984; pp. 823-831.
5. Fordyce WE, Roberts AH, Sternbach RA The behavioral management of chronic pain: a response to critics, Pain, 1985; 22: 113-125.
6. Linton SJ. Behavioral remediation of chronic pain: a status report. Pain, 1986; 24: 125-141.
7. Turk DC, Meichenbaum DH, Genest M. Pain and Behavioral medicine: A Cognitive-Behavioral perspective, Guilford Press, New York, 1983; pp 42.
8. Orne MT, Dinges DF. Hypnosis. In: Wall P.D., Melzack R., Eds., Textbook of Pain, Churchill Livingstone, Edinburgh, 1984; pp. 806-816.

•••

ALTERNATIVE COMPLEMENTARY THERAPY AND HYPNOSIS

81

Alternative Complementary Therapy [ACT] for pain relief includes a vast array of both modalities in which the patient is a passive recipient, as well as self-care techniques. As a result of individuals taking more charge of their health, as well as becoming disenchanted with the costs and outcomes of allopathic care, interest in this area is rapidly growing. These therapies include:[1]

A. Alternative Medical System such as Acupuncture, Needle effect, Cryoanalgesia.

B. Biologically Based Therapy such as Hypnosis, Aromatherapy, Distraction and Music, Chewing gum, Biofeedback, Massage, Psychotherapy.

C. Manipulative and Body Based Therapies such as TENS, Chiropractic, Auriculotherapy, Ice massage, Relaxation techniques etc.

D. Biofield Therapies using Metals such as Copper bracelets, Coin rubbing, Reiki, Vibrational therapies etc.

A survey [1998] of the use of ACT by rehabilitation outpatients showed that one or more ACTs had been used by 29.1% of subjects in the past 12 months for their painful problems, 53% of whom reported some degree of efficacy.

Thus the providers of the pain management services will have to learn the multimodal approach of pain management, using traditional allopathy as well as ACTs. This means that if one type of treatment [Allopathy] is only partially successful in achieving pain relief and increased mobility, ACTs can be added in a systematic manner for maximum patient benefit.

It is beyond the scope of this chapter to cover all modes of ACTs as listed above, but some of the more commonly used ACT modalities are briefly discussed.

A. *Alternative Medical System*[2]

1. **Acupuncture:** Acupuncture refers to the practice of inserting sharp needles into the body to treat pain and disease. Acupuncture can be divided into classical acupuncture, western acupuncture, electrical acupuncture and ear acupuncture. Acupuncture analgesia is of slow onset and long duration, and thus an induction period [2–30 mins.] is required for stimulation. It usually requires a number of sittings on a regular basis and rarely produces complete pain relief.[2]

   The Chinese believe that life energy [Chi] follows specific pathways or meridians in the body upon which the acupuncture points lie. Any pain or disease process can unbalance the circulation of Chi. This can be corrected by the insertion [with or without manual rotation] of acupuncture needles into specific points along the meridians near the body surface. Classically, there are 12 bilaterally symmetrical meridians and 2 non-paired midline control meridians, each representing internal organ. This is classical acupuncture.

   On the contrary, in Westernized acupuncture, standard points are chosen as a priori. Interestingly, many acupuncture points are close to nerves or trigger points. A 30 G stainless steel needle is inserted into these points until the patient experiences tingling, soreness, numbness or heaviness. Acupuncture points can be stimulated by digital pressure [acupressure], electrically and by the use of lasers.

   With electroacupuncture, needles inserted into the acupuncture points apply electrical stimulation with a pulse generator. Most pulse generators deliver pulsed direct current with a square wave. The frequency, pulse width and voltage can be varied. Electroacupuncture produces greater analgesia than manual acupuncture.

   According to ear acupuncture method, all parts of the body and all the inner organs are reflected on well-localized zones on the auricle of the ear. The entire auricle can be viewed as a representation of an inverted foetus in utero. When an organ becomes diseased or painful, the corresponding point on the ear becomes painful.

   In both experimental animal and human studies, both low frequency [2 Hz] and high frequency [100 Hz] electroacupuncture selectively induce the release of enkephalins and endorphins, which may be responsible for the relief of pain.

2. **Needle effect:** In the 1950's, several investigators discovered, independently of one another, that the insertion of a hypodermic needle through the skin at the tender point, without injecting an anaesthetic or injecting only normal saline, often produces a

dramatic relief of myofacial pains associated with musculoskeletal system. The effectiveness of the treatment for acute pain relief is probably related to the intensity of pain produced at the trigger zone, and to the precision with which the needle located the site of maximal tenderness. The needle, in short, must penetrate at the point of maximum pain. The brief shot of pain produced by the needle resulted in striking relief of pain in 86.8% of cases and persistent relief for months or even permanently in about 50% of the cases.

3. **Cryoanalgesia:** It is now well established that freezing a nerve destroys the nerve cell at the site of freezing, perineural collagen and interneural connective tissues are preserved. The perineural collagen provides a scaffold for regenerating capillaries, axons and Schwann cells. The restoration work starts in about 10 days and may be completed by 50 days.

Cryoanalgesia is only suitable for nerves in which the motor component is minimal or unimportant. Freezing intercostal nerves and ilioinguinal nerves under direct vision are very suitable for alleviating post thoracotomy pain and herniorrhaphy pain respectively.

The cryoprobe consists of a fine needle [or an intracath] with a built-in thermocouple [to confirm the temperature at the tip]. The probe temperature falls to –70° C in the distal 5 mm to form a 2-4 mm ice ball, which freezes the nerve. 2-minute freeze cycles separated by a 1-minute warming period, is likely to increase the destructive effect. The patient should be warned about the resulting numbness in the area supplied by the nerve.

B. *Biologically Based Therapy* [2]

Distraction and music: Part of the role of music is distraction. The use of other distraction techniques reduced post-surgical anxiety, but neither these techniques, nor relaxation procedures produced any reduction in post-operative pain. Distraction probably plays a part in the reduction of analgesic requirements in post-operative patients nursed in a ward looking out on trees compared with a ward overlooking a wall.

Audiocontrol: The use of high intensity random noise has been described in the control of acute pain in dental surgery. The patients control the sound, and use it either in anticipation of pain, or when pain is felt. Upto 65% patients obtain adequate pain relief. The patients are advised to listen music for 30 minutes every 2 hours during the first 48 hours after operation. Audio control by music not only reduced the pain scores, but also the B.P. and heart rate.

Chewing gum: This simple remedy after tonsillectomy, has been claimed to reduce pain on swallowing as well as mouth odour, and to cause a thinner fibrin layer to form over the fossa.

Biofeedback: This includes elements of distraction, suggestion, and relaxation, all of which can help to reduce analgesic requirements. In this technique, patients are told, " post-operative pain is primarily due to sustained contraction and tightness of muscles. The goal of this technique is to learn to relax your muscles, so that tension level never gets too high, and you no longer feel pain". Decreased pain scores and morphine requirement have been observed especially on the second and third post-operative days.

Massage: Massage is the systematic stroking, gliding, kneading and percussion of muscles, tendons or ligaments without changing the joint position for pain relief, oedema reduction and minimizing adhesion formation. It is contraindicated in thrombophlebitis, over malignancies, open wounds and inflamed and infected tissues. Massage increases superficial blood flowing the treated area and improves venous and lymph return. The stimulation of peripheral receptors by massage enhances muscle relaxation and well being, sedation and pain relief.

Psychotherapy: Although it is a most useful adjunctive treatment modality, psychological intervention should never be considered a substitute for appropriate medical management. The major goal of psychological intervention is not to eliminate pain, although pain levels may decrease. Instead it is to help patients to regain a sense of control over managing their symptoms and improve their quality of life.

C. *Manipulative and Body Based Therapies*

1. **TENS:** These may be transcutaneous, abbreviated as TCNS or TENS, when electrodes are attached to the skin, or percutaneous [PES] when needle electrodes are used.

The basis of the effectiveness of this method of analgesia is the gate theory of pain proposed by Melzack and Wall in 1965.The pulsed stimulation of large A beta fibres will close the "gate" in the dorsal horn of the spinal cord, and thus inhibit the central transmission of pain stimuli which reach the dorsal horn in small C fibres.

Positioning of electrodes for relief of post-operative pain is very variable. Often one electrode is placed on each side of the incision. Two pairs of electrodes can be used, two being related to the wound site and two elsewhere. One electrode may be placed over the dermatome where pain is perceived, and the other placed on the back over the same spinal cord segment. For relief of labour pain, two pairs of electrodes are required, one pair at T10 – L1 to treat the pain associated with the first stage of labour and a pair at S2 – S4 for the second stage of labour.

The typical range of controls or stimulation suitable for TENS should be: current 0 –15 mA, frequency 0 – 100 Hz, pulse width 0.1 – 0.5 milliseconds. Usually a frequency of 100 Hz and a mid-range current is started. The current is then turned down until the fasciculation stops, after which the patient may adjust the frequency to the most comfortable level. A 20 minutes period of TENS stimulation usually offers pain relief lasting several hours. In a recent trial, TENS was found to have a placebo effect in 33% patients and in 77% actual relief of post-operative pain.

The use of TENS is remarkably free from side effects. The only common problem is an allergic dermatitis to the adhesive tape holding the electrode in position. A mild erythema can occur at the site of stimulation and, if insufficient electrode gel is used, a burning or pricking sensation can occur. The only absolute contraindication is a patient with pacemaker or other implanted electrical device, which may be affected by the field generated by the stimulator.

2. **Auriculotherapy:** The claim by the French physician Nogier [1972] that electrical stimulation at points of the outer ear abolishes pain has led to widespread use of "auriculotherapy". Nogier argued that the body is represented at the ear in the shape of an inverted homunculus. Later, it was shown that auricular electro stimulation in rats produced nalaxone-reversible analgesia accompanied by increased endorphin levels in the CSF. Despite these positive data, auriculotherapy is believed to be no more effective than a placebo in humans in relieving acute pain. However, about a third of the patients report a feeling of warmth, 'glowing feeling' and other sensations in distant parts of the body when the ear is stimulated.
3. **Ice massage:** Ice massage is another way to produce intense sensory inputs. At first, ice massage of an area makes it feel numb. If ice massage is maintained, however, it produces aching, burning pain, and therefore, may act like intense TENS. Acute dental pain has been treated with ice massage of the back of the hand [at the Hoku area between the thumb and index finger] on the same side as the pain. The ice massage decreased the intensity of dental pain by 50% or more in the majority of the patients. In the light of recent evidence, the likely mechanism to explain the effects of distant stimulation on dental pain is the loop involving afferent fibres from the upper limbs to the brain stem inhibitory control structures, and descending control fibres, which go to the trigeminal subnucleus caudalis.
4. **Relaxation training:** Relaxation training teaches patients to become physically and mentally relaxed. It has a number of physiological effects. It may slow heart and respiratory rate, and increase extremity temperature. It can improve sleep, diminish muscle tension and decrease pain. It also enhances coping ability by decreasing anxiety and increasing self-control.

D. *Biofield Therapies*

1. **Reiki :** Reiki is a Japanese word. 'Rei' means universal transcendental spirit and 'Ki' stands for life energy. The belief is that the universe is filled with this invisible life energy and life and health of all living beings is sustained by it. The Reiki energy is there from one's very birth. All one has to do is lay his/her hands on another person and accelerate the process of healing/pain relief using magnetic energy. By touching at various points, various painful conditions and diseases can be tackled. Its role in acute pain management is yet to be properly documented.
2. **Vibrational therapies:** This has been effectively used in patients with severe post-operative dental pain, when both the TENS and drugs have become ineffective.

E. *Bioelectromagnetic Therapy*

1. **Magnetic therapy:** Nociception is influenced by an exposure to magnetic fields. In humans, a significant reduction in pain-related somatosensory evoked potential amplitudes is observed after exposure to oscillating magnetic fields.

Benefits and Limitations of Alternative Complementary Therapy

Benefits : Most of the methods of analgesia described above do not require the administration of drugs. They, therefore, have particular value in situations where drugs are ineffective or may be undesirable. These includes :

1. Post-caesarian section patients, where drugs may be excreted in breast milk and affect the baby, and maternal sedation may inhibit mother-baby bonding.
2. Patients with intercurrent disease; for example, severe respiratory or liver disease.
3. Day case surgery.
4. The duration and degree of relief sometimes become progressively greater over a period of weeks or months. In the occasional fortunate patient, pain may disappear altogether.
5. Sometimes, non-drug ACT methods will provide good analgesia on their own, but even if supplementary drug therapy is required, effective analgesia will often be produced by smaller doses.

Limitations: ACT's has their own limitations such as:

Most of the ACT techniques require time and experienced staff.

More often than not, ACT techniques require more than one sitting for appreciable pain relief.

Pleasant ward surroundings and access to the distraction of people, radio and television needs to be created for maximum effect of ACTs.

ACTs may not work in all patients.

Hypnosis

Hypnosis is an altered state of consciousness slightly different from waking and sleep, characterized by hyper suggestibility. As noninvasive form of treatment, it is useful in psychosomatic diseases. Pain is the psychical adjunct of an imperative protective reflex. Pain is the presenting symptoms in many diseases and psychosomatic problems and a common problem to all practicing doctors. The patient may speak in terms of hurt, pressure, ache, stiffness or cramps rather than pain or he may express something as pain that is really an outward manifestation of anxiety and depression. Anxious and neurotic patients have lower tolerance levels for pain than depressive and schizophrenic patients. Pain is not only a nocuous and disagreeable sensation but is the result of complex interaction of sensory, motivational and cognitive factors involving peripheral receptor, pain pathways, limbic system, thalamus and cortical area of the brain and depends greatly on the pre-existing memories stored in the brain.[1]

Human beings have been struggling hard through the ages to free themselves from the clutches of pain. Laying of hands by kings and priests has relieved pain of primitive people. Hypnosis has been used for the control of organic pain since the time of Mesmer and Esdaile.[3] Iatrogenic pain can be produced by fear tension and anxiety; so one can have freedom from it by the iatrogenic health that may be suggested hypnotically.

Just as drugs, electroshock, psychoanalysis, guidance and group therapy have their role in rounded psychotherapeutic programme, so hypnosis where appropriately applied belongs with these as an additional resource for effecting clinical relief.

Hypotheses of Hypnotic Analgesia

Hypnotic induction is the facilitation of patient's alteration in consciousness for wakefulness to imaginative absorption that supports the acceptance of a clinical suggestion.

1. direct hypnotic suggestions for total abolition of pain;
2. permissive indirect hypnotic abolition of pain;
3. amnesia;
4. hypnotic anaesthesia;
5. hypnotic replacement or substitution of sensation;
6. hypnotic displacement of pain;
7. hypnotic dissociation: Dissociation of part of the body and time can be produced by hypnotic suggestions. In one type of method patient is hypnotically reoriented in time to the earlier stage of his illness. Post hypnotic suggestions help in continuation of the lessened pain feeling through waking state.[4]
8. hypnotic reinterpretation of pain experience;
9. Hypnotic time distortion.

It is suggested that hypnosis bridges the gap between physiological and psychological concepts of pain. It is emphasized that hypnosis promotes a milieu in which effective strategies can be integrated and that hypnotic technique can give patients the needed impetus to recognize their ability to regain control.

There is a need for more extensive participation of clinicians in utilizing hypnosis and in bringing their results to the attention of other physicians, not only through the publications of scientific papers, but also through demonstration, teaching and training at the hospital and medical school level as a way of clearing up misunderstandings about identification of hypnosis with specific modalities of induction and stereotyped patterns of expected behaviour.[5]

Hypnosis is useful in acute pain of labour, dental, cancer, medical, surgical and in burn cases. Besides making the dressing of burnt areas less painful, hypnosis helps those patients to recover rapidly with very little pain experience, increased resistance to infection and great expectation of early return to normal activity.[6] The post hypnotic suggestion can extend the duration of an already achieved temporary pain relief due to dissociation of noxious impulses and neural reorganization after initial analgesia.[7]

Complications: Disorientation, hysterical manifestations, memory contamination specially if the patient is severely depressed, psychotic of pathologically irresponsive.[8]

REFERENCES

1. Loeser JD. Bonica's management of pain. 3rd edi. Philadelphia Lippincott Williams and Wilkins, 2001.
2. Wall PD and Melzack R. Textbook of pain,(3rd) ed Edinburgh Churchill,Livingstone,1994.
3. Esadile J. Hypnosis in medicine and surgery. Introduction and supplementary reports by W S Kroger. New York : Julian 1995.

4. Hilgard E R. A Quantitative study of pain and its reduction through hypnotic suggestions. Proc Natl. Acad sci. 1967;57:1581-1586.

5. Price DD, Barber J. A Quantitative analysis of factors that contribute to the efficacy of hypnotic analgesia. J Abrmorm Psychol 1987;96:46-51.

6. Patterson DR. Non opoid based approaches to burn pain. J Burn Care Rehabil; 1995;16:372-376.

7. Flor H, Elbert T, Knecht S, et al. Phantom limb pain as a perceptual correlative of corical reorganization following an amputation. Nature 1995;375:482-484.

8. Borber J. When hypnosis causes trouble. Int J Clin Exp Hypn, 1998;46:157-170.

•••

SECTION–XIV

Pain Clinic OPD Setup

PAIN CLINIC OPD

82

Chronic pain patient may represent one third of the total population and now is treated as a disease in itself as suggested by Leriche in his classical publication Surgery of Pain, 1930. In 1943, Livingstone published a book and explained mechanism of causalgias which stimulated study and treatment of sympathetic blocks and nerve blocks. During Second World War, Beecher, Bonica and Alexander developed broad view of chronic pain and suggested a multi-modal and interdisciplinary approach to pain management. This led to the set-up of pain clinic or nerve block clinic in USA after the world war. The first multidisciplinary clinic in a teaching hospital was set-up in 1960 by Bonica in University of Washington, Seattle. Bonica was also responsible for foundation of International Association for Study of Pain in 1974. From a 17 pain clinics in USA in 1976 the number rose to 300 in 1977 and 428 in USA and other countries. Bonica suggested 1800 pain clinics in some 36 countries in 1987, while ASA listed 240 pain clinics with a director and its team in 1999.

The Indian Society of Study of Pain was formed in Varanasi by the efforts of Dr. V. Rastogi and Dr. Pramod Kumar under the guidance of Dr. K. Pandey in 1984 and was recognized as Indian chapter of IASP. The number of pain clinics rose from 3-4 centers in 1980 to 70 in 1988 and more than 150 in 1998.

The Pain clinics can either be:

1. Individually run private practice or hospital based services run by a director who coordinates with a group of medical, surgical, psychiatric, and the other support group personnel and services.
2. Community based private pain centre – serves the highly industrialized community for chronic pain and trauma pain.
3. Pain centres in a teaching hospitals – are interdisciplinary in nature providing clinical services as well as training programmes.

Organizing a Pain Centre in a Teaching Hospital

1. Resources assessments – only a few of the clinicians are interested in treating pain patients in a teaching hospital. They start a group or nucleus to start a pain clinic by interacting frequently with physician, surgeons, psychiatrist and physiotherapist. The scope of pain centre and documentation of present and potential future patients is presented to the administrative body of the institution which reviews the needs and the resources and appoints one senior person actively engaged in pain relief as in-charge. The in-charge or director must demonstrate the quality of a scientist, clinician, teacher, and administrator along with his commitment to pain relief and considerable experience in the area. He coordinates and reviews the patient care for quality, manages resources *e.g.*, personnel, equipments, supplies and space. There must be a coordination of education and research activities in the pain centre for all clinical departments. In USA director of Pain services is independent and directly responsible to the Head of the medical college and the hospital.

In India, the pain clinics are run mainly by anaesthesiologists who run OPD and provide nerve block and acute pain services near the operation theatre area. The Medical Council of India has included pain clinic and general intensive care unit as an integral part of anaesthesiology speciality and made it mandatory for UG and PG degree recognization.

The Pain Team : Rawal N suggested an anaesthetist based service run with the help of trained nurses for acute pain services. However, pain clinic centre must have permanent consultants providing treatment and coordinating with other specialties *e.g.*, physiotherapist, psychiatrist, orthopaedician, neurosurgeon, nursing and hospital administration.

Space : The pain clinic OPD should be near the reception area with a waiting area to the consultation room, treatment room and the clerical space. The minor operating room can either be in the OPD or in a nearby OT Complex, equipped like an operation theatre with all monitoring facilities available along with image intensifier and the cardio pulmonary resuscitation facilities.

Evaluation of a Pain patient : A medical, psychosocial and pain conference in case of difficult cases is done regularly, listing following points:

1. Individually:
1. History – Past, pain, family, general medical, drug, occupational, social and psychological histories are documented under separate headings.
2. Physical examination – Pain region, general examination, neurological and orthopaedic.
3. Psychological and Psychiatric evaluation – Psychometric tests (GHQ28), psychiatric interview.
4. Diagnostic procedure – (a) clinical laboratory tests (b) radiological examinations (plain X-ray, CT scan, MRI, nuclear medicine) (c) diagnostic nerve blocks (d) electromyelography (e) EEG (f) ECG.
5. Medical and surgical consultations – needed are well recorded.
6. Interdisciplinary pain conference – for diagnosis, aetiology, pathology and complications and treatment plan (flow chart).

Pain Clinic Flow Chart

- Out patient clinic – Referral from other centres and departments.
- Data collection (History, records, Lab results, X-ray, EMG report).
- Anaesthesia Pain Clinic – Consultations, Psychometric tests, Diagnostics and Therapeutic nerve blocks , Physical therapy, Biofeedback, clinical research, Major blocks, inpatient admissions.
- Neurology and neurosurgery – Complete neurological workup and neurosurgical procedures.
- Oral surgery – Dental evaluation– Dental surgery procedures.
- Staff review conference (disciplinary) – No relief referral to other departments.
- Recommendations for therapy.

Treatment Services used for Pain Relief

1. Medical/ Surgical / Pain consultation services.
2. Biomedical services– nerve blocks, TENS.
3. Nursing care.
4. Social services.
5. Vocational evaluation and counselling.
6. Patient and family education.
7. Individual, group and family psychotherapy.
8. Drug detoxication and pharmacological management.
9. Clinical laboratory and radiology.
10. Dentistry.
11. Dietician.
12. Relaxation modalities-biofeedback, relaxation and imagery.
13. Rehabilitation and social services (NGOs).

Education of Primary Care Physicians

Case discussions, video tape sessions, invitations to attend Pain conferences, CME, residency training, Media coverage of Pain, encouraging self education. The stress is put on removal of common myths prevalent and prerequisites for pain management.

Myths in Chronic Pain Management

1. Chronic pain Myths—The pain is not real, less severe and disabling than other treatable conditions. The same parameters used to evaluate a patient with acute pain are used for chronic pain. The patient does not need a thorough diagnostic evaluation. The chronic pain is always an extension of poorly managed acute pain. Designating chronicity according to duration using 6 months as an arbitrary limit. The myth that chronic pain is always due to psychological reason, there are misconceptions that about treating chronic pain in the same way as acute pain or not treat at all or refer to other speciality.
2. Physicians treating chronic pain should not assure that chronic pain has to be maintained on analgesics, narcotics and tranquilizers, and if medications are not working refer to pain clinics which is taken as a last resort. It is wrong to assume a chronic pain patient as totally and permanently disabled.
3. Chronic Pain patients' myth — Hurt is harmful and the system owes them something. The doctors think that pain is in my head and pain centres are for psychological pain and they are supposed to live with pain. The doctor is supposed to know what is causing the pain and fix it. The patient cannot do anything until pain is present. There is always a notion that another break through will cure them of all ills. It must be understood that chronic pain in a way protects the patients by rendering them inactive allowing the recovery from illness.

General Principles for Chronic Pain Management

1. Establish an early diagnosis.
2. Listen to the patients and create a positive doctor patient relationship.
3. Approach to the patient should be simple, direct without much use of technical words.

4. Educate patients to assure a more active role in managing their problem.
5. Focus less on interrupting pain pathways. Control other systemic diseases.
6. Avoid invasive procedures, polypharmacy.
7. Continue support despite failed therapy.
8. Encourage physical activities, exercises.
9. Treat depression, stress, and psychological problems equally.
10. Emphasis on rehabilitation rather than eradication with single modality.
11. Treatment of whole patient.
12. Decrease the amount of pain.
13. Improve family support.
14. To decrease patient's dependence on medical care and reduce costs.

Cost Effectiveness

Goal of pain clinic is to reduce patient dependence on health care systems and rehabilitation so that they can return to normal work routine, thereby reducing overall costs for the state and the patient.

Table 82.1 : Proforma used in a Medical College Pain Clinic OPD

Dr. Professor Department of Anaesthesiology, Medical College			Department of Anaesthesiology Hospital,			
PAIN RELIEF WORK AND RECORD						
Patient's Name : Address : Ref by Dr.			Pain Clinic Reg. No.: Date : Age : Sex : Race :			
Diagnosis:						
Chief Complainsts :						
Pain : Region :						
Duration :	Continuous	☐	Periodic	☐	Momentory	☐
Intensity of Pain :	Mild	☐	Moderate	☐	Severe	☐
Pain Related to :	Bone :		Soft tissue :			
	Viscera :		Music Spasm :			
	Nerve Compression :		Raised I.C.T. :			
Type of Pain :	Pricking :					
	Cuffing :		Sharp :			
	Dull Aching :		Spasmodic :			
	Burning :		Freezing :			
Sleep Disturbances :						
Past History :			Family History			
General Physical Examination : Facial Expression : Posture : Tremors : Gait :						

Neurological Examination : Higher Functions : GHQ score

Cranial Nerves :

Motor System :

Laboratory Investigations :

Hb : G% T.C. /cmm. D.C. P. L. E. M. B.

Urine examination : Alb : Sug : Micro : Culture :

Dio chemical :	F.B.S.	S. Bilirubin
	P.P.B.S.	S.G.O.T.
	S. Cholestrol	Austr. Antigen
	Bl. Urea	S. Sodium
	Bl. Creatinine	S. Potassium
		Others

Radiological Investigations :

X-ray :	Chest	Abdomen
	Cervical Spine	I.V.P.
	Lumber spine	Ba. Studies
	Skull : A.P. /Lateral	Ba. Enema
	Special Invest - Cr,	Myelogram MRI, Nuclear

Treatment of Pain :

Drug : Technique

Pain Relief Work :

Date	Method	Duration of Relief	Pain Relief				Remarks side effects	GHQ Score /Any other
			None	Slight	Mod.	Complete		

83

GROWTH OF PAIN SERVICES IN INDIA

Though the pain is most common complaint of any patient, not much was known about its mechanisms or cure. Except for opium or spongi somnifera, nothing much has changed till Melzack and Wall's Gate Control Theory, which tried to explain pain mechanisms. Dr. John Bonica of USA first introduced the concept of multidisciplinary management of pain. He laid down the foundation of International Association for Study of Pain (IASP) bringing together the physicians and scientists on a common platform to fight against pain.

Exactly ten years later Indian pain movement started with the formation of Indian Society for Study of Pain. Till then, the pain relief work was done by individuals like Dr. Pritam Singh in Amritsar, Dr. Saini and Dr. Bhattacharya in Delhi, Dr. P. Chari in Chandigarh and Dr. Rastogi in Varanasi. The pain clinic OPD was started in 1984 in Institute of Medical Sciences, Varanasi. Indian Society for Study of Pain was started in 1984, Dr. Rastogi and myself took the responsibility to convince the medical fraternity for the need of pain relief work. Dr. K. Pandey gave a general outline of the constitution of the ISSP, which was later expanded in its present form by Dr. Rastogi and myself. In January 1982, first meeting of ISSP was held under the chairmanship of Prof B.C. Katiyar, Neurologist, in Institute of Medical Sciences Varanasi and it was decided to organize 1st annual conference in Varanasi in February 1985. Among the founders Dr. Akram Lal was appointed as the President, Dr. V. Rastogi as the secretary and Dr. P. Kumar as the Treasurer. ISSP had the blessings and guidance of Dr. K. Pandey, Dr. M.T. Bhatia (Ahmedabad), Dr. S. Yajnik and Dr. Sushila Shah (Mumbai), who guided us throughout and are still our parent figures. I still treasure the moments spent for initial foundation work done in the company of Dr. Rastogi who was the driving force. Simultaneously there was formation of associations in the cities of Ahmedabad by Dr. M. T. Bhatia and ISPRAT from New Delhi by Dr. K.N. Sharma and Dr. P. Bhattacharya. However, since the beginning it was a consensus that there should be only one association of pain. Dr. M.T. Bhatia merged his association with ISSP in 1986. Indian Society for Study of Pain, was recognized as Indian chapter of International Association for Study of Pain in 1987. Indian Journal of Pain was started in 1985 under the editorship of Dr. S. Yajnik. First city branch was started in Varanasi in 1985 and subsequently first regional branch, Vidarbha branch, took the onus of organizing second annual conference at Nagpur in 1986 with Dr. Subhash Sri Rao and myself as the organizing secretaries. The Saurashtra branch of ISSP was formed in Jamnagar in 1986 with myself as its secretary. At the same time Maharashtra branch of ISSP was formed in Mumbai by Dr. S. Saghvi and third conference was held in Hotel Taj Mumbai in 1987. It was my great fortune to be associated with organization of ISSP and its Vidarbha, Saurashtra and Gujarat branches. Probably my migration from Varanasi to Wardha and then to Jamnagar helped in the formation of regional branches and was later instrumental in organizing conferences in Nagpur (1986), AIIMS New Delhi (1989), BYL Nayyar Hospital (1990), ISSP Gujarat state branch in Surat in 1995 and XVII annual conference at Jamnagar (2002).

Dr. Rastogi and myself made a very modest beginning and we were young and ordinary looking, however, it was the greatness of people like Dr. K. Pandey, Dr. A. Lal, Dr. M. Bhatia, Dr. S. Yajnik, Dr. Sushila Shah, Dr. K.N. Sharma who were always encouraging and guiding us. Now at this juncture ISSP has about one thousand five hundred members and state branches in almost all major states. In the beginning there were four centres giving pain relief, the number increased to 70 within 3-4 years. Now every city in India has one or more pain clinic and number is increasing tremendously. As a young man in 1983, I dreamt of a revolution in the pain therapy. But ten years later an assessment of the situation revealed that not much progress has been made in terms of basic science and clinical therapy. Probably a more dedicated approach towards research and therapy is desired instead of just attending conferences and giving lectures from the already existing textbooks.

REFERENCES

1. Kumar. P. Progress of Indian Society for Study of Pain. Souvenir, XXII National conference of ISSP, Jamnagar, 2002.

•••

Epilogue

When Indian Society for Study of Pain was formed in 1984, and was associated with International Association for Study of Pain in 1986, it was a great first step towards care of patients with chronic and acute pain. The enthusiasm slowly died down after 10 years when not much recognition for pain therapy was given. However, the number of pain clinics in India rose to 74 in 1990. In the last decade there has been a surge in the research in pain mechanisms and therapeutics under the guidance of International Association for Study of Pain. Since last 4 years in India, pain clinic OPD, under the Anaesthesiology Department, has been made mandatory for recognition of a medical college by MCI and pain has been included in curriculum of UG and PG medical courses. This increased the interest shown by post graduates and younger generation of specialists specially anaesthesiology, to learn various modalities of pain relief especially in acute pain.

However, the Government has yet not fully recognized the importance of pain relief especially in chronic pain, thereby devoiding the patients of a very cheap morphine tablet which cannot be procured and prescribed by a physician to the cancer pain patient because of complex legalities and documentation. Pain relief clinics are not recognized by hospital administration leading to the use of NSAIDs and peripheral nerve blocks by one or two of the young enthusiasts in anaesthesia department. While anaesthesiologist has taken the lead in the pain relief service, other specialties are still conforming themselves to diagnosis and limiting the cancer tumour spread, overlooking pain and related symptoms. Even in Anaesthesiology department majority of anesthesiologists are apathetic and confine themselves to giving anaesthesia to surgical patients with an inertness. Most of the medical teachers prefer to sit outside OT and in their offices and not teach the UG or PG students. This represents overall rote in the medical education in India where medical college teaching is now left to the mediocres, who could not make it beg in general practice. Sometimes medical college jobs are treated as a safe place where all the work is left to junior doctors. It is the last category who suffers the training of recent modalities in medical sciences. This book has been targeted towards this group who will take the onus of medical treatment and care of the patients. Further, this book guides the physicians of various specialities working with cancer patiants *e.g.*, medicine anaesthesiology ENT, dental, psychiatry and oncologists. Let this book be a clarion call for all young physicians to "Arise", "Awake" and "Care" for the patients' suffering from pain. "Amen"!

Dr. Pramod Kumar

Appendix

APPENDIX-I

Practice Guidelines for Acute Pain Management in the Perioperative Setting

Based on a Report by the American Society of Anaesthesiologists Task Force on Pain Management, Acute Pain Section

Introduction

Practice guidelines are systematically developed recommendations that assist the practitioner and patient in making decisions about health care. These recommendations may be adopted, modified or rejected according to clinical needs and constraints.

A. Definition of Acute Pain in the Perioperative Setting

Acute pain in the perioperative setting is defined as pain that is present in a surgical patient because of pre-existing disease, the surgical procedure (*e.g.*, associated drains, chest or nasogastric tubes, complications) or a combination of disease-related and procedure-related sources.

B. Purpose of Guidelines for Acute Pain Management in the Perioperative Setting

The purpose of these guidelines is to facilitate the efficacy and safety of acute pain management in the perioperative setting and to reduce the risk of adverse outcomes. A number of adverse outcomes can result from undertreatment of post-operative pain. These include (but are not limited to) thromboembolic and pulmonary complications, extension of time spent in an intensive care unit and/or in a hospital, and reduced patient satisfaction. The principal adverse outcomes associated with management of perioperative pain include (but are not limited to) respiratory depression, brain injury, other neurologic injury, sedation, circulatory depression, nausea and /or vomiting, impairment of bowel function, pruritus and urinary retention.

C. Focus

These guidelines focus on modalities of perioperative pain management that require a higher level of expertise and organizational structure than "as needed" intramuscular or intravenous injections of opioids and that generally provide more effective relief of pain. Examples include (but are not limited to) epidural (and intrathecal) analgesia (EA), intravenous patient-controlled analgesia (PCA), and a number of regional analgesic (RA) techniques. The guidelines are not intended as an exhaustive or detailed consideration of specific techniques or all possible approaches.

The speciality of anaesthesiology brings an exceptional level of interest and expertise to the area of perioperative pain management. As a consequence, the anaesthesiologist is in a unique position to provide leadership in integrating pain management into other aspects of perioperative care and thus improve this area of practice. In this leadership role, the anaesthesiologist can contribute further to quality of care by developing and directing institution-wide perioperative analgesia programmes that include collaboration with and participation by others, when appropriate.

The role of anaesthesiologists in managing acute pain extends beyond the perioperative setting. Patients with severe or concurrent medical illness such as sickle cell crisis, pancreatitis or acute pain related to cancer or cancer treatment also benefit from aggressive pain control. Labour pain is another condition of interest to anaesthesiologists. However, the complex interactions of concurrent medical therapies and physiologic alterations make it impractical to address pain management for these populations within the context of this document.

D. Application

These guidelines focus on management of acute pain in the perioperative setting for adult (including geriatric) and paediatric patients. The guidelines apply to inpatient and outpatient surgery. These guidelines are intended for use by anaesthesiologists or by individuals who deliver care under the supervision of anaesthesiologists.

Evidence to support each guideline was carefully sought. The search included a comprehensive review of the published literature, surveys of the opinions of a large panel of consultants with expertise in acute pain management, and the opinions of the members of the Task Force. An indication of the strength of the evidence supporting each guideline is provided.

Guidelines

1. Proactive Planning

The Task Force defines proactive planning as a process of integrating pain management into the perioperative care of patients. The literature, the panel of consultants, and the Task Force members strongly support the use of proactive planning for post-operative pain management. This support is based on recognized associations between pre-operative and intraoperative analgesic techniques for the reduction of pain in the post-operative period.

Recommendations : An individualized proactive plan (*e.g.*, a predetermined strategy for post-operative analgesia) should be considered for all surgical patients. Factors that may influence the formulation of a proactive plan include (but are not limited to) type of surgery and expected severity of post-operative pain, underlying medical conditions (*e.g.*, presence of respiratory or cardiac disease, allergies), the risk-benefit ratio of the techniques available and patients' preferences and/or previous experience with pain. Proactive planning of perioperative pain should be part of the preoperative evaluation by the anaesthesiologist and, in collaboration with others (*e.g.*, nurses, surgeons, pharmacists), should be part of an institution's general plan for patient care.

Activities that are commonly encompassed by proactive planning include (but are not limited to) (1) obtaining a pain history based on patient's experiences, (2) preoperative pain therapy when appropriate and feasible, (3) intraoperative procedures (*e.g.*, wound infiltration) when appropriate and feasible, and (4) intraoperative or postincisional preparation of patients for post-operative pain management (*e.g.*, initiating EA administration before the completion of surgery). Any treatment plan requires regular assessment and refinement based on the changing responses of individual patients.

II. Education and Training of Hospital Personnel

The available literature suggests that training and experience of hospital personnel (*e.g.*, nurses, house-officers, pharmacists, psychologists) may be helpful in reduction of risk. There is strong agreement among the panel of consultants and the Task Force members that such education, training and experience also contribute to improved quality of care.

Recommendations : Anaesthesiologists offering perioperative analgesia services should provide, in collaboration with others as appropriate, ongoing education and training to ensure that hospital personnel are knowledgeable and skilled with regard to the effective and safe use of the available treatment options within the institution. The scope of education should include topics ranging from basic bedside skills for evaluation of acute pain to an understanding of sophisticated pharmacologic techniques (*e.g.*, PCA, EA, and various RA techniques) and nonpharmacologic techniques (*e.g.*, relaxation, imagery, hypnotic methods). The need for education and training is ongoing as new personnel enter an institution and as modifications in therapeutic approaches are made.

Table 1 : Information Recorded on a Bedside Pain Management Flow Sheet

1. Patient assessment at regular intervals
According to institutional protocols (*e.g.*, pain levels, respiratory evaluation, sedation)
2. Medication administration
Intravenous PCA
Incremental dose
Lockout interval
1 to 4 h limit
Rate of continuous infusion (if applicable)
Supplemental doses for breakthrough pain
Total drug use per unit of time (*e.g.*, nursing shift end total)
Epidural analgesia
Bolus dose and time (if applicable)
Infusion rate (if applicable)
Supplemental doses for breakthrough pain

Table 2 : Important Elements of Intravenous PCA Preprinted Orders

1. Drug(s), concentration(s)
2. Pump settings:
Incremental dose
Lockout interval
Other limits (*e.g.*, 4h, 1h)
3. Mode of use:
PCA only
Continuous infusion
4. Initial drug loading instructions
5. Instructions for treating breakthrough pain
6. A statement to eliminate the ordering of CNS depressants by others
7. Monitoring instructions

8. Availability of drugs to treat side effects
9. Instructions for treatment of side effects Respiratory depression Nausea and/or vomiting Pruritus Urinary retention
10. Instructions about concurrent use of other CNS depressants
11. Instructions for whom to contact if problems occur
12. Date, time, signature

Table 3 : Important Elements of Epidural Analgesia Preprinted Orders

1. Drug(s), concentration(s)
2. Instructions for administration If boluses Drug dose Interval between injections If infusion Loading dose Infusion rate
3. Instructions for treating breakthrough pain
4. Maintain IV route and access to drugs for immediate use
5. A statement to eliminate the ordering of CNS depressants by others
6. Monitoring instruction For effects of opioids For effects of local anaesthetics Bradycardia Hypotension Extensive sensory or motor block
7. Observations that should be communicated to the anaesthesiologist (*e.g.*, systolic blood pressure less than ___mmHg)
8. Instructions for treatment of side effects Respiratory depression Nausea and/or vomiting Pruritus Urinary retention
9. Instructions about concurrent use of other CNS depressants
10. Instructions for whom to contact if problems occur
11. Date, time, signature
CNS = Central Nervous System

III. Education and Participation of Patients and Families in Perioperative Pain Control

The panel of consultants and the Task Force members regard the concept of education of patients and families in planning and participation in perioperative pain control as being important to their comfort and well-being.

Recommendations : Anaesthesiologists offering perioperative analgesia services should provide, in collaboration with others as appropriate, education to patients and families regarding their roles in achieving comfort, reporting pain and using the recommended analgesic methods to optimal benefit. Common misconceptions about the risk of side effects and addiction should be dispelled. Educational methods that facilitate optimal care of patients using PCA and other sophisticated methods might include (but are not limited to) discussion of analgesic methods at the time of the preanaesthetic evaluation, brochures and video tapes to educate patients about therapeutic options, and discussion at the bedside during post-operative visits.

IV. Assessment and Documentation of Perioperative Pain Management

The panel of consultants and the Task Force members strongly support the concept of assessment and documentation of response to perioperative pain therapy as important to effective care. Unless the response to pain therapy is regularly evaluated, there is no basis for rational, individualized therapy.

Recommendations : Anaesthesiologists offering perioperative analgesia services should use, in collaboration with others as appropriate, pain assessment instruments to facilitate the regular evaluation and documentation of pain, the effects of pain therapy and side effects caused by the therapy (tables 1 and 6).

Table 4 : Elements of Intravenous PCA Daily Care by Anaesthesiologists

The following items should be included during a bedside evaluation at least once a day while IV PCA is administered.
1. Note the dose of analgesic medication given in the past 24 hours, and parameters of PCA settings (PCA bolus dose, lockout interval, basal infusion [if applicable], hourly or other interval limit).
2. Evaluate pain intensity both at rest and with operation-specific convalescent activity (*e.g.*, passive continuous movement for knee replacement or chest physical therapy for thoracotomy). If pain is out of proportion to the surgical procedure, the number of days elapsed post-operatively, and analgesic therapy given, consider whether another cause is present (*e.g.*, surgical complication, personality disorder, opioid tolerance) and initiate appropriate evaluation, including communication with the surgeon and/or other consultant physicians.
3. Determine whether side effects are present. Assess each side effect in the context of the type

of operation and days elapsed since the operation. Decide whether the side effect is in proportion to the operation, the number of days postoperatively, and the amount of opioid and other medications given. For sedation, as an example, note other concurrent drug therapy and decide whether to undertake additional work-up (*e.g.*, glucose, electrolytes, arterial blood gas, calcium, magnesium, electrocardiogram).

4. Perform a problem-oriented physical examination (*e.g.* surgical site, presence of rates, venous thrombosis). Note the current vital signs (HR, RR, BP) and compare them with the last evaluation. If these are unstable or unsatisfactory (*e.g.*, low BP or irregular pulse), consider suitable diagnostic work-up (*e.g.*, haematocrit, electrocardiogram).
5. Consider whether the patient would benefit from changing the PCA pump settings or the PCA opioid.
6. Note concurrent medications and consider whether the patient would benefit from changing the overall regimen (*e.g.*, simplifying to avert drug interactions), or employing adjuvant analgesic medication or non-pharmacologic therapies, and if so, order these.
7. Evaluate overall patient satisfaction with current care.
8. Evaluate patients response(s) to prior adjustments of pain therapy or addition of adjuvants (*e.g.*, for nausea or anxiety).
9. Evaluate patients suitability for making the transition to simpler alternatives (*e.g.*, oral analgesics).*
10. Discuss the assessment and plan with the patient and the patient's nurse and/or surgeon, when appropriate.
11. Document findings, impression and plan in the hospital chart.
12. Ensure availability of personnel with appropriate expertise to deal with questions or problems at any time.

V. 24-Hour Availability of Anaesthesiologists

The panel of consultants and the Task Force members support the concept of 24-hour availability of anaethesiologists providing perioperative pain management as being important for maximizing patient comfort and safety. The condition of patients after surgery is frequently dynamic, and analgesic needs may change at any time.

Recommendations : Most analgesic techniques place patients at some risk for side effects or complications that require prompt medical evaluation. Anaesthesiologists responsible for perioperative analgesia, in collaboration with others as appropriate, should be available at all times to consult with ward nurses, surgeons or other involved physicians and assist in evaluating patients who are experiencing problems with any aspect of post-operative pain relief.

VI. Use of Standardized Institutional Policies and Procedures for Ordering, Administering, Discontinuing and Transferring Responsibility for Perioperative Pain Management

The available literature suggests that institutional protocols and procedures for ordering, administering, discontinuing and transferring responsibility for pain management are helpful in providing effective and continuous pain control. The Task Force regards the use of institutional policies and procedures as a logical part of interdisciplinary management of perioperative pain, and there is strong agreement from the panel of consultants that this approach is beneficial. The development of hospital-wide policies and procedures help standardize clinical practices using techniques such as PCA, EA and various RA techniques (tables 2 and 3). Standardization promotes safety and creates a framework for customization of care. Routine use of bedside documentation encourages caregivers to continually re-evaluate pain treatment and respond to inadequate therapy in a timely manner. Daily evaluation, planning and written documentation by those who are medically responsible for pain relief help establish the importance of a formal and structured approach to pain management (Tables 4–7).

Recommendations : Anaesthesiologists offering perioperative analgesia services should participate in developing, in collaboration with others as appropriate (especially nurses), standardized institutional policies and procedures for ordering, administering, discontinuing and transferring responsibility for post-operative pain management. Policies (the foundation or "ground rules" for practice) and procedures (outlining the "how to" aspects of applying policies to patient care) should be readily available on each patient care unit. The policies and procedures also serve as ongoing educational and informational references.

Table 5 : Elements of Epidural Analgesia Daily Care by Anesthesiologists

The following items should be included during a bedside evaluation at least once a day while epidural analgesia is administered.

1. Note the dose of analgesic medication given in the past 24 hours, and present parameters of bolus administration or infusion pump settings (if used).

2. Evaluate pain intensity both at rest and with operation-specific convalescent activity (*e.g.* passive continuous movement for knee replacement or chest physical therapy for thoracotomy). If pain is out of proportion to the surgical procedure, the number of days elapsed postoperatively and analgesic therapy given, consider whether another cause is present (*e.g.*, surgical complication, personality disorder, opioid tolerance) and initiate appropriate evaluation, including communication with the surgeon and/or consultant physicians.

3. Determine whether side effects are present. Assess each side effect in the context of the type of operation and days elapsed since the operation. Decide whether the side effect is in proportion to the operation, the number of days post-operatively and amount of opioid and other medications given. For sedation, as an example, note other concurrent drug therapy, as well as the patient's physical status and decide whether to undertake other work-up (*e.g.*, glucose, electrolytes, arterial blood gas, calcium, magnesium, electrocardiogram).

4. Perform a problem-oriented physical examination (*e.g.*, surgical site, presence of rales, venous thrombosis, sensory/motor function). Included in the physical examination should be an examination of the catheter site and brief neurologic evaluation for evidence of Catheter-related complications (*e.g.*, change in position, infection, haematoma), as well as an evaluation for cordiovascular stability (especially in patients receiving local anaesthetics). Note the current vital signs (HR, RR, BP) and compare them with the last evaluation. If these are unstable or unsatisfactory, consider suitable diagnostic work-up (*e.g.*, haematocrit, electrocardiogram).

5. Adjust drug doses, administration interval, infusion pump settings, or change to a different analgesic, as appropriate.

6. Note concurrent medications and consider whether the patient would benefit from changing the overall regimen (*e.g.*, simplifying to avert drug interactions), or employing adjuvant analgesic medications or nonpharmacologic therapies and if so, order these.

7. Evaluate overall patient satisfaction with current care.

8. Evaluate the patient's response(s) to prior adjustments of pain therapy or addition of adjuvants (*e.g.*, for nausea or anxiety). Make changes in pain and adjuvant therapy as indicated.

9. Evaluate the patient's suitability for making the transition to simpler alternatives (*e.g.*, oral analgesics).*

10. Discuss the assessment and plan with the patient and patient's nurse and /or surgeon, when appropriate.

11. Document findings, impression and plan in the hospital chart.

12. Ensure availability of personnel with appropriate expertise to deal with questions or problems at any time.

VII. Use of Three Specific Techniques for Perioperative Pain Management

The literature strongly supports the efficacy and safety of three techniques used by anaesthesiologists for the control of pain in the perioperative setting: (1) PCA with systemic opioids, (2) EA with opioids or opioid/local anaesthetic mixtures (or intrathecal opioids), and (3) RA techniques, including (but not limited to) intercostal blocks, plexus infusions and local anaesthetic infiltration of incisions. The literature indicates that these three techniques used by anaesthesiologists have no higher incidence of side effects than less effective techniques for perioperative pain management. The panel of consultants and the Task Force members strongly support the use of PCA, EA and RA by anaesthesiologists when appropriate and feasible.

Recommendations : To meet the diverse needs of individual patient, anaesthesiologists who manage perioperative pain should make available as appropriate a variety of effective therapeutic options such as PCA, EA and RA.

Table 6 : Preprinted Daily Clinical Note Form

TECHNIQUE

PCA

Opioid : ☐ morphine ☐ meperidine ☐ hydromorphone ☐ other ______

Concentration : ________ mg/mL

Incremental dose ________ mg Lockout ________ min

Infusion ________ mg/h ☐ Continuous ☐ Night only

Total opioid use ________ mg/8h

Epidural

☐ Bolus ________ mg/ ________ h ☐ Infusion ________ mL/h

Opioid

☐ Morphine (1 mg/mL) ☐ Meperidine (2 mg/mL)

☐ Fentanyl (4 μg/mL) ☐ Other ________

Local anaesthetic

☐ Bupivacaine 0.0625% ☐ Bupivacaine 0.125% ☐ Other

Other care ____

Problem-oriented history and physical examination

Pain levels (0–10 scale)

At rest ________ With activity ________ ☐ Patient unable to report

Patient satisfied with current pain management ☐ Yes ☐ No

Epidural catheter Vital signs

Site clean and nontender ☐ Yes ☐ No Satisfactory ☐ Yes ☐ No

☐ Removed intact

Neurologic function

Sensory or motor block is limiting function ☐ Yes ☐ No

Side effects : (0 = absent; 1 = present, no treatment needed; 2 = present, treatment effective; 3 = present, treatment not effective)

Respiratory depression ________ N and V ________ Pruritus ________

Urinary retention ________ Sedation ________

Treatment pain

☐ Continue present therapy to maintain control of severe pain.

☐ Modify present therapy to improve control of severe pain.

☐ Discontinue present therapy; analgesia to be provided by primary care team.

Comments ____

____

Patient seen and examined.

Date ________ Time ________ Signature __________________________ M.D.

VIII. A Multimodality Approach to Perioperative Pain Management

During the administration of anaesthetics for surgery, the needs of many patients may best be met by taking advantage of the combined effects of a number of agents. Similarly, there is growing conviction that a multi-modality approach (*i.e.*, two or more analgesic agents or techniques used in combination) to providing post-operative analgesia has advantages over the use of a single modality.

The literature supports the efficacy of two or more analgesic techniques (including nonpharmacologic methods) used in combination for the control of perioperative pain, especially when different sites and/or mechanisms of action are involved and/or when synergy of effect is achieved. In addition, the literature indicates that multimodality approaches are associated with side effects no greater than those resulting from single analgesic technique for perioperative pain management. The panel of consultants and the Task Force members support the use of multimodality techniques when appropriate and feasible.

Recommendations : Anaethesiologists managing perioperative pain should make available as appropriate a variety of analgesic techniques and should consider their use in combination under appropriate circumstances.

Table 7 : Considerations in Making the Transition of Pain Therapy from More Sophisticated Techniques (*e.g.*, PCA, EA, RA) to Less Sophisticated Techniques (*e.g.*, oral analgesics)

1. Review the efficacy and dose requirement of the sophisticated technique.
2. Consider the pain expected following the transition: type of procedure, level of activity (including physical therapy), and other sources of discomfort (*e.g.*, nasogastric tube).
3. Review the patient's past experience with oral analgesics. What has been effective? What has caused side effects?
4. Based on the above information, use the simple technique with an analgesic drug and dose calculated to provide adequate analgesia. Adjust the dose as needed, based on regular assessment.
5. Overlap therapy during the transition, *i.e.*, do not discontinue the original therapy until the replacement has reached a therapeutic effect.
6. Provide for treatment of "breakthrough" pain during use of the simpler method.
7. If there is to be a change in responsibility for prescribing an analgesic (*e.g.*, the surgeon assumes responsibility for an oral analgesic), be sure the change is clearly understood and that orders are available from the new therapist.

IX. An Organized Interdisciplinary Approach to Perioperative Pain Management

Although dedicated individuals can improve perioperative pain control for the individual patients they treat, comprehensive programmes provide optimal analgesia throughout an institution. Such programmes have been advocated by national and international pain speciality societies[1,2] and the Federal government.* The Task Force strongly believes that, based on training, knowledge, skills, interest and historical innovation, anaesthesiologists are uniquely qualified to provide leadership within their institutions in developing and managing perioperative pain managment programs.

Table 8 : Organizational Aspects of an Anesthesiology based Postoperative Pain Programme

1. Education (initial, updates)
   - Anaesthesiologists
   - Surgeons
   - Nurses
   - Pharmacists
   - Patients and families
   - Hospital administrators
   - Health insurance carriers
2. Areas of regular administrative activity
   - Maintenance of clear lines of communication
   - Human resources: 24-hour a day availability of pain service personnel
   - Evaluation (including safety) of equipment (*e.g.*, pumps)
   - Secretarial support
   - Economic issues
   - Continuing quality improvement (CQI)
   - Resident physician teaching (if applicable)
   - Pain managment-related research (if applicable)
3. Collaboration with nursing services
   - Job description for pain service nurse (if applicable)
   - Nursing policies and procedures
   - Nurse's in-service and continuing education
   - Definition of roles in patient care
   - Institutional administrative activities
   - Continuing quality improvement (CQI)
   - Research activities (if applicable)
4. Elements of documentation
   - Preprinted orders
   - Policies
   - Procedures

Bedside pain management flow sheet
Daily consultation notes
Educational packages

The panel of consultants and the Task Force members regard organized interdisciplinary activities (*e.g.*, anesthesiologists in collaboration with nurses, surgeons, and pharmacists) as important and optimal in providing effective, safe and continuous perioperative pain control (Table 8). An essential feature of such an approach should be an ongoing strong working relationship between anesthesiologists and nurses.

Recommendations : Anesthesiologists who manage perioperative pain should develop (in collaboration with nurses, surgeons, pharmacists and others) an organized, interdisciplinary approach to perioperative pain management within their institutions.

X. Recognition and Management of Special Features of Paediatric Perioperative Pain Management

Paediatric patients (infants and children) present unique problems regarding perioperative pain management for reasons that include differences in the perception of care-givers regarding the need for analgesia, differences in the pharmacology of analgesic medications when used in this group, and the strong emotional components of pain in children. In the past, safe methods for providing analgesia have been underused in paediatric patients because of fear of opioid-induced respiratory depression.

The emotional component of pain is very strong in children. Absence of parents, security objects and familiar surroundings may be perceived by the child to be as painful as the surgical incision. When clear evidence of physical pain is not seen, the tendency of health care providers is to assume that pain is not present and therefore, defer treatment. In addition, young childrens' fear of injections makes intramuscular opioids or other methods, which themselves cause discomfort, less acceptable to this group than to adults. Many children will choose to suffer in silence knowing that an expression of pain will result in a dreaded injection.

Pain assessment is more difficult in children because as they grow and develop, cognitive and emotional responses are different from adults and are constantly changing. Special instruments are available to assist young children in self-reporting of pain and behavioural and physiologic parameters can be employed to assess preverbal children or in those who cannot self-report.

The literaure strongly supports the effectiveness of a variety of techniques in providing analgesia in paediatric patients. Many of these are the same techniques used in adults, although some techniques (*e.g.*, caudal analgesia) are more commonly used in children. There is strong agreement among the panel of consultants and the Task Force members that it is important to recognize that paediatric patients represents a unique population with special features when planning and providing perioperative analgesia.

Recommendations : Anaesthesiologists who treat perioperative pain in paediatric patients should be familiar with the special features of this group. Based on that knowledge, pharmacologic and nonpharmacologic strategies for perioperative analgesia appropriate for the age of the child should be offered in a manner that promotes efficacy and safety.

XI. Recognition and Management of Special Features of Geriatric Perioperative Pain Management

Elderly patients are a unique population facing surgery. They may experience physical and mental limitation and may have different attitudes than younger patients with regard to expressing pain and appropriate therapy for it. Altered physiology with ageing changes the way analgesic drugs and local anaesthetics are distributed and metabolized, frequently necessitating alterations in dosing. There is strong agreement from the panel of consultants and the Task Force members on the importance of recognizing the unique features of geriatric patients in planning and providing perioperative analgesia.

The literature indicates that single and multimodality techniques that have been shown to be effective in younger adult patients are also effective (often with reduced drug dose requirements) in geriatric patients without increasing side effects.

Recommendations: Anaesthesiologists who treat perioperative pain in geriatric patients should be familiar with the special features of this group. In particular, dose reduction for drugs that may cause central nervous system depression should be considered.

XII. Recognition of Special Features of Perioperative Pain Management in Ambulatory Surgery Patients

The increasing trend toward ambulatory surgery poses special problems in perioperative pain management. One of the most common reasons for unanticipated hospital admission in this population is inadequate pain control. Analgesic techniques must provide safe, adequate pain relief for patients who quickly leave the supervised hospital environment. Techniques such as EA and intravenous PCA, which require special nursing and monitoring, are not suitable for such patients, but others such as local anaesthetic wound infiltration and oral nonsteroidal anti-inflammatory drugs may be very effective.

The panel of consultants and the Task Force members strongly agree that the provision of effective analgesia to ambulatory surgery patients is important and beneficial.

A limited search of this evolving literature suggests that planning of perioperative analgesia for ambulatory patients including the use of certain procedures (*e.g.*, local anaesthetic wound infiltration and certain RA techniques) may improve analgesia without increasing the risk of side effects.

Recommendations : Anaesthesiologists who care for ambulatory surgery patients should proactively plan therapeutic strategies appropriate for them, recogniging that they are expected to leave the surgical facility within a few hours after the completion of surgery.

REFERENCES

1. Max MB, Donovan M, Portenoy RK: American Pain Society Quality Assurance Standards for Relief of Acute Pain and Cancer Pain, Committee on Quality Assurance Standards, American Pain Society, Proceedings of the VIth World Congress on Pain. Edited by Bond Mr. Charlton JE, Woolf (GJ), New York, Elsevier, 1991, pp 185-189.
2. Management of Acute Pain : A Practical Guide,Task Force on Acute Pain. International Associate for the Study of Pain. Edited by Ready LB, Edwards WT, Seattle, IASP, 1992.

•••

APPENDIX-II

Practice Guidelines for Chronic Pain Management

Based on a Report by the American Society of Anaesthesiologists Task Force on Pain Management, Chronic Pain Section

The Guidelines provide basic recommendations that are supported by analysis of the current literature and by a synthesis of expert opinion, open forum commentary and clinical feasibility data.

A. Definition of Chronic Pain

For these Guideliens, chronic pain is defined as persistent or episodic pain of a duration or intensity that adversely affects the function or well-being of the patient, attributable to any nonmalignant aetiology. The Task Force has not given preference to literature based on any particular system of definition or classification of chronic pain.

B. Purpose of Guidelines for Chronic Pain Management

The purpose of these Guidelines is to (1) optimize pain control, recognizing that a pain-free state may not be achievable, (2) minimize adverse outcomes and costs, (3) enhance functional abilities and physical and psychological well-being, and (4) enhance the quality of life for patients with chronic pain.

C. Focus

These Guidelines focus on the knowledge base, skills and range of interventions that are the essential elements of effective management of chronic pain and pain-related problems. The Guidelines recognize that the management of chronic pain occurs within the broader context of health care, including psychosocial function and quality of life.

The Guidelines recognize that all anaesthesiologists may not have access to the same knowledge base, skills or range of modalities. However, aspects of these Guidelines may be helpful to anaesthesiologists who manage patients with chronic pain in a variety of practice settings.

The decision to implement a particular management approach should be based on a comprehensive assessment of the patient's overall health. The Guidelines recognize that accurate diagnosis and appropriate therapies used to modify the underlying causes of pain may improve analgesia and outcome. The risks and benefits of therapies designed to modify or correct the underlying cause(s) of pain is outside the scope of these Guidelines. Although headache is included in the definition of chronic pain, these Guidelines are not specifically intended for the management of headache.

D. Application

These Guidelines are intended for use by anaesthesiologists and health care personnel who deliver care under the direct supervision of anaesthesiologists. The Guidelines do not compare the relative effectiveness of different interventions. They are not intended to provide treatment algorithms for specific pain syndromes. Complementary therapies are beyond the scope of these Guidelines.

Guidelines

I. A Comprehensive History and Physical Examination of the Patient with Chronic Pain

The literature suggests that a comprehensive history and physical examination be conducted. The Task Force and panel of consultants support the conduct of a comprehensive pain-related history and physical examination.

Recommendations: General Constructs. The Task Force identifies four fundamental issues that should guide a comprehensive history and physical examination of the patient with chronic pain.

1. The patient's general medical condition and extent of concurrent medical and surgical diagnoses.
2. Knowledge of chronic pain syndromes is a necessary prerequisite for conducting a chronic pain evaluation. Chronic pain syndromes may be related to pathology or dysfunction in one or more organ systems or to psychological

conditions. In addition, knolwedge of other medical or surgical conditions that may present with pain and may mimic chronic pain syndromes also is necessary.

3. Knowledge of the diagnosis and management of painful crises.
4. Knowledge of the diagnosis and management of medical emergencies and complications arising from the underlying cause or treatment.

Elements. The Task Force identifies five essential features of a comprehensive evaluation and treatment plan (Table 1).

1. **History:** A complete pain history includes a general medical history with emphasis on the chronology and symptomatology of the presenting complaint. The data should include information about the onset, quality, intensity, distribution, duration, course and affective components of the pain and details about exacerbating and relieving factors. Additional symptoms (*e.g.*, motor, sensory, and autonomic changes) should be noted. Information regarding previous diagnostic tests, results of previous therapies, and current therapies should be reviewed by the anaesthesiologist (Table 2).
2. **Physical examination.** The physical examination should include an appropriate, directed neurologic and musculoskeletal evaluation, with attention to other systems as indicated. Not only the cause(s) of the pain, but also the effects of the pain, such as physical deconditioning, should be evaluated and recorded.

Table 1 : Algorithm for Comprehensive Evaluation and Longitudinal Assessment of Chronic Pain

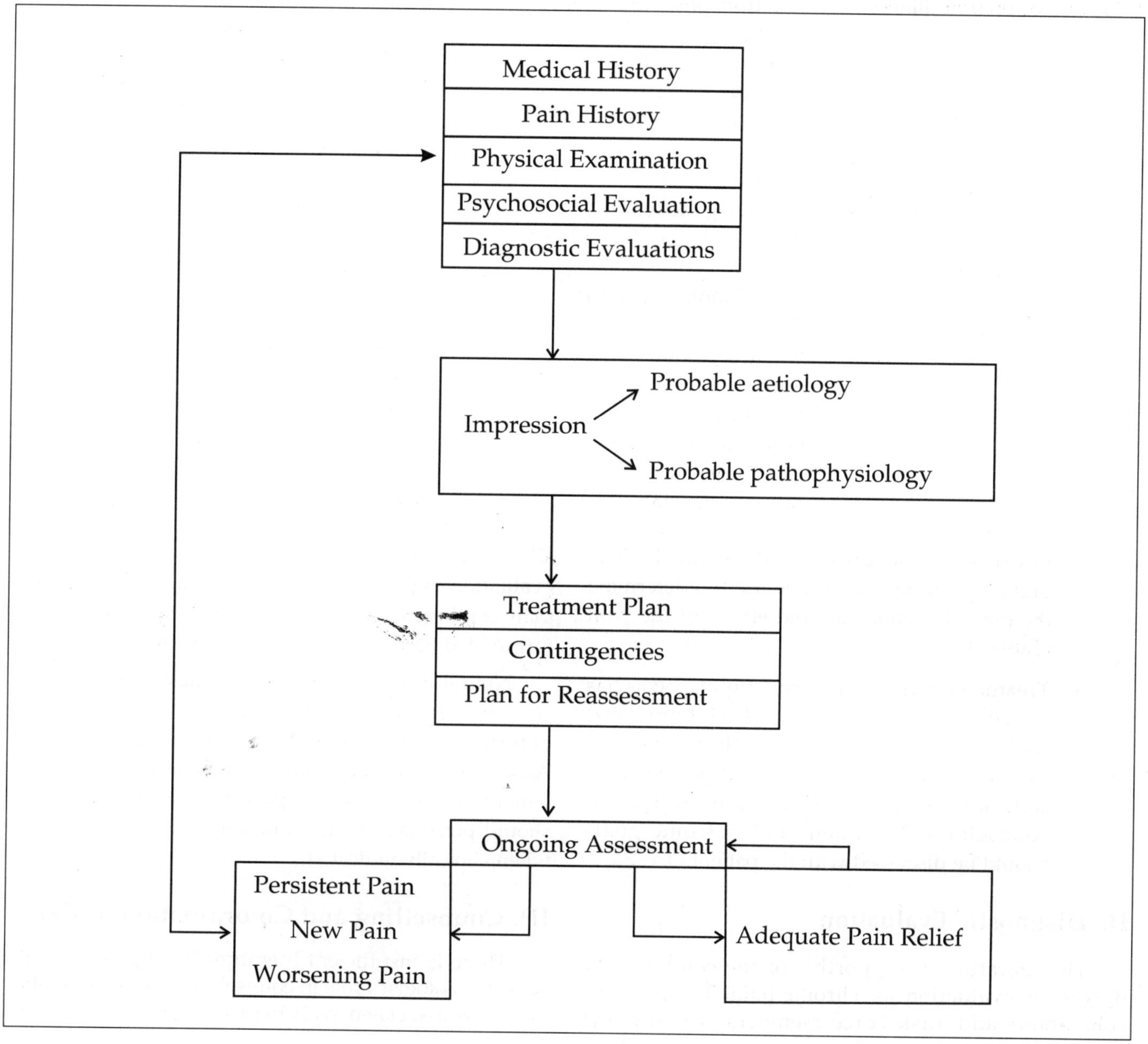

3. **Psychosocial evaluation.** The psychosocial evaluation should include information about the presence of psychological symptoms (*e.g.*, anxiety, depression or anger), psychiatric disorders, personality traits or states, coping mechanisms and the meaning of the pain. Evidence of family, vocational, or legal issues and involvement of rehabilitation agencies should be noted. The expectations of the patient, significant others, employer, attorney and other agencies (*e.g.*, Workers' compensation, Social Security Administration) also should be determined.

diagnostic evaluation for purposes of determining potential aetiologies of chronic pain and for identification of pain sites for treatment. The use of diagnostic local anaesthetic blockade is suggested by the literature and supported by the Task Force.

Recommendations : Anaesthesiologists treating chronic pain should have a working knowledge of the utility and interpretation of diagnostic evaluations, including diagnostic neural blockade, imaging modalities, pharmacodiagnosis, electrodiagnosis, and laboratory studies. Diagnostic evaluation is an essential addition to the history and physical examination in the evaluation of patients with chronic pain. The treatment plan, contingencies and plan for reassessment should be formulated based on these sources of clinical data.

Table 2 : History Review – Sample Form

Patient :		Physician :	
Date :	Referred :	Time in :	Time out :
Chief complaint :			
History of present illiness	Pain from onset to present :		
	Location	Past medical history	
	Quality	Illnesses	
	Severity	Operations	
	Duration	Injuries	
	Timing	Treatments	
	Context	Medications	
	Modifying factors	Family history	
	Associated signs/symptoms	Social history	
Review of symptoms			
	Constitutional symptoms	Integumentary	
	Eyes	Neurologic	
	Ear, nose, mouth, throat	Psychiatric	
	Cardiovascular	Endocrine	
	Respiratory	Haematologic/Lymphatic	
	Gastrointestinal	Allergic/Immunologic	
	Genitourinary		
	Musculoskeletal	Drug reactions	

4. Impression and differential diagnosis. The previous findings should be used to determine the possible aetiologies and effects of the pain (Table 3).

5. **Treatment plan:** Once a working diagnosis has been determined, a treatment plan is formulated with input from patient, other involved professionals, and other involved persons (*e.g.*, significant others or qualified rehabilitation counselors). Treatment and outcome goals should be discussed with the patient.

II. Diagnostic Evaluation

The literature is supportive of the conduct of a diagnostic evaluation for chronic pain. The panel of consultants and Task Force members also support

Neural blockade with local anaesthetic, including somatic and autonomic blocks, may be useful in determining the site and aetiology of chronic pain. Anaesthesiologists have unique skills in this area that may benefit carefully selected patients. Anaesthesiologists should personally review and interpret diagnostic data when clinically indicated.

III. Counselling and Co-ordination of Care

There is insufficient literature to suggest that the anaesthesiologist's role in counselling and co-ordination of care is associated with improved analgesia or other

Table 3 : Elements of Medical Decision-making for Treatment of Chronic Pain

History			
____ Problem focused	____ Expanded problem focused	____ Detailed	____ Comprehensive
Chief complaint	Chief complaint	Chief complaint	Chief complaint
Brief history of present illness or problem	Brief history of present illness or problem	extended history of present illness	extended history of present illness
	Problem pretinent system review	Extended system review	Complete system review
		Pertinent past, family or social history	Complete past, family and social history
Examination			
____ Problem focused	____ Expanded problem focused	____ Detailed	____ Comprehensive
Limited exam of affected body area or organ system	Limited exam of affected body area or organ system and other symptomatic or related organ system(s)	Extended exam of affected body area(s) and other symptomatic or related organ system(s)	Complete single organ system exam OR General multisystem exam

Medical decision-making

Two of the three elements in a category must be met or exceeded for that category to apply

Type of Decision-making	Straight forward	Low Complexity	Moderate Complexity	High Complexity
Number of diagnoses or management options	Minimal	Limited	Multiple	Extensive
Amount or complexity of data reviewed/considered	Minimal or none	Limited	Moderate	Extensive
Risk of complications or morbidity or mortality	Low	Low	Moderate	High

health effects. The Task Force and consultants are supportive of the effectiveness of counselling and appropriate co-ordination of care in improving analgesia and quality of life.

Recommendations : Anaesthesiologists should provide appropriate counselling of the patient regarding the pain syndrome diagnosis, treatment options, rehabilitation and follow-up goals. In addition, the anaesthesiologist should co-ordinate care with other health professionals, rehabilitation and vocational agencies, and social and legal entities. Longitudinal assessments of outcome should be maintained.

IV. Periodic Monitoring and Measurement of Clinical Outcomes

There is insufficient literature to evaluate the effectiveness of periodic pain assessment in chronic pain management. Multiple times of measurements, fluctuating patient and disease status, and variable interventions over time are confounding factors that make useful analysis difficult. The Task Force and consultants support the contention that periodic monitoring of the effects of therapy and patient status will result in improved pain management and reduced adverse health effects from therapy.

Recommendations : Accurate and complete records of pain therapies should be maintained. Reports of pain made by the patient should be the primary source of pain assessment (table 4) and should be obtained at periodic intervals. Periodic monitoring may include, but is not limited to, a patient's verbal report of treatment efficacy, other pain records (*e.g.*, pain diaries), and reports of side effects associated with pain management. Analyses of aggregate outcomes are essential to continuous quality improvement of chronic pain management in the clinical setting.

V. Multidisciplinary Pain Management

For these Guidelines, multidisciplinary care includes, but is not limited to, (1) contributions to patient pain care by more than one health care discipline, (2) a process or programme of pain care by more than one health care discipline, or (3) a combination of 1 and 2.

The literature does not provide a standard definition for multidisciplinary care. The available literature was only sufficient to address multidisciplinary care on a programmatic basis. This literature is supportive of the efficacy of multidisciplinary programmes in providing analgesia and improvement of health status (*e.g.*, functional status, quality of life). The panel of consultants and Task Force members endorse multidisciplinary chronic pain management.

The literature, Task Force, and consultants also support programs that emphasize the reduction or elimination of pain medications as a primary objective of therapy (*i.e.*, through use of physical therapy, biofeedback, behaviour modification, or other psychosocial techniques).

Recommendations: Anaesthesiologists offer a unique contribution to patient care in the context of multidisciplinary chronic pain management. Anaesthesiologists should be involved in patient evaluation, provision and interpretation of diagnostic procedures, clinical pharmacology, provision of alternative drug delivery methods, provision of temporary or long-term neural blockade, and provision of neuromodulatory techniques.

VI. Multimodality Pain Management

For these Guidelines, multimodal therapy is defined as concomitant use of separate therapeutic interventions under the direction of a single practitioner to obtain additive beneficial effects or reduction of adverse effects. Examples include, but are not limited to (1) the use of neural blockade with medications, (2) rehabilitative therapies (*e.g.*, physical therapy) with neural blockade or medications and (3) medications of different categories (Table 5). The literature suggests that concomitant application of separate therapeutic interventions in chronic pain management provides effective analgesia. The literature on other health effects is equivocal. The panel of consultants and Task Force members also are supportive of the efficacy of multimodality techniques for the management of chronic pain.

Table 4 : Pain Intensity Scales

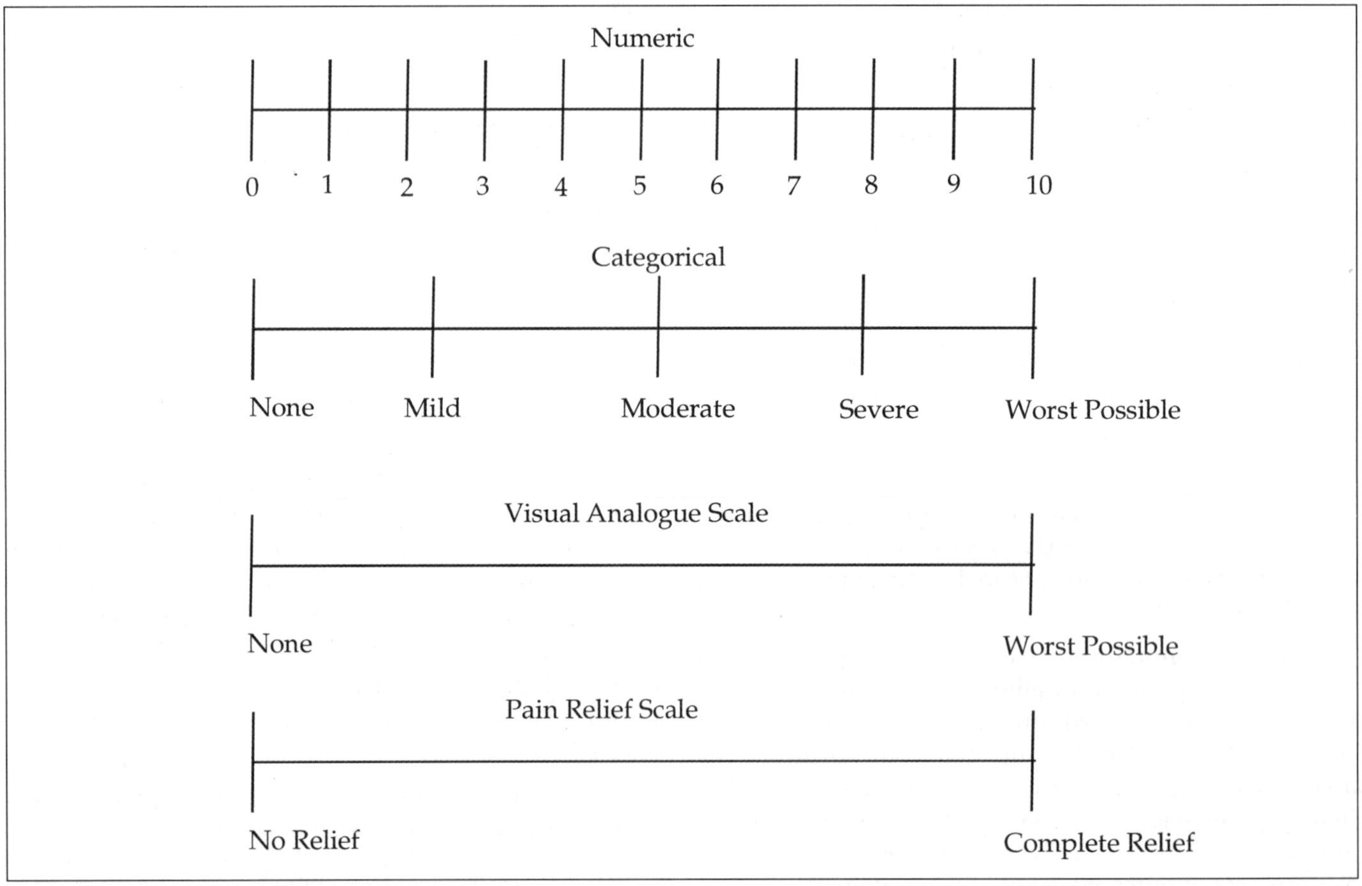

Recommendations: Multiple modalities, such as the combined use of neural blockade, medications, or rehabilitative therapies should be considered when analgesia with acceptable adverse effects is no longer attained with single modality. Ideally, each modality should be administered as appropriate to achieve the desired therapeutic effect. A multimodal approach may reduce the potential for adverse effects arising from either escalating frequency or dosage levels of a single modality.

VII. Adjuvant Analgesics: Antidepressants, Membrane Stabilizing Agents and Nonsteroidal Antiinflammatory Drugs (NSAIDs)

The literature supports the use of antidepressants for reducing chronic pain without notable adverse effects. The literature also supports the use of antidepressants for providing overall health benefits and for improving mood. The literature supports the benefits of membrane stabilizing agents (*i.e.*, anticonvulsants) and NSAIDs for providing analgesia but is equivocal regarding other health effects. The Task Force and consultants are supportive of the use of antidepressants, membrane stabilizing agents and NSAIDs for providing analgesic and health benefits.

Table 5 : Elements of Multimodality Pain Management and Therapeutic Options for Treatment

Elements

1. Comprehensive speciality pain history and physical examination.
2. Personal review of previous consultations, examinations, and diagnostic studies (*e.g.*, radiographs, scans, laboratory data).
3. Discussion or communication with patient's other physicians and allied health care professionals (*e.g.*, rehabilitation counsellor).
4. Indicated laboratory or radiologic diagnostic testing procedures (*e.g.*, radiographs, CT scan, MRI three-phase bone scan, sedimentation rate, ANA).
5. Indicated diagnostic, clinical interventions, procedures, surgical consultation, psychosocial evalutation.
6. Formulation of an appropriate and specific diagnosis.

Options

- Physical therapies
  - Active and passive range of motion
  - Tone and strengthening
  - Desensitization
  - Other.
- Medications
  - NSAIDs
  - Antidepressants
  - α-adrenergic antagonist
  - Membrane stabilizing drugs
  - Opioids.
- Neural blockade
  - Somatic, sympathetic, neuraxial
  - Local single injection technique
  - Continuous infusion-catheter techniques
  - Local anaesthetic, opioid, steroid, other
  - Neuroablation (chemical, thermal).
- Neuroaugmentation
  - Transcutaneous electrical nerve stimulation (TENS)
  - Peripheral nerve stimulation (PNS)
  - Spinal cord stimulation (SCS)
  - Biofeedback-relaxation technique.

Recommendations : Antidepressants are useful medications for the reduction of pain and improvement of sleep. The specific agent and the dosage should be optimized for each patient. The beneficial and adverse effects should be monitored. NSAIDs and membrane stabilizing agents (*e.g.*, anticonvulsants) also may be used for the reduction of pain. As with antidepressants, the specific agent and dosage should be optimized for each patient, with periodic monitoring of beneficial and undesirable health effects.

VIII. Regional Sympathetic Blockade

The literature suggests that regional sympathetic blockade (*e.g.*, lumbar sympathetic block, stellate ganglion block, intravenous regional block) is effective in providing analgesia and is equivocal regarding beneficial or adverse health effects. The Task Force and panel of consultants are supportive of the analgesic benefits of regional sympathetic blockade. The Task Force and panel of consultants are equivocal regarding potentially beneficial or adverse health effects (*e.g.*, hypotension, hyperalgesia, sensory and motor deficit).

Recommendations: The adequacy of sympathetic blockade should be objectively assessed and recorded. Appropriate sympathetic blockade by the anaesthesiologist should be provided within the context of the patient's overall treatment plan. To ensure the judicious use of sympathetic blockade, periodic monitoring should be conducted to assess analgesic benefit and adverse effects (*e.g.*, sensory or motor block; failed blockade of sympathetic outflow, especially to the upper extremity; local anaesthetic toxicity; site infections).

IX. Corticosteroid Injection Therapy

The literature suggests that locally injected corticosteroids are effective in providing analgesia. The literature is equivocal regarding other health effects. The panel of consultants support the importance of locally injected corticosteroids in improving analgesia and enhancing patient functioning and quality of life. The consultants are equivocal regarding the adverse effects of corticosteroids.

Recommendations : Local injection of corticosteroids by the anaesthesiologist should be provided within the context of the patient's overall treatment plan. A directed neurologic evaluation should precede the local injection of corticosteroids. Appropriate follow-up evaluation is necessary to monitor health effects, including analgesia, function, and adverse effects on local tissues and the hypothalamic-pituitary-adrenal axis.

X. Neurostimulation Therapy

The literature is supportive of transcutaneous electrical nerve stimulation (TENS) and spinal cord stimulation (SCS) techniques in providing analgesia and is suggestive of the analgesic benefit of peripheral nerve stimulation (PNS) techniques. The literature is equivocal regarding the beneficial or adverse health effects of TENS, PNS and SCS. The Task Force and panel of consultants are supportive of neurostimulation therapy for analgesia.

Recommendations: An office or home trial of TENS should be considered as an early management option because of its low complexity and low risk. TENS also may be considered as adjunctive therapy.

Peripheral nerve stimulation should be reserved for patients with a peripheral mononeuropathy who have responded to a diagnostic sequence of local neural blockade and a stimulation trial.

Spinal cord stimulation should not be a first-line treatment but may be considered after failure of oral medications. SCS may be effective in the management of patients with peripheral neuropathic pain or with pain arising from the spinal cord (*e.g.*, arachnoiditis, syringomyelia, spinal cord injury, multiple sclerosis). It should be preceded by a trial with a percutaneous electrode system.

XI. Opioid Therapy

Opioid therapy for chronic pain management may be administered by several routes, the most common being systemic delivery (*e.g.*, oral, transdermal or intravenous). Opioids also may be delivered directly to the neuraxis (*e.g.*, epidural, intrathecal). The relative merit of systemic *versus* neuraxial opioid administration for chronic pain management was not addressed in these guidelines.

The literature supports the analgesic efficacy of systemic opioids. However, the literature suggests that systemic use of opioids may be associated with increased risk of adverse sequelae (*e.g.*, tolerance, dependence, pruritus, nausea, and respiratory depression).

The literature suggests that neuraxial delivery of opioids for chronic pain is associated with effective analgesia and is equivocal regarding adverse effects. The consultants are supportive of the analgesic benefits of opioid therapies and are equivocal regarding adverse effects.

Recommendations: Opioid therapy may be considered when analgesia provided by other modalities (*e.g.*, NSAIDs, TENS) is no longer adequate to manage chronic pain. Systemic or neuraxial opioids should be administered on the basis of patient needs. Delivery of opioids should occur within the context of a logistic system that provides the resources and availability of personnel to respond to patient needs and according to applicable local, state and federal regulations. The analgesic benefits of opioids should be balanced against the potential adverse sequelae of long-term opioid use. Patients treated with opioids for chronic pain may require frequent follow-up evaluation. A controlled substance agreement or a second opinion from another provider with expertise in pain management may be considered.

XII. Neuroablative Techniques

Neuroablative techniques destroy neural tissue using chemicals (*e.g.*, alcohol or phenol) or thermal lesions (*e.g.*, radiofrequency or cryoneurolysis). The literature suggests that chemical and thermal neuroablative techniques can provide some control of chronic pain and reduction in regional sympathetic overactivity. Severe adverse health effects from treatment are possible but reported rarely. There is insufficient literature regarding the value of prognostic neural blockade before neuroablative techniques. The Task Force and consultants are supportive of the value of neurolytic techniques in symptom management and are neutral regarding other health effects.

Recommendations : Neuroablation should be preceded by confirmation of needle placement using local anaesthetic, imaging or electrical stimulation. Successful temporary blockade does not guarantee the success of subsequent neuroablation. Although the reported incidence of adverse effects of neuroablative techniques is very low, the impact on the patient may be catastrophic. Reported adverse effects include motor, sensory and autonomic dysfunction (*e.g.*, paralysis, deafferentation pain, loss of sphincter control or impotence), regeneration pain, and neuralgias. Neuroablative techniques should be used as part of a comprehensive approach to managing pain and applied only as a last resort after failure of other therapies. Follow-up assessments of pain and other health effects should be conducted periodically.

REFERENCES

Task Force on Chronic Pain Management.

•••

APPENDIX-III

Practice Guidelines for Sedation and Analgesia by Non-Anaesthesiologists

Based on a Report by the American Society of Anaesthesiologists Task Force on Sedation and Analgesia by Non-Anaesthesiologists

Anaesthesiologists possess specific expertise in the pharmacology, physiology, and clinical management of patients receiving sedation and analgesia. For this reason, they are frequently called on to participate in the development of institutional policies and procedures for sedation and analgesia in nonoperating-room settings. To assist in this process, the American Society of Anaesthesiologists developed these Guidelines for Sedation and Analgesia by Non-Anaesthesiologists.

The practice guidelines enumerated below have been developed using systematic literature summarization techniques. Results of the literature analyses have been supplemented by the opinions of the Task Force members and a panel of more than 60 consultants, drawn from a variety of medical specialities in which sedation and analgesia are commonly provided. In those instances where the literature does not provide conclusive data, there is an explicit statement that the guidelines are based on the opinion of the consultants or the consensus of the Task Force members.

A. Definition

"Sedation and analgesia" describes a state that allows patients to tolerate unpleasant procedures while maintaining adequate cardiorespiratory function and the ability to respond purposefully to verbal command and/ or tactile stimulation. The Task Force decided that the term "sedation and analgesia"(sedation/analgesia) more accurately defines this therapeutic goal than does the commonly used but imprecise term "conscious sedation." Note that patients whose only response is reflex withdrawal from a painful stimulus are sedated to a greater degree than encompassed by "sedation/ analgesia."

B. Purpose

The purpose of these guidelines is to allow clinicians to provide their patients with the benefits of sedation/ analgesia while minimizing the associated risks. Sedation/analgesia provides two general types of benefit: First, sedation/ analgesia allows patients to tolerate unpleasant procedures by relieving anxiety, discomfort, or pain. Second, in children and uncooperative adults, sedation/analgesia may expedite the conduct of procedures that are not particularly uncomfortable but require that the patient does not move. Excessive sedation/analgesia may result in cardiac or respiratory depression that must be rapidly recognized and appropriately managed to avoid the risk of hypoxic brain damage, cardiac arrest, or death. Conversely, inadequate sedation/analgesia may result in undue patient discomfort or patient injury, because of lack of co-operation or adverse physiologic response to stress.

C. Focus

These guidelines have been designed to be applicable to procedures performed in a variety of settings (*e.g.*, hospitals, free-standing clinics, physicians' offices) by practitioners who are not specialists in anaesthesiology. The guidelines specifically exclude the following: (1) patients who are not undergoing a diagnostic or therapeutic procedure (*e.g.*, post operative analgesia, sedation for treatment of insomnia); (2) otherwise healthy patients receiving peripheral nerve blocks, local or topical anaesthesia, and/or no more than 50% N_2O with oxygen and no other sedative or analgesic agents administered by any route; (3) situations when it is anticipated that the required sedation will eradicate the purposeful response to verbal commands or tactile stimulation (as distinct from reflex withdrawal from a painful stimulus); such patients require a greater level of care than recommended by these guidelines; and (4) perioperative management of patients undergoing general anaesthesia or major conduction anaesthesia (spinal or epidural/caudal blockade).

D. Application

These guidelines are intended to be general in their application and broad in scope. The appropriate choice of agents and techniques for sedation/analgesia is dependent on the experience and preference of the individual practitioner, requirements or constraints imposed by the patient or procedures and the likelihood of producing unintended loss of consciousness. Tables are provided as examples to illustrate principles; clinicians and their institutions have ultimate responsibility for selecting patients, procedures, medications, and equipment.

Guidelines

I. Patient Evaluation

Published data suggest and consultant opinion strongly supports the contention that appropriate pre-procedure evaluation of patients' histories and physical findings reduces the risk of adverse outcomes. Additionally, consultant opinion supports the contention that an appropriate history, physical examination, and laboratory evaluation leads to improved patient satisfaction.

Recommendations : Clinicians administering sedation/analgesia should be familiar with relevant aspects of the patient's medical history including : (1) abnormalities of the major organ systems, (2) previous adverse experience with sedation/analgesia, as well as regional and general anaesthesia, (3) current medications and drug allergies, (4) time and nature of last oral intake, and (5) history of tobacco, alcohol, or substance use or abuse. Patients presenting for sedation/analgesia should undergo a focused physical examination including auscultation of the heart and lungs and evaluation of the airway (Table 1). Preprocedure laboratory testing should be guided by the patient's underlying medical condition and the likelihood that the results will affect the management of sedation/analgesia.

Table 1: Example of Airway Assessment Procedures for Sedation and Analgesia

Positive pressure ventilation, with or without endotracheal intubation, may be necessary if respiratory compromise develops during sedation/analgesia. This may be more difficult in patients with atypical airway anatomy. Also, some airway abnormalities may increase the likelihood of airway obstruction during spontaneous ventilation. Factors that may be associated with difficulty in airway management are :

History

- Previous problems with anaesthesia or sedation
- Stridor, snoring, or sleep apnea
- Dysmorphic facial features (*e.g.*, Pierre-Robin syndrome, trisomy 21)
- Advanced rheumatoid arthritis

Physical examination

Habitus

- Significant obesity (especially involving the neck and facial structures)

Head and Neck

- Short neck, limited neck extension, decreased hyoid-mental distance (<3 cm in an adult), neck mass, cervical spine disease or trauma, tracheal deviation

Mouth

- Small opening (<3 cm in an adult); edentulous; protruding incisors; loose or capped teeth; high arched palate; macroglossia; tonsillar hypertrophy; nonvisible uvula

Jaw

- Micrognathia, retrognathia, trismus, significant malocclusion

II. Preprocedure Preparation

Patient Counselling : There is insufficient evidence in the literature to establish the benefit of providing the patient (or her/his guardian, in the case of a child or impaired adult) with preprocedure information about sedation/analgesia. However, the consultants strongly support the contention that appropriate preprocedure counselling improves patient's satisfaction and reduces risks; they also support the view that costs may be reduced. The Task Force members concur that patients undergoing sedation/analgesia should be informed of the benefits, risks, and limitations associated with this therapy, as well as possible alternatives.

***Preprocedure Fasting*:** Because sedatives and analgesics tend to impair airway reflexes in proportion to the degree of sedation/analgesia achieved, members of the Task Force support the concept of preprocedure fasting before sedation/analgesia for elective procedures. However, the literature provides insufficient data to test the hypothesis that preprocedure fasting results in a decreased/incidence of adverse outcomes in patients undergoing sedation/analgesia (as distinct from patients undergoing general anaesthesia).

***Recommendations*:** Patients (or their legal guardians in the case of minors or legally incompetent adults) should be informed of and agree to the administration of sedation/analgesia before the procedure begins. Patients undergoing sedation/analgesia for elective procedures should not drink fluids or eat solid foods for a sufficient period of time to allow for gastric emptying before their procedure (Table 2). In urgent, emergent, or other situations when gastric emptying is impaired, the potential for pulmonary aspiration of gastric contents must be considered in determining the timing of the intervention and the degree of sedation/analgesia.

Table 2 : Fasting Protocol for Sedation and Analgesia for Elective Operations

	Solids and Nonclear Liquids*	Clear Liquids
Adults	6-8 hours or none after midnight	2-3 hours
Children older than 36 months	6-8 hours	2-3 hours
Children aged 6-36 months	6 hours	2-3 hours
Children younger than 6 months	4-6 hours	2 hours

III. Monitoring

Level of Consciousness : The response of patients to commands during procedures performed with sedation/analgesia serves as a guide to their level of consciousness. Spoken responses also provide an indication that the patients are breathing. Patients whose only response is reflex withdrawal from painful stimuli are likely to be deeply sedated, approaching a state of general anaesthesia, and should be treated accordingly. The consultants strongly support the contention that monitoring level of consciousness reduces risks and support the concept that overall costs may be reduced. The members of the Task Force believe that many of the complications associated wth sedation/analgesia can be avoided if adverse drug responses are detected and treated in a timely manner (*i.e.,* before the development of cardiovascular decompensation or cerebral hypoxia); this may pose a special risk to patients given sedatives/analgesics in unmonitored settings in anticipation of a subsequent procedure.

Pulmonary Ventilation : It is the opinion of the Task Force that a primary cause of morbidity associated with sedation/analgesia is drug-induced respiratory depression. The literature suggests and consultant opinion strongly supports the observation that monitoring of ventilatory function reduces the risk of adverse outcomes associated with sedation/analgesia. Ventilatory function usually can be effectively monitored by observation of spontaneous respiratory activity or auscultation of breath sounds. In circumstances where patients are physically separated from the caregiver, the consultants support and the Task Force members concur that automated apnea monitoring (by detection of exhaled carbon dioxide or other means) may decrease risks; the consultants suggest that such monitoring will not reduce overall costs. The Task Force cautions practitioners that impedance plethysmography may fail to detect airway obstruction.

Oxygenation : Published data suggest and the consultants strongly support the view that early detection of hypoxemia through the use of oximetry during sedation/analgesia decreases the likelihood of adverse outcomes, such as cardiac arrest and death. The literature suggests, the consultants strongly support, and Task Force members agree that hypoxemia during sedation and analgesia is more likely to be detected by oximetry than by clinical assessment alone. The Task Force emphasizes that oximetry is not a substitute for monitoring ventilatory function.

Haemodynamics : Although there is insufficient published data to reach a conclusion, it is the opinion of the Task Force that sedative and analgesic agents may blunt the appropriate autonomic compensation for hypovolemia and procedure-related stresses. Early detection of changes in patients' heart rate and blood pressure may enable practitioners to detect problems and intervene in a timely fashion, reducing the risk of cardiovascular collapse. The consultants support the concept that regular monitoring of vital signs reduces risks and suggest that it decreases costs. Although the literature provides no guidance, the consultants suggest the use of continuous electrocardiographic monitoring in patients with hypertension and strongly support its use in patients with significant cardiovascular disease or dysrhythmias; the consultants suggest that electrocardiographic monitoring is not required in patients without cardiovascular disease.

Recommendations : Monitoring of patient's response to verbal commands should be routine, except in patients who are unable to respond appropriately (*e.g.,* young children, mentally impaired or uncooperative patients) or during procedures in which facial movement could be detrimental. During procedures in which a verbal response is not possible (*e.g.,* oral surgery, upper endoscopy), the ability to give a "thumbs up" or other indication of consciousnes in response to verbal or tactile (light tap) stimulation suggests that the patient will be able to control his airway and take deep breaths, if necessary. Note that a response limited to reflex withdrawal from a painful stimulus represents a greater degree of sedation/analgesia than addressed by this document.

Ventilatory function should be continually monitored by observation and/or auscultation. When ventilation cannot be directly observed, exhaled carbon dioxide detection is a useful adjunct to these modalities. All patients undergoing sedation/analgesia should be monitored by pulse oximetry with appropriate alarms. If available, the variable pitch "beep", which gives a continuous audible indication of the oxygen saturation reading, may be helpful. When possible, blood pressure should be determined before sedation/analgesia is initiated. Once sedation/analgesia is established, blood pressure should be measured at regular intervals during the procedure, as well as during the recovery period. Electrocardiographic monitoring should be used in patients with significant cardiovascular disease as well as during procedures in which dysrhythmias are anticipated.

IV. Recording of Monitored Parameters

Both the literature and consultant opinion suggest that contemporaneous recording of patient's level of consciousness, respiratory function, and haemodynamics reduces the risk of adverse outcomes. Although consultant opinion suggests that recording of this information may not improve patient comfort or satisfaction, the consultants suggest that it may reduce costs resulting from adverse events. The consultants strongly support recording of vital signs and respiratory variables before initiating sedation/analgesia, after administration of sedative/analgesic medications, at regular intervals during the procedure, on initiation of recovery, and immediately before discharge. It is the opinion of the Task Force that contemporaneous recording (either automatic or manual) of patient data provides information that could prove critical in determining the cause of any adverse events that might occur. Additionally, manual recording ensures that an individual caring for the patient is aware of changes in patient status in a timely fashion.

Recommendations : Patient's ventilatory and oxygenation status and haemodynamic variables should be recorded at a frequency to be determined by the type and amount of medication administered as well as the length of the procedure and the general condition of the patient. At a minimum, this should be: (1) before the beginning of the procedure, (2) after administration of sedative/analgesic agents, (3) on completion of the procedure, (4) during initial recovery, and (5) at the time of discharge. If recording is performed automatically, device alarms should be set to alert the care team to critical changes in patient status.

V. Availability of a Staff Person Dedicated Solely to Patient Monitoring and Safety

Although there are insufficient data in the literature to provide guidance on this issue, the Task Force recognizes that it is difficult for the individual performing a procedure to be fully cognizant of the patient's condition during sedation/analgesia. The consultants support the contention that the availability of an individual other than the person performing the procedure to monitor the patient's status improves patient comfort and satisfaction; they also strongly support the view that risks are reduced. The consultants support the observation that this would not decrease overall costs. It is the consensus of the Task Force members that the individual monitoring the patient may assist the practitioner with interruptible ancillary tasks of short duration once the patient's level of sedation/analgesia and vital signs have stabilized, provided that adequate monitoring is maintained.

Recommendations : A designated individual, other than the practitioner performing the procedure, should be present to monitor the patient throughout procedures performed with sedation/analgesia. This individual may assist with minor, interruptible tasks.

VI. Training of Personnel

Although there is insufficient literature to determine the effectiveness of training on patient outcomes, the consultants strongly support the observation that providing appropriate training in clinical pharmacology for individuals administering sedative/analgesic medications reduces the risk of adverse outcomes; they also support the views that patient comfort is improved and overall costs are reduced. Specific concerns include: (1) potentiation of sedative-induced respiratory depression by concomitantly administered opioids; (2) inadequate time intervals between doses of sedative or analgesic agents, resulting in a cumulative overdose; and (3) inadequate familiarity with the role of pharmacologic antagonists for sedative and analgesic agents.

Because the primary complications of sedation/analgesia are related to respiratory or cardiovascular depression, it is the consensus of the Task Force that the individual responsible for monitoring the patient should be trained in the recognition of complications associated with sedation/analgesia. In addition, at least one qualified individual, capable of establishing a patient airway and maintaining ventilation and oxygenation, should be present during the procedure.

Recommendations : Individuals responsible for patients receiving sedation/analgesia should understand the pharmacology of the agents that are administered, as well as the role of pharmacologic antagonists for opioids and benzodiazepines. Individuals monitoring patients receiving sedation/analgesia should be able to recognize the associated complications. At least one individual capable of establishing a patent airway and positive pressure ventilation, as well as a means for summoning additional assistance, should be present whenever sedation/analgesia is administered. It is recommended that an individual with advanced life-support skills be immediately available.

VII. Availability of Emergency Equipment

The literature suggests and the consultants strongly support the view that the ready availability of appropriately sized emergency equipment reduces the risk of sedation and analgesia. The consultants also support the contention that overall costs, including those associated with adverse outcomes, may be reduced. The literature does not address the need for cardiac defibrillators during sedation/analgesia. The consultants strongly support the availability of a defibrillator whenever sedation/analgesia is administered.

Recommendations: Pharmacologic antagonists as well as appropriately sized equipment for establishing a patient airway and providing positive pressure ventilation with supplemental oxygen should be present whenever adnubustered sedation/analgesia is administered. Advanced airway equipment and resuscitation medications should be immediately available (Table 3). A defibrillator should be immediately available when sedation/analgesia is administered to patients with significant cardiovascular disease.

Appropriate emergency equipment should be available whenever sedative or analgesic drugs capable of causing cardio-respiratory depression are administered. The table below should be used as a guide, which should be modified depending on the individual practice circumstances. Items in brackets are recommen-ded when infants or children are sedated.

Table 3: Example of Emergency Equipment for Sedation and Analgesia

Intravenous equipment
Gloves
Tourniquets
Alcohol wipes
Sterile gauze pads
Intravenous catheters (24-or 22-G)
Intravenous tubing [paediatric "microdrip" (60 drops/mL)]
Intravenous fluid
Three-way stopcocks
Assorted needles for drug aspiration, intramuscular injection [intraosseous bone marrow needle]
Appropriately sized syringes
Tape
Basic airway management equipment
Source of compressed oxygen (tank with regulator or pipeline supply with flowmeter)
Source of suction
Suction catheters [paediatric suction catheters]
Yankauer-type suction
Face masks [infant/child]
Self-inflating breathing bag-valve set [paediatric]
Oral and nasal airways [infant/child-sized airways]
Lubricant
Advanced airway management equipment (for practitioners with intubation skills)
Laryngoscope handles (tested)
Laryngoscope blades (paediatric)
Endotracheal tubes
Cuffed; 6.0, 7.0, or 8.0 mm ID [Uncuffed; 2.5, 3.0, 3.5, 4.0, 4.5, 5.0, 5.5, or 6.0 mm ID]
Stylet (appropriately sized for endotracheal tubes)
Pharmacologic antagonists
Naloxone
Flumazenil
Emergency medications
Epinephrine
Ephedrine
Atropine
Lidocaine
Glucose, 50% [10% or 25%]
Diphenhydramine
Hydrocortisone, methylprednisolone, or dexamethasone
Diazepam or midazolam
Ammonia spirits

VIII. Use of Supplemental Oxygen

The literature supports the use of supplemental oxygen during sedation/analgesia. There is a decreased incidence and severity of hypoxemia among sedation/analgesia patients given oxygen as compared to those breathing room air. However, it must be appreciated that, by delaying the onset of hypoxemia, supplemental oxygen will delay the detection of apnea by pulse oximetry, emphasizing the importance of monitoring pulmonary ventilation by other means (see above). Consultant opinion supports the view that supplemental oxygen decreases patient risk, while suggesting that routine use of supplemental oxygen may increase costs.

Recommendations : Equipment to administer supplemental oxygen should be present when sedation/analgesia is administered. If hypoxemia is anticipated or develops during sedation/analgesia, supplemental oxygen should be administered.

IX. Use of Multiple Sedative/Analgesic Agents

The literature supports the observation that combinations of agents may be more effective than single agents in certain circumstances. However, the published data also suggest and consultant opinion supports the observation that combinations of sedatives and opioids may increase the likelihood of adverse outcomes, including ventilatory depression and hypoxemia.

Although not evaluated in the literature, it is the consensus of the Task Force that fixed combinations of sedative and analgesic agents may not allow the individual components of sedation/analgesia to be appropriately titrated to meet the individual requirements of the patient and procedure.

Recommendations : Combinations of sedative and analgesic agents should be administered as appropriate for the procedure being performed and the condition of the patient. Ideally, each component should be administered individually to achieve the desired effect (*e.g.*, additional analgesic medication to relieve pain, additional sedative medication to decrease awareness or anxiety). The propensity for combinations of sedative and analgesic agents to potentiate respiratory depression emphasizes the need to appropriately reduce the dose of each component as well as the need to continually monitor respiratory function.

X. Titration of Sedative/Analgesic Medications to Achieve the Desired Effect

The literature suggests that the administration of small, incremental doses of intravenous sedative/analgesic drugs until the desired level of sedation and/or analgesia is achieved is preferable to a single dose based on patient size, weight, or age. The consultants support the concept that incremental drug administration improves patient comfort and decreases costs; they strongly support the contention that the potential risks associated with excessive doses are reduced.

Recommendations : Intravenous sedative/analgesic drugs should be given in small, incremental doses that are titrated to the desired end points of analgesia and sedation. Sufficient time must elapse between doses to allow the effect of each dose to be assessed before subsequent drug administration. When drugs are administered by nonintravenous routes (*e.g.*, oral, rectal, intramuscular), allowance should be made for the time required for drug absorption before supplementation is considered.

XI. Intravenous Access

Published data suggest that, in co-operative patients, administration of sedative/analgesic agents by the intravenous route improves patient comfort and satisfaction.The consultants strongly support the importance of intravenous access in reducing patient risks. In situations when sedative/analgesic medications are to be administered intravenously, it is the consensus of the Task Force that maintaining intravenous access until the patient is no longer at risk for cardiorespiratory depression improves patient safety. In those situations when sedation is begun by nonintravenous routes (*e.g.*, oral, rectal, intramuscular), the need for intravenous access is not sufficiently addressed in the literature. However, initiation of intravenous access after the initial sedation takes effect allows additional sedative/analgesic and resuscitation drugs to be administered, if necessary.

Recommendations: In patients receiving intravenous medications for sedation/analgesia, vascular access should be maintained throughout the procedure and until the patient is no longer at risk for cardiorespiratory depression. In patients who have received sedation/analgesia by nonintravenous routes or whose intravenous line has become dislodged or blocked, practitioners should determine the advisability of establishing or re-establishing intravenous access on a case-by-case basis. In all instances, an individual with the skills to establish intravenous access should be immediately available.

XII. Reversal Agents

Specific antagonist agents that are available for the opioids (*e.g.*, naloxone) and benzodiazepines (*e.g.*, flumazenil). The literature supports the ability of naloxone to reverse opioid-induced sedation and ventilatory depression during sedation/analgesia. However, the Task Force reminds practitioners that acute reversal of opioid-induced analgesia may result in pain, hypertension, tachycardia, or pulmonary oedema. The literature supports the ability of flumazenil to reverse benzodiazepine-induced sedation and its effectiveness in reversing ventilatory depression in patients who have received benzodiazepines alone. In patients who have received benzodiazepines and opioids, published data support the ability of flumazenil to reverse sedation; however, there are insufficient data to establish the effectiveness of flumazenil in reversing ventilatory depression under these circumstances. The consultants strongly support the contention that the availability of reversal agents is associated with decreased risk. It is the consensus of the Task Force that respiratory depression should be initially treated with supplemental oxygen and, if necessary, positive pressure ventilation by mask.

Recommendations : Specific antagonists should be available whenever opioid analgesics or benzodiazepines are administered for sedation/analgesia. Naloxone and/or flumazenil may be administered to improve spontaneous ventilatory efforts in patients who have received opioids or benzodiazepines respectively. This may be especially helpful in cases in which airway control and positive pressure ventilation are difficult. Before or concomitantly with pharmacologic reversal, patients who become hypoxemic or apneic during sedation/analgesia should : (1) be encouraged or stimulated to breathe deeply, (2) receive positive pressure ventilation, if spontaneous ventilation is inadequate, and (3) receive supplemental oxygen. After pharmacologic reversal, patients should be observed long enough to ensure that cardiorespiratory depression does not recur.

XIII. Recovery Care

Patients may continue to be at significant risk for complications after their procedure is completed. Decreased procedural stimulation, prolonged drug absorption after oral or rectal administration, and post-procedure haemorrhage may contribute to cardio-respiratory depression. When sedation/analgesia is administered to outpatients, one must assume there will be no medical supervision once the patient leaves the medical facility. Although there is not sufficient literature to examine the effects of postprocedure monitoring on patient outcomes, the consultants suggest that appropriate monitoring of patients during the recovery period will improve patient comfort and strongly support the view that adverse outcomes may be reduced. It is the consensus of the Task Force that discharge criteria should be established that minimize the risk for cardiorespiratory depression after patients are released from observation by trained personnel.

Recommendations : After sedation/analgesia, patients should be observed until they are no longer at increased risk for cardiorespiratory depression. Vital signs and respiratory function should be monitored at regular intervals until patients are suitable for discharge. Discharge criteria should be designed to minimize the risk of central nervous system or cardiorespiratory depression after discharge from observation by trained personnel (Table 4).

Table 4 : Example of Recovery and Discharge Criteria after Sedation and Analgesia

Each patient-care facility in which sedation/analgesia is administered should develop recovery and discharge criteria that are suitable for its specific patients and procedures. Some of the basic principles that might be incorporated in these criteria are enumerated.

General Principles

1. All patients receiving sedation/analgesia should be monitored until appropriate discharge criteria are satisfied. The duration of monitoring must be individualized depending on the level of sedation achieved, overall condition of the patient, and nature of the intervention for which sedation/analgesia was administered.
2. The recovery area should be equipped with appropriate monitoring and resuscitation equipment.
3. A nurse or other trained individual should be in attendance until discharge criteria are fulfilled. An individual capable of establishing a patent airway and providing positive pressure ventilation should be immediately available.
4. Level of consciousness and vital signs (including frequency and depth of respiration in the absence of stimulation) should be recorded at regular intervals during recovery. The responsible practitioner should be notified if vital signs fall outside of the limits previously established for each patient.

Guidelines for discharge

1. Patients should be alert and oriented; infants and patients whose mental status was initially abnormal should have returned to their baseline. Practitioners must be aware that paediatric patients are at risk for airway obstruction should the head fall forward while the child is secured in a car seat.
2. Vital signs should be stable and within acceptable limits.
3. Sufficient time (upto 2 hour) should have elapsed after the last administration of reversal agents (naloxone, flumazenil) to ensure that patients do not become resedated after reversal effects have abated.
4. Outpatients should be discharged in the presence of a responsible adult who will accompany them home and be able to report any post procedure complications.
5. Outpatients should be provided with written instructions regarding post procedure diet, medications and activities and a phone number to use in case of emergency.

XIV. Special Situations

The literature suggests, the consultants strongly support, and the Task Force members concur that certain classes of patients (*e.g.*, uncooperative patients; extremes of age; severe cardiac, pulmonary, hepatic, renal, or central nervous system disease; morbid obesity; sleep apnea; pregnancy; drug or alcohol abuse) are at increased risk for developing complications related to sedation/analgesia unless special precautions are taken. However, the consultants support the view that risks may be reduced by preprocedure consultation with appropriate specialists (*e.g.*, cardiologist, pulmonologist, nephrologist, obstetrician, paediatrician, anaesthesiologist) before administering sedation/analgesia to these individuals. The consultants support the concept that patient comfort is improved and risks are reduced by consultation with an anaesthesiologist before administering sedation/analgesia to patients who are likely to develop complications (*e.g.*, inadequate spontaneous ventilation, loss of airway control, cardiovascular compromise) or in whom sedation/analgesia alone is not expected to provide adequate conditions (*e.g.*, young children, unco-operative patients). However, the consultants also support the contention that such consultation will not reduce costs.

Recommendations: Whenever possible, appropriate medical specialists should be consulted before administration of sedation/analgesia to patients with significant underlying conditions. The choice of specialists depends on the nature of the underlying condition and the urgency of the situation. For significantly compromised patients (*e.g.*, severe obstructive pulmonary disease, coronary artery disease, congestive heart failure) or if it appears likely that sedation to the point of unresponsiveness or general anaesthesia will be necessary to obtain adequate conditions, practitioners who are not specifically qualified to provide these modalities should consult an anaesthesiologist.

REFERENCE

Task Force on sedation and Analgesia by Non Anaesthesiologists. American Society of Anaesthesio-logists, 1996;84:459-71.

INDEX

A

B

C

K

L

M

N

O

P

R

S